CANCELLED 24 MAY

Health Fitness Instructor's Handbook

Fourth Edition

Edward T. Howley, PhD
University of Tennessee at Knoxville

B. Don Franks, PhD
University of Maryland at College Park

Human Kinetics

Library of Congress Cataloging-in-Publication Data

Howley, Edward T., 1943-
Health fitness instructor's handbook / Edward T. Howley, B. Don Franks. -- 4th ed.
p. ; cm.
Includes bibliographical references and index.
ISBN 0-7360-4210-5 (hard cover)
1. Physical fitness--Handbooks, manuals, etc. 2. Physical fitness--Testing--Handbooks, manuals, etc. 3. Exercise--Physiological aspects--Handbooks, manuals, etc. 4. Health. I. Franks, B. Don. II. Title
[DNLM: 1. Exercise--physiology. 2. Health Behavior. 3. Nutrition. 4. Physical Fitness--physiology. QT 255 H865h 2003]
GV481.H734 2003
613.7--dc21

2002010983

ISBN: 0-7360-4210-5

The Web addresses cited in this text were current as of *9/24/2002*, unless otherwise noted.

Acquisitions Editor: Michael S. Bahrke, PhD; **Developmental Editor:** Rebecca Crist; **Assistant Editor:** Sandria M. Washington; **Copyeditor:** Julie Anderson; **Proofreader:** Sarah Wiseman; **Indexer:** Craig Brown; **Permission Manager:** Dalene Reeder; **Graphic Designer:** Nancy Rasmus; **Graphic Artist:** Angela K. Snyder; **Photo Manager:** Leslie A. Woodrum; **Cover Designer:** Keith Blomberg; **Photographer (cover):** Dan Wendt; **Photographer (interior):** Leslie A. Woodrum; **Art Manager:** Kelly Hendren; **Illustrator:** Mic Greenberg; **Printer:** Creative USA

We thank the staff of Gold's Gym in Champaign, Illinois, for their assistance with photos on pages 228 and 254, and the staff of the Mettler Center in Urbana, Illinois, for assistance with the cover photo.

Printed in Hong Kong 10 9 8 7 6 5 4 3 2 1

Human Kinetics
Web site: www.HumanKinetics.com

United States: Human Kinetics
P.O. Box 5076
Champaign, IL 61825-5076
800-747-4457
e-mail: humank@hkusa.com

Canada: Human Kinetics
475 Devonshire Road Unit 100
Windsor, ON N8Y 2L5
800-465-7301 (in Canada only)
e-mail: orders@hkcanada.com

Europe: Human Kinetics
107 Bradford Road
Stanningley
Leeds LS28 6AT, United Kingdom
+44 (0) 113 255 5665
e-mail: hk@hkeurope.com

Australia: Human Kinetics
57A Price Avenue
Lower Mitcham, South Australia 5062
08 8277 1555
e-mail: liahka@senet.com.au

New Zealand: Human Kinetics
P.O. Box 105-231, Auckland Central
09-523-3462
e-mail: hkp@ihug.co.nz

To Ann and Elizabeth

preface

Are you sitting down?

You probably are, in order to read this book most comfortably. And that's probably a good idea. But every year, new statistics show that people are doing a lot more sitting. Despite a multi-billion dollar fitness industry in the United States, a startling percentage of the population gets little or no regular physical activity.

There is also good news, however. Exercise scientists and fitness professionals are becoming ever more knowledgeable about the best ways to evaluate fitness, prescribe exercise to improve health and performance, and motivate the inactive to participate in regular activity. These recent advances prompted this revision, the fourth edition of *Health Fitness Instructor's Handbook.*

We've updated the entire text to include the latest research you'll need to know, whether you're a current practitioner, a professional preparing for the ACSM Health/Fitness Instructor$_{SM}$ exam, or a college student just beginning your career study. A few distinctions of this edition include:

- Expanded information on calibrating exercise testing equipment
- New and reorganized information on assessing muscular fitness, and guidelines for strength and muscular endurance training
- A new focus on timely and pivotal research, showcased in the *Research Insight* spotlights that identify new theories and current issues in the field

In addition, we've greatly expanded information on exercise prescription for special populations. In this edition, we'll take a closer look at the benefits and limitations of exercise for

- children and youth,
- older adults,
- coronary heart disease,
- obesity,
- diabetes,
- asthma and pulmonary disease, and
- women's health.

Lastly, we have fully updated the text to reflect the most recent American College of Sports Medicine guidelines and positions. This update will be of certain use to those studying for the HFI certification exam, but is equally crucial to anyone interested in staying well informed amid ongoing research advances.

By choosing to become involved in health fitness instruction, you are providing a great service to the health of our communities. We're pleased to be a part of that, and hope that you find this text a valuable resource along the way.

contents

Part IV Special Populations

Part V Exercise Programming

part one

Activity, Fitness, and Health

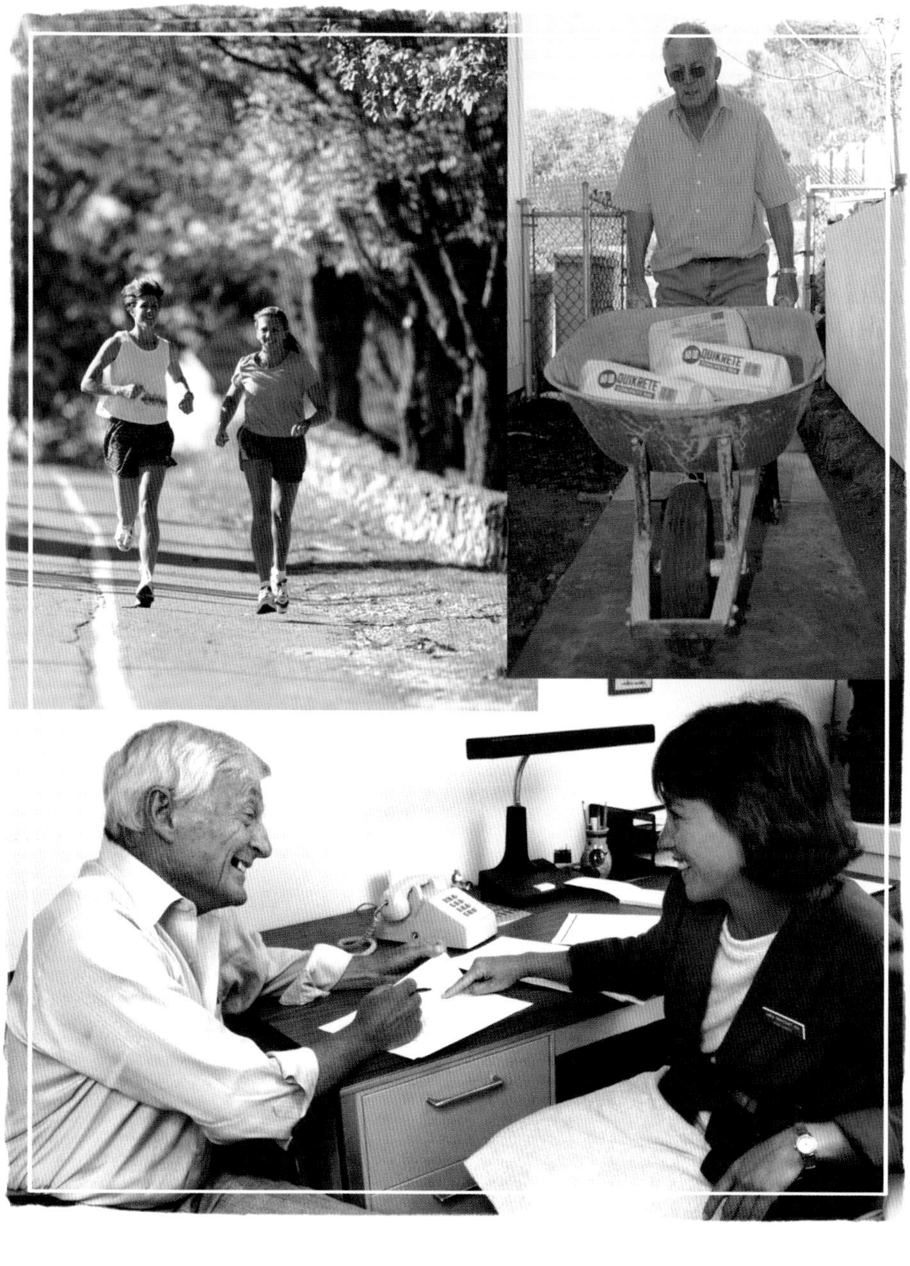

Physical activity is an important and essential element in human health and well-being. With that in mind, we wrote this book for current and future health fitness instructors (HFIs) and personal fitness trainers (PFTs), who help individuals, communities, and groups gain the benefits of regular physical activity in a positive and safe environment.

The chapters of **part I** explain the foundations underlying the study of physical activity and its relevance to fitness. In **chapter 1,** we summarize the current evidence regarding physical activity and health. Next, we describe the relationships among health, fitness, and performance in **chapter 2**. Finally, in **chapter 3** we provide a process for screening potential fitness participants and recommend criteria to be used for medical referrals and the development of supervised and unsupervised programs.

This part is followed by two primary responsibilities of health fitness instructors: fitness evaluation **(part II)** and recommendations for physical activity and exercise **(part III)**. The new section in this fourth edition—special populations **(part IV)**—is an increasing element in fitness programs. **Part V** completes the programming aspects for HFIs, and **part VI** reviews the physiological and biomechanical bases for fitness.

one

Physical Activity and Health

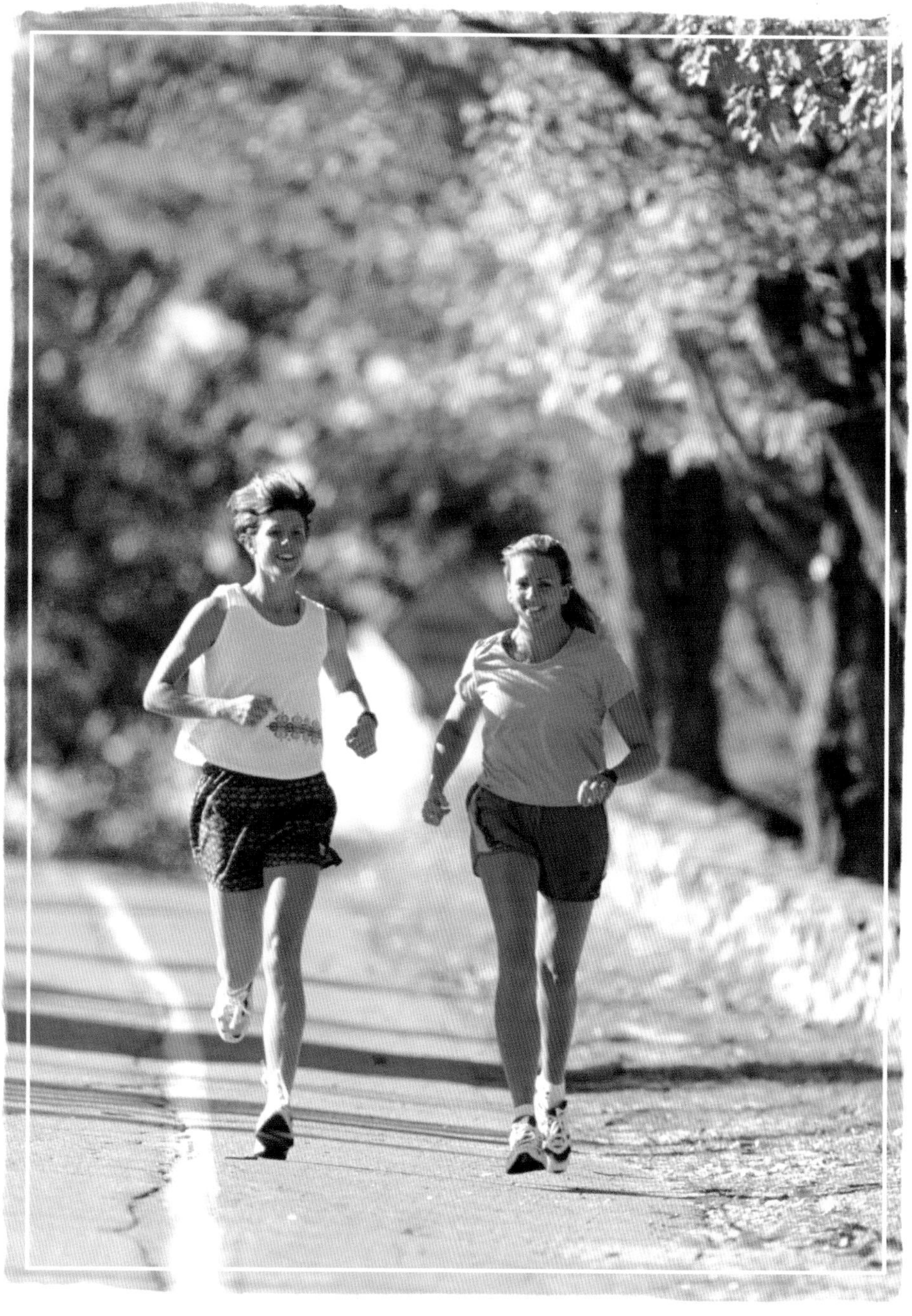

© ImageState/Dennis W. Welsch

Objectives

The reader will be able to do the following:

1. Provide evidence that the importance of physical activity is widely recognized.
2. Describe some of the barriers that prevent physical activity from improving the health of the overall population.
3. Describe the relationship of physical activity to health.
4. Describe the elements of total fitness.
5. Understand the role of physical activity in quality of life.
6. Describe the goals and behaviors of a healthy life.
7. Describe the link between physical activity and lowered risk of premature health problems.
8. Understand the pathophysiology of arteriosclerosis and other cardiovascular problems.
9. Identify risk factors for coronary heart disease and designate those that may be favorably modified by regular and appropriate physical activity habits.
10. Differentiate between the amount and type of exercise required for various health benefits and that required for fitness development.
11. Identify the short-term and long-term benefits associated with fitness
12. Be aware of the risks associated with exercise participation.
13. Describe three key elements of promoting physical activity.

From the beginning of recorded history, philosophers and health professionals have observed that regular physical activity is an essential part of a healthy life. Hippocrates wrote the following in *Regimen*, about 400 B.C.:

> *Eating alone will not keep a man [woman] well; he [she] must also take exercise. For food and exercise, while possessing opposite qualities, yet work together to produce health. . . . And it is necessary, as it appears, to discern the power of various exercises, both natural exercises and artificial, to know which of them tends to increase flesh and which to lessen it; and not only this, but also to proportion exercise to bulk of food, to the constitution of the patient, to the age of the individual . . . (19)*

The Best of Times and Worst of Times for Physical Activity Professionals

In the past two decades, the public, professional organizations, and the medical community have accepted the importance of physical activity. It seems that almost everyone recognizes the overwhelming evidence, accumulated by exercise scientists over the past five decades, that points to the importance of regular physical activity for quality of life, health, and prevention and rehabilitation of many health problems. The information at the top of the box on page 5 (*The Good News*) illustrates this widespread acceptance.

1 In Review

Professional groups, such as the American College of Sports Medicine (ACSM) and the American Heart Association (AHA), and governmental agencies, such as the Centers for Disease Control and Prevention (CDC), the National Institutes of Health (NIH), the President's Council on Physical Fitness and Sports (PCPFS), and the Surgeon General's Office, have released reports emphasizing the importance of physical activity to good health.

Public recognition of the importance of physical activity for good health is a major accomplishment for fitness scholars and professionals who for many years have conducted research and disseminated their findings related to the importance of physical activity. To have so many statements promoting physical activity appear within the space of a few years indicates the excitement felt by all those involved with physical activity; however, there are many challenges left for health fitness instructors (HFIs) who wish to promote the connections between physical activity and health benefits of physical activity for everyone (see *The Bad News* at the bottom of the box below).

Good News and Bad News for Physical Activity Professionals

The Good News

People know that physical activity is important for good health: Surveys indicate that women and men of all ages, races, and socioeconomic status believe that regular physical activity is important for health.

- The *Healthy People 2010* objectives (37) list physical activity and fitness as one of the priority areas. In addition, physical activity is listed as one of the 10 top health indicators!
- The AHA (5) included physical inactivity and low fitness levels as primary risk factors along with smoking, hypertension, and high cholesterol.
- The NIH (25) released a consensus statement on the importance of physical activity for cardiovascular health.
- The CDC, Division of Adolescent School Health, issued guidelines for healthy levels of nutrition (10) and physical activity (11) for adolescents.
- The United States Department of Agriculture and United States Department of Health and Human Services published its sixth edition of the *Dietary Guidelines for the Nation* (34), which includes a statement on the importance of physical activity.
- The Office of the Surgeon General released its report on physical activity and health, which strongly supports the role of physical activity for good health and prevention of major health problems (36).

The Bad News

Forty percent of Americans are sedentary: Although there was a general increase in the number of individuals who participated in physical activity in the 1960s and 1970s, there was little change during the 1980s and early 1990s. In 1997, 40% of Americans had no leisure-time physical activity (37).

The public is confused about what physical activity is recommended for health and fitness. There is still confusion about what recommendations for different types, amounts, and intensities of activities are relevant for specific individuals.

The resources allocated for physical activity have lagged far behind money spent for other aspects of health: The resources for physical education, community physical activity programs, and prevention of health problems are inadequate to provide safe and quality programs.

Safe, attractive, and well-supervised facilities for participation in activity are not available for many individuals: Bike and walking trails are an exception rather than a rule in communities. Low-cost recreation programs for the masses are simply not sufficient to accommodate all who could benefit.

In the schools, health and physical education are low on the priority list and are often among the first curricular components cut during budget crises.

2 In Review

Resources for and access to safe and supervised quality physical activities lag far behind the position statements on physical activity's importance. The public is confused regarding what exactly is recommended for physical activity to improve health and fitness.

Connections Between Physical Activity and Health

Starting in the 1940s with such fitness pioneers as T.K. Cureton, Bruno Balke, and Peter Karpovich, numerous experimental studies explored the effects of regular physical activity on components of fitness, especially cardiorespiratory fitness and body composition. These studies led to the 1978 ACSM position statement, with Michael Pollock as senior author, concerning the amount and type of physical activity needed to improve fitness (1). It appeared from these studies that doing a little bit of activity had little effect on cardiorespiratory fitness; in fact, results for groups assigned to perform less than the ACSM recommendations often were not different from the sedentary control groups.

Epidemiological studies explore risk factors for various health problems, especially heart disease. The major findings of the earlier studies showed that smoking, high total cholesterol, and high blood pressure were strongly related to the development of heart disease. More recently, it has been recognized that physical inactivity is also a major risk factor for heart disease (25).

Haskell (16) was one of the first scholars to observe the apparent contradiction of the relationship of physical activity to fitness and health outcomes. The 1978 ACSM statement was a good summary of findings from the experimental studies on what was needed to make fitness changes over a few months, but the large population studies spanning several years appeared to show that individuals with activity levels below the ACSM recommendations had reduced risk of heart disease and other health problems. Two of the major population studies had sufficient data to analyze different levels of physical activity (26) and different levels of cardiorespiratory fitness (7) to determine the relative risks of heart disease and all-cause mortality. Both the behavior (physical activity) and the outcome (cardiorespiratory fitness) appear to be important in reducing the risk of heart disease. Figures 1.1 and 1.2 (18) show the relationship between activity level, fitness level, and risk of coronary heart disease (CHD). A substantial reduction in risk is shown when an individual moves from the lowest activity or fitness level to a slightly increased level of activity or fitness. These studies also show additional benefit from higher levels of activity and fitness.

Drawing on these and other studies, the ACSM, the CDC, and the PCPFS (27) issued a position statement that supplemented the earlier ACSM recommendation. This ACSM/CDC statement proclaimed that sedentary individuals could greatly reduce their risk of developing heart disease and other health problems simply by participating in 30

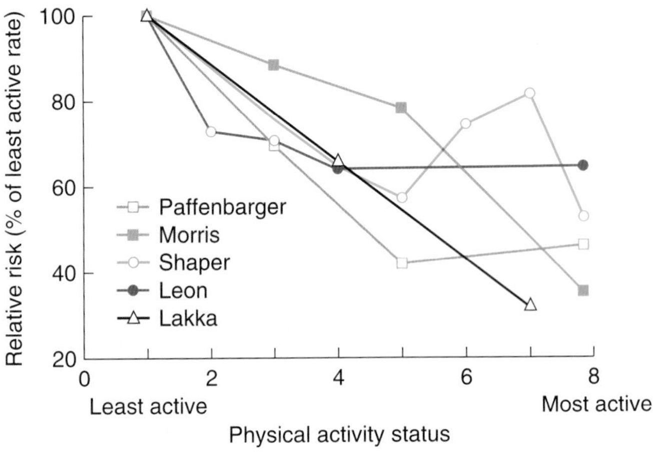

Figure 1.1 Physical activity and risk of coronary heart disease.

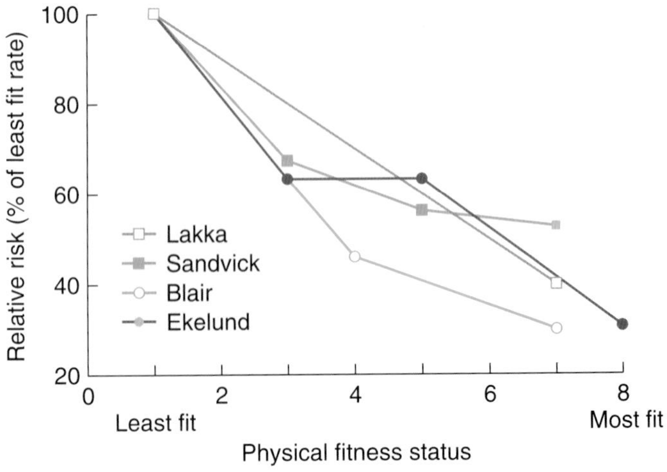

Figure 1.2 Physical fitness and risk of coronary heart disease.

min of moderate activity most, preferably all, days of the week. Additional fitness benefits can result from going beyond that to the 3 to 5 days per week of vigorous aerobic activity specified in the original ACSM position statement, but the greatest boost in improving the health of our nation would come from sedentary individuals beginning to do just a little bit of exercise every day! This position is reflected in the revised ACSM position statements (2, 3, 4), which continue to be the gold standard for fitness improvement (see part III). *Healthy People 2000* and *2010* (35, 37) include objectives for both daily moderate and regular vigorous activity. The NIH Consensus Conference on Physical Activity and Cardiovascular Health (25) drew the same conclusions.

3 In Review

An active lifestyle enhances the quality of life. An increase in the total amount of moderate physical activity is associated with decreased risk of heart disease. Regular vigorous exercise increases cardiorespiratory fitness.

What We Know About Physical Activity, Fitness, and Health

For many people, it would be impossible to describe the highest level of positive, dynamic health without including physical activity. Physical activity is essential to optimal physical and mental health. Consistent with the link between activity and positive health, a sedentary lifestyle is a major element in poor health for a large number of individuals. Just adding regular physical activity to the lifestyle of sedentary individuals substantially increases overall health.

Elements Involved in Total Fitness

Although we can recognize individuals who have that special optimal quality of life, it is difficult to describe it in concise and precise terms. Many individuals and groups have used the term wellness to emphasize that positive health is much more than simply being free from illness, that there is an added quality to being well. We use the term total fitness to try to capture this same concept. Total fitness is a condition reached through striving for optimal quality of life in all aspects of life—social, mental, psychological, spiritual, and physical. This dynamic, multidimensional state has a positive health base and includes individual performance goals. The highest quality of life includes all these components: mental alertness and curiosity, positive emotional feelings, meaningful relationships with others, awareness and involvement in societal strivings and problems, recognition of the broader forces of life, and the physical capacity to accomplish personal goals with vigor. These aspects of total fitness are interrelated; a high level in one area enhances the other areas, and, conversely, a low level in any area restricts the accomplishments possible in other areas. Although physical activity plays a major role in the physical dimension, it also can contribute to learning, relationships, and a sense of our human limitations within the broader perspective. An optimal quality of life requires a person to strive, grow, and develop, but the highest level of fitness may never be achieved. The totally fit person nevertheless continually reaches for the highest quality of life possible.

Heredity

People can achieve fitness goals up to their genetic potential, but it is not possible to establish the relative portion of a person's health or performance that is determined by heredity and development. Although heredity influences physical activity, fitness status, and health (8), most people can lead healthy or unhealthy lives regardless of their genetic makeup. Thus, genetic background neither dooms a person to poor health nor guarantees a high fitness level.

Environmental Factors

We are born not only with fixed genetic potentials but also into environments that affect our development in many ways. An environment includes physical factors (e.g., climate, altitude, pollution) and social factors (e.g., networks of friends, parental values, characteristics of the workplace) that affect activity, fitness, and health. Some elements, such as nutrition or the air we breathe and water we drink, affect us directly. Other elements, such as the values and behaviors of people we admire, influence our lifestyles indirectly.

Certain aspects of our environments can be controlled—many of the mental and physical activities we undertake are a matter of choice. However, our past and current environments affect us all in various ways. For example, some children have inadequate food as a part of their environments and obviously cannot think about other aspects of fitness until that basic need is fulfilled.

Individual Interests

A major ingredient in total fitness involves individual choices for discretionary use of time. These selected activities are important in two ways: the nature of the activity and preparation for enjoyable participation. One of the purposes of education is to provide people a positive exposure to a wide variety of activities that enrich life. Thus, a well-educated person has many mentally and physically healthy activities from which to choose.

The long-term interests that are developed may require additional preparation for their enjoyment. For example, someone may enjoy reading and tennis as a result of early positive involvement in both. In addition to becoming involved in groups interested in literature, the individual will need to pay attention to proper posture, lighting, and so on while reading. The person will need to develop underlying fitness components and specific skills to continue to enjoy playing tennis.

Research Insight

In a comprehensive review of the research related to quality of life and independent living in older adults, Spirduso and Cronin (32) found that physical activity postponed disability and enhanced independent living. Regular physical activity enhances physical function in individuals with chronic disease; however, there was insufficient evidence to differentiate between aerobic and resistance training. In addition, there did not appear to be evidence for a dose-response relationship for exercise intensity related to these results.

The energy and physical, mental, psychological, and social well-being that can result from appropriate physical activity are reasons enough to promote activity. The reduced risk of developing premature health problems and the potential of a longer life are additional benefits.

4 In Review

Total fitness is striving for the highest level of existence, including mental, psychological, social, spiritual, and physical components. It is dynamic, multidimensional, and related to heredity, environment, and individual interests.

5 In Review

Physical activity is an important ingredient in the quality of life because it increases energy and promotes physical, mental, and psychological well-being in addition to conferring worthy health benefits.

Quality of Life

The purpose of the opening section of the chapter dealing with global notions of health is to emphasize that the importance of physical activity goes beyond whether it can prolong life or prevent heart disease. Later in this chapter we explore the evidence that activity is linked to longevity and reduced risk of heart disease; however, the point here is that regular physical activity would be important for quality of life even if activity had no relationship to length of life or premature disease. Several studies have explored the relationship between physical activity and the overall quality of life, including such variables as mental, psychological, and social well-being. Although the type and amount of physical activity essential for global quality of life are not as easily described, interest in and evidence related to the role that physical activity plays in one's quality of life are increasing (31) (see the Research Insight).

Goals and Behaviors for a Healthy Life

Health is defined as being alive with no major health problem. The two primary health goals are to delay death and to avoid disease. Although these goals provide a minimum basis for health, they are not the optimal goals for total fitness. These health goals are desirable first steps, but they fall far short of the optimal level of fitness.

Delaying Death

The death rate for humans is 100%! Death cannot be avoided, but beyond your inherited characteristics, there are some things that you can do to postpone death. Most generally, you can practice a healthy lifestyle in a healthy and safe environment.

Avoiding Disease

Along with delaying death, the other minimum health goal for all of us is to be free from disease (i.e., to be apparently healthy). We try to prevent illness and known diseases through awareness, health checks, and healthy habits. You probably have assisted at or attended health fairs that help people identify signs, symptoms, and test scores that might indicate possible medical problems.

Positive activities and habits are related to total fitness and low risk of developing major health problems. These behaviors include exercising regularly, maintaining healthy nutrition, getting adequate sleep, relaxing and coping with stressors, practicing safety habits, and abstaining from tobacco, excess alcohol, and nonessential drugs (table 1.1).

6 In Review

The primary health goals are to avoid premature death and to avoid preventable disease. Components related to these goals include heredity, environment, habits, and health status. Behaviors that contribute to a healthy life are regular exercise, proper nutrition, adequate sleep, relaxation, and abstinence from tobacco, excess alcohol, and nonessential drugs.

Physical Activity and Prevention of Premature Health Problems

If one lives long enough, health problems will develop, leading to an inability to function independently and eventually causing death. One aspect of an individual's quality of life is to prevent or delay the premature development of these health problems, prolonging the healthy and independent living portions of life. There is evidence that physical activity is related to lower risk of premature development of many health problems including atherosclerosis (24), back pain (28), some cancers (23), chronic lung disease (39), coronary heart disease (17), diabetes (21), hypertension (13), mental health problems (22), obesity (38), osteoporosis (30), and stroke (20). An active lifestyle also is related to estimates of prolonged quality of life (31) and independent living in the elderly (12, 32) and individuals with disabilities (29). In fact, *the Surgeon General's Report on Physical Activity and Health* (36) reviewed the evidence relating physical activity to reduced risks of a variety of health problems and concluded that physical activity reduces the risks of colon

Table 1.1 Health Goals, Components, and Behaviors

Goal	Component	Behavior
Delay death	Heredity	
	Healthy habits	Nutrition Physical activity No smoking/drugs Limited alcohol Relaxation Sleep Coping with stressors
	Safe habits	Seat belts Avoid high risks
	Environment	Clean air and water
Avoid disease	Heredity	
	Prevention	Medical/dental exams Immunization
	Awareness of symptoms	Check with health provider
	Lower CHD risk	Daily moderate activity
	Nutrition	Balance different foods Low fat, cholesterol, salt Intake = expenditure High complex carbohydrates

Note. CHD = coronary heart disease.

cancer, coronary heart disease, non-insulin-dependent diabetes, hypertension, obesity, osteoporosis, and all-cause mortality, and it enhances mental health.

7 In Review

Regular physical activity helps prevent and delay premature development of a variety of major health problems.

Pathophysiology of Arteriosclerosis and Other Cardiovascular Problems

Cardiovascular problems cause the majority of premature deaths in the United States (37). In addition, many who survive with these problems have severe limitations in their lives. These heart health problems take many different forms:

- arteriosclerosis
- atherosclerosis
- coronary artery thrombosis
- coronary heart disease (CHD)
- embolism
- hypertension
- myocardial infarction (MI)
- stroke
- thrombosis
- cholesterol

CHD is the single leading cause of premature death in the United States (37). Cholesterol is predominant in the plaques that clog up the arteries. As the coronary arteries become narrowed and hardened, the arteries may not be able to supply the oxygen needed by the heart muscle (myocardium). This inability to supply the myocardium with oxygen is likely to occur when more oxygen is needed (e.g., during stress or strenuous activity). The resulting imbalance between the need for and supply of oxygen may lead to pain in the chest (angina), neck, jaw, or left shoulder and arm. The narrowed section of the artery may close or become totally occluded, which will lead to an MI. (See chapter 3 for standards that define abnormal levels of cholesterol and blood pressure.)

High blood pressure (hypertension) is the most common cardiovascular disease (37). Hypertension is related to CHD and stroke. Stroke is the result of obstructions in or hemorrhages of blood vessels in the brain. It usually results in an abrupt disruption of bodily function and loss of consciousness and may cause partial paralysis. There is some evidence that regular physical activity reduces the risk of stroke.

8 In Review

Cardiovascular problems cause the majority of premature deaths in the United States. Coronary heart disease is linked to the buildup of fatty deposits in the coronary arteries, limiting oxygen delivery to the myocardium.

Risk Factors for Cardiovascular Disease

Large-population epidemiological studies of cardiovascular problems have found that several characteristics (risk factors) are highly related to the premature development of cardiovascular disease. See the Surgeon General's report (36) for a comprehensive review of epidemiological studies and risk factors.

One way to classify risk factors is to distinguish between inherited risk factors that cannot be altered and unhealthy lifestyle behaviors that can be modified. The risk factors that cannot be altered include the family history of premature cardiovascular disease (4), sex (15) (men are at greater risk), race (37) (African-Americans have higher risk), and age (4) (the risk increases for all of us as we grow older).

Part of the risk associated with family history and age cannot be changed. The good news, however, is that some of the family history risks can be changed. These alterable family history risks include an unhealthy diet, sedentary lifestyle, smoking, and poor stress-coping behaviors that tend to be transmitted from parents to children. These types of behaviors can be corrected with proper attention throughout life, especially in early childhood.

In terms of aging, many fitness characteristics (e.g., maximum cardiovascular function and amount of body fat) worsen with age; that is, if people from 20 to 80 years of age were tested and the results were plotted against age, a steady deterioration (i.e., decreased cardiovascular function, increased fat) would occur with each decade. This decline, starting in the mid-20s, has been called the aging curve. However, the lack of participation in optimal levels of physical activity as individuals age contributes to a portion of the deterioration seen in aging curves. People who maintain active lifestyles slow down the decline in fitness seen in typical aging curves.

Modifiable characteristics that increase risk include smoking (4), high levels of serum cholesterol (4), high blood pressure (4), low levels of physical activity (4) and cardiorespiratory fitness (7), glucose intolerance (4), high fibrinogen (25), obesity (4), psychosocial factors (15), and low socioeconomic status (15). Fortunately, many of these characteristics can be favorably altered with healthy habits. (See chapter 3 for use of risk factors in screening for fitness programs.)

Numerous studies have shown that more active people have a lower risk of heart disease than sedentary individuals; however, in the past, physical inactivity was viewed as less important than control of serum cholesterol, blood pressure, and smoking. Studies indicate that both physical activity, such as expending 2000 kcal per week in various types of activities (26), and high levels of cardiorespiratory fitness, such as being able to go longer on a treadmill test (7), are major factors that reduce the relative risk of heart disease and all-cause mortality. Physical inactivity and low levels of fitness deserve the same emphasis as the traditional primary risk factors. Regular exercise also affects many of the CHD risk factors, improving serum cholesterol levels, blood pressure, glucose tolerance, fibrinogen, and body fat (25). Activity also helps people learn to cope with stressors. See the summary in table 1.2 of how physical activity affects disease risk factors.

Although these risk factors have normally been linked with some form of cardiovascular disease, many of them are also related to pulmonary (e.g., chronic obstructive pulmonary disease) and metabolic (e.g., diabetes) health problems.

Low Back Problems

Clinical evidence indicates that several risk factors are associated with low back problems (see chapters 9 and 13):

- Lack of abdominal muscle endurance
- Lack of flexibility in the midtrunk and hamstrings
- Poor posture—while lying, sitting, standing, and moving
- Poor lifting habits
- Injury of low back
- Overuse of low back muscles
- Inability to cope with stressors

Regular activities that strengthen the abdominal muscles and increase flexibility in the low back and hamstrings are highly recommended to prevent low back problems.

Table 1.2 Effect of Physical Activity on Risk Factors

	Effect of regular physical activity		
Risk factor	**Improve**	**May improve**	**No effect**
Older age			X
Smoking		X	
High total cholesterol	X		
High low-density cholesterol	X		
African American			X
Low high-density cholesterol	X		
Fibrinogen	X		
Male			X
High very low-density cholesterol	X		
Family history			X
High blood pressure	X		
Physical inactivity	X		
Low cardiorespiratory fitness	X		
High-fat diet		X	
Obesity	X		
Insulin needs, glucose tolerance	X		
Inability to cope with stress		X	

9 In Review

Some inherited characteristics and behaviors place an individual at higher risk of premature health problems (such as cardiovascular disease and low back problems) and death. Risk factors of high serum cholesterol levels, high blood pressure, glucose intolerance, high fibrinogen, obesity, and mechanisms for stress reduction can be reduced or eliminated through physical activity.

Implications for Fitness Professionals

Fitness professionals need to keep up with the constantly evolving recommendations for health and physical fitness that have direct application for fitness programs and exercise recommendations. Because the media use brief headlines and TV sound bites that provide only limited and confusing information about the latest fitness recommendations, it is important to provide more in-depth explanations to help individuals put each new study or report into perspective in terms of overall recommendations for a healthy life.

Exercise Prescription

One of the most controversial and confusing areas for the public is how much and what type of physical activity should be done for health and fitness benefits. One reason for this confusion is that recommendations differ for individuals depending on their current activity levels and their fitness, health, and performance goals (14) (appropriate screening for different individuals is discussed in chapter 3). It is not surprising that headlines and 20-s sound bites provide conflicting messages when one recommendation is for functional living in the frail elderly, another is for improving cardiorespiratory health in active adults, and yet another involves how to train for a marathon. Any set of guidelines for exercise recommendations that does not address activity status and health and fitness goals will add to the confusion. It is possible to have clear and consistent recommendations for physical activity (see activity pyramid in figure 1.3).

This section provides an overview of how fitness professionals can deal with questions about exercise prescription. A more comprehensive treatment of exercise prescription is found in the chapters in part III. As the past few years have illustrated so clearly, providing exercise recommendations is a dynamic process that should be in tune with new research findings. Thus, although we are confident that the recommendations in this book are appropriate for the beginning of the 21st century, there is a need to continually review research findings and to periodically update these recommendations.

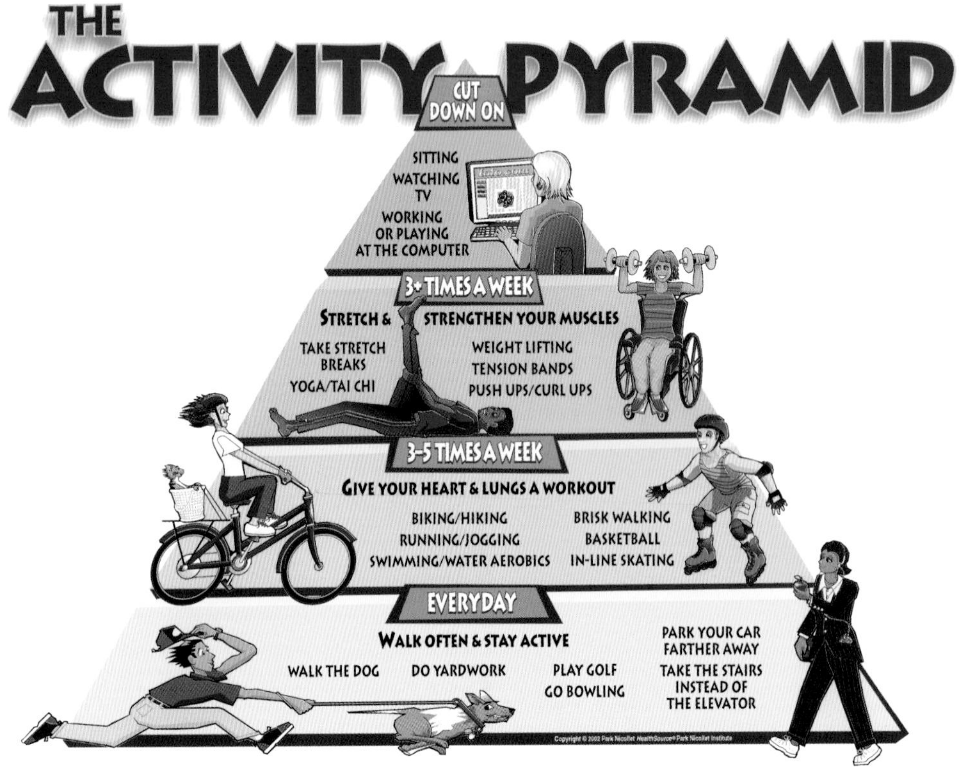

Figure 1.3 Activity pyramid.

Physical activity includes movement of the whole body, or large parts of it, whereas exercise is using physical activity in ways that increase components of physical fitness. Everyone should be encouraged to include physical activity as part of daily life, by using stairs instead of elevators, walking or cycling for visits or errands, and including active leisure-time pursuits with family and friends. Sedentary individuals should accumulate at least 30 min of some type of physical activity every day. Everything counts, from housework to yard work to the types of activities mentioned previously for everyone. Additional 10- to 15-min exercise breaks during the day would be a good way to start.

Persons who are already active for 30 min daily can enhance their fitness and health by including 20 min of vigorous physical activity 3 to 5 days per week (cardiovascular fitness and health), engaging in daily activities that use large amounts of energy with attention to nutritional habits (body composition and obesity), emphasizing weight-bearing activities (bone health), resistance training 2 to 3 days/week (muscular strength/endurance and bone health), engaging in regular stretching (flexibility and low back health), and choosing activities done in an enjoyable atmosphere (enhanced adherence and psychological health).

Persons with high levels of fitness can increase their exercise levels and work on skills for a variety of performance goals (see chapter 2).

Intensity

One of the major differences in recommendations based on current activity status is the intensity of exercise. Table 10.1 describes intensity levels, but in general, the daily activities for the general population and sedentary individuals are light intensity. Fitness activities are hard (vigorous) intensity, with performance intensity being very hard.

10 In Review

Exercise prescription must consider the individual's current activity status and desired outcomes. By making some simple changes, everyone can include more physical activity as part of their daily lives. Sedentary individuals should include at least 30 min of daily light-intensity activity. Moderately active individuals can improve their overall health and fitness by incorporating regular hard aerobic, resistance, and flexibility activities in an enjoyable atmosphere.

Benefits of Physical Activity

The long-term benefits of regular activity in terms of health and fitness are well known, including reduced risk of major health problems and improvement in cardiorespiratory function, muscular strength and endurance, flexibility, and body composition (fat content). Although we normally focus on the long-term (chronic) effects of regular physical activity, part of the benefit of physical activity is the repeated acute (or short-term) activity. For example, chronic activity reduces resting blood pressure, but there is some additional lowering of blood pressure after each acute bout of exercise. A single bout of activity has positive psychological effects for many individuals, such as a positive mood change after exercise. Finally, the time spent in physical activity is not being spent in unhealthy behaviors, such as smoking or eating unhealthy snacks. Table 1.3 summarizes some of the acute and chronic effects of physical activity.

11 In Review

The short- and long-term benefits of physical activity are summarized in table 1.3.

Exercise-Related Risks

Exercise and fitness tests involve risk of injury, cardiovascular problems, or death. High-intensity exercise and competition in many sports place extreme demands on the cardiovascular system and increase the risk of musculoskeletal injury. In addition, some fitness participants become obsessed with exercise and overtrain, which decreases fitness and leads to frequent injuries.

Moderate-intensity exercise is a very low-risk activity. There is an increased risk of MI or sudden death with vigorous exercise, but these risks are still very low. In the general population, it is estimated that there are seven deaths and 56 MIs for every 100,000 exercisers (33). In the postcardiac population, there is one death for every 784,000 patient-hours of exercise and one MI for every 294,000 patient-hours of exercise (33). Because of the decreased risk of heart disease in active or fit persons, the overall risk of a cardiovascular problem is greater for those who maintain sedentary habits (36).

Table 1.3 Short- and Long-Term Benefits of Physical Activity

Variable	Short-term benefits	Long-term benefits
Heart rate	+, then –	– (except max)
Stroke volume		+
Ejection fraction		+
Lactate threshold		+
Fibrinogen	–	–
Fibrinolysis	+	+
Blood pressure	+, then –	–
Oxygen uptake, max		+
Muscle mass		+
Strength/endurance		+
Fat		–
Cholesterol, HDL		+
LDL, VLDL		–
Flexibility		+
Appetite	–	+
Use of leisure time	+	+
Positive mood	+	
Anxiety	–	–
Depression	–	–
Self-esteeem		+
Stress	+, then –	–
Overreaction to stress		–

Note. + = increases; – = decreases; HDL = high-density lipoprotein; LDL = low-density lipoprotein, VLDL = very low-density lipoprotein.

The risks from exercise testing are also quite low, with 0.01% risk of death, 0.04% risk of having an MI, and 0.2% risk of a complication requiring hospitalization during or immediately after the test (4).

Exertion-related deaths are uncommon and generally are related to congenital heart defects (e.g., hypertrophic cardiomyopathy, Marfan's syndrome, severe aortic-valve stenosis, prolonged QT syndromes, cardiac conduction abnormalities) or to acquired myocarditis. The NIH consensus statement on physical activity and cardiovascular health (25) recommends that individuals with these conditions remain active but not participate in vigorous or competitive athletics.

The tendency is to deal with the question of risk by identifying various classes of individuals for whom a certain type of medical examination or test is recommended before initiation of an exercise program (see chapter 3). Per Olof Åstrand, a well-known Swedish physiologist, has offered another view. He stated that consulting a physician is advisable if there are any doubts about health, but that there is less risk in being active than in continuous inactivity. He stated that it is more advisable to pass a careful medical examination if one intends to be sedentary to detemine whether one's state of health is good enough to stand the inactivity! (6). This view is consistent with recent evidence that physical activity and a high level of cardiorespiratory fitness are related directly to a lower risk of heart disease and death (37).

12 In Review

Exercise carries some risk of injury, cardiovascular problems, and death. The health risk of an inactive lifestyle is higher than the risk associated with the kind of fitness activities and tests recommended in this book.

What Is Necessary to Promote Physical Activity

The obvious need is for communities, schools, states, and the nation to endorse the importance of regular physical activity for the nation's health by working with fitness professionals and allocating resources to encourage everyone to choose activity as part of a healthy lifestyle. Three elements of a strategy to enhance our nation's health through physical activity are clarity, access, and safety.

Clarity

Fitness scholars and professionals must clearly interpret and explain the evidence about physical activity as it relates to various health, fitness, and performance variables. New evidence must be viewed and interpreted within a clearly articulated model that indicates what type of physical activity is related to which outcomes for particular groups of individuals. In addition, we must become more adept at providing short and simple explanations for the media's use that are accurate and easy to understand.

Access

The issue of access is largely outside our direct control. We must nonetheless work continually with public and private partners to provide an environment that makes regular physical activity available and attractive to people of all ages and every socioeconomic status. This includes good health and physical education programs in the schools for all children and youth; community activity programs that are convenient and open to everyone; and programs at the worksite, in preschool programs, and in facilities serving older adults. Qualified fitness professionals are an essential part of these programs.

Safety

We also must advocate that participation in all physical activities take place in a positive and safe environment. Safe equipment, activities appropriate to each individual's age and fitness level, and careful monitoring of signs and symptoms of participants are all part of a quality program. For example, helmets should be worn for cycling, skating, and other activities; pregnant women should avoid intense activity in hot environments; and older adults should be monitored carefully for any signs of cardiovascular problems.

13 In Review

HFIs must provide clear guidelines for physical activity recommendations combined with adequate resources so that everyone can participate in quality physical activity in an enjoyable and safe atmosphere.

Case Studies

You can check your answers by referring to appendix A.

1.1

You have just presented a speech on physical fitness to a local service club. One of the members says that he knows of two men who have died in incidents related to exercise during the past 5 years, and he has read that there have been other exercise-related deaths. He has decided that it will be safer to lead a quiet life and not take the risk of exercising. How would you respond?

1.2

A client calls you and complains that he has been deceived by all the exercise recommendations you have given him over the past several years. He just read a report from the CDC indicating that a person has to only do moderate exercise (walking) to achieve health benefits. He wants to know if he should continue his vigorous exercise program in which he exercises at his target heart rate for 30 min 3 to 4 times per week, or whether he should switch to a walking program. How would you respond?

Source List

1. American College of Sports Medicine. (1978). The recommended quality and quantity of exercise for developing and maintaining fitness in healthy adults. *Medicine and Science in Sports and Exercise, 10,* vii-x.
2. American College of Sports Medicine. (1990). The recommended quantity and quality of exercise for developing and maintaining cardiorespiratory and muscular fitness in healthy adults. *Medicine and Science in Sports and Exercise, 22,* 265-274.
3. American College of Sports Medicine. (1995). *ACSM's guidelines for exercise testing and prescription* (5th ed.). Baltimore: Williams & Wilkins.
4. American College of Sports Medicine. (2000). *ACSM's guidelines for exercise testing and prescription* (6th ed.). Philadelphia: Lippincott Williams & Wilkins.
5. American Heart Association. (1992). Statement on exercise. *Circulation, Internal Medicine, 103,* 994-995.
6. Åstrand, P-O., & Rodahl, K. (1986). *Textbook of work physiology* (3rd ed.). New York: McGraw-Hill.
7. Blair, S.N., Kohl, H.W., III, Paffenbarger, R.S., Jr., Clark, D.G., Cooper, K.H., & Gibbons, L.W. (1989). Physical fitness and all-cause mortality. *Journal of the American Medical Association, 262,* 2395-2401.
8. Bouchard, C., & Perusse, L. (1994). Heredity, activity level, fitness, and health. In C. Bouchard, R.J. Shephard, & T. Stephens (Eds.), *Physical activity, fitness, and health* (pp. 106-118). Champaign, IL: Human Kinetics.
9. Caspersen, C.J., Powell, K.E., & Christensen, G.M. (1985). Physical activity, exercise, and physical fitness: Definition and distinctions for health-related research. *Public Health Reports, 100,* 126-131.
10. Centers for Disease Control and Prevention. (1996). *Guidelines for nutrition for adolescents.* Atlanta: Author.
11. Centers for Disease Control and Prevention. (1996). *Guidelines for physical activity for adolescents.* Atlanta: Author.
12. Chodzko-Zajko, W.J. (1998). Physical activity and aging: Implications for health and quality of life in older persons. *PCPFS Research Digest, 3*(4).
13. Fagard, R.H., & Tipton, C.M. (1994). Physical activity, fitness, and hypertension. In C. Bouchard, R.J. Shephard, & T. Stephens (Eds.), *Physical activity, fitness, and health* (pp. 633-655). Champaign, IL: Human Kinetics.
14. Franks, B.D. (1997). Personalizing physical activity prescription. *PCPFS Research Digest, 2*(9).
15. Gordon, N.F. (1998). Conceptual basis for coronary artery disease risk factor assessment. In J.L. Roitman (Ed.), *ACSM's resource manual for guidelines for exercise testing and prescription* (3rd ed.). Philadelphia: Lippincott Williams & Wilkins.
16. Haskell, W.L. (1984). The influence of exercise on the concentrations of triglyceride and cholesterol in human plasma. *Exercise and Sport Sciences Reviews, 12,* 205-244.
17. Haskell, W.L. (1996). Background and definitions. In S. Blair (Ed.), *Surgeon General's report: Physical activity and health.* Washington, DC: U.S. Department of Health and Human Services.
18. Haskell, W.L. (1996). Personal communication.
19. Jones, W.H.S. (Trans.). (1953). *Regimen (Hippocrates).* Cambridge, MA: Harvard University Press.
20. Kohl, H.W., & McKenzie, J.D. (1994). Physical activity, fitness, and stroke. In C. Bouchard, R.J. Shephard, & T. Stephens (Eds.), *Physical activity, fitness, and health* (pp. 609-621). Champaign, IL: Human Kinetics.
21. Kriska, A. (1997). Physical activity and the prevention of Type II diabetes. *PCPFS Research Digest, 2*(10).
22. Landers, D.M. (1997). The influence of exercise on mental health. *PCPFS Research Digest, 2*(12).
23. Lee, I.M. (1995). Physical activity and cancer. *PCPFS Research Digest, 2*(2).
24. Moore, S. (1994). Physical activity, fitness, and atherosclerosis. In C. Bouchard, R.J. Shephard, & T. Stephens (Eds.), *Physical activity, fitness, and health* (pp. 570-578). Champaign, IL: Human Kinetics.
25. National Institutes of Health. (1996). *Physical activity and cardiovascular health.* Rockville, VA: Author.
26. Paffenbarger, R.S., Hyde, R.T., & Wing, A.L. (1986). Physical activity, all-cause mortality, and longevity of college alumni. *New England Journal of Medicine, 314,* 605-613.
27. Pate, R.R., Pratt, M., Blair, S.N., Haskell, W.L., Marcera, C.A., & Bouchard, C. (1995). Physical activity and public health: A recommendation from the Centers for Disease Control and Prevention and the American College of Sports Medicine. *Journal of the American Medical Association, 273,* 402-407.
28. Plowman, S.A. (1993). Physical fitness and healthy low back function. *PCPFS Research Digest, 1*(3).
29. Seaman, J.A. (1999). Physical activity and fitness for persons with disabilities. *PCPFS Research Digest, 3*(5).
30. Shaw, J.M., & Snow-Harter, C. (1995). Osteoporosis and physical activity. *PCPFS Research Digest, 2*(3).
31. Shephard, R. (1996). Exercise, independence, and quality of life in the elderly. *Quest, 48,* 354-365.
32. Spirduso, W.W., & Cronin, D.L. (2001). Exercise dose-response effects on quality of life and independent living in older adults. *Medicine and Science in Sports and Exercise, 33*(Suppl. 6), S598-S608.
33. Thompson, P.D., & Fahrenbach, M.C. (1994). Risks of exercising: Cardiovascular including sudden cardiac death. In C. Bouchard, R.J. Shephard, & T. Stephens (Eds.), *Physical activity, fitness, and health* (pp. 1019-1028). Champaign, IL: Human Kinetics.
34. United States Department of Agriculture and United States Department of Health and Human Services. (2000). *Dietary guidelines for American adults* (6th ed.). Washington, DC: U.S. Government Printing Office.
35. United States Department of Health and Human Services. (1991). *Healthy people 2000: National health promotion and disease prevention objectives* (Publication No. PHS 91-50212). Washington, DC: Author.
36. United States Department of Health and Human Services. (1996). *Surgeon General's report on physical activity and health.* Washington, DC: Author.
37. United States Department of Health and Human Services. (2000). *Healthy people 2010: National health promotion and disease prevention objectives.* Washington, DC: Author.
38. Welk, G.J., & Blair, S.N. (2000). Physical activity protects against the health risks of obesity. *PCPFS Research Digest, 3*(12).
39. Whipp, B.J., & Casaburi, R. (1994). Physical activity, fitness, and chronic lung disease. In C. Bouchard, R.J. Shephard, & T. Stephens (Eds.), *Physical activity, fitness, and health* (pp. 749-761). Champaign, IL: Human Kinetics.

two

Physical Fitness and Performance

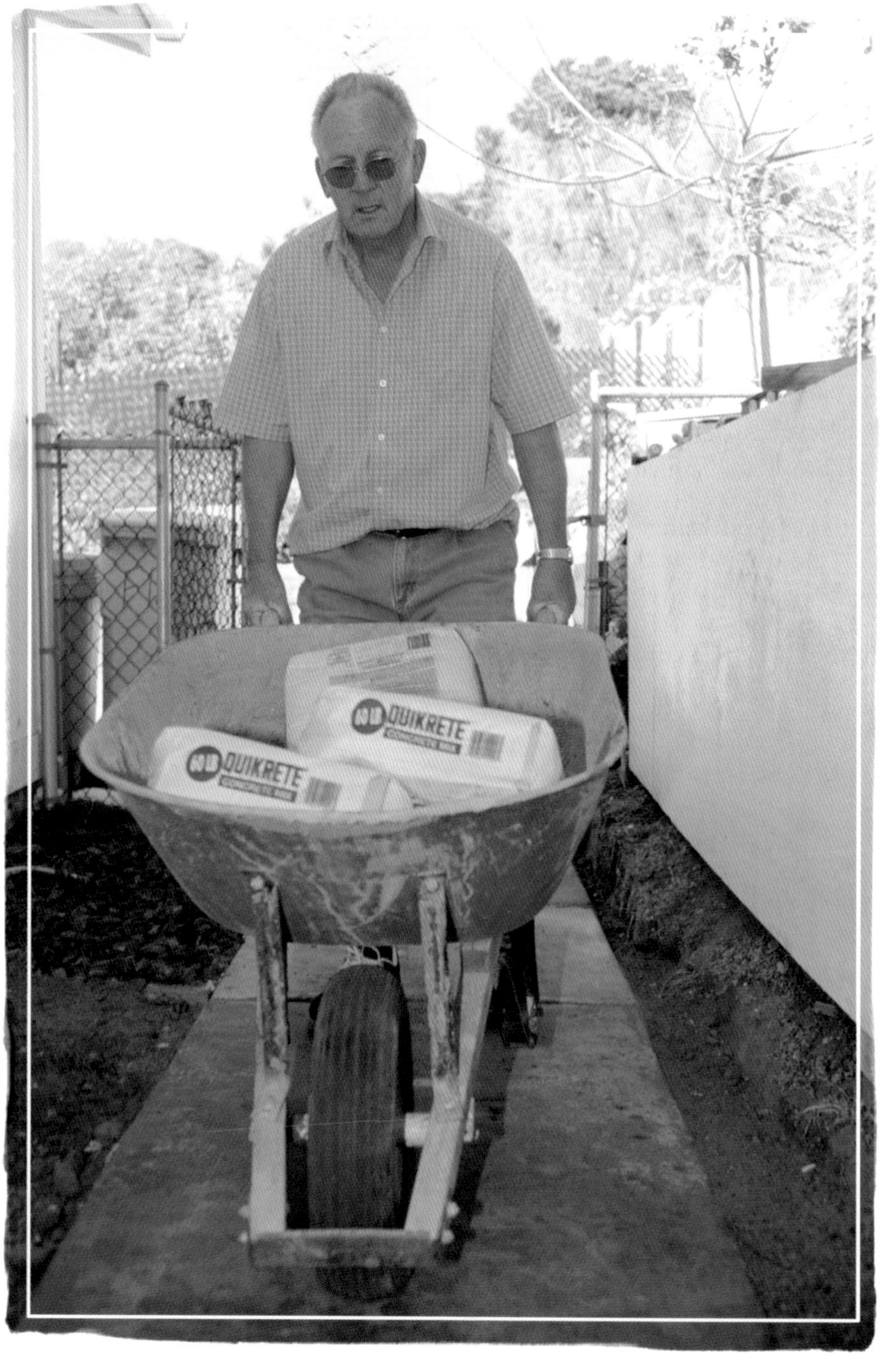

© I.G. Vorster

Objectives

The reader will be able to do the following:

1. Describe the goals of fitness and performance.
2. Demonstrate an understanding of the components of fitness.
3. Define and differentiate among terms related to fitness and performance.
4. Define the major components of performance.
5. Describe healthy behaviors related to fitness.
6. Describe factors related to setting individual fitness goals.
7. Explain the role of fitness professionals in encouraging healthy behavior.

Chapter 1 dealt with the importance of physical activity for total fitness, health, and prevention of premature health problems. It presented the two-prong recommendation for moderate- and vigorous-intensity activity. The first part of the physical activity recommendation emphasizes the importance of sedentary individuals doing some regular moderate-intensity activity to achieve health goals. The second part of the recommendation is to provide vigorous activity (exercise) to enhance fitness benefits and to provide the basis for participation in a variety of performance activities that also enrich life for many individuals. Using recommended definitions, the first chapter dealt with physical activity and health, whereas this chapter explores exercise, physical fitness, and performance. We continue the discussion of activity, fitness, and health by comparing the goals, components, and behaviors related to **physical fitness** (1, 2) and **performance**.

Physical Fitness Goals

The physical fitness goals are to lower risks of developing health problems and to maintain positive physical health. You are undoubtedly familiar with the components of these goals.

To Lower Risks of Developing Health Problems

This goal is an extension of the health goal to avoid disease (chapter 1). Many of the health problems responsible for premature deaths can be prevented with careful screening and preventive action (e.g., immunization). There are still many people in the world who need this basic health care, and medical science can provide this service. The solution to this aspect of health care is finding the resources and political will to make it available to everyone.

In more affluent sectors of societies, where preventive health care is routine, another set of health problems has emerged (e.g., cardiovascular diseases) that cause premature death or disability. As discussed in chapter 1, physical activity plays a major role in preventing the development of premature health problems.

To Maintain Physical Well-Being

Many of the same characteristics that lower our risk for developing serious health problems also provide a higher quality of life. In other words, having high levels of functional capacity and optimal levels of body fat help us feel good and have the energy to do things that enrich our lives. In addition, good muscular endurance and flexibility in the midtrunk area are related to a healthy low back. Weight-bearing activities enhance bone density, helping prevent osteoporosis. As people increase their levels of physical fitness, they move toward a better life, whereas decreases in physical fitness lead to health problems and decreased quality of life.

Performance Goals

The primary performance goals are to complete daily tasks efficiently and to achieve desired levels in selected sports. These goals also involve a number of components.

To Complete Daily Tasks Efficiently

To get through the day efficiently, we must have fundamental motor skills to be able to accomplish various tasks. We must be able to move from place to place and push, pull, pick up, carry, and do a number of other tasks requiring use of the hands and arms. Moderate levels of muscular strength and endurance, flexibility, and cardiorespiratory function are essential for these routine tasks. In addition, we need special abilities to perform the unique activities related to work or home.

This goal also is related to the positive health goal of independent functional living. It is an extension of the physical fitness goal of having healthy levels of cardiorespiratory function, relative leanness, muscular strength and endurance, and flexibility.

To Achieve Desired Levels of Sport Performance

Many individuals also engage in selected games, sports, and high-level performance. In addition to requiring high levels of physical fitness, these activities require specific kinds and levels of motor abilities (such as agility, balance, coordination, power, and speed related to the sport) as well as the particular skills of the sport.

1 In Review

The goals of physical fitness are to have a positive physical health base with a low risk of health problems. Performance goals include the ability to engage in daily tasks with adequate energy and to participate successfully in selected sports.

Components of Physical Fitness and Performance

The components of physical fitness and performance are derived directly from their goals. The physical fitness goals are achieved through exercise that improves and maintains cardiorespiratory function, a healthy level of body fat, muscular strength and endurance, and flexibility. The performance goals are enhanced by specific conditioning to achieve and maintain high levels of aerobic and anaerobic energy; muscular strength, endurance, and power; speed; agility; coordination; balance; and sport skills.

Physical Fitness Components

Components of physical fitness are **cardiorespiratory function**, **relative leanness**, **muscular strength and endurance**, and **flexibility**.

Cardiorespiratory function is essential not only for the health and physical fitness goals of preventing premature cardiovascular problems but also for providing the energy to accomplish other elements related to quality of life. Chapter 28 explains the physiology underlying this component, chapter 5 describes ways to test it, and chapter 10 deals with exercise prescription for improving cardiorespiratory function.

The importance of healthy levels of body fat relates to numerous health and psychological problems. One of the major negative trends reported in the *Healthy People 2010* objectives (3) is the substantial increase in obesity in all ages since the mid-1980s. This is a complex area involving nutrition, physical activity, and behavior modification, which are covered in chapters 6, 7, 11, and 22.

The activities that improve and maintain muscular strength and endurance appear to be important for bone density, thus helping prevent osteoporosis, a problem of decreasing bone mass that affects older women in particular. Chapter 27 provides the basic anatomy, chapter 8 describes ways to assess strength and endurance, and chapter 12 deals with exercise prescription for increasing strength and endurance.

Midtrunk strength, endurance, and flexibility are essential elements in maintaining a healthy low back. Flexibility and low back function are covered in chapters 9 and 13.

2 In Review

Physical fitness components are cardiorespiratory function, relative leanness, muscular strength and endurance, and flexibility. These fitness elements are related to a higher quality of life and prevention of major health problems.

Performance Components

Appropriate levels of cardiorespiratory function, body composition, muscular strength and endurance, and flexibility are important for achieving performance goals. In the first place, modest levels of these fitness components increase the efficiency with which we can do daily tasks around the home, in the yard, and at work. Although this is important at all ages, it is a top priority for elderly individuals because it allows them to continue to live independently for a longer time.

Second, higher levels of these fitness components also provide the basis for successful participation in a variety of sport and performance activities. Although an individual can attain health and fitness goals by doing nonsporting activities, participation in sports and games provides enjoyable health and fitness supplements. In addition to requiring the fitness components, each sport has unique demands for energy, body composition, strength, endurance, and flexibility, along with skill requirements specific to each particular sport. Many sports demand high levels of **agility**, **balance**, **coordination**, **power**, and **speed** that are directly related to the sport.

3 In Review

The definitions provided in the glossary differentiate among terms related to fitness and performance.

Examples of Performance Goals

Because most of this book deals with health and fitness, the following example illustrates the differing needs for the two performance goals. The first performance goal is to complete daily tasks efficiently. Most individuals move around during the day, doing some bending, lifting, carrying, pushing, and pulling, all of which require appropriate levels of cardiorespiratory function, muscular strength and endurance, flexibility, and body fat. In addition to those common needs, a person's lifestyle adds other needs. Contrast, for example, a computer programmer, a firefighter, and a parent staying at home with an infant. The computer programmer will need some stretching and relaxation activities to prevent low back and postural problems and can benefit from short activity breaks. The firefighter is sedentary for most of the time but must be able to respond quickly with near-maximal levels of anaerobic energy and muscular strength and endurance, in an adverse environment with heavy equipment. This person must engage in regular vigorous aerobic, anaerobic, and resistance exercise to maintain the conditioning necessary to respond to emergencies. The parent needs flexibility, strength, and endurance to lift and carry the infant and other items through an obstacle course of toys, clothes, and so on, in addition to learning to perform under conditions of sleep deprivation.

The second performance goal is to achieve desired levels in selected sports, games, and competitions. Although high fitness levels are desirable as a base, individuals here also have very different needs. Compare, for example, 10K runners, basketball players, and golfers. The runners rely on high levels of aerobic power that comes from lots of distance running, with careful stretching before and after. Basketball players depend on a combination of aerobic and anaerobic energy, coordination, and very specific passing, shooting, and defensive skills. Golfers require a moderate cardiorespiratory base, some muscular power, and coordination of a complex skill used in a variety of settings (e.g., fairway, bunker, woods).

Page 21 provides recommendations for performance of sports or work tasks. This box extends that idea to those vigorously active individuals who want to engage in sports and endurance performance. These individuals should enhance fitness components related to their selected sports and increase the skills directly related to the sport.

4 In Review

Performance components include a general fitness base. Specific levels of fitness components and unique skills related to the sport or game are needed for performance.

Behaviors That Support Fitness and Performance Components

The first two sections of this chapter discussed definitions, goals, and components related to physical fitness and performance. To achieve the components of physical fitness, a person must adopt healthy behaviors.

Recommendations for Vigorously Active Individuals Performing Specific Sports or Work Tasks

A vigorously active individual is able to jog 3 miles at moderate to vigorous intensity (e.g., 60-80% maximal oxygen uptake or heart rate reserve) 3 to 5 times/week without discomfort or undue fatigue.

Activity goal:

To engage successfully in selected work or sport performance activities.

Fitness goal:

To have the underlying levels of fitness and the specific skills needed to perform the tasks at the desired level with minimum risks of health problems or injury.

Screening prior to activity:

If the training involves maximal exertion, a medical examination including a maximal exercise test is recommended.

Recommended activities:

Do fitness activities as base (see Part III).

Add additional training related to specific requirements of sport or activity. You may need to exceed total work, intensity, duration, and/or frequency of fitness workouts.

Develop and maintain skills related to the sport or work tasks.

Be aware of safety concerns in performance.

Increase time for warm-up, including moderate-intensity activities directly related to performance of the sport or work tasks.

Behaviors that contribute to fitness goals include adopting healthy eating habits; exercising regularly; avoiding smoking, illegal drug use, and excessive alcohol use; getting adequate sleep and managing stress; and adopting a stretching and strength training regimen. Performance goals can be achieved by adopting healthy behaviors such as developing a resistance training program, using static stretching exercises, participating in regular vigorous exercise, practicing specific sport-related movements, using interval training, and practicing skills in gamelike conditions. The box on the next page summarizes the goals, components, and behaviors for physical fitness and performance.

We have tried to show both the common and unique elements of health, fitness, and performance in these first two chapters. You have probably noticed that there is some repetition in the behaviors recommended for delaying death, avoiding disease, providing low risk of major health problems, and developing high levels of positive health. Although individuals need to be educated about signs, symptoms, and risk factors, the major emphasis of a fitness program should be on the behaviors given in the Health and Fitness Behaviors list (see box on page 23).

Common Behaviors for Fitness and Health

Although behaviors for fitness and health can be differentiated, they are interrelated. People who exercise and exhibit other healthy behaviors are more likely to be fit. Achieving fitness standards leads to a healthy, longer life. On the other hand, sedentary existence is related to low levels of fitness and major health problems that shorten life.

5 In Review

Although there are some differences between health and fitness goals, many of the recommended behaviors are common to both goals. Health and fitness are enhanced with regular exercise and sleep, nutritious diet, no smoking or drug abuse, limited alcohol, ability to cope with stressors, ability to relax, preventive checkups, and safe habits.

Physical Fitness and Performance Goals, Components, and Behaviors

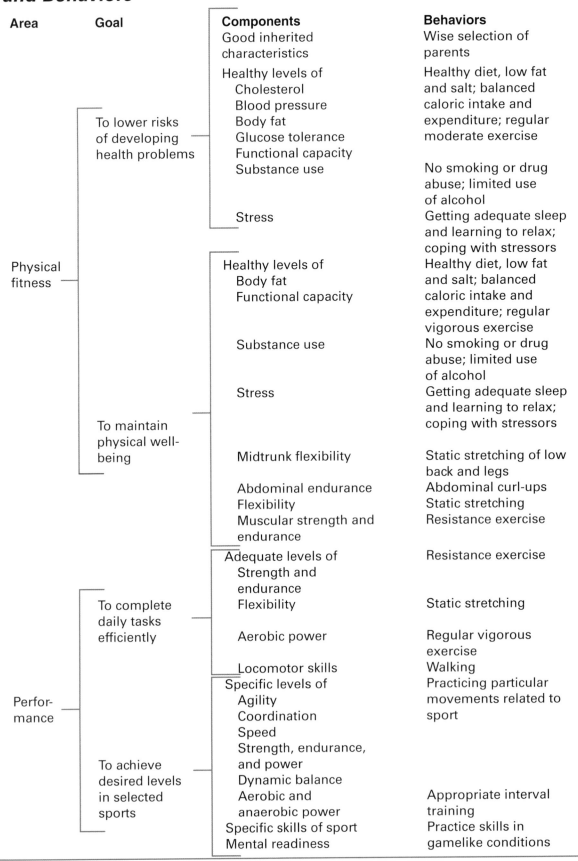

Area	Goal	Components	Behaviors
Physical fitness	To lower risks of developing health problems	Good inherited characteristics	Wise selection of parents
		Healthy levels of Cholesterol Blood pressure Body fat Glucose tolerance Functional capacity	Healthy diet, low fat and salt; balanced caloric intake and expenditure; regular moderate exercise
		Substance use	No smoking or drug abuse; limited use of alcohol
		Stress	Getting adequate sleep and learning to relax; coping with stressors
	To maintain physical well-being	Healthy levels of Body fat Functional capacity	Healthy diet, low fat and salt; balanced caloric intake and expenditure; regular vigorous exercise
		Substance use	No smoking or drug abuse; limited use of alcohol
		Stress	Getting adequate sleep and learning to relax; coping with stressors
		Midtrunk flexibility	Static stretching of low back and legs
		Abdominal endurance	Abdominal curl-ups
		Flexibility	Static stretching
		Muscular strength and endurance	Resistance exercise
Performance	To complete daily tasks efficiently	Adequate levels of Strength and endurance	Resistance exercise
		Flexibility	Static stretching
		Aerobic power	Regular vigorous exercise
		Locomotor skills	Walking
	To achieve desired levels in selected sports	Specific levels of Agility Coordination Speed Strength, endurance, and power Dynamic balance	Practicing particular movements related to sport
		Aerobic and anaerobic power	Appropriate interval training
		Specific skills of sport Mental readiness	Practice skills in gamelike conditions

Health and Fitness Behaviors

Regular physical activity
Low-intensity activity
Moderate-intensity exercise
Abdominal curl-ups
Static stretching for low-back flexibility
Whole-body flexibility and strength/endurance exercise
Healthy diet
Proper proportions of fat, carbohydrates, and proteins
Balance between energy expenditure and intake
Balance among food groups
High levels of complex carbohydrates
Low saturated and total fat
Low salt
Substance use
No smoking
No drugs (except as prescribed by physician)
Limited alcohol use
Stress
Learn to cope with stressors
Learn to relax
Regular sleep
Regular tests for fitness and health
Health risk appraisal
Healthy habits
Fitness status

Setting Fitness Goals

People entering your fitness class or asking you to be their personal trainer have taken an important first step toward improving their fitness levels. It is your responsibility to help them

- understand the components of fitness,
- analyze their current fitness status,
- begin or continue appropriate exercise habits,
- determine other health behaviors that need to be changed, and
- take appropriate steps to change unhealthy behavior.

Chapter 22 suggests ways to help participants start changing unhealthy behaviors. Chapter 14 provides tips for leading fitness programs, as well as specific types of activities that can be used.

6 In Review

Information presented in chapters 1 and 2 will help HFIs and personal fitness trainers (PFTs) to assist individuals in setting appropriate health, fitness, and performance goals.

Taking Control of Personal Health Status

One of the most frustrating and exciting aspects of dealing with current health problems is that individuals can modify their health status and control major health risks. The frustrating aspect is that many people find it difficult to change unhealthy lifestyles. The exciting element is that they can gain control of their health. The HFI and PFT are at the cutting edge of health, in much the same way in which the scientist discovering vaccines for major health problems was at the turn of the 20th century. This opportunity to help people who wish to alter their unhealthy lifestyles carries the responsibility for making recommendations based on the best evidence available. The HFI and PFT can help people gain control of their lives through an evaluation of their risk factors and behaviors related to health. Chapter 3 examines this type of health appraisal.

7 In Review

Physical activity professionals live in an exciting time because of the increasing evidence and recognition that regular physical activity is an essential element for the good life. Nevertheless, it will be a worthwhile challenge to motivate people to begin and continue an active lifestyle when there is so much competition for everyone's time.

Case Study

You can check your answers by referring to appendix A.

2.1

Two people come to you and say they want to "get in shape." After talking with them, you discover that Fred seems to be free from major health problems, but he hasn't done any regular activity for 20 years. Susan, also apparently healthy, has been jogging and doing exercise to music 2 to 4 times per week for the past 5 years. She has just joined an adult soccer league and wants to be able to compete at a higher level. How would you help them formulate and achieve their goals?

Source List

1. Caspersen, C.J., Powell, K.E., & Christensen, G.M. (1985). Physical activity, exercise, and physical fitness: Definition and distinctions for health-related research. *Public Health Reports, 100,* 126-131.
2. Corbin, C.B., Pangrazi, R.P., & Franks, B.D. (2000). Definitions: Health, fitness, and physical activity. *PCPFS Research Digest, 3*(9).
3. U.S. Department of Health and Human Services. (2000). *Healthy people 2010: National health promotion and disease prevention objectives.* Washington, DC: Author.

three

Health Appraisal

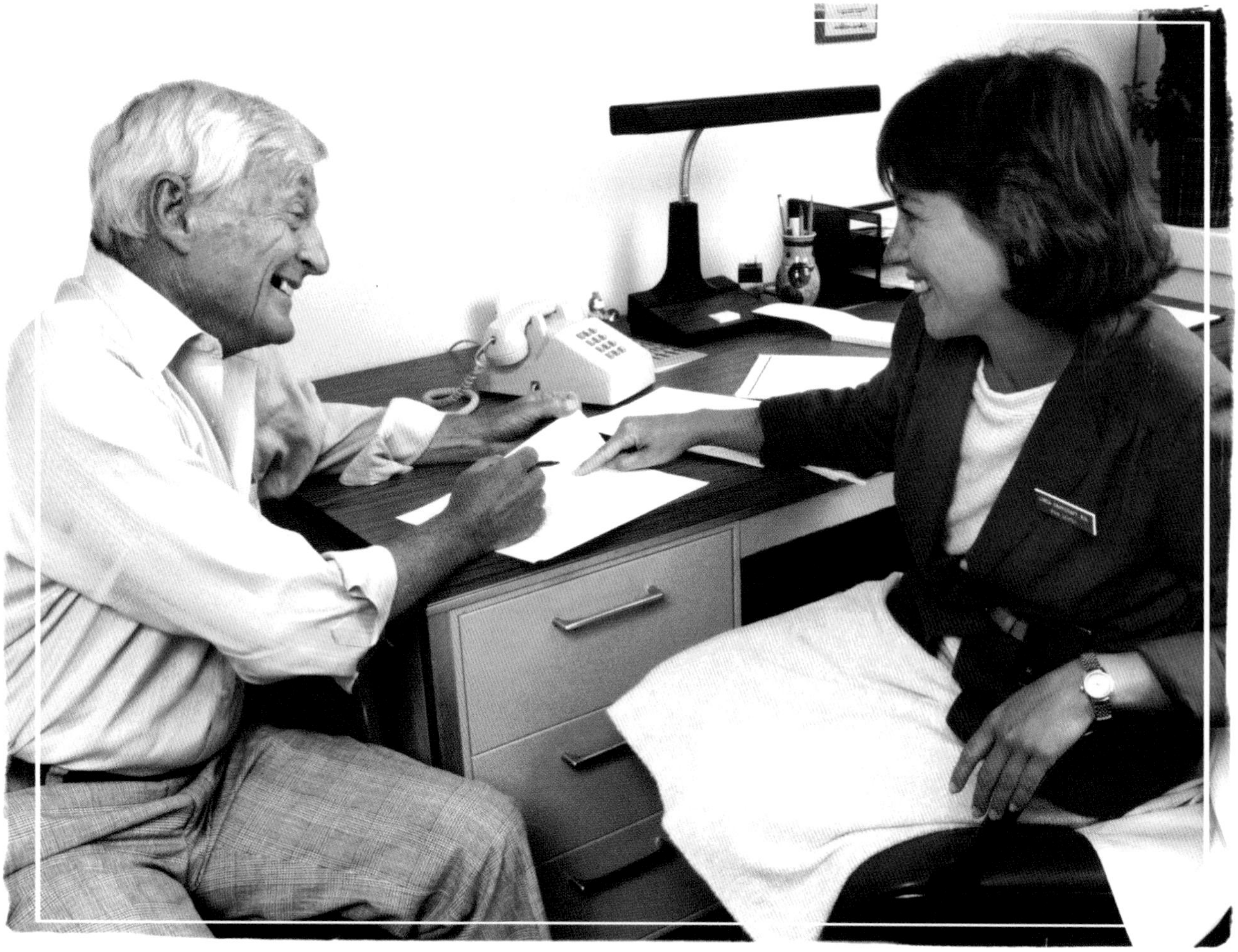

© Getty Images

Objectives

The reader will be able to do the following:

1. Understand the purpose of evaluating the health status of potential fitness participants and identify appropriate instruments for health appraisal.
2. Describe appropriate screening for moderate- and vigorous-intensity exercise.
3. Make recommendations for the type of fitness program participants should develop based on their health status, describe the categories of participants who should receive medical clearance before administration of an exercise test or participation in an exercise program, and identify relative and absolute contraindications to exercise testing or participation.
4. List the conditions and test scores that may indicate the need for a supervised program or special attention during exercise.
5. Identify individuals who need educational material.
6. Identify conditions that would require a change in exercise recommendations and describe the signs and symptoms for participants (including special populations) to defer, delay, or terminate the exercise session.

An important responsibility of the HFI or PFT is to help potential fitness participants determine their current health status. If the person has a major health problem that has been diagnosed and is being treated, then you must rely on guidance from the fitness program director and medical professionals for appropriate fitness programs. If physicians and health professionals have carefully analyzed an individual's health status and found no health problems or unhealthy behaviors, then the individual can start or continue a fitness program, making modifications based on his or her personal interests. Most people, however, are somewhere in between these two extremes. They do not have a known major health problem, but their health status has not been thoroughly checked.

Evaluating Health Status

The HFI or PFT can assist individuals in evaluating their health status by examining five major categories:

- Diagnosed medical problems
- Characteristics that increase the risk of health problems
- Signs or symptoms indicative of health problems
- Lifestyle behaviors related to positive or negative health
- Fitness test results

The health status of the individual is evaluated to provide the person with information concerning health status and healthy and unhealthy behaviors. Health status also is used to make decisions concerning appropriate physical activity recommendations for health and fitness improvement. This chapter includes some forms and charts to use with fitness participants. Forms and charts also are included in the *Health Fitness Handbook* (5). Encourage participants in your fitness program to complete these forms and submit them to you so you can assist them in their programs.

Health Status Questionnaire

The Health Status Questionnaire (HSQ; form 3.1) provides information concerning the first four categories in the preceding list. Part 1 of the HSQ provides personal and emergency information about the individual. You should keep the emergency information readily available in case you need to call the participant's physician or family. Part 2 of the HSQ includes a medical history of the participant and her or his family. This information will help the director of the fitness program decide on appropriate physical activity and educational programs. Part 3 deals with behaviors known to be related to safety and health. You might be able to help the participant modify these behaviors for a healthier lifestyle. Part 4 addresses health-related attitudes associated with a healthy life. Individual questions and parts of questions are coded to help the HFI and PFT use the information. The key to the codes appears at the end of the HSQ.

1 In Review

Evaluating a participant's health status provides the basis for recommended physical activity programs. The HSQ helps appraise medical conditions, characteristics, symptoms, and behaviors.

Fitness Testing

Testing is the other source of information concerning an individual's health status. Items included in fitness testing are listed in table 3.1. Chapters in part II of this book include detailed recommendations for fitness testing.

People of all ages with varying levels of fitness can be encouraged to engage in moderate-intensity activities without either medical clearance or fitness testing. The walking program found in chapter 14 is a good example of the type of exercise that can be recommended almost universally. The Physical Activity Readiness Questionnaire (PAR-Q; figure 3.1) can be used to screen individuals beginning moderate-intensity exercise (3). It has been shown to be useful in referring those who need additional medical screening and advice while not excluding the majority of people who will benefit from participation in daily moderate-intensity exercise. The rest of this chapter deals primarily with the screening procedures used for people interested in vigorous-intensity exercise.

The ACSM (1) recommends that all men over 45 years of age and women over 55 years of age have a maximal graded exercise test (GXT), with a physician present, before beginning vigorous-intensity exercise. The maximal GXT, with a physician present, is also recommended for those who have a high risk of heart disease (e.g., two or more risk factors, one or more signs or symptoms) and those with known cardiac, pulmonary, or metabolic disease. Qualified testers can administer submaximal tests, without a physician, to individuals without disease or symptoms to determine cardiorespiratory fitness and to

Table 3.1 Components of Fitness Testing

Minimum battery	Additional variables
Rest	
HR (beats · min^{-1})	12-lead ECG[a]
BP (mmHg)	Blood profile[b]
% fat	Flexibility for specific joints
Waist circumference	Pulmonary function
Sit-and-reach (cm)	
Submaximal	
HR	ECG
BP	Blood profile
RPE	
Maximal	
BP	$\dot{V}O_2max$
RPE	Blood profile
Time to max (min)	ECG
Functional capacity (METs)	Modified pull-ups
Curl-ups	

Note. HR = heart rate; ECG = electrocardiogram; BP = blood pressure; RPE = rating of perceived exertion: METs = metabolic equivalents.

[a]ECG abnormalities are medically evaluated to determine appropriate referral or placement.

[b]Includes total cholesterol, high-density lipoprotein cholesterol, triglycerides, and glucose. See Ref. (1), table 3.5, p. 48, for other blood variables.

form
3.1

Health Status Questionnaire

Instructions

Complete each question accurately. All information provided is confidential if you choose to submit this form to your fitness instructor.

Part 1. Information about the individual

1. Social Security number ______________________ Date ______________

2. Legal name ______________________ Nickname ______________

3. Mailing address ______________________________________

   Home phone ______________________ Business phone ______________

4. *EI* ______________________________________
   Personal physician Phone

   Address ______________________________________

5. *EI* ______________________________________
   Person to contact in emergency Phone

6. Sex (circle one): Female Male (*RF*)

7. *RF* Date of birth: ______________________________________
   Month Day Year

8. Number of hours worked per week: Less than 20 20-40 41-60 Over 60

9. *SLA* More than 25% of time spent on job (circle all that apply)
   Sitting at desk Lifting or carrying loads Standing Walking Driving

Part 2. Medical history

10-A. *RF* Circle any who died of heart attack before age 55:

Father Brother Son

10-B. *RF* Circle any who died of heart attack before age 65:

Mother Sister Daughter

11. Date of

    Last medical physical exam ______________________
    Year

    Last physical fitness test ______________________
    Year

From Edward T. Howley and B. Don Franks, 2003, *Health Fitness Instructor's Handbook,* 4th ed. (Champaign, IL: Human Kinetics).

(continued)

12. Circle operations you have had:

Back *SLA*	Heart *MC*	Kidney *SLA*	Eyes *SLA*	Joint *SLA*	Neck *SLA*
Ears *SLA*	Hernia *SLA*	Lung *SLA*	Other		

13. Please circle any of the following for which you have been diagnosed or treated by a physician or health professional:

Alcoholism *SEP*	Diabetes *SEP*	Kidney problem *MC*
Anemia, sickle cell *SEP*	Emphysema *SEP*	Mental illness *SEP*
Anemia, other *SEP*	Epilepsy *SEP*	Neck strain *SLA*
Asthma *SEP*	Eye problems *SLA*	Obesity *RF*
Back strain *SLA*	Gout *SLA*	Phlebitis *MC*
Bleeding trait *SEP*	Hearing loss *SLA*	Rheumatoid arthritis *SLA*
Bronchitis, chronic *SEP*	Heart problem *MC*	Stroke *MC*
Cancer *SEP*	High blood pressure *RF*	Thyroid problem *SEP*
Cirrhosis, liver *MC*	Hypoglycemia *SEP*	Ulcer *SEP*
Concussion *MC*	Hyperlipidemia *RF*	Other
Congenital defect *SEP*	Infectious mononucleosis *MC*	

14. Circle all medicine taken in last 6 months:

Blood thinner *MC*	Epilepsy medication *SEP*	Nitroglycerin *MC*
Diabetic *SEP*	Heart rhythm medication *MC*	Other
Digitalis *MC*	High blood pressure medication *MC*	
Diuretic *MC*	Insulin *MC*	

(continued)

15. Any of these health symptoms that occurs frequently is the basis for medical attention. Circle the number indicating how often you have each of the following:

5 = Very often
4 = Fairly often
3 = Sometimes
2 = Infrequently
1 = Practically never

a. Cough up blood *MC*
1 2 3 4 5

b. Abdominal pain *MC*
1 2 3 4 5

c. Low-back pain *MC*
1 2 3 4 5

d. Leg pain *MC*
1 2 3 4 5

e. Arm or shoulder pain *MC*
1 2 3 4 5

f. Chest pain *RF MC*
1 2 3 4 5

g. Swollen joints *MC*
1 2 3 4 5

h. Feel faint *MC*
1 2 3 4 5

i. Dizziness *MC*
1 2 3 4 5

j. Breathless with slight exertion *MC*
1 2 3 4 5

k. Palpitation or fast heart beat *MC*
1 2 3 4 5

l. Unusual fatigue with normal activity *MC*
1 2 3 4 5

Part 3. Health-related behavior

16. *RF* Do you now smoke (or have smoked in last 6 months)? Yes No

17. *RF* If you are a smoker, indicate number smoked per day:

Cigarettes: 40 or more 20-39 10-19 1-9

Cigars or pipes only: 5 or more or any inhaled Less than 5, none inhaled

18. *RF* Do you exercise regularly (i.e., accumulate at least 30 min per day, at least five days/week)? Yes No

19. How many days per week do you accumulate 30 minutes of moderate activity?

0 1 2 3 4 5 6 7 days per week

20. How many days per week do you normally spend at least 20 minutes in vigorous exercise?

0 1 2 3 4 5 6 7 days per week

21. Can you walk 4 miles briskly without fatigue? Yes No

22. Can you jog 3 miles continuously at a moderate pace without discomfort? Yes No

23. Weight now: _________ lb. One year ago: _________ lb. Age 21: _________ lb.

From Edward T. Howley and B. Don Franks, 2003, *Health Fitness Instructor's Handbook,* 4th ed. (Champaign, IL: Human Kinetics).

(continued)

Part 4. Health-related attitudes

24. *RF*These are traits that have been associated with coronary-prone behavior. Circle the number that corresponds to how you feel:

    6 = Strongly agree
    5 = Moderately agree
    4 = Slightly agree
    3 = Slightly disagree
    2 = Moderately disagree
    1 = Strongly disagree

    I am an impatient, time-conscious, hard-driving individual.

    1 2 3 4 5 6

25. List everything not already included on this questionnaire that might cause you problems in a fitness test or fitness program:

    ____
    ____
    ____
    ____
    ____
    ____
    ____
    ____
    ____
    ____

Code for Health Status Questionnaire
The following code will help you evaluate the information in the Health Status Questionnaire.
EI = Emergency Information—must be readily available.
MC = Medical Clearance needed—do not allow exercise without physician's permission.
SEP = Special Emergency Procedures needed—do not let participant exercise alone; make sure the person's exercise partner knows what to do in case of an emergency.
RF = Risk Factor for CHD (educational materials and workshops needed).
SLA = Special or Limited Activities may be needed—you may need to include or exclude specific exercises.
OTHER (not marked) = Personal information that may be helpful for files or research.

Physical Activity Readiness
Questionnaire - PAR-Q
(revised 1994)

PAR - Q & YOU

(A Questionnaire for People Aged 15 to 69)

Regular physical activity is fun and healthy, and increasingly more people are starting to become more active every day. Being more active is very safe for most people. However, some people should check with their doctor before they start becoming much more physically active.

If you are planning to become much more physically active than you are now, start by answering the seven questions in the box below. If you are between the ages of 15 and 69, the PAR-Q will tell you if you should check with your doctor before you start. If you are over 69 years of age, and you are not used to being very active, check with your doctor.

Common sense is your best guide when you answer these questions. Please read the questions carefully and answer each one honestly: check YES or NO.

YES	NO		
☐	☐	1.	Has your doctor ever said that you have a heart condition and that you should only do physical activity recommended by a doctor?
☐	☐	2.	Do you feel pain in your chest when you do physical activity?
☐	☐	3.	In the past month, have you had chest pain when you were not doing physical activity?
☐	☐	4.	Do you lose your balance because of dizziness or do you ever lose consciousness?
☐	☐	5.	Do you have a bone or joint problem that could be made worse by a change in your physical activity?
☐	☐	6.	Is your doctor currently prescribing drugs (for example, water pills) for your blood pressure or heart condition?
☐	☐	7.	Do you know of any other reason why you should not do physical activity?

If you answered

YES to one or more questions

Talk with your doctor by phone or in person BEFORE you start becoming much more physically active or BEFORE you have a fitness appraisal. Tell your doctor about the PAR-Q and which questions you answered YES.

- You may be able to do any activity you want — as long as you start slowly and build up gradually. Or, you may need to restrict your activities to those which are safe for you. Talk with your doctor about the kinds of activities you wish to participate in and follow his/her advice.
- Find out which community programs are safe and helpful for you.

NO to all questions

If you answered NO honestly to all PAR-Q questions, you can be reasonably sure that you can:

- start becoming much more physically active — begin slowly and build up gradually. This is the safest and easiest way to go.
- take part in a fitness appraisal — this is an excellent way to determine your basic fitness so that you can plan the best way for you to live actively. It is also highly recommended that you have your blood pressure evaluated. If your reading is over 144/94, talk with your doctor before you start becoming much more physically active.

DELAY BECOMING MUCH MORE ACTIVE:

- if you are not feeling well because of a temporary illness such as a cold or a fever — wait until you feel better; or
- if you are or may be pregnant — talk to your doctor before you start becoming more active.

Please note: If your health changes so that you then answer YES to any of the above questions, tell your fitness or health professional. Ask whether you should change your physical activity plan.

Informed Use of the PAR-Q: The Canadian Society for Exercise Physiology, Health Canada, and their agents assume no liability for persons who undertake physical activity, and if in doubt after completing this questionnaire, consult your doctor prior to physical activity.

You are encouraged to copy the PAR-Q but only if you use the entire form

NOTE: If the PAR-Q is being given to a person before he or she participates in a physical activity program or a fitness appraisal, this section may be used for legal or administrative purposes.

I have read, understood and completed this questionnaire. Any questions I had were answered to my full satisfaction.

NAME ______________________________

SIGNATURE ______________________________ DATE ______________________

SIGNATURE OF PARENT ______________________________ WITNESS ______________________
or GUARDIAN (for participants under the age of majority)

Supported by: Health Canada Santé Canada

Figure 3.1 PAR-Q. Encourage individuals of various fitness levels to complete this form prior to beginning moderate-intensity exercise.

serve as a baseline for exercise prescription. Table 3.2 summarizes the ACSM recommendations (1) concerning who should have medical clearance and submaximal or maximal GXTs before participation and who should have medical supervision while taking exercise tests.

Regular medical examinations are encouraged for everyone. Obviously, seeing a physician is appropriate whenever special medical problems exist. Table 3.3 presents guidelines for the frequency of medical examinations recommended by the National Conference on Preventive Medicine (8). The Expert Panel on Detection, Evaluation, and Treatment of High Blood Cholesterol in Adults (4) recommends that healthy adults get cholesterol screened every 5 years.

2 In Review

Moderate-intensity exercise can be recommended for anyone who has self-screened with the PAR-Q. All aspects of health status—medical problems, health-related characteristics, signs, symptoms, behaviors, and fitness tests—should be evaluated before vigorous-intensity exercise. GXTs are recommended as the first part of a fitness program.

Table 3.3 Recommended Frequency of Medical Exams

Age	Frequency of medical examination
0-1	At least 4 times
2, 5, 8, 15, 18, 25	At each age listed
35 to 65	Every 5 years
Over 65	Every 2 years

Making Decisions Based on Health Status

Health status information, informed consent of the potential participant, and the goals and interests of the individual are all part of making decisions about appropriate physical activities. The following guidelines based on health status must be tempered with consideration of participants' long-term goals and interests. We discuss the decision-making process in terms of a structured fitness program/center; however, PFTs working with individuals can use the same guidelines.

Table 3.2 ACSM Recommendations for (A) Medical Examination* and Exercise Testing Before Participation and (B) Physician Supervision of Exercise Tests

	Low risk	Moderate risk	High risk
A.			
Moderate exercise†	Not necessary‡	Not necessary	Recommended
Vigorous exercise§	Not necessary	Recommended	Recommended
B.			
Submaximal test	Not necessary	Not necessary	Recommended
Maximal test	Not necessary	Recommended‖	Recommended

*Within the past year.

†Absolute moderate exercise is defined as activities that are approximately 3-6 METs or the equivalent of brisk walking at 3 to 4 mph for most healthy adults (13). Nevertheless, a pace of 3 to 4 mph might be considered to be "hard" to "very hard" by some sedentary, older persons. Moderate exercise may alternatively be defined as an intensity well within the individual's capacity, one which can be comfortably sustained for a prolonged period of time (~45 min), which has a gradual initiation and progression, and is generally noncompetitive. If an individual's exercise capacity is known, relative moderate exercise may be defined by the range 40-60% maximal oxygen uptake.

‡The designation of "Not necessary" reflects the notion that a medical examination, exercise test, and physician supervision of exercise testing would not be essential in the preparticipation screening; however, they should not be viewed as inappropriate.

§Vigorous exercise is defined as activities of >6 METs. Vigorous exercise may alternatively be defined as exercise intense enough to represent a substantial cardiorespiratory challenge. If an individual's exercise capacity is known, vigorous exercise may be defined as an intensity of >60% maximal oxygen uptake.

‖When physician supervision of exercise testing is "Recommended," the physician should be in close proximity and readily available should there be an emergent need.

Reprinted, by permission, from American College of Sports Medicine 2000.

Making Fitness Program Decisions

A fitness program might not use all of the items on the HSQ—the program director should decide what items are relevant for a specific fitness program. Each item on the HSQ is coded to help you identify emergency information and the items that are related to major health problems or require special attention (see HSQ code at the end of form 3.1). The health status form and fitness testing allow the fitness program director to recommend one of the following actions concerning the person's request to enter a fitness program:

- Denial of request for entry to fitness program or immediate referral for medical attention
- Admission to one of the following fitness programs:

  Medically supervised exercise

  Exercise carefully prescribed and supervised by an exercise leader

  Vigorous-intensity exercise

  Any unsupervised physical activity
- Educational information, workshops, or professional help

The fitness director needs to decide whether a potential fitness participant should get medical clearance before beginning a fitness program. The standards in this area are changing. In the 1960s and 1970s it was recommended that everyone get a complete medical examination before beginning a fitness program. Three factors, however, have caused that standard to change. First, it was increasingly recognized that being active is healthier than being inactive. Second, there was increasing evidence that beginning a good fitness program involved a very low risk of health problems for the vast majority of people. And third, the expense and time could not be justified for healthy individuals—medical examinations were needed more for individuals with known or suspected health problems.

Each fitness program should determine its policy with regard to medical clearance and testing before a participant begins an exercise program. The information in table 3.2 can serve as guidelines for the development of policy.

Guidelines for Determining Necessary Supervision

Table 3.4 summarizes the criteria for determining the level of supervision needed by an individual participating in or beginning an exercise program. This section discusses the criteria more thoroughly. Selecting specific test scores as an indication of high, moderate, or low risk is somewhat arbitrary. In most cases, it would be more accurate to view the variable as going from low to high risk. For example, it is better to have lower total cholesterol (the sum of all forms of cholesterol). Although 240 mg/dl has been set as a high-risk level (4), a person with 239 mg/dl is not really different from someone with 242 mg/dl. Nor is a person with 202 mg/dl really different from someone with 198 mg/dl, even though 200 mg/dl is set as a target goal. We should encourage all participants to decrease their total cholesterol; as it decreases, they will have lower risk. There is nothing magical about getting below 240 mg/dl or 200 mg/dl—these are only goals that have been set along the continuum of high to low risk.

Note that the values listed for medical referral and for supervised programs are guidelines to be used along with other information by the individual and fitness program director. For example, the risk of the same total cholesterol would be viewed differently for people with different levels of high-density lipoprotein cholesterol (HDL-C). Some of the variables may be influenced by pretest activities and reaction to the testing situation itself (especially in the person who is not accustomed to being tested). Borderline scores, especially at rest and during light work, should be replicated before medical referral. For example, if a high resting heart rate (HR) or blood pressure (BP) is measured, it may have been because the participant ate, smoked, or participated in physical exercise just before the test. Was the person anxious about taking the test itself? Were there unusual conditions during the test (e.g., lots of people, noise)? The individual should relax for a few minutes, be reassured about the purpose and safety of the test, and then be measured again. On the other hand, a test session might be scheduled for another day. If the questionable test result is repeated, the program director may refer that individual to a physician.

There may be other factors that would cause a person with the characteristics we have listed under *supervised* programs to be medically referred (e.g., multiple risk factors close to the referral value). Or the medical consultant may recommend that someone in our *referral* category be in the supervised program, based on a recent medical examination or conversation with the personal physician. Programs with excellent and accessible medical and emergency personnel may want to use higher values for referral than a program that is isolated from medical

Table 3.4 Conditions and Test Score Criteria for Physical Activity Decisions

Basis for medical referral

Conditions

Breathless with slight exertion	Heart operation, disease, or problem
Cirrhosis	Pain in the abdomen, leg, arm, shoulder, or chest
Concussion	Phlebitis
Coughing up blood	Stroke
Current medication for heart, blood pressure, or diabetes	Swollen joints
Faintness or dizziness	

Test scores[a]

Resting HR > 100 bpm	LDL > 130 mg/dl
Resting SBP > 160 mmHg	
Resting DBP > 100 mmHg	Fasting glucose > 120 mg/dl
% fat > 40 female; > 30 male	Vital capacity < 75% predicted
Cholesterol > 240 mg/dl	FEV_1 < 75%

Basis for a supervised program

Conditions (currently under control)[b]

Alcoholism	Diabetes
Allergy	Emphysema
Anemia	Epilepsy
Asthma	Hypoglycemia
Bleeding trait	Mental illness
Bronchitis	Peptic ulcer
Cancer	Pregnancy
Colitis	Thyroid problem

Test scores[c]

Hypertension 140-155/90-95 mmHg	Waist circumference > 100 cm
Hyperlipidemia (cholesterol) 200-239 mg/dl	Smoking > 20 cigarettes/day
LDL > 100 mg/dl	Exercise < 1.5 hr/week at or above moderate intensity
Obesity 32-38% female; 25-28% male	

Basis for special attention

Conditions

Arthritis	Hearing loss
Back, eye, joint, lung, or neck operations	Hernia
Eye problems	Lengthy time spent driving, lifting, sitting, or standing
Gout	Low-back pain

Test scores

Values of risk factors approaching those in supervised programs	% fat < 15% or > 30% females; < 6% or > 25% males[d]
Any of the reasons for stopping a maximal test that occur at light to moderate work	Curl-ups < 10
Max RPE < 5 (15 on 6-20 scale)	Sit-and-reach < 15 cm
Max METs < 8	Modified pull-ups < 5
Max $\dot{V}O_2$ < 30	Push-ups < 10

Note. Any condition or test value that causes the person or the HFI to be concerned for the person's health or safety is the basis for medical referral. HR = heart rate; LDL = low-density lipoprotein; SBP = systolic blood pressure; DBP = diastolic blood pressure; FEV_1 = forced expiratory volume in 1 s; RPE = rating of percceived exertion.

[a]Any of these individual scores would be the basis for referral. A person might also be referred if more than one test score approached these values.

[b]Severe or uncontrolled levels should be referred for medical attention.

[c]Persons with higher scores should be referred for medical attention.

[d]Participants who have either too little fat or too much fat may have health problems that need special attention. If there is any question, refer them to the program director.

and emergency facilities. It is recommended that each program, in consultation with its medical advisors, establish its own standards.

Medical Referral

All people indicating illness, characteristics, or symptoms coded MC (medical clearance) in the HSQ are referred to appropriate medical personnel. With permission of the appropriate physician, the individual can be placed in a medically supervised, or HFI-supervised, fitness program. The items that fall into those categories, as well as the test scores from the fitness tests that would be the basis for medical referral, are shown in table 3.4.

The values selected for medical referral or supervised programs are somewhat arbitrary, but they are based on the recommendations of experts in these areas. All of the variables (with the exception of high HR) have been listed as risk factors for CHD at these levels. The values for medical referral are considered very high (with substantial risk of CHD). The minimal level indicating problems in these areas (with greater risk of CHD than normal values) is reflected in our values for supervised programs.

A high resting HR indicates severe stress, which may have a physical or emotional base. Extreme amounts of fat put the individual at high risk for a variety of health problems (see chapter 6). A high level of serum glucose is related to diabetes. High BP has been the subject of numerous reports and conferences. For example, the sixth report of the Joint National Committee on Detection, Evaluation, and Treatment of High Blood Pressure (6) identifies mild, moderate, and severe hypertension as systolic BP of 140, 160, or 180 mmHg, respectively, with diastolic BP of 90, 100, or 110 mmHg as mild, moderate, or severe hypertension, respectively. These values are based on repeated measurements.

The role of serum lipids in the atherosclerotic process has been investigated extensively. Cholesterol and triglycerides are carried in the bloodstream in lipoproteins, with the following subdivisions:

- very low density lipoproteins (VLDL)
- low density lipoprotein cholesterol (LDL-C)
- high density lipoprotein cholesterol (HDL-C)
- total cholesterol
- total cholesterol/HDL-C ratio

The third report of the Expert Panel on Detection, Evaluation, and Treatment of High Blood Cholesterol in Adults (4) selected 200 mg/dl and below as a desirable total cholesterol goal, with 240 mg/dl and higher as high risk. LDL-C levels 130 mg/dl and over are high risk, with 100 mg/dl and below being low risk. HDL-C values 40 mg/dl and below are considered a high risk for CHD. In addition, the ACSM (1) lists HDL-C greater than 60 mg/dl (1.6 mmol/L) as a negative risk factor for CHD.

Pulmonary function frequently is evaluated as a part of the screening aspect of a fitness program. Although many of these variables change little during a typical fitness program, the HFI or PFT can provide a service to participants by suggesting that people with low values participate in additional testing. Both vital capacity (VC) forced expiratory volume in 1 second (FEV_1) should be tested.

3 In Review

Based on evaluation of participants' health status, HFIs can advise people to seek medical attention, begin moderate-intensity exercise, or participate in vigorous-intensity exercise with or without supervision. The items listed in table 3.4 for medical referral or supervised programs are guidelines to be used with other information about the individual in making a decision concerning safe and appropriate physical activity. Individuals with medical conditions or characteristics, symptoms, behaviors, or test scores that place them at a high risk for major health problems should have medical clearance before increasing their level of physical activity.

Supervised Program

The conditions and test scores listed in table 3.4 may be the basis for medical referral if they are severe; however, individuals with mild or moderate levels can participate in moderate-intensity exercise or in carefully supervised fitness programs. A person indicating items on the HSQ coded special emergency procedure (SEP) or with risk factors for CHD (coded RF) can be placed in a carefully supervised fitness program, with the necessary emergency procedures readily available, or can participate in moderate-intensity exercise with education about what to do in case of an emergency. It is important that the program director determine whether any of the participants have these or other conditions that might affect their ability to exercise.

Numerous conditions and fitness test scores call for special or limited activities. Your recommended adaptation of activities will be based on common sense regarding the condition, talking with the participant about how to deal with the situation, and consulting with the fitness director or physician about appropriate limitations. You should encourage these individuals to include special activities aimed at improving the fitness components for which they obtained the low scores.

Although we recommend that all fitness participants be screened before participation in a vigorous-intensity exercise program, we know that exercise leaders are often in a position to lead vigorous-intensity exercise (such as an aerobic dance class) for people who have not been screened. The PAR-Q can be completed either by each individual before exercise (in writing or orally) or by the exercise leader asking for answers from the group as the first part of the exercise session. We suggest that you refer all those who answer yes to any of these questions to the director of the fitness program prior to exercise. The director should decide whether to make a medical referral, recommend moderate-intensity exercise, or allow participation in the vigorous-intensity supervised program. For example, individuals who have been active in the past without problems may be allowed in the exercise program even if they have high cholesterol or smoke, whereas previously sedentary individuals with the same risk factors might be directed to a walking and stretching program.

4 In Review

Individuals with moderate risk of major health problems or conditions that require special attention or emergency procedures may be directed by qualified instructors or medical personnel to participate in supervised physical activities. Exercise leaders who have unevaluated individuals in a group program should include some screening as part of the class.

Unsupervised Program

People without any of the problems coded under MC, SEP, or RF in the HSQ can participate in an unsupervised program and be admitted to any of the fitness activities offered by a fitness center. If they have not been active in the past few months, it is recommended that they begin with moderate-intensity activities, but they will be able to progress quickly to other activities of interest and greater intensity.

Education

The HSQ and fitness test results also provide the fitness leader with information about needed education and workshops. All people with risk factors for CHD should be given information about their increased risk. Sufficient evidence allows you to indicate areas of potential health problems, assist individuals in becoming aware of the risk characteristics that cannot be changed, and help people to change those health-related behaviors that can be modified. Chapter 22 provides information to assist the fitness leader in using behavior modification for desired behavior changes. Also, a number of questions on the HSQ indicate a need for education in terms of exercise, nutrition, alcohol, smoking, or stress management. This information will be useful for the program director in deciding what workshops and educational materials should be offered to the participants.

5 In Review

Individuals who have moderate risk of CHD, conditions that might be affected by exercise, or borderline fitness scores should receive education about their problems and know what to do in emergencies.

Change of Health/ Fitness Status

This chapter has dealt with the initial screenings and the resulting decisions concerning appropriate fitness programs. The HFI and PFT need to understand that people who are in exercise programs may have changes in their health/fitness status that require a change in their program. One of the purposes of periodic testing is to determine whether people should be reassigned to different programs. It is common for individuals to make improvements that will safely allow additional exercise options as part of their fitness programs. In other cases, negative changes might occur that need your attention. For example, if an individual in an unsupervised program develops chronic symptoms such as pain in the chest or legs during exercise, he or she should be referred to a physician, retested, or placed in the supervised program, depending on the severity of the problem. Temporary symptoms such as unusual fatigue may suggest a modification of the exercise (e.g., lowering the arms to lower HR) or a temporary deferment of the exercise session.

There are reasons to discontinue a vigorous-intensity exercise program, including severe psychological, medical, or drug- or alcohol-abuse problems that are not responding to therapy, or problems that are aggravated by activity (7). Other reasons to temporarily defer exercise include excessive heat, humidity, or pollution (see chapter 10); sunburn; overindulgence in food, alcohol, stimulating beverages, or drugs such as decongestants, bronchodilators, or atropine; dehydration; or anything that causes unusual discomfort with exercise. Exercise should be deferred with major changes in resting BP or emotional problems (adapted from 2 and 7).

6 In Review

The HFI should be alert to temporary or chronic conditions, such as the ones discussed in this section, that will change an individual's health status, resulting in an increase or decrease in exercise options, a postponement of exercise, a reevaluation of the degree of supervision needed during exercise, or a medical referral.

Case Studies

You can check your answers by referring to appendix A.

3.1

You are teaching an exercise-to-music class open to the public. Everyone in the class answered no to all the questions on the checklist for walk-in, vigorous-intensity exercisers, except for one obese woman who answered that she becomes breathless after mild exercise. When you talk to her, it is obvious that she does not know her BP or cholesterol levels. She has never done any fitness or sport activities and cannot climb a flight of stairs or walk two blocks without getting out of breath. She has been reading about the importance of exercise and decided that she should become active. What advice would you give her?

3.2

An African-American male letter carrier for the post office, age 42, has just signed up for the fitness program. He appears to be a little nervous. According to his HSQ, he can engage in unsupervised exercise. You are checking his resting HR and BP before a GXT and measure HR = 110 and BP = 180/86. What would you do?

3.3

John is a 50-year-old white male and is employed as an executive with a large computer firm. He is responsible for marketing new computer systems in a very competitive environment. He is married and has three children, ages 14, 18, and 22. He feels the financial pressures associated with college bills and the need to keep up with the neighbors. His father died of a heart attack last year at age 72; his mother is 70 and suffered a stroke 3 months after her husband's death. John smokes a pack of cigarettes a day and, recently, he experienced dizziness when climbing stairs. He decided to get a physical exam. The following values were obtained: resting BP = 148/96 mm Hg; total cholesterol = 198 mg/dl; HDL-C = 25 mg/dl; glucose = 90 mg/dl; height = 70 in.; weight = 198 lb; % fat = 32%.

a. List his risk factors.
b. What kind of nonpharmacological intervention programs do you think his physician might recommend?

Source List

1. American College of Sports Medicine. (2000). *ACSM's guidelines for exercise testing and prescription* (6th ed.). Philadelphia: Lippincott Williams & Wilkins.
2. American Heart Association Science Advisory. (1997). Guide to primary prevention of cardiovascular diseases. A statement for healthcare professionals from the task force on risk reduction. *Circulation, 95*, 2-4.
3. Canadian Society for Exercise Physiology. (1994). *PAR-Q and you*. Gloucester, ON: Canadian Society for Exercise Physiology.
4. Expert Panel on Detection, Evaluation, and Treatment of High Blood Cholesterol in Adults. (2001). *Journal of the American Medical Association*, 285(19), 2486-97.
5. Franks, B.D., Howley, E.T., & Iyriboz, Y. (1999). *Health fitness handbook*. Champaign, IL: Human Kinetics.
6. Joint National Committee on Prevention, Detection, Evaluation, and Treatment of High Blood Pressure. (2001). *Sixth report* (NIH Publication No. 98-4080). Bethesda, MD: National Institutes of Health.
7. Painter, P., & Haskell, W.H. (1988). Decision making in programming exercise. In S.N. Blair, P. Painter, R.R. Pate, L.K. Smith, & C.B. Taylor (Eds.), *Resource manual for guidelines for exercise testing and prescription* (pp. 256-262). Philadelphia: Lea & Febiger.
8. Sharkey, B.J. (1990). *Physiology of fitness* (3rd ed.). Champaign, IL: Human Kinetics.

part two

Evaluation of Fitness

An important responsibility of HFIs and PFTs is to answer the question, "what does it mean?" This question is often raised regarding fitness test scores. In the chapters in **Part II,** we examine evaluation of energy cost **(chapter 4)**, cardiorespiratory fitness **(chapter 5)**, body composition and nutrition **(chapters 6 and 7)**, muscular strength and endurance **(chapter 8)**, and flexibility and low back function **(chapter 9)**.

Before you begin, you may want to review or acquaint yourself with the general principles supporting fitness testing. How do you select appropriate tests? How can you obtain more accurate results? What is the best way to analyze results? For a complete introduction to the general topic of fitness evaluation, please see appendix E.

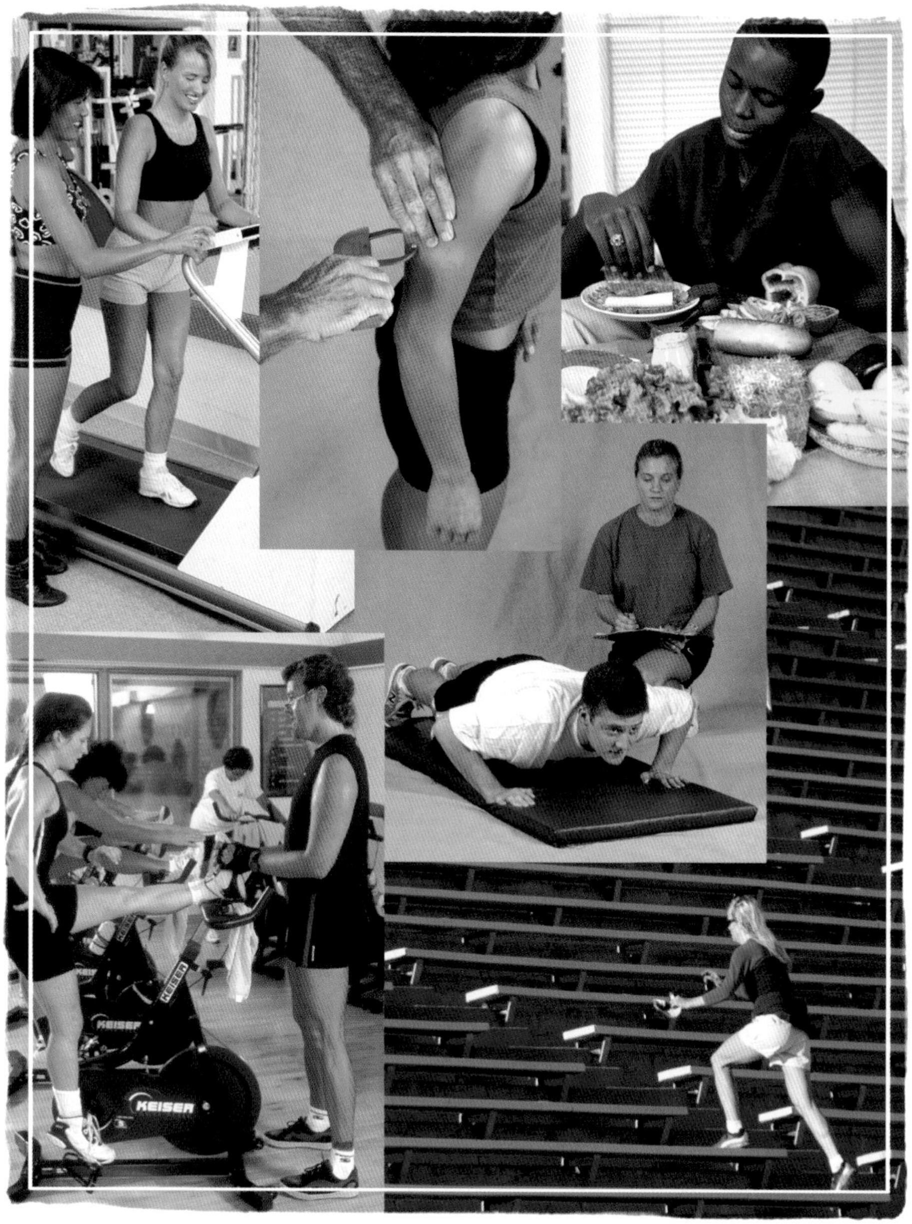

four

Energy Costs of Physical Activity

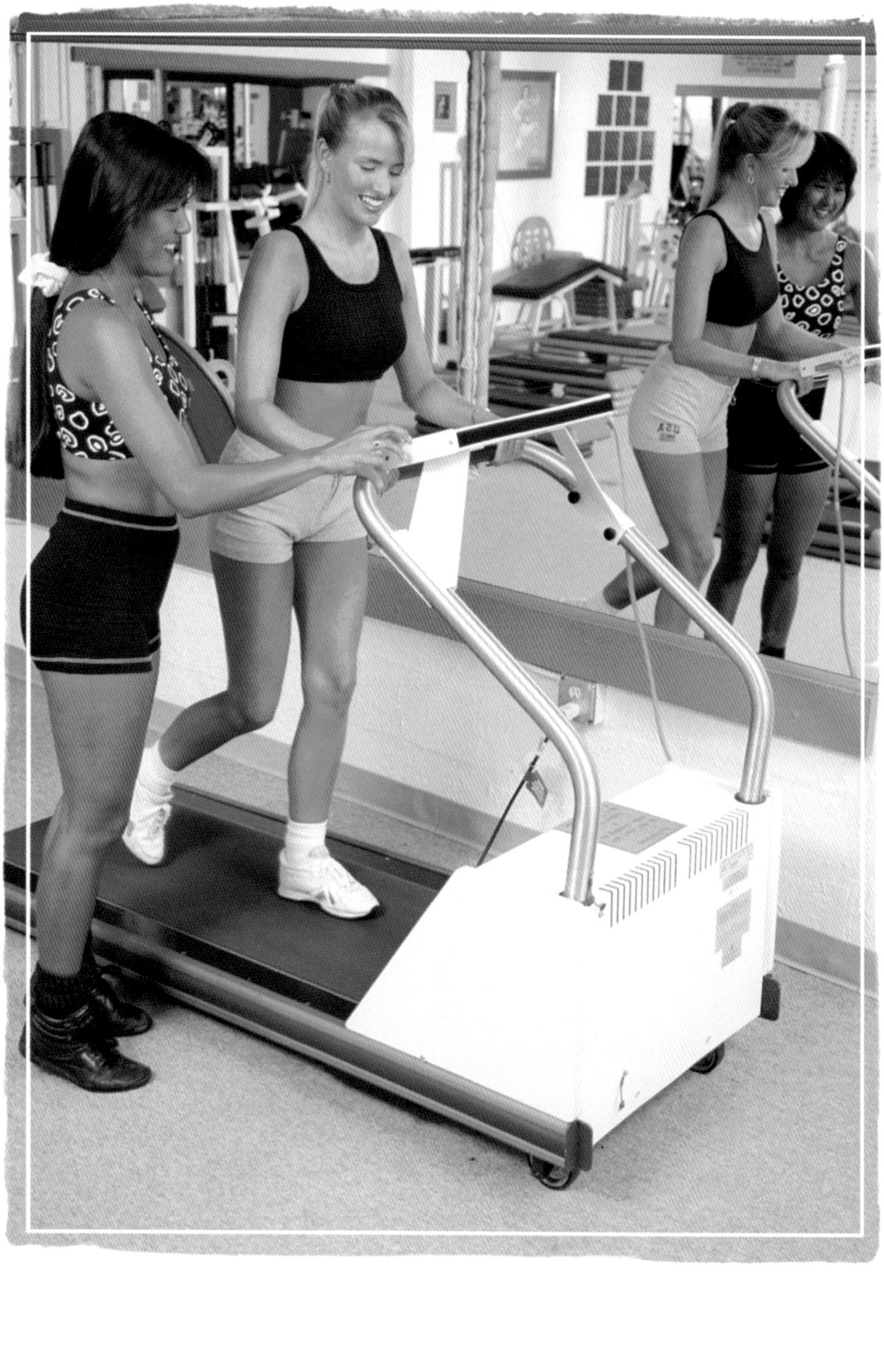

© ImageState/Chuck Mason

Objectives

The reader will be able to do the following:

1. Describe how oxygen consumption measurements can be used to estimate energy production, and list the number of calories derived per liter of oxygen and per gram of carbohydrate, fat, and protein.
2. Express energy expenditure as $L \cdot min^{-1}$, $kcal \cdot min^{-1}$, $ml \cdot kg^{-1} \cdot min^{-1}$, metabolic equivalents (METs), and $kcal \cdot kg^{-1} \cdot hr^{-1}$.
3. Estimate the oxygen cost of walking, jogging, and running, including the cost of walking and running 1 mile.
4. Estimate the oxygen cost of cycle ergometry exercise for both arm and leg work.
5. Estimate the oxygen cost of bench stepping.
6. Identify the approximate energy cost of recreational, sport, and other activities, and describe the effect of environmental factors on the HR response to a fixed work rate.

HFIs are usually concerned about the following two questions when they recommend specific physical activities to participants:

1. Are the activities appropriate, in terms of exercise intensity, to achieve the target HR (see chapter 10)?
2. Is the combination of intensity and duration appropriate for achieving an energy expenditure goal to balance or exceed caloric intake (see chapter 11)?

To answer these questions, the HFI should become familiar with the energy costs of various activities. The purpose of this chapter is to offer some basic information about how to estimate the energy requirement of various physical activities and to summarize the values associated with common recreational activities.

Ways to Measure Energy Expenditure

Energy expenditure can be measured by direct and indirect calorimetry. **Direct calorimetry** requires that the person perform an activity within a specially constructed chamber that is insulated and has water flowing through its walls. The water is warmed by the heat given off by the subject, and heat production can be calculated by knowing the volume of water flowing through the chamber per minute and the change in the water temperature from entry to exit. For example, a person does bench-stepping exercises in the chamber at the rate of 30 steps $\cdot$ min^{-1} using a 20-cm bench. The water flows through the walls of the chamber at 20 $L \cdot min^{-1}$, and the increase in the temperature of the water from entry to exit is 0.5° C. Because it takes approximately 1 kcal to raise the temperature of 1 L of water 1° C, the following calculation yields the approximate energy expenditure.

$$\frac{20\ L}{min} \cdot \frac{1\ kcal}{^\circ C} \cdot 0.5^\circ C = \frac{10\ kcal}{min}$$

Additional heat is lost from the subject by evaporation of water from the skin and respiratory passages. This heat loss can be measured and added to that picked up by the water to yield the rate of energy produced by the individual for that task.

Indirect calorimetry estimates energy production by measuring oxygen consumption, the procedures of which are described in chapter 28. These procedures rely on certain constants to convert liters of oxygen consumption to calories expended. The constants are derived from measurements made in a bomb calorimeter, a heavy metal chamber into which carbohydrate, fat, or protein can be placed with 100% oxygen under pressure. The chamber is immersed in a water bath, and the foodstuff is oxidized to CO_2 and H_2O when an electric spark sets the process in motion. The heat given off by the combustion warms the water, and it has been determined that carbohydrates, fats, and proteins give off approximately 4, 9, and 5.6 kcal of heat per gram, respectively. Because the nitrogen in protein cannot be completely oxidized in the body and is excreted as urea, the physiological value for protein is actually 4.0 kcal $\cdot$ g^{-1}.

Knowing how much oxygen is required to oxidize 1 g of carbohydrate, fat, and protein allows one to calculate the number of calories of energy produced when 1 L of oxygen is consumed. This is called the **caloric equivalent of oxygen**. Values for carbohydrate, fat, and protein are listed in table 4.1. The table shows that carbohydrates give about 6% more energy per liter of oxygen than fats (5.0 vs. 4.7 kcal $\cdot$ L^{-1}), whereas fats give more than twice as much energy per gram than carbohydrate (9 vs. 4 kcal $\cdot$ g^{-1}). If a person is deriving energy from a 50/50 mixture of carbohydrates and fats during exercise, the caloric equivalent is approximately 4.85 kcal $\cdot$ L^{-1}, halfway between the value of 4.7 for fat and 5.0 for carbohydrates (18). The ratio of carbon dioxide produced to oxygen consumed at the cell is called the respiratory quotient (RQ). The same ratio, when measured by conventional gas exchange procedures, is called the respiratory exchange ratio (R) and is used as an indicator of fuel use (carbohydrate vs. fat) during exercise (see chapter 28 for details).

Indirect calorimetry employs two techniques to measure oxygen consumption: **closed-circuit** and **open-circuit spirometry**. In the closed-circuit technique, the subject usually breathes 100% oxygen from a spirometer, and the exhaled air passes through a chemical to absorb the carbon dioxide. Over time, the volume of oxygen contained in the spirometer decreases, giving a measure of the oxygen consumption in ml $\cdot$ min^{-1}. Because the carbon dioxide is absorbed, one cannot calculate R, so a caloric equivalent of 4.82 kcal $\cdot$ L^{-1} is used to indicate that a mixture of carbohydrates, fats, and proteins is used. This closed-circuit technique has been used extensively to measure basal metabolic rate (18).

The open-circuit technique for measuring oxygen consumption and carbon dioxide production is the most common indirect calorimetry technique. In this procedure, oxygen consumption is calculated by simply subtracting the volume of oxygen exhaled from the volume of oxygen inhaled. The difference is taken as the oxygen uptake or oxygen consumption (see chapter 28 for details). Carbon dioxide production is calculated in the same manner. This makes it possible to calculate R. One can then determine which substrate, fat or carbohydrate, provided the most energy during work and also determine what value to use for the caloric equivalent of 1 L of oxygen in the calculation of energy expenditure (i.e., 5.0 kcal $\cdot$ L^{-1} for carbohydrates and 4.7 kcal $\cdot$ L^{-1} for fats). However, as described in the Research Insight, an average value of 5.0 kcal $\cdot$ L^{-1} is typically used to convert oxygen uptake to kilocalories.

Table 4.1 Caloric Density, Caloric Equivalent, and Respiratory Quotient Associated With Oxidation of Carbohydrate, Fat, and Protein

Measurement	Carbohydrate	Fat	Protein[a]
Caloric density (kcal $\cdot$ g^{-1})	4.0	9.0	4.0
Caloric equivalent of 1 L of O_2 (kcal $\cdot$ L^{-1})	5.0	4.7	4.5
Respiratory quotient	1.0	0.7	0.8

[a]Does not include the energy derived from the oxidation of nitrogen in the amino acids because the body excretes this as urea.

Adapted from "Energy Metabolism" by L.K. Koebel (18). In *Physiology* (5th edition) by E. Selkurt (Ed.), 1984, Boston: Little Brown & Co.

Research Insight

As we described, carbohydrates yield about 6% more energy (5 kcal) per liter of oxygen than fat (4.7 kcal), making carbohydrates a better fuel to use at high intensities of exercise when oxygen delivery to the working muscles is limited. However, with rare exceptions, carbohydrates make up at least 50% of the fuel used during a workout in the range of 60% to 80% of maximal oxygen uptake, a typical intensity range for individuals with average levels of cardiorespiratory fitness (see chapter 10). Consequently, the range of values that might be used to convert oxygen uptake to kilocalories is reduced to 4.85 to 5.0 kcal · L^{-1}, or about a 3% difference. Therefore, there is little error involved in converting oxygen uptake to kilocalories when using a constant value of 5 kcal · L^{-1}.

1 In Review

Oxygen consumption ($\dot{V}O_2$) is a measure of how much energy (calories) is produced by the body. When we know how many calories are generated per gram of carbohydrate and fat and how much oxygen is used to do that, liters of oxygen used can be converted to calories of energy produced. The following values are the number of calories per gram of food when metabolized in the body: carbohydrates = 4 kcal · g^{-1}, fats = 9 kcal · g^{-1}, and protein = 4 kcal · g^{-1}. Knowing how much oxygen is used in the metabolism of a food, we know that we obtain 4.7 kcal · L^{-1} when fat is oxidized and 5.0 kcal · L^{-1} when carbohydrate is oxidized. When a 50/50 mixture of carbohydrates and fats is used for energy, we obtain 4.85 kcal · L^{-1}.

Ways to Express Energy Expenditure

The energy requirement for an activity is calculated on the basis of a subject's steady-state oxygen uptake ($\dot{V}O_2$) measured during an activity. Once the steady-state (leveling off) oxygen uptake is reached, the energy (adenosine triphosphate, or ATP) supplied to the muscles is derived from the aerobic metabolism of the various substrates. The measured oxygen uptake then can be used to express energy expenditure in different ways. The five most common expressions follow:

1. **$\dot{V}O_2$ (L · min^{-1}).** The calculation of oxygen uptake (see chapter 28) yields a value expressed in liters of oxygen used per minute. For example, the following data were collected during a submaximal run on a treadmill by an 80-kg man: ventilation (STPD) = 60 L · min^{-1}; inspired O_2 = 20.93%; expired O_2 = 16.93%.

$$\dot{V}O_2\ (L \cdot min^{-1}) = 60\ L \cdot min^{-1} \cdot (20.93\%\ O_2 - 16.93\%\ O_2)$$
$$= 2.4\ L \cdot min^{-1}$$

2. **kcal · min^{-1}.** Oxygen uptake can be expressed in kilocalories used per minute. The caloric equivalent of 1 L of O_2 ranges from 4.7 kcal · L^{-1} for fats to 5.0 kcal · L^{-1} for carbohydrates. For practical reasons, and with little loss in precision, 5 kcal per liter of O_2 is used to convert the oxygen uptake to kilocalories per minute. Energy expenditure is calculated by multiplying the kilocalories expended per minute (kcal · min^{-1}) by the duration of the activity in minutes. For example, if the 80-kg man mentioned previously runs on the treadmill for 30 min at a $\dot{V}O_2$ = 2.4 L · min^{-1}, the total energy expenditure can be calculated as follows.

$$\frac{2.4\ \text{L}\ O_2}{\text{min}} \cdot \frac{5\ \text{kcal}}{\text{L}\ O_2} = \frac{12\ \text{kcal}}{\text{min}}$$

$$\frac{12\ \text{kcal}}{\text{min}} \cdot 30\ \text{min} = 360\ \text{kcal}$$

3. $\dot{V}O_2$ (ml · kg^{-1} · min^{-1}). If the measured oxygen uptake, expressed in liters per minute, is multiplied by 1000 to yield milliliters per minute and then divided by the subject's body weight in kilograms, the value is expressed in milliliters of O_2 per kilogram of body weight per minute, or ml · kg^{-1} · min^{-1}. This facilitates comparisons among people of different body sizes. For example, for the 80-kg man with a $\dot{V}O_2$ = 2.4 L · min^{-1},

$$\frac{2.4\ \text{L}}{\text{min}} \cdot \frac{1000\ \text{ml}}{\text{L}} \div 80\ \text{kg} = 30\ \text{ml} \cdot \text{kg}^{-1} \cdot \text{min}^{-1}$$

4. METs. The resting metabolic rate (oxygen uptake) is approximately 3.5 ml · kg^{-1} · min^{-1}. This is called 1 MET. Activities are expressed in terms of multiples of the MET unit. For example, using the values presented previously,

$$30\ \text{ml} \cdot \text{kg}^{-1} \cdot \text{min}^{-1} \div 3.5\ \text{ml} \cdot \text{kg}^{-1} \cdot \text{min}^{-1} = 8.6\ \text{METs}$$

5. kcal · kg^{-1} · hr^{-1}. The MET expression of energy expenditure carries a special bonus; the value also indicates the number of calories the subject uses per kilogram of body weight per hour. In the example mentioned previously, the subject is working at 8.6 METs, or about 30 ml · kg^{-1} · min^{-1}. When this value is multiplied by 60 min · hr^{-1}, it equals 1800 ml · kg^{-1} · hr^{-1}, or 1.8 L · kg^{-1} · hr^{-1}. If the person is using a mixture of carbohydrates and fats as the fuel, then this oxygen consumption is multiplied by 4.85 kcal per liter of O_2 to give 8.7 kcal · kg^{-1} · hr^{-1}. The following steps show the detail.

$$8.6\ \text{METs} \cdot \frac{3.5\ \text{ml} \cdot \text{kg}^{-1} \cdot \text{min}^{-1}}{\text{MET}} = 30\ \text{ml} \cdot \text{kg}^{-1} \cdot \text{min}^{-1}$$

$$30\ \text{ml} \cdot \text{kg}^{-1} \cdot \text{min}^{-1} \cdot 60\ \text{min} \cdot \text{hr}^{-1} = 1800\ \text{ml} \cdot \text{kg}^{-1} \cdot \text{hr}^{-1} = 1.8\ \text{L} \cdot \text{kg}^{-1} \cdot \text{hr}^{-1}$$

$$1.8\ \text{L} \cdot \text{kg}^{-1} \cdot \text{hr}^{-1} \cdot 4.85\ \text{kcal} \cdot \text{L}\ O_2^{-1} = 8.7\ \text{kcal} \cdot \text{kg}^{-1} \cdot \text{hr}^{-1}$$

2 In Review

Energy expenditure can be expressed in L · min^{-1}, kcal · min^{-1}, ml · kg^{-1} · min^{-1}, METs, and kcal · kg^{-1} · hr^{-1}. To convert L · min^{-1} to kcal · min^{-1}, multiply by 5.0 kcal · L^{-1}. To convert L · min^{-1} to ml · kg^{-1} · min^{-1}, multiply by 1000 and divide by body weight in kilograms. To convert ml · kg^{-1} · min^{-1} to METs or kcal · kg^{-1} · hr^{-1}, divide by 3.5 ml · kg^{-1} · min^{-1}.

Equations for Estimating the Energy Cost of Activities

In the mid-1970s, the ACSM identified some simple equations to estimate the steady-state energy requirement associated with common modes of activities used in GXTs: walking, stepping, running, and cycle ergometry (2). Over the years the equations have been modified based on the best information available, and this chapter represents the current thinking in the sixth edition of that text (3). The oxygen uptake calculated from these equations is an estimate, and a typical standard deviation associated with the actual measured average value is about 7 to 9% of the value (3, 10). This normal variation in the energy cost of activities is important to remember when you use these equations in prescribing exercise.

The ACSM equations have been applied to GXTs to estimate maximal aerobic power. This application has been shown to give reasonable estimates when the subjects are healthy and the rate at which the GXT progresses is slow enough to allow a steady-state oxygen uptake to be achieved at each stage (20, 21). When the increments in the stages of the GXT are large or the individual being tested is somewhat unfit, his or her oxygen uptake will not keep pace with each stage of the test. In these cases, the equations overestimate the actual measured oxygen uptake (14). The fact that this overestimation is more likely to happen in diseased populations (e.g., cardiac patients) suggests that the GXTs used may be too aggressive. A test that progresses at a slower rate and allows the subject to reach the steady-state $\dot{V}O_2$ at each stage reduces the chance of an overestimation of functional capacity and still requires the subject to work at an appropriate metabolic rate to overload the system (see chapter 10). The previous information is presented to clarify the usefulness of the following equations. The equations estimate the steady-state energy requirements for activities.

When the ACSM equations were developed, an attempt was made to use a true physiological oxygen cost for each type of work. Each activity is broken down into the energy components. That is, in estimating the total oxygen cost of grade walking, add the net oxygen cost of the horizontal walk to the net oxygen cost of the vertical (grade) walk to the resting metabolic rate, which is taken to be 1 MET (3.5 ml · kg^{-1} · min^{-1}).

$$\text{Total } O_2 \text{ cost} = \text{net oxygen cost of activity} + 3.5 \text{ ml} \cdot \text{kg}^{-1} \cdot \text{min}^{-1}$$

Note that for the equations to estimate the oxygen cost of the activity, the subject must follow instructions carefully (e.g., do not hold on to the treadmill railing, maintain the pedal cadence), and the work instruments (treadmill, cycle ergometer) must be calibrated so the settings are correct (see chapter 5).

Energy Requirements of Walking, Running, Cycle Ergometry, and Stepping

The following sections provide equations to estimate the energy cost of walking, running, cycle ergometry, and stepping. These activities are common to cardiac rehabilitation and adult fitness programs. Examples are provided to show how the equations are used in designing exercise programs.

Oxygen Cost of Walking

Equations to determine the oxygen cost of walking differ depending on the walking speed and whether the walker is on a horizontal or a graded surface.

Walking on a Horizontal Surface

One of the most common activities used in an exercise program and in GXTs is walking. The following equation can be used to estimate the energy requirement between the walking speeds of 50 and 100 m · min^{-1}, or 1.9 to 3.7 miles · hr^{-1}. (Multiply miles per hour by 26.8 to obtain meters per minute. Divide meters per minute by 26.8 to obtain miles per hour.) Dill (12) showed that the net cost of walking 1 m · min^{-1} on a horizontal surface is 0.100 to 0.106 ml · kg^{-1} · min^{-1}. A value of 0.1 ml · kg^{-1} · min^{-1} is used in the ACSM equations to simplify calculations without the loss of too much precision. The equation for calculating the oxygen cost (ml · kg^{-1} · min^{-1}) of walking on a flat surface is as follows:

$$\dot{V}O_2 = 0.1 \text{ ml} \cdot \text{kg}^{-1} \cdot \text{min}^{-1} \text{ (horizontal velocity)} + 3.5 \text{ ml} \cdot \text{kg}^{-1} \cdot \text{min}^{-1}$$

QUESTION: What are the estimated steady-state $\dot{V}O_2$ and METs for a walking speed of 90 m · min^{-1} (3.4 miles · hr^{-1})?

Answer:

$$\dot{V}O_2 = 90\ \text{m} \cdot \text{min}^{-1} \cdot \frac{0.1\ \text{ml} \cdot \text{kg}^{-1} \cdot \text{min}^{-1}}{\text{m} \cdot \text{min}^{-1}} + 3.5\ \text{ml} \cdot \text{kg}^{-1} \cdot \text{min}^{-1}$$

$$= 9.0\ \text{ml} \cdot \text{kg}^{-1} \cdot \text{min}^{-1} + 3.5\ \text{ml} \cdot \text{kg}^{-1} \cdot \text{min}^{-1} = 12.5\ \text{ml} \cdot \text{kg}^{-1} \cdot \text{min}^{-1}$$

$$\text{METs} = 12.5\ \text{ml} \cdot \text{kg}^{-1} \cdot \text{min}^{-1} \div 3.5\ \text{ml} \cdot \text{kg}^{-1} \cdot \text{min}^{-1} = 3.6$$

The equations also can be used to predict the level of activity required to elicit a specific energy expenditure.

QUESTION: An unfit participant is told to exercise at 11.5 ml · kg^{-1} · min^{-1} to achieve the proper exercise intensity. What walking speed would you recommend?

Answer:

$$11.5\ \text{ml} \cdot \text{kg}^{-1} \cdot \text{min}^{-1} = ?\,\text{m} \cdot \text{min}^{-1} \cdot \frac{0.1\ \text{ml} \cdot \text{kg}^{-1} \cdot \text{min}^{-1}}{\text{m} \cdot \text{min}^{-1}} + 3.5\ \text{ml} \cdot \text{kg}^{-1} \cdot \text{min}^{-1}$$

Subtract the resting metabolic rate of 3.5 ml · kg^{-1} · min^{-1} from both sides of the equation. Subtracting 3.5 ml · kg^{-1} · min^{-1} from 11.5 ml · kg^{-1} · min^{-1} gives you the net oxygen cost of the activity (8.0 ml · kg^{-1} · min^{-1}).

$$8\ \text{ml} \cdot \text{kg}^{-1} \cdot \text{min}^{-1} = ?\,\text{m} \cdot \text{min}^{-1} \cdot \frac{0.1\ \text{ml} \cdot \text{kg}^{-1} \cdot \text{min}^{-1}}{\text{m} \cdot \text{min}^{-1}}$$

The net cost (8 ml · kg^{-1} · min^{-1}) is divided by 0.1 ml · kg^{-1} · min^{-1} per m · min^{-1} to yield 80 m · min^{-1} (3 miles · hr^{-1}). Next, to obtain miles per hour, divide meters per minute by 26.8.

$$80\ \text{m} \cdot \text{min}^{-1} = 8\ \text{ml} \cdot \text{kg}^{-1} \cdot \text{min}^{-1} \div \frac{0.1\ \text{ml} \cdot \text{kg}^{-1} \cdot \text{min}^{-1}}{\text{m} \cdot \text{min}^{-1}}$$

$$3.0\ \text{mi} \cdot \text{hr}^{-1} = 80\ \text{m} \cdot \text{min}^{-1} \div \frac{26.8\ \text{m} \cdot \text{min}^{-1}}{\text{mi} \cdot \text{hr}^{-1}}$$

Walking Up a Grade

The oxygen cost of grade walking is the sum of the oxygen cost of horizontal walking, the oxygen cost of the vertical component, and the resting metabolic rate of 3.5 ml · kg^{-1} · min^{-1}. Studies have shown that the oxygen cost of moving (walking or stepping) 1 m · min^{-1} vertically is 1.8 ml · kg^{-1} · min^{-1} (7, 22). The vertical component (velocity) is calculated by multiplying the grade (expressed as a fraction) times the speed in meters per minute. A person walking at 80 m · min^{-1} on a 10% grade is walking 8 m · min^{-1} vertically (0.10 times 80 m · min^{-1}). The equation for calculating the oxygen cost (ml · kg^{-1} · min^{-1}) of walking on a grade is

$$\dot{V}O_2 = 0.1\ \text{ml} \cdot \text{kg}^{-1} \cdot \text{min}^{-1}\ (\text{horiz. velocity}) + 1.8\ \text{ml} \cdot \text{kg}^{-1} \cdot \text{min}^{-1}\ (\text{vert. velocity}) + 3.5\ \text{ml} \cdot \text{kg}^{-1} \cdot \text{min}^{-1}$$

QUESTION: What is the total oxygen cost of walking 90 m · min^{-1} up a 12% grade?

Answer: Horizontal component: Calculated as in preceding equation for walking on a horizontal surface and equals 9 ml · kg^{-1} · min^{-1}.

$$\dot{V}O_2 = 0.12\ (\text{grade}) \cdot 90\ \text{m} \cdot \text{min}^{-1} \cdot \frac{1.8\ \text{ml} \cdot \text{kg}^{-1} \cdot \text{min}^{-1}}{\text{m} \cdot \text{min}^{-1}} = 19.4\ \text{ml} \cdot \text{kg}^{-1} \cdot \text{min}^{-1}$$

$$\dot{V}O_2\ (\text{ml} \cdot \text{kg}^{-1} \cdot \text{min}^{-1}) = 9.0\ (\text{horiz.}) + 19.4\ (\text{vert.}) + 3.5\ (\text{rest}) = 31.9\ \text{ml} \cdot \text{kg}^{-1} \cdot \text{ml}^{-1}, \text{ or } 9.1\ \text{METs}$$

Vertical component:
As indicated earlier, the equations can be used to estimate the settings needed to elicit a specific oxygen uptake.

QUESTION: Set the treadmill grade to achieve an energy requirement of 6 METs (21.0 ml · kg^{-1} · min^{-1}) when walking at 60 m · min^{-1}.

Answer: The net oxygen cost of the activity is 21 – 3.5, or 17.5, ml · kg^{-1} · min^{-1}.

$$\text{Horizontal component} = 60 \text{ m} \cdot \text{min}^{-1} \cdot \frac{0.1 \text{ ml} \cdot \text{kg}^{-1} \cdot \text{min}^{-1}}{\text{m} \cdot \text{min}^{-1}}$$

$$= 6.0 \text{ ml} \cdot \text{kg}^{-1} \cdot \text{min}^{-1}$$

$$\text{Vertical component} = 17.5 - 6.0 = 11.5 \text{ ml} \cdot \text{kg}^{-1} \cdot \text{min}^{-1}$$

$$11.5 \text{ ml} \cdot \text{kg}^{-1} \cdot \text{min}^{-1} = \text{fractional grade} \cdot 60 \text{ m} \cdot \text{min}^{-1} \cdot \frac{1.8 \text{ ml} \cdot \text{kg}^{-1} \cdot \text{min}^{-1}}{\text{m} \cdot \text{min}^{-1}}$$

$$= \text{fractional grade} \cdot 108 \text{ ml} \cdot \text{kg}^{-1} \cdot \text{min}^{-1}$$

$$\text{Fractional grade} = 11.5 \div 108 = 0.106 \cdot 100\% = 10.6\% \text{ grade}$$

Walking at Different Speeds

The preceding equations are useful within the range of walking speeds of 50 to 100 m · min^{-1} (1.9-3.7 miles · hr^{-1}); beyond that, the oxygen requirement for walking increases in a curvilinear manner (10). Because many people choose to walk at a fast speed rather than jog, knowledge of the energy requirements for walking at these higher speeds is useful in prescribing exercise. Values for the energy requirement for walking on the level and at various grades at these faster speeds (4.0 to 5.0 miles · hr^{-1}) are included in table 4.2.

Table 4.2 Energy Requirement, in METs, for Walking at Various Speeds (miles · hr^{-1} or m · min^{-1}) and Grades (%)

	Miles · hr^{-1}/meters · min^{-1}						
% Grade	2.0/54	2.5/67	3.0/80	3.5/94	4.0/107	4.5/121	5.0/134
0	2.5	2.9	3.3	3.7	4.9	6.2	7.9
2	3.1	3.6	4.1	4.7	5.9	7.4	9.3
4	3.6	4.3	4.9	5.6	7.1	8.7	10.6
6	4.2	5.0	5.8	6.6	8.1	9.9	12.0
8	4.7	5.7	6.6	7.5	9.3	11.1	13.4
10	5.3	6.3	7.4	8.5	10.4	12.4	14.8
12	5.8	7.1	8.3	9.5	11.4	13.6	16.6
14	6.4	7.7	9.1	10.4	12.6	14.9	17.5
16	6.9	8.4	9.9	11.4	13.6	16.1	18.9
18	7.5	9.1	10.7	12.4	14.8	17.4	20.3
20	8.1	9.8	11.6	13.3	15.9	18.6	21.7
22	8.6	10.3	12.4	14.3	17.0	19.9	23.1
24	9.1	11.1	13.2	15.3	18.1	21.1	
26	9.7	11.9	14.0	16.2	19.2	22.3	
28	10.3	12.5	14.9	17.2	20.3	23.6	
30	10.8	13.2	15.7	18.2	21.4		

Note. Based on *ACSM's Guidelines for Exercise Testing and Prescription* (3) and Bubb et al. (10).

One of the most common and useful ways that the energy cost of walking can be expressed is in kilocalories per minute. In this way, the HFI can simply locate the walking speed in a table, identify the number of calories used per minute, and calculate the total energy expenditure, depending on the duration of the walk. Table 4.3 presents the energy cost (in kcal · min^{-1}) for walking at speeds of 2 to 5 miles · hr^{-1} and includes values for people of different body weights. It is no surprise that the energy cost of walking increases with the speed of the walk; however, the rate of increase is higher at the higher speeds. For example, when walking speed increases from 2 to 3 miles · hr^{-1} for a 170-lb participant, the energy cost increases from 3.2 to 4.2 kcal · min^{-1}. But going from 4 to 5 miles · hr^{-1} requires an increase from 6.3 to 10.2 kcal · min^{-1}. It is clear that the very sedentary individual can walk at slow speeds and achieve the desired exercise intensity, and the relatively fit individual can walk at high speeds at which the elevated energy requirement provides the necessary stimulus for a training effect. As a participant loses weight, the energy cost of walking at a certain speed decreases because the energy cost is dependent on body weight. One can compensate by walking for a longer period of time or for a greater distance.

Table 4.3 Energy Costs of Walking (kcal · min^{-1})

Body weight		Miles · hr^{-1}						
kg	lb	2.0	2.5	3.0	3.5	4.0	4.5	5.0
50.0	110	2.1	2.4	2.8	3.1	4.1	5.2	6.6
54.5	120	2.3	2.6	3.0	3.4	4.4	5.6	7.2
59.1	130	2.5	2.9	3.2	3.6	4.8	6.1	7.8
63.6	140	2.7	3.1	3.5	3.9	5.2	6.6	8.4
68.2	150	2.8	3.3	3.7	4.2	5.6	7.0	9.0
72.7	160	3.0	3.5	4.0	4.5	5.9	7.5	9.6
77.3	170	3.2	3.7	4.2	4.8	6.3	8.0	10.2
81.8	180	3.4	4.0	4.5	5.0	6.7	8.4	10.8
86.4	190	3.6	4.2	4.7	5.3	7.0	8.9	11.4
90.9	200	3.8	4.4	5.0	5.6	7.4	9.4	12.0
95.4	210	4.0	4.6	5.2	5.9	7.8	9.9	12.6
100.0	220	4.2	4.8	5.5	6.2	8.2	10.3	13.2

Note. Multiply value by the duration of the activity to obtain total calories expended. Based on *ACSM's Guidelines for Exercise Testing and Prescription* (3) and Bubb et al. (10).

Oxygen Cost of Jogging and Running

Jogging and running are common activities used in fitness programs for apparently healthy individuals. It is possible to use the ACSM equations to estimate the oxygen cost of these activities for a broad range of speeds, generally from 130 to 350 m · min^{-1}. The equations are also useful at speeds below 130 m · min^{-1} as long as the person is really jogging. The fact that a person can walk or jog at speeds below 130 m · min^{-1} complicates the issue. The oxygen cost of walking is less than that of jogging at slow speeds; however, at approximately 140 m · min^{-1} (5.2 mph), the oxygen cost of jogging and walking are about the same. Above this speed, the oxygen cost of walking exceeds that of jogging (5).

Jogging and Running on a Horizontal Surface

The net oxygen cost of jogging or running 1 m · min^{-1} on a horizontal surface is about twice that of walking, 0.2 ml · kg^{-1} · min^{-1} per m · min^{-1} (6, 9, 19). Remember that the equation will, in general, yield a reasonable estimate of the oxygen cost of running for average individuals. However, it is well known that trained runners are more economical (in terms of energy expenditure) than the average person and also that running economy varies within any specific group, trained or untrained (9, 11, 21). The equation used to estimate the oxygen cost ($ml \cdot kg^{-1} \cdot min^{-1}$) of running on a flat surface is as follows:

$$\dot{V}O_2 = 0.2\ ml \cdot kg^{-1} \cdot min^{-1}\ (\text{horizontal velocity}) + 3.5\ ml \cdot kg^{-1} \cdot min^{-1}$$

QUESTION: What is the oxygen requirement for running a 10K race on a track in 60 min?

Answer:

$$10{,}000\ m \div 60\ min = 167\ m \cdot min^{-1}$$

$$\dot{V}O_2 = 167\ m \cdot min^{-1} \cdot \frac{0.2\ ml \cdot kg^{-1} \cdot min^{-1}}{m \cdot min^{-1}} + 3.5\ ml \cdot kg^{-1} \cdot min^{-1}$$

$$= 36.9\ ml \cdot kg^{-1} \cdot min^{-1},\ \text{or } 10.5\ \text{METs}$$

QUESTION: A 20-year-old female distance runner with a $\dot{V}O_2max$ of 50 $ml \cdot kg^{-1} \cdot min^{-1}$ wants to run intervals at 90% of $\dot{V}O_2max$. At what speed should she run on a track given that 1 mile equals 1610 m?

Answer: 90% of 50 = 45 $ml \cdot kg^{-1} \cdot min^{-1}$, and the net cost of the run is equal to 45 $ml \cdot kg^{-1} \cdot min^{-1}$ – 3.5 $ml \cdot kg^{-1} \cdot min^{-1}$, or 41.5 $ml \cdot kg^{-1} \cdot min^{-1}$.

$$41.5\ ml \cdot kg^{-1} \cdot min^{-1} \div \frac{0.2\ ml \cdot kg^{-1} \cdot min^{-1}}{m \cdot min^{-1}} = 207\ m \cdot min^{-1}$$

$$1610\ m \cdot min^{-1} \div 207\ m \cdot min^{-1} = 7.78\ min,\ \text{or } 7{:}47\ (\text{min:s})\ \text{mile pace}$$

Jogging and Running Up a Grade

There is not as much information about the oxygen cost of grade running as there is about the previous activities. But one thing is clear—the oxygen cost of running up a grade is about one half that of walking up a grade (8, 19). Some of the vertical lift associated with running on a flat surface is used to accomplish some grade work during inclined running, lowering the net oxygen requirement for the vertical work. The oxygen cost of running 1 $m \cdot min^{-1}$ vertically is about 0.9 $ml \cdot kg^{-1} \cdot min^{-1}$. As in grade walking, the vertical velocity is calculated by multiplying the fractional grade times the horizontal velocity. The following equation is used for calculating the oxygen cost of grade running.

$$\dot{V}O_2 = 0.2\ ml \cdot kg^{-1} \cdot min^{-1}\ (\text{horiz. velocity}) + 0.9\ ml \cdot kg^{-1} \cdot min^{-1}\ (\text{vert. velocity}) + 3.5\ ml \cdot kg^{-1} \cdot min^{-1}$$

QUESTION: What is the oxygen cost of running 150 $m \cdot min^{-1}$ up a 10% grade?

Answer:
Horizontal component:

$$\dot{V}O_2 = 150\ m \cdot min^{-1} \cdot \frac{0.2\ ml \cdot kg^{-1} \cdot min^{-1}}{m \cdot min^{-1}} = 30\ ml \cdot kg^{-1} \cdot min^{-1}$$

Vertical component:

$$\dot{V}O_2 = 0.10\ (\text{fractional grade}) \cdot 150\ m \cdot min^{-1} \cdot \frac{0.9\ ml \cdot kg^{-1} \cdot min^{-1}}{m \cdot min^{-1}}$$

$$= 13.5\ ml \cdot kg^{-1} \cdot min^{-1}$$

$$\dot{V}O_2 = 30.0\ (\text{horizontal}) + 13.5\ (\text{vertical}) + 3.5\ (\text{rest}) = 47\ ml \cdot kg^{-1} \cdot min^{-1}$$

QUESTION: The oxygen cost of running 350 m · min^{-1} on a flat surface is about 73.5 ml · kg^{-1} · min^{-1}. What grade should be set on a treadmill for a speed of 300 m · min^{-1} to achieve the same $\dot{V}O_2$?

Answer:
Horizontal component:

$$\dot{V}O_2 = 300 \text{ m} \cdot \text{min}^{-1} \cdot \frac{0.2 \text{ ml} \cdot \text{kg}^{-1} \cdot \text{min}^{-1}}{\text{m} \cdot \text{min}^{-1}} = 60 \text{ ml} \cdot \text{kg}^{-1} \cdot \text{min}^{-1}$$

Vertical component:

$$\text{Net } \dot{V}O_2 = 73.5 \text{ (total)} - 60 \text{ (horizontal)} - 3.5 \text{ (rest)} = 10.0 \text{ ml} \cdot \text{kg}^{-1} \cdot \text{min}^{-1}$$

$$10.0 \text{ ml} \cdot \text{kg}^{-1} \cdot \text{min}^{-1} = \text{fractional grade} \cdot 300 \text{ m} \cdot \text{min}^{-1} \cdot \frac{0.9 \text{ ml} \cdot \text{kg}^{-1} \cdot \text{min}^{-1}}{\text{m} \cdot \text{min}^{-1}}$$

$$\text{Fractional grade} = 10 \text{ ml} \cdot \text{kg}^{-1} \cdot \text{min}^{-1} \div 270 \text{ ml} \cdot \text{kg}^{-1} \cdot \text{min}^{-1}$$

$$= .037 \text{ or } 3.7\% \text{ grade}$$

Table 4.4 summarizes the values for oxygen cost of running on the level and up a grade.

Table 4.4 Energy Requirement, in METs, for Jogging/Running at Various Speeds (miles · hr^{-1} or m · min^{-1}) and Grades

	Miles · hr^{-1}/m · min^{-1}							
% Grade	**3/80**	**4/107**	**5/134**	**6/161**	**7/188**	**8/215**	**9/241**	**10/268**
0	5.6	7.1	8.7	10.2	11.7	13.3	14.8	16.3
1	5.8	7.4	9.0	10.6	12.2	13.8	15.4	17.0
2	6.0	7.7	9.3	11.0	12.7	14.4	16.0	17.7
3	6.2	7.9	9.7	11.4	13.2	14.9	16.6	18.4
4	6.4	8.2	10.0	11.9	13.7	15.5	17.3	19.1
5	6.6	8.5	10.4	12.3	14.2	16.1	17.9	19.8
6	6.8	8.8	10.7	12.7	14.6	16.6	18.5	20.4
7	7.0	9.0	11.0	13.1	15.1	17.1	19.1	21.1
8	7.2	9.3	11.4	13.5	15.6	17.7	19.7	21.8
9	7.4	9.6	11.7	13.9	16.1	18.3	20.3	22.5
10	7.6	9.9	12.1	14.3	16.6	18.8	21.0	23.2

Note. Based on equations published in *ACSM's Guidelines for Exercise Testing and Prescription* (3).

Jogging and Running at Different Speeds

In contrast to walking, the energy cost of jogging and running increases in a linear and predictable manner with increasing speed. Table 4.5 shows the caloric cost of running, in kilocalories per minute, for participants of different body weights. If we consider the 170-lb participant, the energy cost increases from 7.2 to 11.2 kcal · min^{-1} when increasing speed from 3 to 5 miles · hr^{-1}; the increase is also 4 kcal · min^{-1} when increasing the speed from 7 to 9 miles · hr^{-1}. As with walking, the energy cost is higher for heavier individuals.

Table 4.5 Energy Costs of Jogging and Running ($kcal \cdot min^{-1}$)

Body weight		Miles · hr^{-1}							
kg	lb	3.0	4.0	5.0	6.0	7.0	8.0	9.0	10.0
50.0	110	4.7	5.9	7.2	8.5	9.8	11.1	12.3	13.6
54.5	120	5.1	6.4	7.9	9.3	10.6	12.1	13.4	14.8
59.1	130	5.5	7.0	8.6	10.0	11.5	13.1	14.6	16.1
63.6	140	5.9	7.5	9.2	10.8	12.4	14.1	15.7	17.3
68.2	150	6.4	8.1	9.9	11.6	13.3	15.1	16.8	18.5
72.7	160	6.8	8.6	10.5	12.4	14.2	16.1	17.9	19.8
77.3	170	7.2	9.1	11.2	13.1	15.1	17.1	19.1	21.0
81.8	180	7.6	9.7	11.8	13.9	15.9	18.1	20.2	22.2
86.4	190	8.1	10.2	12.5	14.7	16.8	19.1	21.3	23.5
90.9	200	8.5	10.8	13.2	15.4	17.7	20.1	22.4	24.7
95.4	210	8.9	11.3	13.8	16.2	18.6	21.1	23.5	25.9
100.0	220	9.3	11.8	14.5	17.0	19.5	22.2	24.7	27.2

Note. Multiply value by the duration of the activity to obtain total calories expended.

Oxygen Cost of Walking and Running 1 Mile

Despite the vast amount of information available regarding the costs of walking and running, a good deal of misunderstanding still exists. We hear claims that the energy cost of walking 1 mile is equal to that of running the same distance. In general, this is not the case (16). The equations for estimating the energy cost of walking and running can be used to estimate the caloric cost of walking and running 1 mile, a piece of information that is useful in achieving energy expenditure goals.

If a person walks at 3 miles · hr^{-1} (80 m · min^{-1}), 1 mile will be completed in 20 min. The caloric cost for walking 1 mile for a 70-kg person is calculated as follows:

$$\dot{V}O_2 = 80\ m \cdot min^{-1} \cdot 0.1\ ml \cdot kg^{-1} \cdot min^{-1} + 3.5\ ml \cdot kg^{-1} \cdot min^{-1}$$

$$\dot{V}O_2 = 11.5\ ml \cdot kg^{-1} \cdot min^{-1}$$

$$\dot{V}O_2(ml \cdot mile^{-1}) = 11.5\ ml \cdot kg^{-1} \cdot min^{-1} \cdot 70\ kg \cdot 20\ min \cdot mile^{-1} = 16\ 100\ ml \cdot mile^{-1}$$

$$\dot{V}O_2(L \cdot min^{-1}) = 16\ 100\ ml \cdot mile^{-1} \div 1000\ ml \cdot L^{-1} = 16.1\ L \cdot mile^{-1}$$

At about 5.0 kcal per liter of O_2, the gross caloric cost per mile of walking is 80.5 kcal (5 kcal · L^{-1} · 16.1 L · $mile^{-1}$). The net caloric cost for the mile walk can be calculated by subtracting the oxygen cost of 20 min of rest from the gross cost of the 3 mile · hr^{-1} walk. For example, 20 min of rest · 70 kg · (3.5 ml · kg^{-1} · min^{-1}) = 4900 ml, or 4.9 L. At 5 kcal · L^{-1}, this equals 24.5 kcal for 20 min of rest. The net cost of the mile walk is 80.5 kcal – 24.5 kcal, or 56 kcal per mile.

If the same 70-kg individual ran the mile at 6 miles · hr^{-1} (161 m · min^{-1}), the oxygen cost could be calculated by the following method.

$$\dot{V}O_2 = 161\ m \cdot min^{-1} \cdot 0.2\ ml \cdot kg^{-1} \cdot min^{-1} + 3.5\ ml \cdot kg^{-1} \cdot min^{-1}$$

$$\dot{V}O_2 = 35.7\ ml \cdot kg^{-1} \cdot min^{-1}$$

$$\dot{V}O_2(ml \cdot mile^{-1}) = 35.7\ ml \cdot kg^{-1} \cdot min^{-1} \cdot 70\ kg \cdot 10\ min \cdot mile^{-1} = 25\ 000\ ml \cdot mile^{-1}$$

$$\dot{V}O_2(L \cdot min^{-1}) = 25\ 000\ ml \cdot mile^{-1} \div 1000\ ml \cdot L^{-1} = 25\ L \cdot mile^{-1}$$

At about 5 kcal per liter of O_2, 125 kcal is used to jog or run 1 mile (5 kcal · L^{-1} · 25 L · $mile^{-1}$). The gross caloric cost per mile is about 50% higher for jogging than for walking (125 vs. 80 kcal). The net caloric cost of jogging or running 1 mile (calories used above resting), however, is relatively independent of speed and is about twice that of walking. For example, when we subtract the caloric cost for 10 min of rest (12 kcal) from the gross caloric cost of the run (125 kcal), the net cost is 113 kcal, or twice that for the walk (56 kcal). Table 4.6 lists values for the net and gross caloric costs of walking and running 1 mile for a variety of body weights, with the values expressed in kilocalories per mile.

For weight control it is important to use the net cost of the activity, because it measures the energy used over and above that of sitting around. When a person is moving at slow to moderate speeds (2-3.5 miles · hr^{-1}), the net cost of walking a mile is about half that of jogging or running the mile. This means that a person who jogs a mile at 3 miles · hr^{-1} will

Table 4.6 Gross and Net (Gross/Net) Cost in Kilocalories per Mile for Walking and Running

Walking

Body weight		Miles · hr^{-1}						
kg	lb	2.0	2.5	3.0	3.5	4.0	4.5	5.0
50.0	110	64/39	58/39	54/39	53/39	60/48	68/57	79/67
54.5	120	69/42	63/42	59/42	57/42	66/52	75/63	86/75
59.1	130	75/45	68/45	64/45	62/45	71/57	81/68	93/81
63.6	140	80/49	73/49	69/49	67/49	77/61	87/73	100/88
68.2	150	87/52	79/52	74/52	72/52	82/65	93/78	108/94
72.7	160	92/56	84/56	79/56	76/56	88/70	100/84	115/100
77.3	170	98/59	90/59	84/59	81/59	93/74	106/89	122/107
81.8	180	104/63	95/63	89/63	86/63	99/78	112/94	139/113
86.4	190	110/66	100/66	94/66	91/66	104/83	118/99	136/119
90.9	200	115/70	105/70	99/70	95/70	110/87	124/104	144/125
95.4	210	121/73	111/73	104/73	100/73	115/92	131/110	151/132
100.0	220	127/77	116/77	109/77	105/77	121/96	137/115	158/138

Running

Body weight		Miles · hr^{-1}							
kg	lb	3.0	4.0	5.0	6.0	7.0	8.0	9.0	10.0
50.0	110	93/77	89/77	86/77	84/77	84/77	83/77	82/77	81/77
54.5	120	101/83	97/83	94/83	92/83	92/83	90/83	89/83	89/83
59.1	130	110/90	105/90	102/90	100/90	99/90	98/90	97/90	96/90
63.6	140	118/97	113/97	110/97	108/97	107/97	106/97	104/97	104/97
68.2	150	127/104	121/104	118/104	115/104	114/104	113/104	112/104	111/104
72.7	160	135/111	129/111	125/111	123/111	122/111	121/111	119/111	119/111
77.3	170	144/118	137/118	133/118	131/118	130/118	128/118	127/118	126/118
81.8	180	152/125	146/125	141/125	138/125	137/125	136/125	134/125	133/125
86.4	190	161/132	154/132	149/132	146/132	145/132	143/132	141/132	141/132
90.9	200	169/139	162/139	157/139	154/139	153/139	151/139	149/139	148/139
95.4	210	177/146	170/146	165/146	161/146	160/146	158/146	156/146	155/146
100.0	220	186/153	178/153	173/153	169/153	168/153	166/153	164/153	163/153

Note. Multiply value by the number of miles walked or run to obtain the total (gross/net) calories expended.

be working at a higher metabolic rate than someone who walks at the same speed, and of course the HR response will be higher as well. Because many people walk at these slower speeds, it is important to remember that the net energy cost of the mile is half that of running. If we look at very high walking speeds (5 miles $\cdot$ hr^{-1}, or 1 mile in 12 min), however, we see that the net energy cost of walking 1 mile is only slightly less than that of running.

Table 4.6 shows that the net cost of running a mile is independent of speed. It does not matter whether participants jog at 3 miles $\cdot$ hr^{-1} or run at 6 miles $\cdot$ hr^{-1}—the net caloric cost is the same. At 6 miles $\cdot$ hr^{-1} the individual will be expending energy at about twice the rate measured at 3 miles $\cdot$ hr^{-1}, but because the mile is finished in half the time, the net energy expenditure is about the same. HR will, of course, be higher in the 6 mile $\cdot$ hr^{-1} run in order to deliver the oxygen to the muscles at the higher rate.

3 In Review

The oxygen cost of walking increases linearly between the speeds of 50 and 100 m $\cdot$ min^{-1}; it increases faster at higher walking speeds. The oxygen cost of jogging or running increases linearly with speed from slow jogging (3 miles $\cdot$ hr^{-1}) to fast running. The net caloric cost of jogging or running a mile is twice that of walking a mile at a moderate pace.

Oxygen Cost of Cycle Ergometry

Cycle ergometry exercise is a popular exercise done at a sport club, at home, or as part of a rehabilitation program. Generally, energy expenditure is accomplished with less trauma to ankle, knee, and hip joints compared with jogging. Cycle ergometers are used for conventional leg-exercise programs, but they are also adapted for arm exercise (by placing the ergometer on a table). The following sections describe how to estimate the energy costs of leg and arm cycle ergometry.

Leg Ergometry

In the previous activities the individual was carrying his or her body weight, and the oxygen requirement was therefore proportional to body weight (ml $\cdot$ kg^{-1} $\cdot$ min^{-1}). This is not the case in cycle ergometry, in which an individual's body weight is supported by the cycle seat and the work rate is determined primarily by the pedal rate and the resistance on the wheel. The oxygen requirement, in liters per minute, is approximately the same for people of different sizes for the same work rate. Thus, when a light person is doing the same work rate as a heavy person, the relative $\dot{V}O_2$ (ml $\cdot$ kg^{-1} $\cdot$ min^{-1}), or MET level, is higher for the lighter person.

The work rate is set on the simple, mechanically braked cycle ergometers by varying the force (weight, or load) on the wheel and the number of pedal revolutions per minute (rev $\cdot$ min^{-1}). On the Monark cycle ergometer, the wheel travels 6 m per pedal revolution; on the Tunturi ergometer, the wheel travels only 3 m per revolution. If we use the Monark ergometer as an example, a pedal rate of 50 rev $\cdot$ min^{-1} causes the wheel to travel a distance of 300 m (6 m per pedal revolution times 50 rev $\cdot$ min^{-1}). If a 1-kg force (1-kg weight) were applied to the wheel, the work rate would be 300 kilogram-meters (kgm) per minute (300 kgm $\cdot$ min^{-1}). Work rates also are expressed in watts (W), where 6.1 kgm $\cdot$ min^{-1} is equal to 1 W; the 300 kgm $\cdot$ min^{-1} work rate would be expressed as 50 W. The work rate can be doubled by changing the force from 1 to 2 kg or by changing the pedal rate from 50 to 100 rev $\cdot$ min^{-1}. In contrast, some cycle ergometers are electronically controlled to deliver a specific work rate somewhat independent of pedal rate; as the pedal rate decreases, the load on the wheel is increased proportionally to maintain the work rate (4).

The total oxygen cost of doing leg cycle ergometry exercise is the sum of the resting oxygen uptake, the cost of unloaded cycling (movement of the legs against no resistance), and the cost of the work itself. The oxygen cost of doing 1 kgm of work is 1.8 ml. The energy required to move the pedals against no resistance has been estimated to be 1 MET or 3.5 $ml \cdot kg^{-1} \cdot min^{-1}$, and as with the other equations, resting oxygen uptake is 3.5 $ml \cdot kg^{-1} \cdot min^{-1}$ (3). The latter two terms are combined in the equation to yield 7 $ml \cdot kg^{-1} \cdot min^{-1}$. The estimates from the following equations are reasonable for work rates between approximately 150 and 1200 $kgm \cdot min^{-1}$ (see table 4.7). The equations for work rates expressed in $kgm \cdot min^{-1}$ and watts follow.

$$\dot{V}O_2\ (ml \cdot kg^{-1} \cdot min^{-1}) = (kgm \cdot min^{-1} \cdot 1.8\ ml\ O_2 \cdot kgm^{-1})/\text{body weight (kg)} + 7\ ml \cdot kg^{-1} \cdot min^{-1}$$

$$\dot{V}O_2\ (ml \cdot kg^{-1} \cdot min^{-1}) = (W \cdot 10.8\ ml\ O_2 \cdot W^{-1})/\text{body weight (kg)} + 7\ ml \cdot kg^{-1} \cdot min^{-1}$$

Table 4.7 Energy Expenditure, in METs, for Cycle Ergometry for for Legs and Arms

Body weight		Work rate in $kgm \cdot min^{-1}$ and /watts						
kg	**lb**	**300/50**	**450/75**	**600/100**	**750/125**	**900/150**	**1050/175**	**1200/2000**
50	110	5.1(6.1)*	6.6(8.7)	8.2(11.3)	9.7(13.9)	11.3(–)	12.8(–)	14.3(–)
60	132	4.6(5.3)	5.9(7.4)	7.1(9.6)	8.4(11.7)	9.7(–)	11.0(–)	12.3(–)
70	154	4.2(4.7)	5.3(6.5)	6.4(8.3)	7.5(10.2)	8.6(12.0)	9.7(–)	10.8(–)
80	176	3.9(4.2)	4.9(5.8)	5.9(7.4)	6.8(9.0)	7.8(10.6)	8.8(12.3)	9.7(–)
90	198	3.7(3.9)	4.6(5.3)	5.4(6.7)	6.3(8.1)	7.1(9.6)	8.0(11.0)	8.9(12.4)
100	220	3.5(3.6)	4.3(4.9)	5.1(6.1)	5.9(7.4)	6.6(8.7)	7.4(10.0)	8.2(11.3)

Note. Values in ( ) are for arm work. Table is based on equations for estimating the oxygen cost of arm and leg work published in *ACSM's Guidelines for Exercise Testing and Prescription* (6th ed.) 2000.

QUESTION: What is the oxygen cost of doing 600 $kgm \cdot min^{-1}$ (100 W) on a cycle ergometer for 50-kg and 100-kg subjects?

Answer:
For the 50-kg subject:

$$\dot{V}O_2\ (ml \cdot kg^{-1} \cdot min^{-1}) = (600\ kgm \cdot min^{-1} \cdot 1.8\ ml\ O_2 \cdot kgm^{-1})/50\ kg + 7\ ml \cdot kg^{-1} \cdot min^{-1}$$

$$= 28.6\ ml \cdot kg^{-1} \cdot min^{-1} \text{ or } 8.2 \text{ METs}$$

For the 100-kg subject:

$$\dot{V}O_2\ (ml \cdot kg^{-1} \cdot min^{-1}) = (600\ kgm \cdot min^{-1} \cdot 1.8\ ml\ O_2 \cdot kgm^{-1})/100\ kg + 7\ ml \cdot kg^{-1} \cdot min^{-1}$$

$$= 17.8\ ml \cdot kg^{-1} \cdot min^{-1} \text{ or } 5.1 \text{ METs}$$

In some exercise programs, a participant might use a variety of exercise equipment to achieve a training effect and might like to be able to set about the same intensity on each. In this regard, the equation for the cycle ergometer can be used to set the load to achieve a particular MET value on the cycle ergometer and bring it in balance with what is done during walking or jogging.

QUESTION: A 70-kg participant must work at 6 METs ($21\ ml \cdot kg^{-1} \cdot min^{-1}$) to match the intensity of his walking program. What force (load) should be set on a Monark cycle ergometer at a pedal rate of $50\ rev \cdot min^{-1}$?

Answer:

$$21\ ml \cdot kg^{-1} \cdot min^{-1} = (?\ kgm \cdot min^{-1} \cdot 1.8\ ml\ O_2 \cdot kgm^{-1})/70\ kg + 7\ ml \cdot kg^{-1} \cdot min^{-1}$$

$$\text{Net cost of cycling} = 21 - 7\ ml \cdot kg^{-1} \cdot min^{-1} = 14\ ml \cdot kg^{-1} \cdot min^{-1}$$

$$14\ ml \cdot kg^{-1} \cdot min^{-1} = (?\ kgm \cdot min^{-1} \cdot 1.8\ ml\ O_2 \cdot kgm^{-1})/70\ kg$$

Multiply each side by 70 kg.

$$980\ ml \cdot min^{-1} = ?\ kgm \cdot min^{-1} \cdot 1.8\ ml\ O_2 \cdot kgm^{-1}$$

Divide each side by $1.8\ ml\ O_2 \cdot kgm^{-1}$ to obtain the work rate.

$$\text{Work rate} = 544\ kgm \cdot min^{-1}$$

Because the Monark wheel travels $300\ m \cdot min^{-1}$ at 50 rpm, the load on the wheel should be $544\ kgm \cdot min^{-1} / 300\ m \cdot min^{-1} = 1.8\ kg$.

Arm Ergometry

A cycle ergometer can be used to exercise the arms and shoulder-girdle muscles by modifying the pedals and placing the cycle on a table. Arm ergometry is used on a limited basis as a GXT to evaluate cardiovascular function. It is used more generally as a routine exercise in rehabilitation programs (13).

There are a variety of factors to keep in mind when considering arm ergometry:

- $\dot{V}O_2max$ for the arms is only 70% of that measured with the legs in a normal healthy population and less in an unfit, elderly, or diseased population.
- The natural endurance of the muscles used in this work is less than that of the legs.
- The HR and BP responses are higher for arm work compared with leg work at the same $\dot{V}O_2$.
- There is no need to account for unloaded arm cycling, but the oxygen cost of doing 1 kgm of work is about $3\ ml\ O_2 \cdot kgm^{-1}$ for arm work because of the action's inefficiency (3).

The equations for estimating the oxygen cost of arm work for work rates expressed in $kgm \cdot min^{-1}$ or watts are as follows:

$$\dot{V}O_2\ (ml \cdot kg^{-1} \cdot min^{-1}) = (kgm \cdot min^{-1} \cdot 3\ ml\ O_2 \cdot kgm^{-1})/\text{body weight (kg)} + 3.5\ ml \cdot kg^{-1} \cdot min^{-1}$$

$$\dot{V}O_2\ (ml \cdot kg^{-1} \cdot min^{-1}) = (W \cdot 18\ ml\ O_2 \cdot W^{-1})/\text{body weight (kg)} + 3.5\ ml \cdot kg^{-1} \cdot min^{-1}$$

See table 4.7 for estimates of the oxygen cost of arm work on a cycle ergometer.

QUESTION: What is the oxygen requirement of doing $150\ kgm \cdot min^{-1}$ on an arm ergometer for a 70-kg man?

Answer:

$$\dot{V}O_2\ (ml \cdot kg^{-1} \cdot min^{-1}) = (150\ kgm \cdot min^{-1} \cdot 3\ ml\ O_2 \cdot kgm^{-1})/70\ kg + 3.5\ ml \cdot kg^{-1} \cdot min^{-1}$$

$$= 9.9\ ml \cdot kg^{-1} \cdot min^{-1} \text{ or } 2.8\ \text{METs}$$

4 In Review

The oxygen cost of cycle ergometry is primarily dependent on the work rate because body weight is supported. The net oxygen cost of leg ergometry is 1.8 $ml \cdot kgm^{-1}$ versus 3 $ml \cdot kgm^{-1}$ for arm ergometry. Physiological responses (HR, BP) are exaggerated for arm work compared with leg work at the same work rate because the oxygen cost is higher and represents a higher percentage of the arm $\dot{V}O_2max$.

Oxygen Cost of Bench Stepping

One of the most useful and inexpensive forms of exercise is bench stepping. The activity can be done at home and requires little or no equipment. The work rate is adjusted easily by simply increasing step height or cadence (number of lifts per minute).

The total oxygen cost of this exercise is the sum of the costs of (a) stepping up, (b) stepping down, (c) moving back and forth on a level surface at the specified cadence, and (d) resting oxygen uptake (3.5 $ml \cdot kg^{-1} \cdot min^{-1}$). The oxygen cost of stepping up is 1.8 $ml \cdot kg^{-1} \cdot min^{-1}$ per $m \cdot min^{-1}$, as in walking (22). The oxygen cost of stepping down is a third of the cost of stepping up; therefore, the oxygen cost of stepping up and down is 1.33 times the cost of stepping up. The oxygen cost of stepping back and forth on a flat surface is equal to 0.2 ml O_2 for the four-cycle step per kilogram of body mass (3). The number of meters moved up or down per minute is calculated by multiplying the number of lifts per minute by the height of the step; for example, if the step height is 0.2 m (20 cm) and the cadence is 30 $steps \cdot min^{-1}$, then the total lift or descent per minute is 30 times 0.2 m, or 6 $m \cdot min^{-1}$. To determine step height, multiply inches by 2.54 to obtain centimeters, and divide centimeters by 100 to obtain meters. The equation for estimating the energy requirement for stepping follows:

$$\dot{V}O_2\ (ml \cdot kg^{-1} \cdot min^{-1}) = (0.2 \cdot \text{step rate}) + (1.8 \cdot 1.33 \cdot \text{step rate} \cdot \text{step height in meters}) + 3.5\ ml \cdot kg^{-1} \cdot min^{-1}$$

QUESTION: What is the oxygen requirement for stepping at a rate of 20 $steps \cdot min^{-1}$ on a 20-cm bench?

Answer:

$$\dot{V}O_2 = \left(\frac{0.2\ ml \cdot kg^{-1} \cdot min^{-1}}{steps \cdot min^{-1}} \cdot 20\ steps \cdot min^{-1}\right) + \left(\frac{1.8\ ml}{kgm} \cdot 1.33 \cdot \frac{0.2\ m}{step} \cdot \frac{20\ steps}{min}\right) + 3.5\ ml \cdot kg^{-1} \cdot min^{-1}$$

$$= 4.0\ ml \cdot kg^{-1} \cdot min^{-1} + 9.6\ ml \cdot kg^{-1} \cdot min^{-1} + 3.5\ ml \cdot kg^{-1} \cdot min^{-1}$$

$$= 17.1\ ml \cdot kg^{-1} \cdot min^{-1} \text{ or } 4.9\ \text{METs}$$

Table 4.8 summarizes the energy requirement of stepping at different rates.

Table 4.8 Energy Expenditure in Metabolic Equivalents (METs) During Stepping at Different Rates on Steps of Different Heights

Step height		Steps · min^{-1}			
cm	**in.**	**12**	**18**	**24**	**30**
0	0	1.7	2.0	2.4	2.7
4	1.6	2.0	2.5	3.0	3.5
8	3.2	2.3	3.0	3.7	4.4
12	4.7	2.7	3.5	4.3	5.2
16	6.3	3.0	4.0	5.0	6.0
20	7.9	3.3	4.5	5.7	6.8
24	9.4	3.7	5.0	6.3	7.6
28	11.0	4.0	5.5	7.0	8.5
32	12.6	4.3	6.0	7.6	9.3
36	14.2	4.6	6.5	8.3	10.1
40	15.8	5.0	7.0	8.9	10.9

Note. The table is based on equations published in *ACSM's Guidelines for Exercise Testing and Prescription* (6th ed.) 2000.

5 In Review

The oxygen cost of bench stepping includes the cost of stepping up and down, moving horizontally back and forth, and resting oxygen uptake. The oxygen cost of stepping up is the same as in walking. The oxygen cost of stepping down is 1.33 times the cost of stepping up. The oxygen cost of stepping back and forth is proportional to the cadence.

Energy Requirements of Other Activities

Many activities are available to you when designing a fitness program (see chapter 14). These include exercising to music, rope skipping, swimming, and playing games. Not surprisingly, the energy expenditure associated with these activities is difficult to predict compared with walking or running, in which the energy cost between people is similar because of the natural movements associated with those activities. In contrast, many activities have variable energy costs depending on the skill level of the participants and the motivation they bring to the activity. This will be clear in the following examples. Estimates of the energy requirements of some common aerobic activities also are presented.

Exercising to Music

Exercising to music is a fun alternative to walking and running. The energy requirement depends on whether the session is high or low impact; done at a low, medium, or high intensity; and done with or without hand weights (24). A person who is starting out might simply walk through the movements, whereas an experienced person might go through the full range of motion with each step. Thus, the energy costs of this activity vary considerably. Values might range from as low as 4 METs for someone walking through the routine to 10 METs for the experienced participant working at a high intensity in either a low- or high-impact session (24). Remember that this activity often involves small-muscle groups and includes some static (stabilizing) muscle contractions; as a result, HR response is higher for the same oxygen uptake measured in walking and running. Table 4.9 summarizes the caloric expenditure associated with exercise to music at low, moderate, and high intensities.

Table 4.9 Gross Energy Cost of Exercise to Music (kcal · min^{-1})

kg	lb	Low intensity	Moderate intensity	High intensity
50.0	110	3.3	5.8	8.3
54.5	120	3.6	6.4	9.1
59.1	130	3.9	6.9	9.8
63.6	140	4.2	7.4	10.6
68.2	150	4.5	7.9	11.3
72.7	160	4.8	8.5	12.1
77.3	170	5.1	9.0	12.8
81.8	180	5.4	9.5	13.6
86.4	190	5.7	10.1	14.3
90.9	200	6.0	10.6	15.1
95.4	210	6.3	11.1	15.9
100.0	220	6.6	11.7	16.7

Note. Multiply value by the duration of the aerobic phase of the exercise-to-music class to obtain total calories expended.

Rope Skipping

In walking and running, the energy requirement is proportional to the rate at which the person moves. But the energy requirement for rope skipping at only 60 to 80 turns per minute (about as slow as the rope can be turned) is about 9 METs. At 120 turns per minute, the energy cost increases to only 11 METs (17). Consequently, rope skipping is not a graded activity as are walking and running. Second, the HR response is higher than expected from the oxygen cost of the activity. This, again, may be because a small-muscle mass (lower leg) is the primary muscle group involved in the activity. Despite this, rope skipping can be included as an effective part of a fitness program when done intermittently using target HR (THR) as the guide (see chapter 14). Rope skipping should not be used, however, in the early part of a fitness program because the energy cost and loading on ankle, knee, and hip joints are relatively high. Table 4.10 presents a summary of the energy costs of skipping rope at two speeds.

Table 4.10 Gross Energy Cost of Rope Skipping ($kcal \cdot min^{-1}$)

		Body weight	
kg	lb	Slow skipping	Fast skipping
50.0	110	3.3	5.8
54.5	120	3.6	6.4
59.1	130	8.9	10.9
63.6	140	9.5	11.7
68.2	150	10.2	12.5
72.7	160	10.9	13.4
77.3	170	11.6	14.2
81.8	180	12.3	15.0
86.4	190	13.0	15.9
90.9	200	13.6	16.7
95.4	210	14.3	17.5
100.0	220	15.0	18.4

Note. Multiply value by the duration of the rope-skipping session to obtain total calories expended.

Swimming

Swimming is a preferred activity for many people because of the dynamic, large-muscle nature of the task and because little joint trauma is associated with it. The limitation is in finding a convenient facility that allows lap swimming and, of course, having enough skill to do the activity. The energy requirement depends on the velocity of movement and the stroke being used, but it is also influenced by the skill of the swimmer. A skilled swimmer requires less energy to move through the water, so the skilled swimmer has to swim a greater distance than an unskilled person to achieve the same caloric expenditure.

The energy cost of simply treading water can be as high as 1.5 $L \cdot min^{-1}$ (7.5 $kcal \cdot min^{-1}$). Elite swimmers use this same number of kilocalories per minute to swim at 36 $m \cdot min^{-1}$, whereas an unskilled swimmer might require twice that to maintain the same velocity. For elite swimmers, the front and back crawl are the most economical and the butterfly is the least economical. The net caloric cost per mile of swimming has been estimated to be more than 400 kcal, or about 4 times that of running 1 mile and about 8 times that of walking 1 mile. However, the actual caloric cost per mile of swimming varies greatly, depending on skill and gender. Table 4.11 is a summary of the values presented by Holmer (15) for men and women.

The HR response measured during swimming at a specific $\dot{V}O_2$ is lower than that measured during running at the same $\dot{V}O_2$. In fact, the maximal HR response is about 14 $beats \cdot min^{-1}$ lower for swimming (see chapter 17). With this in mind, you should instruct participants to decrease the THR range when you prescribe swimming activities.

Table 4.11 Caloric Cost Per Mile ($kcal \cdot mile^{-1}$) of Swimming the Front Crawl

Skill level	Women	Men
Competitive	180	280
Skilled	260	360
Average	300	440
Unskilled	360	560
Poor	440	720

Adapted from "Physiology of swimming man" by I. Holmer. In *Exercise and Sport Sciences Review, 7,* by R.S. Hutton and D.I. Miller (Eds.), 1970.

Estimation of Energy Expenditure Without Equations

Appendix C contains a tabular summary of the energy requirements for a wide variety of physical activities, including exercises, sports, occupations, and home-related tasks (1). This is helpful in estimating the energy expenditure associated with an individual's structured physical activity program; however, there is considerable variability in many of these estimates. There is an easier way to estimate the energy costs of an exercise session without using equations.

The HFI selects activities that cause the fitness participant to exercise in the range of 40 to 85% of his or her $\dot{V}O_2max$, the intensity needed to improve or maintain cardiorespiratory fitness (see chapter 10). It should be possible, therefore, to estimate the energy expenditure for each individual on the basis of the subject's $\dot{V}O_2max$ and the portion of the THR range at which the person is working. If a person has a $\dot{V}O_2max$ of 10 METs, energy expenditure can be estimated in the following way. Ten METs is equivalent to about 10 kcal $\cdot$ kg^{-1} $\cdot$ hr^{-1}. If a person is working at the bottom portion of the THR range for young healthy persons, at about 60% $\dot{V}O_2max$, then the energy expenditure should be about 6 METs (60% of 10 METs). If the person weighs 70 kg, then 420 kcal are expended per hour (70 kg $\cdot$ 6 kcal $\cdot$ kg^{-1} $\cdot$ hr^{-1}). A 30-min workout would require half this, or about 210 kcal. These simple calculations assume that the person is performing a large-muscle activity. Table 4.12 shows the estimated calorie expenditure for a 30-min workout at 70% $\dot{V}O_2max$ for a variety of fitness levels ($\dot{V}O_2max$ expressed as METs) and body weights (23).

Table 4.12 Estimated Energy Expenditure for a 30-Min Workout at 70% Functional Capacity for People of Various Fitness Levels ($\dot{V}O_2max$) and Body Weights

$\dot{V}O_2max$ (METs) (kcal · kg^{-1} · hr^{-1})	70% max METs (kcal · kg^{-1} · hr^{-1})	50 kg/110 lb	70 kg/154 lb	90 kg/198 lb
20	14.0	350	490	630
18	12.6	315	441	567
16	11.2	280	392	504
14	9.8	245	343	441
12	8.4	210	294	378
10	7.0	175	245	315
8	5.6	140	196	252
6	4.2	105	147	189

Note. MET = metabolic equivalent.

Environmental Concerns

Although changes in temperature, relative humidity, pollution, and altitude do not change the energy requirements for submaximal exercise, they do change the participant's response to the exercise bout. Remember that a person's HR response is the best indicator of the relative stress being experienced due to the interaction of exercise intensity, duration, and environmental factors. The participant should be instructed to cut back on the intensity of the activity when environmental factors increase the HR response. The duration of the activity can be increased to accommodate any energy expenditure goal.

6 In Review

The energy cost of exercise to music varies from 4 to 10 METs, depending on effort and whether the exercise is high or low impact. Rope skipping requires about 10 METs, whereas the oxygen cost of swimming is inversely related to skill. Energy expenditure can be estimated without equations. If a person is working at 60% of $\dot{V}O_2max$ and has a $\dot{V}O_2max$ of 10 METs, the person is expending energy at 6 METs, or 6 kcal · kg^{-1} · hr^{-1}. If the person weighs 80 kg, 480 kcal are expended per hour. Environmental factors such as heat, humidity, altitude, and pollution can increase the HR response to work while not affecting the energy cost very much. HR should be monitored more frequently in these settings to adjust the intensity of the activity downward to keep the person in the appropriate HR range.

Case Studies

You can check your answers by referring to appendix A.

4.1

A 75-kg man walks at 3.5 miles · hr^{-1} for 30 min. How many calories does he expend?

4.2

A 60-kg woman rides a cycle ergometer at a work rate of 100 W. What is her oxygen uptake?

4.3

A 70-kg college student runs 3 miles in 24 min. How many calories did he expend?

4.4

An 85-kg man with a functional capacity of 12 METs works at 70% of his capacity for 30 min. How many calories did he expend?

4.5

A client has read that he can expend the same number of calories per mile whether he walks it at 3 mi · hr^{-1} or jogs it at 6 mi · hr^{-1}. How would you respond?

Source List

1. Ainsworth, B.E., Haskell, W.L., Whitt, M.C., Irwin, M.L., Swartz, A.M., Strath, S.J., O'Brien, W.L., Bassett, D.R., Jr., Schmitz, K.H., Emplaincourt, P.O., Jacobs, D.R., Jr., & Leon, A.S. (2000). Compendium of physical activities: An update of activity codes and MET intensities. *Medicine and Science in Sports and Exercise, 32,* S498-S516.
2. American College of Sports Medicine. (1980). *Guidelines for graded exercise testing and exercise prescription* (2nd ed.). Philadelphia: Lea & Febiger.
3. American College of Sports Medicine. (2000). *ACSM's guidelines for exercise testing and prescription* (6th ed.). Baltimore: Lippincott Williams & Wilkins.
4. Åstrand, P-O. (1979). *Work tests with the bicycle ergometer.* Verberg, Sweden: Monark-Crescent AB.
5. Åstrand, P-O., & Rodahl, K. (1986). *Textbook of work physiology* (3rd ed.). New York: McGraw-Hill.
6. Balke, B. (1963). A simple field test for assessment of physical fitness. In *Civil Aeromedical Research Institute report* (pp. 63-66). Oklahoma City: Civil Aeromedical Research Institute.
7. Balke, B., & Ware, R.W. (1959). An experimental study of "physical fitness" of Air Force personnel. *Armed Forces Medical Journal, 10,* 675-688.
8. Bassett, D.R., Jr., Giese, M.D., Nagle, F.J., Ward, A., Raab, D.M., & Balke, B. (1985). Aerobic requirements of overground versus treadmill running. *Medicine and Science in Sports and Exercise, 17,* 477-481.
9. Bransford, D.R., & Howley, E.T. (1977). The oxygen cost of running in trained and untrained men and women. *Medicine and Science in Sports, 9,* 41-44.
10. Bubb, W.J., Martin, A.D., & Howley, E.T. (1985). Predicting oxygen uptake during level walking at speeds of 80 to 130 meters per minute. *Journal of Cardiac Rehabilitation, 5*(10), 462-465.
11. Daniels, J.T. (1985). A physiologist's view of running economy. *Medicine and Science in Sports and Exercise, 17,* 332-338.
12. Dill, D.B. (1965). Oxygen cost of horizontal and grade walking and running on the treadmill. *Journal of Applied Physiology, 20,* 19-22.
13. Franklin, B.A. (1985). Exercise testing, training, and arm ergometry. *Sports Medicine, 2,* 100-119.
14. Haskell, W.L., Savin, W., Oldridge, N., & DeBusk, R. (1982). Factors influencing estimated oxygen uptake during exercise testing soon after myocardial infarction. *American Journal of Cardiology, 50,* 299-304.
15. Holmer, I. (1979). Physiology of swimming man. *Exercise and Sport Sciences Reviews, 7,* 87-123.
16. Howley, E.T., & Glover, M.E. (1974). The caloric costs of running and walking 1 mile for men and women. *Medicine and Science in Sports, 6,* 235-237.
17. Howley, E.T., & Martin, D. (1978). Oxygen uptake and heart-rate responses measured during rope skipping. *Tennessee Journal of Health, Physical Education and Recreation, 16,* 7-8.
18. Knoebel, L.K. (1984). Energy metabolism. In E. Selkurt (Ed.), *Physiology* (5th ed., pp. 635-650). Boston: Little, Brown.
19. Margaria, R., Cerretelli, P., Aghemo, P., & Sassi, J. (1963). Energy cost of running. *Journal of Applied Physiology, 18,* 367-370.
20. Montoye, H.J., Ayen, T., Nagle, F., & Howley, E.T. (1986). The oxygen requirement for horizontal and grade walking on a motor-driven treadmill. *Medicine and Science in Sports and Exercise, 17,* 640-645.
21. Nagle, F.J., Balke, B., Baptista, G., Alleyia, J., & Howley, E. (1971). Compatibility of progressive treadmill, bicycle, and step tests based on oxygen-uptake responses. *Medicine and Science in Sport, 3,* 149-154.
22. Nagle, F.J., Balke, B., & Naughton, J.P. (1965). Gradational step tests for assessing work capacity. *Journal of Applied Physiology, 20,* 745-748.
23. Sharkey, B.J. (1990). *Physiology of fitness* (3rd ed.). Champaign, IL: Human Kinetics.
24. Williford, H.N., Scharff-Olson, M., & Blessing, D.L. (1989). The physiological effects of aerobic dance—A review. *Sports Medicine, 8,* 335-345.

five

Cardiorespiratory Fitness

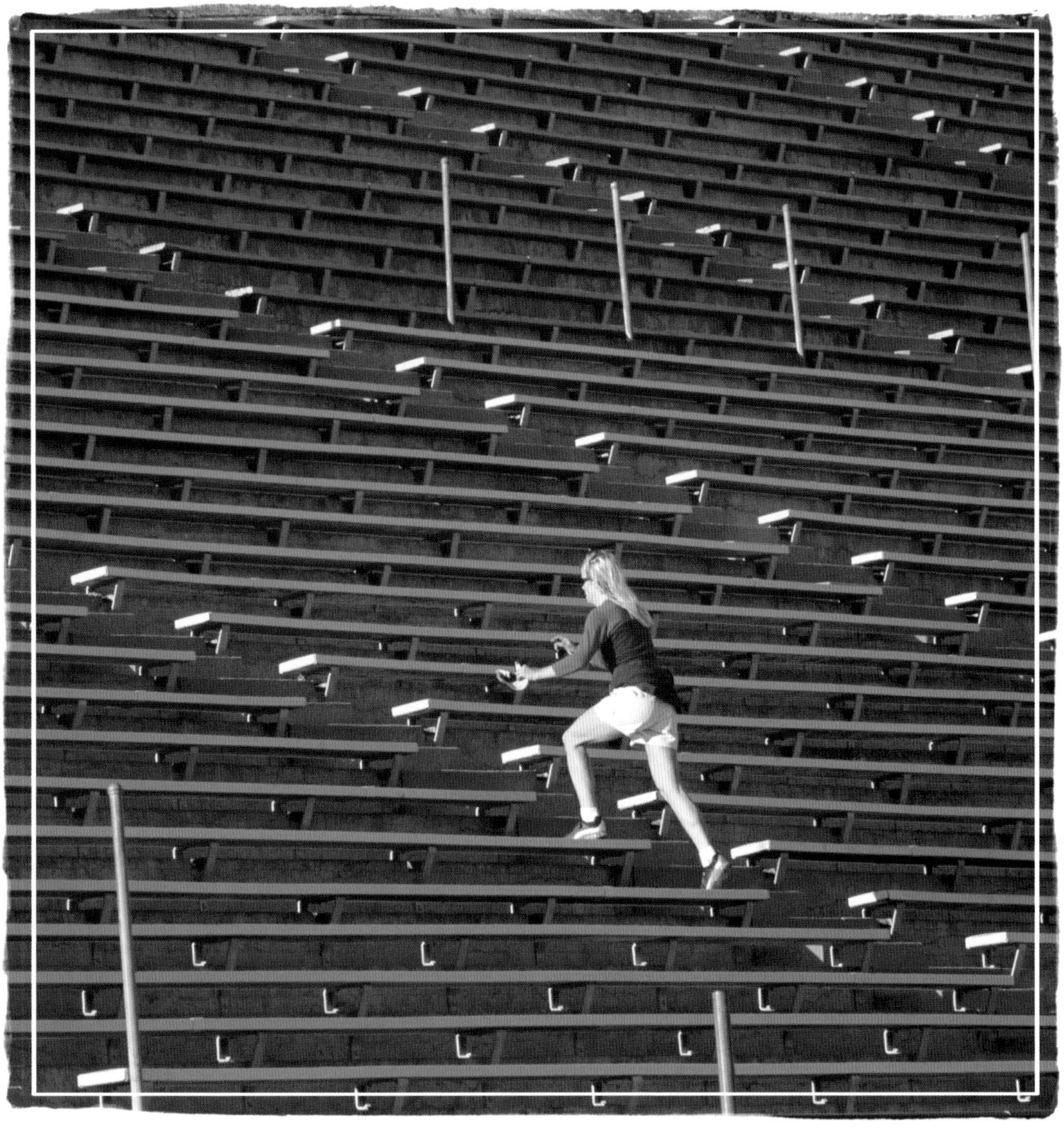

© I.G. Vorster

Objectives

The reader will be able to do the following:

1. Describe the relationship of cardiorespiratory fitness (CRF) to health and list reasons for testing CRF as well as risks associated with CRF testing.
2. Present a logical sequence of testing.
3. Describe procedures for conducting walking and jogging/running field tests to estimate CRF.
4. Contrast the treadmill, cycle ergometer, and bench step as instruments to use for GXTs.
5. List variables measured during a GXT.
6. Describe procedures used before, during, and after testing.
7. Contrast submaximal and maximal GXTs.
8. Describe the HR extrapolation procedures to estimate $\dot{V}O_2max$ using submaximal treadmill, cycle, and bench step GXTs.
9. Calibrate a treadmill, a Monark cycle ergometer, and a sphygmomanometer.

The usual introduction to cardiorespiratory fitness (CRF) delineates heart disease as the major cause of death and proceeds to describe the role of exercise in prevention and rehabilitation programs. It is also important, however, to focus attention on a high level of CRF as a normal, lifelong goal that makes life more enjoyable. That alone merits the inclusion of CRF in any discussion about positive health. Cardiorespiratory fitness, also called cardiovascular or aerobic fitness, is a good measure of the heart's ability to pump oxygen-rich blood to the muscles. Although the terms **cardio-** (heart), **vascular** (blood vessels), **respiratory** (lungs and ventilation), and **aerobic** (working with oxygen) differ technically, they all reflect different aspects of this component of fitness. The person with a healthy heart can pump great volumes of blood with each beat and will have a high level of CRF. CRF values are expressed in the following ways:

- Liters of oxygen used by the body per minute ($L \cdot min^{-1}$)
- Milliliters of oxygen used per kilogram of body weight per minute ($ml \cdot kg^{-1} \cdot min^{-1}$)
- METs, multiples of resting metabolic rate, where 1 MET = $3.5\ ml \cdot kg^{-1} \cdot min^{-1}$

A person with the ability to use $35\ ml \cdot kg^{-1} \cdot min^{-1}$ during maximal exercise is said to have a CRF equal to 10 METs ($35 \div 3.5 = 10$). Aerobic training programs increase the heart's ability to pump blood, so it is no surprise that CRF improves as a result of such programs.

Chapter 28 describes how CRF variables respond to acute or short-term exercise and the effect of endurance training on those responses. Chapter 10 explains how to recommend activities to clients to improve their CRF. This chapter emphasizes the evaluation of CRF. The reader is referred to other resources for additional details (1, 33).

Historically, measurements of HR, BP, and electrocardiogram (ECG) taken at rest were used to evaluate CRF. In addition, some static pulmonary function tests (e.g., vital capacity) were used to characterize respiratory function. It became clear, however, that measurements made at rest reveal little about the way a person's cardiorespiratory system responds to physical activity. We are now familiar with the use of a GXT to evaluate HR, ECG, BP, ventilation, and oxygen uptake responses during work.

Why Test Cardiorespiratory Fitness?

The measurements obtained from cardiorespiratory fitness tests are used to write exercise recommendations and allow the HFI or physician to evaluate positive or negative changes in CRF as a result of physical conditioning, aging, illness, or inactivity. Given the recent increase in obesity and inactivity in persons of all ages, it makes good sense to evaluate CRF throughout life, from early childhood to old age. This information can indicate where the individual stands relative to health-criterion test scores, and it will alert the individual to subtle changes in lifestyle that may compromise positive health. The nature of the tests and the level of monitoring should vary across age groups to reflect the type of information that is needed.

CRF testing depends on the purposes of the test, the type of person to be evaluated, and the work tasks available. Reasons for testing include

- determining physiological responses at rest and during **submaximal** and/or **maximal** work,
- providing a basis for exercise programming,
- screening for CHD, and
- determining one's ability to perform a specific work task.

The choice of an appropriate test depends on several factors. People differ in age, fitness levels, known health problems, and risks of CHD. Also, financial considerations determine the amount of time that can be devoted to each individual and the type of work tasks available.

Risks of CRF Testing

As indicated in chapter 1, the risks associated with exercise testing are quite low. Health professionals should emphasize that the overall risk of a cardiovascular problem is greater for those who maintain sedentary habits than for those who take an exercise test and then embark on a regular exercise program (1). This is consistent with evidence showing that low levels of cardiorespiratory fitness are related directly to a higher risk of heart disease and death (10).

1 In Review

CRF is an important aspect of quality of life for healthy individuals as well as a risk factor for CHD. The ability to use oxygen during exercise is the basis for this fitness component and can be expressed in $L \cdot min^{-1}$, $ml \cdot kg^{-1} \cdot min^{-1}$, and METs. CRF testing is used for exercise programming, screening for heart disease, and determining one's ability to do a specific work task. The risk of death attributable to exercise testing is very low.

Testing Sequence

A logical sequence for fitness testing (and activities) can be followed when people attend the same fitness center over a substantial period of time. This sequence progresses from the initial screening to fitness testing and programming, with opportunities for periodic retesting and revision of the program as fitness gains are made. The box below lists the sequence of testing and activity prescription. The rest of this section describes the process in detail. For people who request fitness testing but do not have continuing involvement with the fitness center, the submaximal and maximal tests are usually a part of the same GXT protocol.

Informed Consent

Fitness participants should be informed volunteers. The fitness program should clearly describe all of its procedures and the potential risks and benefits of the fitness tests and activities. The participants should understand that their individual data will be

Sequence of Testing and Activity Prescription

1. Informed consent
2. Health history
3. Screening
4. Resting CRF, body composition, and psychological tests
5. Submaximal CRF
6. Tests for low back function
7. Begin light activity program here
8. Tests for muscular strength and endurance
9. Maximal CRF
10. Revise activity program; include games and sports here
11. Periodic retest (and activity revision)

confidential and that any test or activity can be terminated at any time should they feel uncomfortable. A written **informed consent** form should be signed by the participant after reading a description of the program and having all questions answered. A sample consent form is included in chapter 26.

Health History

Chapter 3 describes procedures for determining current health status. This information can be used to determine appropriate testing protocol and activity recommendations. In addition, follow-up testing should be advised for people with symptoms of health problems. Referrals to other professionals might be warranted based on the person's history.

Screening

We recommended in chapter 3 that individuals have regular medical examinations and health screenings and engage in moderate-intensity exercise. Fitness programs need to determine whether the person needs medical permission to be in a fitness program involving vigorous-intensity activities. Older individuals and those with CHD or other known major health problems must have medical supervision or clearance before embarking on any fitness testing or program that goes beyond moderate-intensity exercise.

We've listed on page 69 the conditions (absolute contraindications) that the ACSM has identified in which the risk of testing outweighs the possible benefits. Other conditions (relative contraindications) may increase the risk of exercise testing; people with these conditions should only be tested if a doctor determines that the need for the test outweighs the potential risk.

Apparently healthy people who have no known major health problems or symptoms can be tested or begin the type of fitness program recommended in this book with minimal risk. Chapter 3 identifies the people who need medical clearance, a carefully supervised program, and educational information about health problems and behaviors.

Resting Measurements

Typical resting tests may include CRF measures (e.g., 12-lead ECG, HR, BP, blood chemistry profile) as well as other fitness variables such as body composition and psychological traits. Evaluation of the ECG by a physician determines whether any abnormalities require further medical attention. People with extreme BP or blood chemistry values (see chapter 3) should also be referred to their personal physicians.

Submaximal Tests to Estimate CRF

If the resting tests reflect normal values, then a submaximal test is administered. (See table 3.2 for level of medical supervision needed for submaximal and maximal testing.) The submaximal test usually provides the HR and BP responses to different intensities of work, from light intensity up to a predetermined point (usually 85% of predicted maximum HR). This test can use a bench step, cycle ergometer, or treadmill. Once again, if unusual responses to the submaximal test appear, then the person is referred for further medical tests. If the results appear normal, then an activity program is begun at intensities less than those reached on the test (e.g., a person goes to 85% of maximum HR on the test and starts the fitness program at 70%). After the person has become accustomed to regular exercise and appears to be adjusting to fitness activities, a maximal test can be administered.

Submaximal testscan also be used to estimate maximal functional capacity (maximal oxygen uptake) by extrapolating HR to a predicted maximum and then using the linear relationship between HR and oxygen uptake to estimate maximal oxygen uptake. Although this estimated maximum is useful for evaluating a person's current status and prescribing or revising exercise, there is considerable error involved in the estimation (±15%). In addition to submaximal CRF, flexibility and muscular strength and endurance (especially related to low back function) are often measured at this stage (see chapters 8 and 9).

Maximal Tests to Estimate or Measure CRF

If no problems occur up to this point, a maximal test is administered. Two basic types of maximal tests are used to estimate CRF: laboratory tests that measure physiological responses (e.g., HR, BP) to increasing levels of work, and all-out endurance performance tests (e.g., time on a 1-mile run). The results of the maximal test can be used to revise the activity program (i.e., the person's maximal functional capacity provides a new basis for selection of fitness activities). The person's measured maximal HR (instead of the estimated maximal HR) should now be used to determine THR.

Contraindications to Exercise Testing

Absolute

- A recent significant change in the resting ECG suggesting significant ischemia, recent myocardial infarction (within 2 days), or other acute cardiac event
- Unstable angina
- Uncontrolled cardiac arrhythmias causing symptoms or hemodynamic compromise
- Severe symptomatic aortic stenosis
- Uncontrolled symptomatic heart failure
- Acute pulmonary embolus or pulmonary infarction
- Acute myocarditis or pericarditis
- Suspected or known dissecting aneurysm
- Acute infections

Relative*

- Left main coronary stenosis
- Moderate stenotic valvular heart disease
- Electrolyte abnormalities (e.g., hypokalemia, hypomagnesemia)
- Severe arterial hypertension (i.e., systolic BP of >200 mm Hg and/or a diastolic BP of >110 mm Hg) at rest
- Tachyarrhythmias or bradyarrhythmias
- Hypertrophic cardiomyopathy and other forms of outflow tract obstruction
- Neuromuscular, musculoskeletal, or rheumatoid disorders that are exacerbated by exercise
- High-degree atrioventricular block
- Ventricular aneurysm
- Uncontrolled metabolic disease (e.g., diabetes, thyrotoxicosis, or myxedema)
- Chronic infectious disease (e.g., mononucleosis, hepatitis, AIDS)

Note. This list was modified from Gibbons, R.A., Balady, G.J., Beasely, J.W., et al. (1997). ACC/AHA guidelines for exercise testing. *Journal of the American College of Cardiology, 30,* 260-315.

*Relative contraindications can be superseded if benefits outweigh risks of exercise. In some instances, these individuals can be exercised with caution and/or using low-level end points, especially if they are asymptomatic at rest.

Reprinted from ACSM (2000).

Program Modification and Periodic Retests

After a minimum level of fitness has been achieved, a wider variety of activities (e.g., games and sports) can be included in the fitness program. All of the tests should be retaken periodically to determine the progress being made and to revise the program in areas where the gains are not as great as desired.

2 In Review

A logical sequence of steps to follow in fitness testing includes informed consent, health history, screening, resting CRF, submaximal CRF and other tests, light activity prescription, maximal CRF, program modification, and periodic retesting (see box on page 67).

Field Tests

A variety of field tests can be used to estimate CRF. These are called "field tests" because they require very little equipment, can be done just about anywhere, and use the simple activities of walking and running. Because these tests involve running or walking as fast as possible over a set distance, they are not recommended at the start of an exercise program. Instead, we recommend that participants complete the graduated walking program before taking the walking test and the graduated jogging program before taking the running test. The walk/jog programs are found in chapter 14. The graduated nature of the fitness program allows participants to start at a low and safe level of activity and gradually improve. It is then appropriate to administer an endurance run test to evaluate fitness status.

Field tests rely on the observation that for one to walk or run at high speeds over long distances, the heart must pump great volumes of oxygen to the muscles. In this way, the average speed maintained in these walk/run tests gives an estimate of CRF. The higher the CRF score, the greater the heart's capacity to transport oxygen. An endurance run of a set distance for a given time, or a set time for a given distance, provides information about a person's CR endurance as long as it is 1 mile or more. The advantages of an endurance run test include its moderately high correlation to maximum oxygen uptake, the use of a natural activity, and the large numbers of participants who can be tested in a short period of time. The disadvantages of endurance running are that it is difficult to monitor physiological responses, other factors affect the outcome (e.g., motivation), endurance running cannot be used for graded or submaximal testing, and the SEE is about 5 ml · kg^{-1} · min^{-1} (31).

1-Mile Walk Test

A 1-mile walk test to predict CRF has been developed to accommodate individuals of different ages and fitness levels. Follow the steps on page 71 to administer the 1-mile walk test.

In this test, the individual walks as fast as possible on a measured track, and HR is measured at the end of the mile. The following equation is used to calculate $\dot{V}O_2max$ (ml · kg^{-1} · min^{-1}):

$$\dot{V}O_2max = 132.853 - 0.0769\ (weight) - 0.3877\ (age) + 6.315\ (sex) - 3.2649\ (time) - 0.1565\ (HR)$$

where weight is body weight in pounds, age is in years, sex equals 0 for female and 1 for male, time is in minutes and hundredths of minutes, and HR is in beats · min^{-1}. The formula was developed and validated on men and women ages 30 to 69 years (24), and the SEE is about 5 ml · kg^{-1} · min^{-1} (1, 24).

QUESTION: What is the CRF of a 25-year-old, 170-lb man who walks the mile in 20 min and has an immediate postexercise HR of 140 beats · min^{-1}?

Answer:

$$\dot{V}O_2max = 132.853 - 0.0769\ (weight) - 0.3877\ (age) + 6.315\ (sex) - 3.2649\ (time) - 0.1565\ (HR)$$

$$= 132.853 - 0.0769\ (170) - 0.3877\ (25) + 6.315\ (1) - 3.2649\ (20.0) - 0.1565\ (140)$$

$$= 29.2\ ml \cdot kg^{-1} \cdot min^{-1}$$

To simplify the steps in using this 1-mile walk test, table 5.1 was generated on the basis of the preceding formula for men weighing 170 lb and women weighing 125 lb. For each 15 lb above (or below) these weights, subtract (or add) 1 ml · kg^{-1} · min^{-1}.

To use table 5.1, find the part of the table for the individual's sex and age, then go across the top until you find the time (to the nearest minute) that person took to walk a mile, and then go down that column until it intersects with the person's postexercise HR (listed on the left side). The number at which the mile time and postexercise HR meet is the CRF value in terms of ml · kg^{-1} · min^{-1}. For example, a 25-year-old man who walked the mile in 20 min and had a postexercise HR of 140 would have an estimated maximal oxygen uptake of 29.2 ml · kg^{-1} · min^{-1}. You can evaluate CRF by using that number to compare with the standards presented in table 5.2. In the example of the 25-year-old man, his maximal oxygen uptake is less than 30, indicating a need for improvement. The standards in table 5.2 represent the levels of oxygen uptake for females and males with regard to health-related fitness. Those wishing to focus on performance should strive for higher values.

Jog/Run Test

One of the most common CRF field tests is the 12-min or 1.5-mile run popularized by Cooper (14). This test is very much like the walk test mentioned previously: jog or run as fast as possible for 12 min or for 1.5 miles. This test is based on original work by Balke (7), who showed that 10- to 20-min running tests could be used to estimate $\dot{V}O_2max$. Balke found the optimal duration to be 15 min. The test is based

Steps to Administer the 1-Mile Walk Test

Before Test Day

1. Arrange to have the following elements at the test site:
   - A person to start and read the time from a stopwatch
   - A partner with a watch (with a second hand) for each walker (perhaps with a sheet to mark off laps)
   - A stopwatch for the timer (with a spare ready)
   - A score sheet or scorecard
2. Explain the purpose of the test (i.e., to determine how fast the participants can walk a mile, which reflects the endurance of their cardiovascular system).
3. Select and mark off (if needed) a level area for the walk.
4. Explain to people being tested that they are to walk the mile in the fastest time possible. Only walking is allowed, and the goal is to cover the distance as fast as possible.

Test Day

1. Participants warm up with stretching and slow walking.
2. Several people will walk at the same time.
3. Explain the procedure again. Remind the participants not to speed up at the end of the walk but to maintain a fast and steady pace throughout.
4. The timer says, "Ready, go," and starts the stopwatch.
5. Each individual has a partner with a watch with a second hand.
6. The partner counts the laps and tells the individual at the end of each lap how many more laps to walk.
7. The timer calls out the minutes and seconds as each person finishes the mile walk.
8. The partner listens for the time when his or her walker finishes the mile and records it (to the nearest second) immediately on a scorecard.
9. The walker takes a 10-s HR immediately after the end of the mile walk while the partner times.

Table 5.1 Estimated Maximal Oxygen Uptake (ml · kg^{-1} · min^{-1}) for Men and Women, 20-69 Years Old

	Min · $mile^{-1}$										
HR	**10**	**11**	**12**	**13**	**14**	**15**	**16**	**17**	**18**	**19**	**20**
Men (20-29)											
120	65.0	61.7	58.4	55.2	51.9	48.6	45.4	42.1	38.9	35.6	32.3
130	63.4	60.1	56.9	53.6	50.3	47.1	43.8	40.6	37.3	34.0	30.8
140	61.8	58.6	55.3	52.0	48.8	45.5	42.2	39.0	35.7	32.5	29.2
150	60.3	57.0	53.7	50.5	47.2	43.9	40.7	37.4	34.2	30.9	27.6
160	58.7	55.4	52.2	48.9	45.6	42.4	39.1	35.9	32.6	29.3	26.1
170	57.1	53.9	50.6	47.3	44.1	40.8	37.6	34.3	31.0	27.8	24.5
180	55.6	52.3	49.0	45.8	42.5	39.3	36.0	32.7	29.5	26.2	22.9
190	54.0	50.7	47.5	44.2	41.0	37.7	34.4	31.2	27.9	24.6	21.4
200	52.4	49.2	45.9	42.7	39.4	36.1	32.9	29.6	26.3	23.1	19.8
Women (20-29)											
120	62.1	58.9	55.6	52.3	49.1	45.8	42.5	39.3	36.0	32.7	29.5
130	60.6	57.3	54.0	50.8	47.5	44.2	41.0	37.7	34.4	31.2	27.9
140	59.0	55.7	52.5	49.2	45.9	42.7	39.4	36.1	32.9	29.6	26.3
150	57.4	54.2	50.9	47.6	44.4	41.1	37.8	34.6	31.3	28.0	24.8
160	55.9	52.6	49.3	46.7	42.8	39.5	36.3	33.0	29.7	26.5	23.2
170	54.3	51.0	47.8	44.5	41.2	38.0	34.7	31.4	28.2	24.9	21.6
180	52.7	49.5	46.2	42.9	39.7	36.4	33.1	29.9	26.6	23.3	20.1
190	51.2	47.9	44.6	41.4	38.1	34.8	31.6	28.3	25.0	21.8	18.5
200	49.6	46.3	43.1	39.8	36.5	33.3	30.0	26.7	23.5	20.2	16.9
Men (30-39)											
120	61.1	57.8	54.6	51.3	48.0	44.8	41.5	38.2	35.0	31.7	28.4
130	59.5	56.3	53.0	49.7	46.5	43.2	39.9	36.7	33.4	30.1	26.9
140	58.0	54.7	51.4	48.2	44.9	41.6	38.4	35.1	31.8	28.6	25.3
150	56.4	53.1	49.9	46.6	43.3	40.1	36.8	33.5	30.3	27.0	23.8
160	54.8	51.6	48.3	45.0	41.8	38.5	35.2	32.0	28.7	25.5	22.2
170	53.3	50.0	46.7	43.5	40.2	36.9	33.7	30.4	27.1	23.9	20.6
180	51.7	48.4	45.2	41.9	38.6	35.4	32.1	28.8	25.6	22.3	19.1
190	50.1	46.9	43.6	40.3	37.1	33.8	30.5	27.3	24.0	20.8	17.5
Women (30-39)											
120	58.2	55.0	51.7	48.4	45.2	41.9	38.7	35.4	32.1	28.9	25.6
130	56.7	53.4	50.1	46.9	43.6	40.4	37.1	33.8	30.6	27.3	24.0
140	55.1	51.8	48.6	45.3	42.1	38.8	35.5	32.3	29.0	24.7	22.5
150	53.5	50.3	47.0	43.8	40.5	37.2	34.0	30.7	27.4	24.2	20.9
160	52.0	48.7	45.4	42.2	38.9	35.7	32.4	29.1	25.9	22.6	19.3
170	50.4	47.1	43.9	40.6	37.4	34.1	30.8	27.6	24.3	21.0	17.8
180	48.8	45.6	42.3	39.1	35.8	32.5	29.3	26.0	22.7	19.5	16.2
190	47.3	44.0	40.8	37.5	34.2	31.0	27.7	24.4	21.2	17.9	14.6
Men (40-49)											
120	57.2	54.0	50.7	47.4	44.2	40.9	37.6	34.4	31.1	27.8	24.6
130	55.7	52.4	49.1	45.9	42.6	39.3	36.1	32.8	29.5	26.3	23.0
140	54.1	50.8	47.6	44.3	41.0	37.8	34.5	31.2	28.0	24.7	21.4

Table 5.1 (continued)

HR	10	11	12	13	14	15	16	17	18	19	20
						Min · mile^{-1}					
150	52.5	49.3	46.0	42.7	39.5	36.2	32.9	29.7	26.4	23.1	19.9
160	51.0	47.7	44.4	41.2	37.9	34.6	31.4	28.1	24.8	21.6	18.3
170	49.4	46.1	42.9	39.6	36.3	33.1	29.8	26.5	23.3	20.0	16.7
180	47.8	44.6	41.3	38.0	34.8	31.5	28.2	25.0	21.7	18.4	15.2
Women (40-49)											
120	54.4	51.1	47.8	44.6	41.3	38.0	34.8	31.5	28.2	25.0	21.7
130	52.8	49.5	46.3	43.0	39.7	36.5	33.2	29.9	26.7	23.4	20.1
140	51.2	48.0	44.7	41.4	38.2	34.9	31.6	28.4	25.1	21.8	18.6
150	49.7	46.4	43.1	39.9	36.6	33.3	30.1	26.8	23.5	20.3	17.0
160	48.1	44.8	41.6	38.3	35.0	31.8	28.5	25.2	22.0	18.7	15.5
170	46.5	43.3	40.0	36.7	33.5	30.2	26.9	23.7	20.4	17.2	13.9
Men (50-59)											
120	53.3	50.0	46.8	43.5	40.3	37.0	33.7	30.5	27.2	23.9	20.7
130	51.7	48.5	45.2	42.0	38.7	35.4	32.2	28.9	25.6	22.4	19.1
140	50.2	46.9	43.7	40.4	37.1	33.9	30.6	27.3	24.1	20.8	17.5
150	48.6	45.4	42.1	38.8	35.6	32.3	29.0	25.8	22.5	19.2	16.0
160	47.1	43.8	40.5	37.3	34.0	30.7	27.5	24.2	20.9	17.7	14.4
170	45.5	42.2	39.0	35.7	32.4	29.2	25.9	22.6	19.4	16.1	12.8
Women (50-59)											
120	50.5	47.2	43.9	40.7	37.4	34.1	30.9	27.6	24.3	21.1	17.8
130	48.9	45.6	42.4	39.1	35.8	32.6	29.3	26.0	22.8	19.5	16.2
140	47.3	44.1	40.8	37.5	34.3	31.0	27.7	24.5	21.2	17.9	14.7
150	45.8	42.5	39.2	36.0	32.7	29.4	26.2	22.9	19.6	16.4	13.1
160	44.2	40.9	37.7	34.4	31.1	27.9	24.6	21.3	18.1	14.8	11.5
170	42.6	39.4	36.1	32.8	29.6	26.3	23.0	19.8	16.5	13.2	10.0
Men (60-69)											
120	49.4	46.2	42.9	39.6	36.4	33.1	29.8	26.6	23.3	20.0	16.8
130	47.9	44.6	41.3	38.1	34.8	31.5	28.3	25.0	21.7	18.5	15.2
140	46.3	43.0	39.8	36.5	33.2	30.0	26.7	23.4	20.2	16.9	13.6
150	44.7	41.5	38.2	34.9	31.7	28.4	25.1	21.9	18.6	15.3	12.1
160	43.2	39.9	36.6	33.4	30.1	26.8	23.6	20.3	17.0	13.8	10.5
Women (60-69)											
120	46.6	43.3	40.0	36.8	33.5	30.2	27.0	23.7	20.5	17.2	13.9
130	45.0	41.7	38.5	35.2	31.9	28.7	25.4	22.2	18.9	15.6	12.4
140	43.4	40.2	36.9	33.6	30.4	27.1	23.8	20.6	17.3	14.1	10.8
150	41.9	38.6	35.3	32.1	28.8	25.5	22.3	19.0	15.8	12.5	9.2
160	40.3	37.0	33.8	30.5	27.2	24.0	20.7	17.5	14.2	10.9	7.7

Note. Calculations assume 170 lb for men and 125 lb for women. For each 15 lb beyond these values, subtract 1 ml · kg^{-1} · min^{-1}. HR = heart rate.

Adapted from Kline et al. 1987.

on the relationship between running velocity and the oxygen uptake required to run at that velocity (figure 5.1). The greater the running speed, the greater the oxygen uptake required. The reason for the duration of 12 to 15 min is that the running test has to be long enough to diminish the contribution of anaerobic sources of energy (immediate and short-term) to the average velocity. In essence, the average velocity that can be maintained in a 5- or 6-min run overestimates $\dot{V}O_2max$ because the anaerobic energy sources contribute substantially to total energy production in a 5-min run compared with a 12- to 15-min run. If the run is too long, the person is not able to run close to 100% of $\dot{V}O_2max$, and the estimate is too low (figure 5.2).

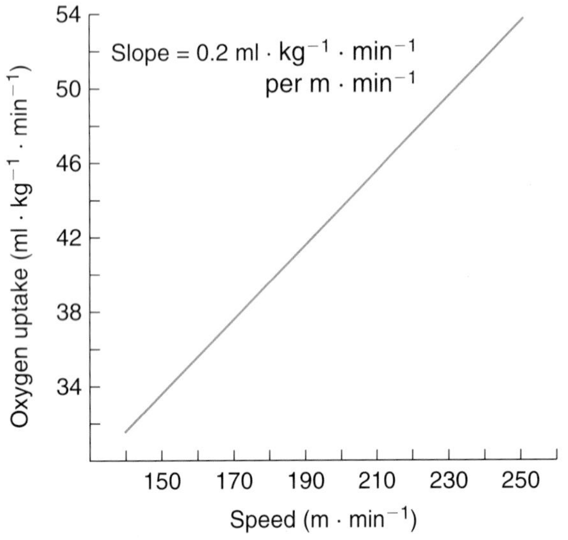

Figure 5.1 Relationship between steady-state oxygen uptake and running speed (12).

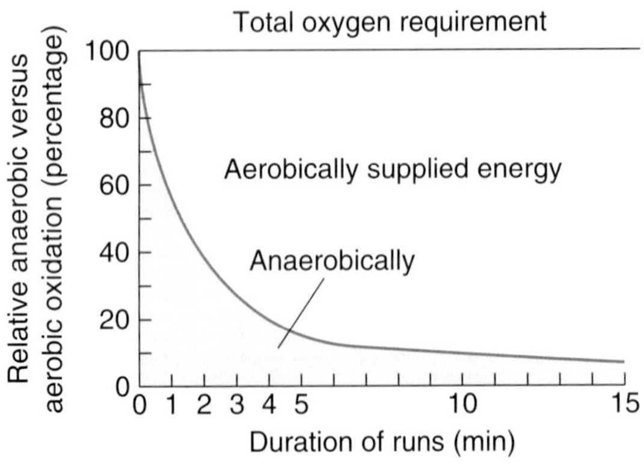

Figure 5.2 The relative role of aerobic and anaerobic energy sources in best-effort runs of various durations.

Reprinted from Balke 1963.

The $\dot{V}O_2$ associated with a specific running speed can be calculated using the following formula (see chapter 4 for details):

$$\dot{V}O_2 = \text{horizontal velocity } (\text{m} \cdot \text{min}^{-1}) \cdot 0.2 \text{ ml} \cdot \text{kg}^{-1} \cdot \text{min}^{-1} / (\text{m} \cdot \text{min}^{-1}) + 3.5 \text{ ml} \cdot \text{kg}^{-1} \cdot \text{min}^{-1}$$

These estimates are reasonable for adults who jog/run the entire 12 min or 1.5 miles. The formula will underestimate $\dot{V}O_2max$ in children because of the higher oxygen cost of running in children (17). In contrast, the formula will overestimate $\dot{V}O_2max$ in trained runners because of their better running economy (16) and in those who walk through the test because the net oxygen cost of walking is half that of running (see chapter 4).

QUESTION: A 20-year-old woman takes the Cooper 12-min run test following a 15-week walk/jog program and completes six laps on a 440-yd (402.3-m) track. What is her $\dot{V}O_2max$?

Answer:

$$402.3 \text{ m} \cdot \text{lap}^{-1} \cdot 6 \text{ laps} = 2414 \text{ m}$$

$$2414 \text{ m} \div 12 \text{ min} = 201 \text{ m} \cdot \text{min}^{-1}$$

$$\dot{V}O_2 = 201 \text{ m} \cdot \text{min}^{-1} \cdot 0.2 \text{ ml} \cdot \text{kg}^{-1} \cdot \text{min}^{-1} / (\text{m} \cdot \text{min}^{-1}) + 3.5 \text{ ml} \cdot \text{kg}^{-1} \cdot \text{min}^{-1}$$

$$= 43.7 \text{ ml} \cdot \text{kg}^{-1} \cdot \text{min}^{-1}$$

Applying the 12-Min Run Test

The advantage of the 12-min run is that it can be used regularly to evaluate CRF without expensive equipment. It is easily adapted to cyclists and swimmers, who can evaluate their progress by determining how far they can ride or swim in 12 min. Although no equations exist that can relate cyclists' and swimmers' respective performances to $\dot{V}O_2max$, each participant is able to make a personal judgment about her or his current state of CRF and improvement attributable to training.

As Cooper (14) and others agree, an endurance run should not be used for testing at the beginning of an exercise program. A person new to exercise should progress through the jogging program at low intensities to make some fitness improvements before using an endurance-run field test.

Table 5.2 lists values for CRF as *good*, *adequate*, *borderline*, and *needs extra work*. The table takes age and sex into consideration. For example, a 40-year-old woman who runs 1.5 miles in 14 min and 15 s (14:15) would rate between adequate and good. Her time of 14:15 corresponds to a CRF value of about 37 to 40 ml · kg^{-1} · min^{-1}. We recommend that you

Table 5.2 Standards for Maximal Oxygen Uptake and Endurance Runs

Age[a]	$\dot{V}O_2max$ (ml · kg^{-1} · min^{-1}) Female[b]	Male	1.5-mile run (min:s) Female	Male	12-min run (miles) Female	Male
Good						
15–30	>40	>45	<12	<10	>1.5	>1.7
35–50	>35	>40	<13:30	<11:30	>1.4	>1.5
55–70	>30	>35	<16	<14	>1.2	>1.3
Adequate for most activities						
15–30	35	40	13:30	11:50	1.4	1.5
35–50	30	35	15	13	1.3	1.4
55–70	25	30	17:30	15:30	1.1	1.3
Borderline						
15–30	30	35	15	13	1.3	1.4
35–50	25	30	16:30	14:30	1.2	1.3
55–70	20	25	19	17	1.0	1.2
Needs extra work on CRF						
15–30	<25	<30	>17	>15	<1.2	<1.3
35–50	<20	<25	>18:30	>16:30	<1.1	<1.2
55–70	<15	<20	>21	>19	<0.9	<1.0

Note. These standards are for fitness programs. People wanting to do well in endurance performance need higher levels. For those at the "good" level, the emphasis is on maintaining this level the rest of their lives. For those in the lower levels, emphasis is on setting and reaching realistic goals.

[a]CRF declines with age.

[b]Women have lower standards because they have a larger amount of essential fat.

Reprinted from Howley and Franks 1986.

encourage participants to achieve and maintain the "good" value for age and sex. If people are not at that level, help them to plan on making small and systematic progress toward that goal by using the walking and jogging programs in chapter 14.

Administrating an Endurance-Run Test

The 1-mile run is used in many youth fitness programs (15, 32). The steps to administering the 1-mile run are listed on page 76. They can be used for other endurance runs (e.g., 1.5-mile or 12-min run). The 1-mile run is used as an example.

> **3 In Review**
>
> A 1-mile walking test can be used to estimate CRF. The time for the mile as well as the HR measured at the end of the walk are used in a formula to calculate $\dot{V}O_2max$. A 1.5-mile run test also can be used to estimate CRF. The time for the 1.5 miles is used to determine average velocity, and a formula (see chapter 4) is used to calculate $\dot{V}O_2max$.

Graded Exercise Tests

Many fitness programs use a **graded exercise test (GXT)** to evaluate CRF. These multilevel tests can be administered by using a bench, cycle ergometer, or treadmill.

Bench Step

Bench stepping is very economical. It can be used for both submaximal and maximal testing. The disadvantages include the limited number of stages that feasibly can be included for any one bench height and individual fitness level and the difficulty of taking certain measurements during the test (e.g., BP). The oxygen cost for stepping at different rates on steps of different heights was presented in chapter 4.

Steps to Administer the 1-Mile Run

Before Test Day

1. Arrange to have the following elements at the test site:
   - A person to start and read the time from a stopwatch
   - A partner for each runner (perhaps with a sheet to mark off laps)
   - A stopwatch for the tester (with a spare ready)
   - A score sheet or scorecard
2. Explain the purpose of the test (i.e., to determine how fast participants can run a mile, which reflects the endurance of their cardiovascular system).
3. Do not administer the test until participants have had several fitness sessions, including some with running.
4. Have participants practice running at a set submaximal pace for one lap, then two, and so on, several times before the test day.
5. Select and mark off (if needed) a level area for the run.
6. Explain to people being tested that they are to run the mile in the fastest time possible. Walking is allowed, but the goal is to cover the distance as fast as possible.

Test Day

1. Participants warm up with stretching, walking, and slow jogging.
2. Several people will run at the same time.
3. The procedure is explained again.
4. The timer says, "Ready, go," and starts the stopwatch.
5. Each individual has a partner with a watch with a second hand.
6. The partner counts the laps and tells the individual at the end of each lap how many more laps to run.
7. The timer calls out the minutes and seconds as the runner finishes the mile run.
8. The partner listens for the time when the runner finishes the mile and records it (to the nearest second) immediately on a scorecard.
9. The runners continue to walk one lap after finishing the run.

Cycle Ergometer

Cycle ergometers are portable, moderately priced work instruments that allow measurements to be made easily because the upper body is essentially stationary. Among their disadvantages, however, are that the exercise load is self-paced and that leg-muscle fatigue may be a limiting factor. On mechanically braked cycle ergometers such as the Monark models, altering the pedal rate or the resistance on the flywheel can change the work rate. Generally, the pedal rate is maintained constant during a GXT at a rate appropriate to the individuals being tested: 50 to 60 rev · min^{-1} for individuals of low to average fitness and 70 to 100 rev · min^{-1} for the highly fit and competitive cyclists (22). The pedal rate is maintained by having the individual use a metronome or some other source of feedback such as a speedometer. The resistance (load) on the wheel is increased sequentially to systematically overload the cardiovascular system. The starting work rate and the increment from one stage to the next depend on the fitness of the person being tested and the purpose of the test. $\dot{V}O_2$ can be estimated from a formula (1) that gives reasonable estimates of $\dot{V}O_2$ up to work rates of about 1200 kgm · min^{-1} or 200 W (see chapter 4 for details):

$$\dot{V}O_2\ (ml \cdot kg^{-1} \cdot min^{-1}) = (kgm \cdot min^{-1} \cdot 1.8\ ml\ O_2 \cdot kgm^{-1}) / \text{body weight (kg)} + 7\ ml \cdot kg^{-1} \cdot min^{-1}$$

$$\dot{V}O_2\ (ml \cdot kg^{-1} \cdot min^{-1}) = (W \cdot 10.8\ ml\ O_2 \cdot W^{-1}) / \text{body weight (kg)} + 7\ ml \cdot kg^{-1} \cdot min^{-1}$$

The cycle ergometer differs from the treadmill in that the seat supports the body weight and the work rate depends primarily on pedal rate and the load on the wheel. This means that the relative $\dot{V}O_2$ at any work rate is higher for a small person than for a big person.

QUESTION: What is the relative difficulty of a work rate of 900 kgm · min^{-1} for two individuals, one weighing 60 kg and the other 90 kg?

Answer: For the 60-kg subject:

$$\dot{V}O_2\ (ml \cdot kg^{-1} \cdot min^{-1}) = (900\ kgm \cdot min^{-1} \cdot 1.8\ ml\ O_2 \cdot kgm^{-1}) / 60\ kg + 7\ ml \cdot kg^{-1} \cdot min^{-1}$$

$$\dot{V}O_2\ (ml \cdot kg^{-1} \cdot min^{-1}) = 34\ ml \cdot kg^{-1} \cdot min^{-1} \text{ or } 9.7 \text{ METs}$$

For the 90-kg subject:

$$\dot{V}O_2\ (ml \cdot kg^{-1} \cdot min^{-1}) = (900\ kgm \cdot min^{-1} \cdot 1.8\ ml\ O_2 \cdot kgm^{-1}) / 90\ kg + 7\ ml \cdot kg^{-1} \cdot min^{-1}$$

$$\dot{V}O_2\ (ml \cdot kg^{-1} \cdot min^{-1}) = 25\ ml \cdot kg^{-1} \cdot min^{-1} \text{ or } 7.1 \text{ METs}$$

In addition, the increments in the work rate, by demanding a fixed increase in the $\dot{V}O_2$ (e.g., an increment of 150 kgm · min^{-1} is equal to a $\dot{V}O_2$ change of 270 ml · min^{-1}), force the small or unfit subject to make larger cardiovascular adjustments than a large or highly fit subject. As we will see, these factors are considered in selecting work rates when a cycle ergometer test is used to evaluate CRF. Table 5.3 summarizes the effects that differences in body weight have on the metabolic responses to weight-supported (e.g., cycle ergometry) and weight-carrying (e.g., bench stepping, jogging) work tasks. Thus, a larger person achieves a greater absolute $\dot{V}O_2$ (L · min^{-1}) but has the same MET level for tasks in which the body weight provides the resistance (weight-carrying tasks). In cycling (a weight-supported task), a similar absolute $\dot{V}O_2$ is achieved, but the larger person has a lower MET level.

Treadmill

Treadmill protocols are very reproducible because they set the appropriate pace for the subject, whereas the subject may go too slow or too fast on either the bench step or the cycle ergometer. Treadmill tests can accommodate the least to the most fit individuals and use the natural activities of walking and running, with the running tests placing the greatest potential load on the cardiovascular system. Treadmills, however, are expensive, are not portable, and make some measurements (BP and blood sampling) difficult. The type of treadmill test influences the measured $\dot{V}O_2$max, with the graded running test giving the highest value, a running test at 0% grade the next highest value, and the walking test protocols the lowest value (6, 26).

For estimates of $\dot{V}O_2$ to be obtained from grade and speed considerations, the grade and speed settings must be calibrated correctly (see details on how to calibrate a treadmill and other equipment later in this chapter). Furthermore, the subject must not hold onto the treadmill railing during the test if the estimated $\dot{V}O_2$ values are going to be reasonable. For example, it has been observed that HR decreased 17 beats · min^{-1} when a subject who was walking on a treadmill at 3.4 miles · hr^{-1} and a 14% grade held onto the treadmill railing (4). This would result in an overestimation of the $\dot{V}O_2$max because the HR would be lower at any stage of the test and test duration would be extended. In addition,

Table 5.3 Work Differences Based on Body Weight in Work Tasks

Work task	$\dot{V}O_2$max L · min^{-1}	$\dot{V}O_2$max ml · kg^{-1} · min^{-1}	Total work (kcal)	METs
A heavier person will respond with the following differences compared with a lighter person when doing the task at the same rate:				
Bench	↑	=	↑	=
Walk	↑	=	↑	=
Jog	↑	=	↑	=
Body weight supported				
Cycle	=	↓	=	↓

Note. MET = metabolic equivalent.

there is no need to adjust the $\dot{V}O_2$ calculation for differences in body weight, because treadmill tests require the person being tested to carry his or her own weight; therefore, the $\dot{V}O_2$ ($ml \cdot kg^{-1} \cdot min^{-1}$) is proportional to body weight (27).

4 In Review

CRF responses to different levels of exercise can be determined with a bench-stepping, cycle ergometer, or treadmill protocol. The oxygen uptake values (expressed in $ml \cdot kg^{-1} \cdot min^{-1}$) are similar for most adults at specific stages of a treadmill or step test because the energy cost is proportional to the body weight, which is carried along. In contrast, the absolute oxygen uptake (expressed in $L \cdot min^{-1}$) is similar for most adults at each stage of a cycle ergometer test; however, the relative cost ($ml \cdot kg^{-1} \cdot min^{-1}$) is higher for the lighter participant.

Common Variables Measured During a GXT

The variables that are commonly measured for resting and submaximal tests include HR, BP, and rating of perceived exertion (RPE). For maximal testing, $\dot{V}O_2$max and the final stage achieved on a GXT are often measured.

Heart Rate

Heart rate (HR) often is used as a fitness indicator at rest and during a standard submaximal work task. Maximal HR is useful for determining the THR for fitness workouts (see chapter 10), but it is not a good fitness indicator because it changes very little with training. Table 5.4 summarizes the effects of aerobic exercise or conditioning on HR in different situations.

Table 5.4 Effects of Conditioning on HR

Condition	Effects of fitness on HR
Rest	↓
Standard submaximal work (same external work rate)	↓
Maximal work	no change
Set % of maximal	no change

Note. HR = heart rate.

When an ECG is being recorded, the HR can be taken from the ECG strip (see chapter 24). When an ECG is not obtained, HR can be taken by an HR watch, a stethoscope, or manual palpation of an artery at the wrist or neck. HR watches have been found to be accurate and are the easiest way to measure HR. Fingers (not the thumb) should be used to take HR, preferably at the wrist (radial artery). If a person takes HR at the neck (carotid artery), caution should be used not to apply too much pressure because it could trigger a reflex that slows the HR. Reliable measures are obtained, however, when people are trained in this procedure (30). The HR at rest or during a steady-state exercise should be taken for 30 s for higher reliability. However, when HRs are taken after exercise, the measurement should begin soon after termination of exercise (e.g., 5 s) and should be taken for 10 or 15 s because the HR changes so rapidly. The 10-s or 15-s rate is multiplied by 6 or 4, respectively, to calculate beats per minute. For example, if a 10-s postexercise HR is 20 beats $\cdot$ min^{-1}, the HR is 120 beats $\cdot$ min^{-1} (6×20).

Blood Pressure

Systolic blood pressure (SBP) and diastolic blood pressure (DBP) are often determined at rest, during work, and after work. The proper size of the cuff (in which the bladder overlaps two thirds of the arm) and a sensitive stethoscope are required to get accurate values at rest and during work. At rest, the person should have both feet flat on the floor and be in a relaxed position with the arm supported. The cuff should be wrapped securely around the arm at heart level, usually with the tube on the inside of the arm. The stethoscope should be below (not under) the cuff—the placement will depend on where the sound can be most easily heard, often toward the inside of the arm (20). The first and fourth Korotkoff sounds (the first sound heard and the sound when the tone changes or becomes muffled) should be used for SBP and DBP, respectively, during exercise. The fifth Korotkoff sound (disappearance of sound) is used for classification purposes at rest (1). If SBP fails to increase or the DBP increases excessively (>115 mm Hg) with increased work, the test should be stopped.

Rating of Perceived Exertion

Borg introduced the **rating of perceived exertion (RPE)**, that is, how hard the participant perceives his or her workout to be, using a scale from 6 to 20 (roughly based on resting to maximal HR, i.e., 60-200 beats · min^{-1}). Table 5.5 presents this scale as well as Borg's revised 10-point RPE scale (11). Either can be used with a GXT to provide useful information during the test as the person approaches exhaustion and to serve as a reference point for exercise prescription. When you administer the RPE scale, we recommend that you provide participants with the following instructions (1, p. 79):

"During the exercise test we want you to pay close attention to how hard you feel the exercise work rate is. This feeling should reflect your total amount of exertion and fatigue, combining all sensations and feelings of physical stress, effort, and fatigue. Don't concern yourself with any one factor such as leg pain, shortness of breath, or exercise intensity, but try to concentrate on your total, inner feeling of exertion. Try not to underestimate or overestimate your feeling of exertion; be as accurate as you can."

Estimating Versus Measuring Functional Capacity

Functional capacity is defined as the highest work rate (oxygen uptake) reached in a GXT during which time HR, BP, and ECG responses are within the normal range for heavy work. For cardiac patients, the highest work rate normally does not reflect a measure of the maximal capacity of the cardiorespiratory systems because the GXT might be stopped for ECG changes, angina, claudication pain, and so on. For the apparently healthy person, functional capacity can be called maximal aerobic power or maximal oxygen uptake ($\dot{V}O_2max$) (see chapter 28 for procedures for measuring oxygen uptake).

Oxygen uptake increases with each stage of the GXT until the upper limit of CRF is reached. At that point, $\dot{V}O_2$ does not increase further when the test moves to the next stage; the person's $\dot{V}O_2max$ has been reached. Given the complexity and cost of these procedures, $\dot{V}O_2max$ usually is estimated with equations relating the stage of the GXT to a specific oxygen uptake.

As discussed in chapter 4, a variety of formulas may be used to estimate oxygen uptake on the basis of the stage reached in a GXT. In general, these formulas give reasonable estimates of the $\dot{V}O_2$ achieved in a GXT if the test has been suited to the individual. However, if the increments in the stages

Table 5.5 Category and Category-Ratio Scales for Ratings of Perceived Exertion (RPE)

Category Scale		Category-Ratio Scale		
6		0	Nothing at all	"No I"
7	Very, very light	0.3		
8		0.5	Extremely weak	Just noticeable
9	Very light	0.7		
10		1	Very weak	
11	Fairly light	1.5		
12		2	Weak	Light
13	Somewhat hard	2.5		
14		3	Moderate	
15	Hard	4		
16		5	Strong	Heavy
17	Very hard	6		
18		7	Very Strong	
19	Very, very hard	8		
20		9		
		10	Extremely strong	"Strongest I"
		11		
		•	Absolute maximum	Highest possible

Note. Copyright Gunnar Borg. Reproduced with permission.

On the Category-Ratio Scale, "I" represents intensity.

For correct usage of the Borg scales, it is necessary to follow the administration and instructions given in G. Borg's Perceived Exertion and Pain Scales. Champaign, IL: Human Kinetics, 1998.

of the GXT are too large relative to the person's CRF, or if the time for each stage is too short, then the person might not be able to reach the steady-state oxygen requirement associated with that stage (28). Failure to achieve the oxygen requirement for a GXT stage results in an overestimation of the $\dot{V}O_2$ at each stage of the test, with the overestimation growing larger with each stage. Inability to reach the oxygen requirement is a common problem with less fit individuals (e.g., cardiac patients). This inability suggests that more conservative (i.e., smaller increments between stages) GXT protocols should be used to allow the less fit individual to reach the oxygen demand at each stage. A more complete explanation of this problem is found in chapter 28.

In contrast, shorter stages and larger increments between stages in a GXT can be used if the purpose of the test is to screen for ECG abnormalities (rather than to estimate $\dot{V}O_2$max). In addition, changes in CRF over time can be determined by periodically using the same GXT on an individual.

5 In Review

Common variables measured during a resting or submaximal GXT include HR, BP, and RPE. Oxygen uptake can be measured at each stage of a test and at maximal exertion; however, $\dot{V}O_2$max usually is estimated from the final stage achieved by using the formulas described in chapter 4.

Procedures for Graded Exercise Testing

This section provides information about how to administer a GXT and uses examples of different testing protocols. Before administering any GXT, the tester should

- calibrate the equipment,
- check supplies and data forms,
- select the appropriate test protocol for the participant,
- obtain informed consent,
- provide instruction in the task, including the cool-down procedure,
- have the participant practice the task, if needed, and
- check to see that pretest instructions were followed.

Because HR, BP, and RPE responses to submaximal work are influenced by a variety of factors, care must be taken to minimize the variation in each from one testing period to the next. These factors include, but are not limited to,

- temperature and relative humidity of the room;
- number of hours of sleep before testing;
- emotional state;
- hydration state;
- medication;
- time of day;
- time since last meal, cigarette smoking, caffeine intake, and exercise; and
- psychological environment for the test (i.e., the participant's comfort level with his or her surroundings during testing).

Attention to these factors increases the likelihood that changes in HR, BP, or RPE from one test to the next actually are caused by changes in physical fitness and physical activity habits. A form such as the Pretest Instructions for a Fitness Test (see form 5.1) is helpful in ensuring that the client will be ready for testing.

Typical procedures to follow during GXTs are shown on page 82, Steps to Administering a GXT.

A series of end points should be used to stop a GXT (see box on page 83) (1). These guidelines are for nondiagnostic testing performed without direct physician involvement or electrocardiographic monitoring.

6 In Review

Equipment to measure and record CRF variables should be checked for availability and calibration before testing. Careful attention to procedures before and during a test will enhance the safety and accuracy of the test. The tester should know when to stop a test, based on signs, symptoms, or CRF measurements.

When to Use Submaximal and Maximal Tests

GXTs have been used to evaluate CRF in fitness programs for healthy populations and in the clinical assessment of ischemic heart disease—a condition in which an inadequate blood flow to the heart muscle can alter the ECG. Exercise is used to place a load on the heart to determine the cardiovascular response and to see if changes occur in the ECG (18).

form 5.1

Pretest Instructions for a Fitness Test

Name ______________________________________ Test date _________ Time _______

Report to ____________________________________

Instructions

Please observe the following:

1. Wear running shoes, shorts, and a loose-fitting shirt.
2. No food, drink (except water), tobacco, or medication for 3 hours prior to test.
3. Minimal physical activity on day of test.

Cancellation

If you cannot keep this appointment, please call ______________ or ______________ .

From Edward T. Howley and B. Don Franks, 2003, *Health Fitness Instructor's Handbook,* 4th ed. (Champaign, IL: Human Kinetics).

Steps to Administering a GXT

1. Greet the patient/client.
2. Obtain consent (oral and written).
3. Record age and measure height and weight. Calculate and record estimated HRmax and 70% to 85% HRmax.
4. Obtain resting HR and BP.
5. Instruct participants how to do a step test.
   - Instruct participant to step all the way up and all the way down.
   - Tell participant to keep pace with the metronome.

   OR

   Instruct participant in how to use the cycle ergometer.
   - Tell participant to adjust seat height so the knee is slightly flexed when the foot is at the bottom of the pedal swing and parallel to the floor.
   - Instruct participant to keep pace with the metronome.
   - Tell participant not to hold tightly onto the handlebars; release hold when BP is taken.

   OR

   Instruct participant in how to walk on the treadmill.
   - Have the participant hold onto railing and get the "feel" of the belt speed by putting one foot on the belt, keeping up with belt speed.
   - Instruct participant to step on, keeping eyes ahead and back straight; walk relaxed with arms swinging.
   - Initially, the person can hold on for balance and then use just a finger or the back of the hand to touch the railing lightly.
6. Follow test protocol.
   - Advise the person to talk during the test about how he or she feels.
   - Follow criteria for termination of the test.

Note. For fitness evaluations HR, BP, and RPE are the usual variables measured.

Adapted from Howley 1988.

Some controversy has arisen concerning whether to use submaximal or maximal tests. On the basis of thousands of exercise stress tests conducted since the mid-1950s, it generally is recommended that a maximal exercise test be used to determine the presence of ischemic heart disease in asymptomatic individuals (1). Although submaximal exercise tests are not as effective in identifying disease conditions, they are appropriate for evaluating CRF before and after exercise programs.

When a fitness center is responsible for both fitness testing and the fitness program, the sequence of testing and activity recommended earlier provides the advantages of each while minimizing the disadvantages. The main objection to maximal tests is the stress they put on a person who has been inactive. Although the risk of a maximal GXT is very small with adequate screening and qualified testing personnel, the discomfort of going to one's maximum without prior conditioning may discourage some people from participating in a fitness program. Objections to the submaximal test include finding fewer abnormal responses to exercise and inaccurately estimating $\dot{V}O_2max$ from submaximal data. In a fitness program for apparently healthy people, the objections against either maximal or submaximal tests given alone are overcome by administering the submaximal test early in the fitness program and waiting until the participant has been involved in a regular exercise program to administer the maximal test. Any of the GXT protocols can be used for submaximal or maximal testing—the only difference is the criteria for stopping the test. Either test is stopped if any of the abnormal responses listed in

General Indications for Stopping an Exercise Test in Low-Risk Adults

- Onset of angina or angina-like symptoms.
- Significant drop (20 mm Hg) in systolic blood pressure or a failure of the systolic blood pressure to rise with an increase in exercise intensity.
- Excessive rise in blood pressure: systolic pressure > 260 mm Hg or diastolic pressure > 115 mm Hg.
- Signs of poor perfusion: light-headedness, confusion, ataxia, pallor, cyanosis, nausea, or cold and clammy skin.
- Failure of heart rate to increase with increased exercise intensity.
- Noticeable change in heart rhythm.
- Subject requests to stop.
- Physical or verbal manifestations of severe fatigue.
- Failure of the testing equipment.

Note. "Low Risk" assumes the testing is nondiagnostic and is being performed without direct physician involvement or electrocardiographic monitoring.

Reprinted, by permission, from American College of Sports Medicine 2000.

the box above occur. In the absence of abnormal responses, the submaximal test is usually terminated when the person reaches a certain HR (often 85% of maximum HR), and the maximal test is stopped when the person reaches a state of voluntary exhaustion.

Maximal Exercise Test Protocols

No one GXT protocol is appropriate for all types of people. The duration, starting points, and increments between stages should vary with the type of person. Young active people, normal sedentary people, and people with questionable health status should start at 6, 4, and 2 METs, respectively. The same three groups should increase 2 to 3, 1 to 2, and 0.5 to 1 METs, respectively, for progressive stages of the test. If the test is being used to compare CRF at different times, then 1 or 2 min per stage can be used. If one is trying to predict $\dot{V}O_2max$, however, the time per stage should be 2 to 3 min. Table 5.6 illustrates how these criteria might be used for a bench, cycle, or treadmill test for different fitness levels.

The following testing protocols are examples of tests that could be used for different populations. The first protocol, shown in table 5.7, could be used with deconditioned subjects, who would start at a very low MET level, walk slowly, and increase 1 MET per 3-min stage (29). The Balke standard protocol (8) could be used for typical inactive adults by progressing at 1 MET per 2-min stage and starting at a higher MET level. More active or younger people could be tested on the Bruce protocol (13), which starts at a moderate MET level and goes up 2 or 3 METs per 3-min stage. Unfortunately, some testing centers attempt to use the same testing protocol for all people, with the result that the initial stage is often too high or too low and the work increments for each stage are either too small or too large for the individual being tested. Estimating $\dot{V}O_2max$ from the final stage of a maximal GXT has an SEE of about 3 $ml \cdot kg^{-1} \cdot min^{-1}$ (31).

Submaximal Exercise Test Protocols

Any GXT protocol can be used for submaximal or maximal testing. The HFI typically uses a submaximal GXT to estimate a person's $\dot{V}O_2max$ or to simply show before-and-after changes in selected variables attributable to the exercise program. Predicting maximal oxygen uptake from any submaximal test involves substantial error (see Research Insight on page 84). However, it can provide useful information in a fitness program to estimate a person's functional capacity and to determine in what fitness category the person belongs and what exercise programming therefore would be most appropriate. The only way to determine an individual's true functional capacity is to measure it during a maximal test. Changes in HR, BP, and RPE as a result of an exercise conditioning program make a submaximal test a good mechanism for showing improvements in CRF. Estimating $\dot{V}O_2max$ from

Table 5.6 Testing Protocol for Different Groups

Stage	METs	Bench: Height (cm)	Bench: Steps · min^{-1}	Cycle: Work rate (kpm · min^{-1})	Cycle: RPM	Treadmill: Speed (km · hr^{-1})	Treadmill: Grade (%)
Individuals with questionable health							
1	2	0	24	0	50	3.2	0
2	3	16	12	150	50	4.8	0
3	4	16	18	300	50	4.8	2.5
4	5	16	24	450	50	4.8	5.0
5	6	16	30	600	50	4.8	7.5
"Normal" sedentary individuals							
1	4	16	18	360	60	4.8	2.5
2	6	16	30	540	60	4.8	7.5
3	7–8	36	18–24	720–900	60	4.8–5.5	10.0
4	9	36	27	900–1080	60	5.5	12.0
5	10–11	36	30–33	1080–1260	60	9.7	0–1.75
Young active individuals							
1	6	16	30	630	70	4.8	7.5
2	9	36	27	1060	70	5.5	12.0
3	12	36	36	1270	70	9.7	3.5
4	15	50	33	1900	70	11.3	7.0
5	17	50	39	2110	70	11.3	11.0

Note. MET = metabolic equivalent.

Reprinted from Franks 1979.

submaximal exercise test protocols has an SEE of about 5 ml · kg^{-1} · min^{-1} (31).

7 In Review

GXT protocols can be used for submaximal tests (early in the testing sequence) or maximal tests (for active persons who have reached minimal fitness levels). Submaximal and maximal tests can use the same GXT protocol; however, the criteria for test termination differ. Maximal tests are more effective in determining the presence of ischemic heart disease. Submaximal tests are useful in assessing fitness and are relatively inexpensive to administer. Although the $\dot{V}O_2$max value estimated from a submaximal test is not as accurate as that obtained from a maximal test, the information is useful in evaluating CRF before and after an exercise program.

Research Insight

As each test has been introduced, we have provided a measure of the SEE associated with estimating $\dot{V}O_2$max. If the standard error is 4 ml · kg^{-1} · min^{-1}, it means that 68% of the true $\dot{V}O_2$max values are within ±4 ml · kg^{-1} · min^{-1} of the estimated $\dot{V}O_2$max value, and 95% of the true values are within ±8 ml · kg^{-1} · min^{-1} of the estimated value. The problem is that for any individual you test, you don't know where the individual is within that ±8 ml ·kg^{-1} · min^{-1}. Consequently, if you estimate a person's $\dot{V}O_2$max as being 38 ml · kg^{-1} · min^{-1}, it is probably between 30 and 46 ml · kg^{-1} · min^{-1}. For that reason, HFIs must interpret the test results with caution, especially when comparing them with norms. On the other hand, the fact that the HR response to submaximal work (or performance in a distance run or walk) is altered easily by endurance training, the submaximal tests and field tests are good educational and motivation devices to use in working with fitness participants.

Table 5.7 Treadmill Protocols for Various Categories

Stage	METS	Speed (km · hr^{-1})	Grade %	Time (min)
For deconditioned people[a]				
1	2.5	3.2	0	3
2	3.5	3.2	3.5	3
3	4.5	3.2	7	3
4	5.4	3.2	10.5	3
5	6.4	3.2	14	3
6	7.3	3.2	17.5	3
7	8.5	4.8	12.5	3
8	9.5	4.8	15	3
9	10.5	4.8	17.5	3
For normal inactive people[b]				
1	4.3	4.8	2.5	2
2	5.4	4.8	5	2
3	6.4	4.8	7.5	2
4	7.4	4.8	10	2
5	8.5	4.8	12.5	2
6	9.5	4.8	15	2
7	10.5	4.8	17.5	2
8	11.6	4.8	20	2
9	12.6	4.8	22.5	2
10	13.6	4.8	25	2
For young active people[c]				
1	5	2.7	10	3
2	7	4	12	3
3	9.5	5.4	14	3
4	13	6.7	16	3
5	16	8	18	3

Note. MET = metabolic equivalent.

[a]From "Methods of Exercise Testing" by J.P. Naughton and R. Haider. In *Exercise Testing and Exercise Training in Coronary Heart Disease,* by J.P. Naughton, H.R. Hellerstein, and L.C. Mohler (Eds.), 1973, New York: Academic Press.

[b]From "Advanced Exercise Procedures for Evaluation of the Cardiovascular System," *Monograph,* by B. Balke, 1970, Milton, WI: The Burdick Corporation.

[c]From "Multi-Stage Treadmill Test of Maximal and Submaximal Exercise" by R.A. Bruce. In American Heart Association, *Exercise Testing and Training of Apparently Healthy Individuals: A Handbook for Physicians* (pp. 32–34), 1972, New York: American Heart Association.

Submaximal Treadmill Test Protocol

The initial stage and rate of progression of the GXT should be selected on the basis of the criteria mentioned earlier. In the following example, a Balke standard protocol (3 miles · hr^{-1}, 2.5% grade increase every 2 min) was used; HR was monitored in the last 30 s of each stage. The test was terminated at 85% of age-adjusted maximal HR (with the equation 220 – age). Maximal aerobic power was estimated by extrapolating the HR response to the person's estimated maximal HR. Figure 5.3 presents the results of this test with a graph showing the HR response at each work rate. Note that the HR response is rather flat between the 0% and 5% grades. This is not an uncommon finding (see the discussion that follows of the YMCA test); perhaps the subject is too excited, or perhaps the stroke volume changes are accounting for the changes in cardiac output at these low work rates. The HR response is usually quite linear between 110 beats · min^{-1} and the subject's 85% of maximal HR cutoff.

To estimate $\dot{V}O_2$max, the procedures of Maritz et al. (25) are followed. A line is drawn through the HR points from 7.5% grade to the final work rate. The line is extended (extrapolated) to the person's estimated maximal HR (183 beats · min^{-1}). A vertical line is dropped from the last point to the baseline to estimate the subject's maximal aerobic power, which is 11.8 METs, or 41.3 ml · kg^{-1} · min^{-1}. Any formula used to estimate maximal HR has an SEE of about ±10 beats · min^{-1}. Consequently, any estimate of maximal oxygen uptake derived from an extrapolation of HR to an estimated maximal HR will be influenced by this possible inaccuracy. If this person's true (measured) maximal HR were 173 or 193 beats · min^{-1}, the estimated maximal MET level would have been 11.0 METs and 12.6 METs, respectively.

Submaximal Cycle Ergometer Test Protocol

The steps in administering submaximal cycle ergometer tests are provided on page 86. One of the most common submaximal cycle ergometer protocols (figure 5.4) is taken from the *YMCA Physical Fitness Testing and Assessment Manual* (21). This protocol relies on the observation that there is a linear relationship between HR and work rate ($\dot{V}O_2$) once

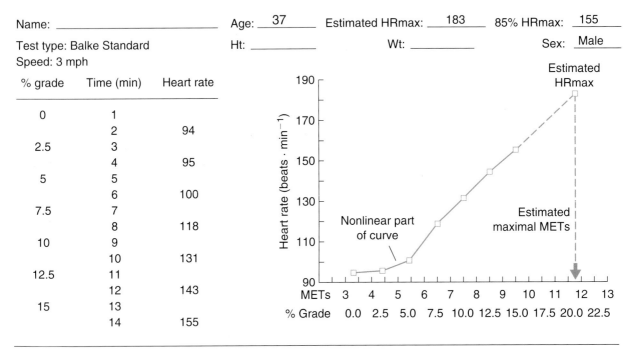

Name: ______________________ Age: 37 Estimated HRmax: 183 85% HRmax: 155

Test type: Balke Standard Ht: ________ Wt: ________ Sex: Male

Speed: 3 mph

% grade	Time (min)	Heart rate
0	1	
	2	94
2.5	3	
	4	95
5	5	
	6	100
7.5	7	
	8	118
10	9	
	10	131
12.5	11	
	12	143
15	13	
	14	155

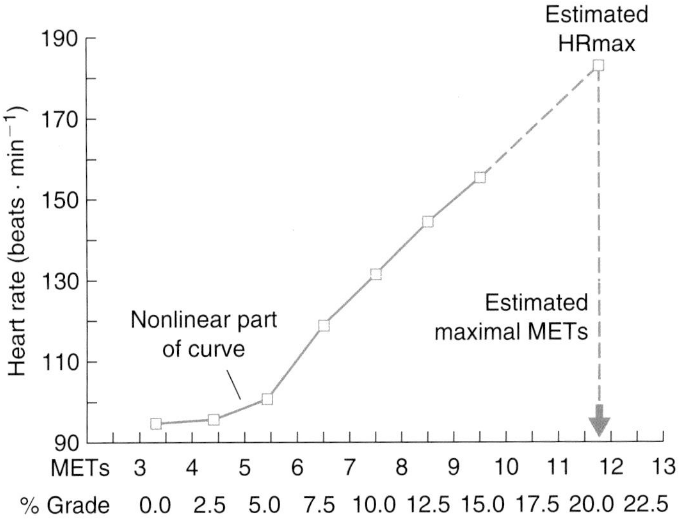

Figure 5.3 Maximal aerobic power estimated by measuring the HR response to a submaximal GXT on a treadmill.

Steps to Administering a Submaximal Cycle Ergometer Test

1. Complete pretest items.
2. Select the test protocol.
3. Estimate the participant's HRmax (220 – age = beats · min^{-1}).
4. Determine 85% of participant's HRmax (HRmax × 0.85 = 85% HRmax).
5. Review the procedure with participant.
6. Set and record the seat height (leg should be slightly bent at the knee when foot is at the bottom of the pedaling stroke).
7. Start the metronome (set at 100 beats · min^{-1} so that one foot is at the bottom of the pedaling stroke on each beat, resulting in 50 complete rev · min^{-1}).
8. Have the participant begin pedaling in rhythm with the metronome.
9. As soon as the correct pace is achieved, set the resistance according to the protocol chosen.
10. Start the timer for the beginning of the 3-min stage.
11. Check the resistance setting (it may drift) and observe the participant for signs or symptoms that require terminating the test.
12. At 1:30 into the stage, measure and record BP and HR.
13. At 2:30, measure and record HR.
14. At 2:50, ask for and record the participant's RPE.
15. At 2:55, ask the participant, "How are you doing?"
16. At 3:00, if HR is less than 85% of HRmax, BP is responding normally, and participant is all right, increase resistance to the next stage. Note: If the two HR values (from minutes 2 and 3) are not within 5 beats · min^{-1}, the YMCA protocol calls for adding another minute to the stage to obtain a steady-state value.
17. Repeat steps 10 through 16 until the participant reaches 85% of HRmax or there is another reason to stop the test. Go back to Stage 1 (for cool-down) and repeat steps 10 through 15, stopping at 3:00 in the cool-down stage.
18. Talk with the participant and check out any problems.

Reprinted from Franks and Howley 1989.

an HR of approximately 110 beats · min^{-1} is reached. The test requires the person to complete one more stage past the one that induces an HR of 110 beats · min^{-1}. The intent of the test is to extrapolate the line describing the HR-work rate relationship out to the person's age-adjusted maximal HR (as was done for the treadmill protocol) to estimate the person's $\dot{V}O_2$max. Each stage of the test lasts 3 min, unless a person's HR has not yet reached a steady state (>5 beats · min^{-1} difference between 2nd- and 3rd-min HR). In that case, an extra minute is added to that stage. The pedal rate is maintained at 50 rev · min^{-1}, so that, on a Monark cycle ergometer, a 0.5-kg increase in load is equal to 150 kgm · min^{-1} (25 W). Seat height is adjusted so that the knee is slightly bent (5°) when the pedal is at the bottom of the swing through 1 revolution. The seat height is recorded for future reference. HR is monitored during the later half of the 2nd and 3rd min of each stage.

Proper selection of the initial work rate and the rate of progression of the work rate on the cycle ergometer should take into consideration body weight, sex, age, and level of fitness. In general, absolute $\dot{V}O_2$max (L · min^{-1}) is lower in smaller people; women have lower absolute $\dot{V}O_2$max values than men; $\dot{V}O_2$max decreases with age; and inactivity is associated with low $\dot{V}O_2$max values. The YMCA test addresses the concerns of body weight, fitness, and so on by starting everyone at 150 kgm · min^{-1} and using the HR response to that specified work rate to set subsequent stages in the test (see figure 5.4). Large or fit individuals would have a low HR response to this work rate and would use the most strenuous sequence of work rates (far left boxes in the figure). A small or unfit individual would have a high HR response to the 150 kgm · min^{-1} work rate and would follow a sequence of work rates with the smallest increments in the power output. People

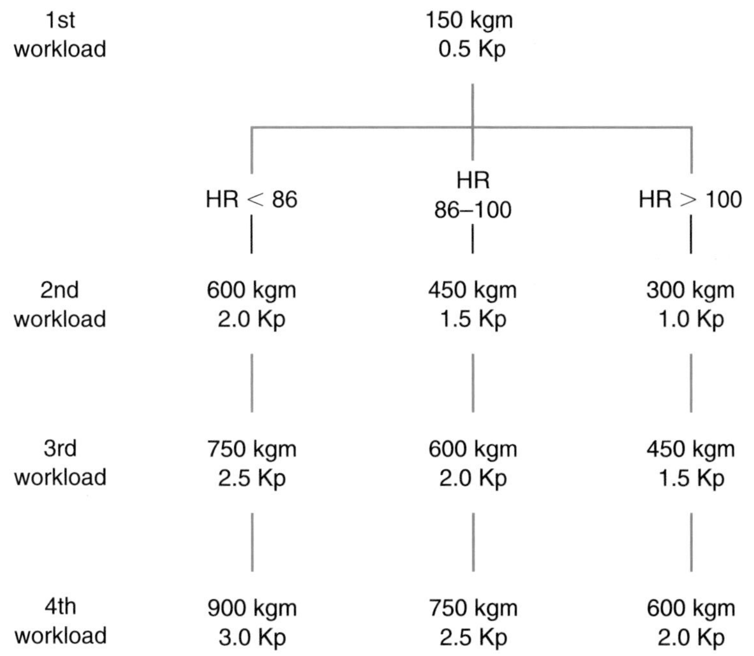

Directions:

1. Set the first workload at 150 kgm/min (0.5 kp).
2. If the HR in the third minute is
   - less than 86, set the second load at 600 kgm (2.0 kp);
   - 86 to 100, set the second load at 450 kgm (1.5 kp);
   - greater than 100, set the second load at 300 kgm (1.0 kp).
3. Set the third and fourth (if required) loads according to the loads in the boxes below the second loads.

Figure 5.4 Guide for setting power outputs (workloads) on YMCA submaximal cycle ergometer test.

Reprinted from *YMCA fitness testing and assessment manual.* Champaign, IL: Human Kinetics., 4th ed., with permission of the YMCA of the USA

being tested should complete only one additional work rate beyond the one demanding an HR of 110 beats · min^{-1}.

The HR values for the 2nd and 3rd min of each work rate are recorded, and directions are followed to estimate $\dot{V}O_2$max in liters per minute. The YMCA protocol directions and an example are presented in figure 5.5 for a 50-year-old woman who weighs 59 kg. The stages followed the pattern dictated by the HR response to the initial work rate of 150 kgm · min^{-1}. A line was drawn through the last two HR values and extrapolated to the estimated maximal HR. A vertical line, dropped from the last point to the baseline, estimated the subject's maximal work rate to be 750 kgm · min^{-1}. With the formula described earlier (and in chapter 4) for the cycle ergometer, $\dot{V}O_2$max was estimated to be ~30 ml · kg^{-1} · min^{-1}, or about 1.77 L · min^{-1}.

In contrast to the YMCA test, the Åstrand and Rhyming cycle ergometer test (5) requires the subject to complete only one 6-min work rate demanding an HR between 125 and 170 beats · min^{-1}. These investigators observed that for young (18-30 years) subjects, the average HR was 128 beats · min^{-1} for males and 138 beats · min^{-1} for females at 50% $\dot{V}O_2$max, and at 70% $\dot{V}O_2$max the average HRs were 154 and 164 beats · min^{-1}, respectively. Using these observations, if you know from an HR response that a person is at 50% $\dot{V}O_2$max at a work rate equal to 1.5 L · min^{-1}, then the estimated $\dot{V}O_2$max would be twice that, or 3.0 L · min^{-1}. Table 5.8 is used to estimate $\dot{V}O_2$max based on the subject's HR response to one 6-min work rate (3).

Using the data collected for the YMCA test displayed earlier, we can see how $\dot{V}O_2$max is estimated in the Åstrand and Rhyming protocol. The 50-year-old woman had an HR of 140 beats · min^{-1} at a work rate of 450 kgm · min^{-1}. Using table 5.8, for women, look down the leftmost column to an HR of 140, and look across to the second column (450 kgm · min^{-1}). The estimated $\dot{V}O_2$max is 2.4 L · min^{-1}. Because maximal HR decreases with increasing age, however, and the data in table 5.8 were collected on young subjects, I. and P.O. Åstrand (2, 3) established the following correction factors with which one could multiply the estimated $\dot{V}O_2$max to correct for the lower maximal HR:

Name: ______________

Sex: Female Age: 50

Estimated HRmax: 170 Ht: ____ in. Wt: ____ lb

85% HRmax: 145 ____ cm 59 kg

Work rate kpm · min^{-1}	Heart rate 2nd min	3rd min
150	95	96
300		
450	138	140
600	153	154

YMCA Protocol

1. Plot 3rd min HR for each work rate.
2. Draw line though points starting at HR > 110.
3. Extrapolate line to subject's estimated HRmax.
4. Drop vertical line from HRmax to baseline.
5. Record estimated maximal work rate.

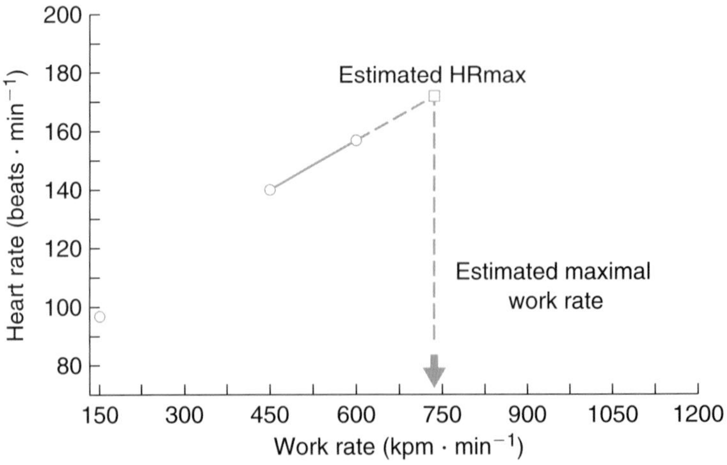

Figure 5.5 Maximal aerobic power estimated by measuring the HR response to a submaximal GXT on a cycle ergometer, using the *YMCA Physical Fitness Testing and Assessment Manual* (21) protocol.

Table 5.8 Predicting Maximal Oxygen Uptake From Heart Rate and Work Load During a 6-Min Cycle Ergometer Test

	Values for women $\dot{V}O_2$max (L · min^{-1})						Values for men $\dot{V}O_2$max (L · min^{-1})				
Heart rate	300 kgm/min	450 kgm/min	600 kgm/min	750 kgm/min	900 kgm/min	Heart rate	300 kgm/min	600 kgm/min	900 kgm/min	1200 kgm/min	1500 kgm/min
120	2.6	3.4	4.1	4.8		120	2.2	3.5	4.8		
121	2.5	3.3	4.0	4.8		121	2.2	3.4	4.7		
122	2.5	3.2	3.9	4.7		122	2.2	3.4	4.6		
123	2.4	3.1	3.9	4.6		123	2.1	3.4	4.6		
124	2.4	3.1	3.8	4.5		124	2.1	3.3	4.5	6.0	
125	2.3	3.0	3.7	4.4		125	2.0	3.2	4.4	5.9	
126	2.3	3.0	3.6	4.3		126	2.0	3.2	4.4	5.8	
127	2.2	2.9	3.5	4.2		127	2.0	3.1	4.3	5.7	
128	2.2	2.8	3.5	4.2	4.8	128	2.0	3.1	4.2	5.6	
129	2.2	2.8	3.4	4.1	4.8	129	1.9	3.0	4.2	5.6	
130	2.1	2.7	3.4	4.0	4.7	130	1.9	3.0	4.1	5.5	
131	2.1	2.7	3.4	4.0	4.6	131	1.9	2.9	4.0	5.4	
132	2.0	2.7	3.3	3.9	4.5	132	1.8	2.9	4.0	5.3	
133	2.0	2.6	3.2	3.8	4.4	133	1.8	2.8	3.9	5.3	
134	2.0	2.6	3.2	3.8	4.4	134	1.8	2.8	3.9	5.2	
135	2.0	2.6	3.1	3.7	4.3	135	1.7	2.8	3.8	5.1	
136	1.9	2.5	3.1	3.6	4.2	136	1.7	2.7	3.8	5.0	
137	1.9	2.5	3.0	3.6	4.2	137	1.7	2.7	3.7	5.0	
138	1.8	2.4	3.0	3.5	4.1	138	1.6	2.7	3.7	4.9	
139	1.8	2.4	2.9	3.5	4.0	139	1.6	2.6	3.6	4.8	
140	1.8	2.4	2.8	3.4	4.0	140	1.6	2.6	3.6	4.8	6.0
141	1.8	2.3	2.8	3.4	3.9	141		2.6	3.5	4.7	5.9
142	1.7	2.3	2.8	3.3	3.9	142		2.5	3.5	4.6	5.8
143	1.7	2.2	2.7	3.3	3.8	143		2.5	3.4	4.6	5.7
144	1.7	2.2	2.7	3.2	3.8	144		2.5	3.4	4.5	5.7
145	1.6	2.2	2.7	3.2	3.7	145		2.4	3.4	4.5	5.6
146	1.6	2.2	2.6	3.2	3.7	146		2.4	3.3	4.4	5.6
147	1.6	2.1	2.6	3.1	3.6	147		2.4	3.3	4.4	5.5
148	1.6	2.1	2.6	3.1	3.6	148		2.4	3.2	4.3	5.4
149		2.1	2.6	3.0	3.5	149		2.3	3.2	4.3	5.4
150		2.0	2.5	3.0	3.5	150		2.3	3.2	4.2	5.3
151		2.0	2.5	3.0	3.4	151		2.3	3.1	4.2	5.2
152		2.0	2.5	2.9	3.4	152		2.3	3.1	4.1	5.2
153		2.0	2.4	2.9	3.3	153		2.2	3.0	4.1	5.1
154		2.0	2.4	2.8	3.3	154		2.2	3.0	4.0	5.1
155		1.9	2.4	2.8	3.2	155		2.2	3.0	4.0	5.0
156		1.9	2.3	2.8	3.2	156		2.2	2.9	4.0	5.0
157		1.9	2.3	2.7	3.2	157		2.1	2.9	3.9	4.9
158		1.8	2.3	2.7	3.1	158		2.1	2.9	3.9	4.9
159		1.8	2.2	2.7	3.1	159		2.1	2.8	3.8	4.8
160		1.8	2.2	2.6	3.0	160		2.1	2.8	3.8	4.8
161		1.8	2.2	2.6	3.0	161		2.0	2.8	3.7	4.7
162		1.8	2.2	2.6	3.0	162		2.0	2.8	3.7	4.6
163		1.7	2.2	2.6	2.9	163		2.0	2.8	3.7	4.6
164		1.7	2.1	2.5	2.9	164		2.0	2.7	3.6	4.5
165		1.7	2.1	2.5	2.9	165		2.0	2.7	3.6	4.5
166		1.7	2.1	2.5	2.8	166		1.9	2.7	3.6	4.5
167		1.6	2.1	2.4	2.8	167		1.9	2.6	3.5	4.4
168		1.6	2.0	2.4	2.8	168		1.9	2.6	3.5	4.4
169		1.6	2.0	2.4	2.8	169		1.9	2.6	3.5	4.3
170		1.6	2.0	2.4	2.7	170		1.8	2.6	3.4	4.3

Reprinted from Åstrand 1979.

Age	Factor
15	1.10
25	1.00
35	0.87
40	0.83
45	0.78
50	0.75
55	0.71
60	0.68
65	0.65

One of the correction factors is multiplied by the estimated $\dot{V}O_2max$ to calculate the corrected $\dot{V}O_2max$. For our 50-year-old subject, the correction factor is 0.75, and the corrected $\dot{V}O_2max$ is $0.75 \cdot 2.4\ L \cdot min^{-1} = 1.8\ L \cdot min^{-1}$. This value compares well with that estimated by the YMCA protocol. The Åstrand and Rhyming calculations can be simplified by using formulas developed by Shephard (34).

Submaximal Step Test Protocol

A multistage step test can be used to estimate $\dot{V}O_2max$ and to show changes in CRF with training or detraining. As always, attention must be given to the initial stage and rate of progression of the stages so that the test is suited to the individual. Table 5.6 presented three examples of step test protocols. The subject must be instructed to follow the metronome (4 counts per cycle, i.e., up-up-down-down) and step all the way up and all the way down. Each stage should last at least 2 min, with HR monitored in the last 30 s of each 2-min period.

HR is more difficult to monitor during a step test protocol if the palpation technique is used. The HR watch simplifies the process, but when one is not available, a BP cuff can be used. When an HR measure is needed, pump the cuff up just above diastolic pressure (around 80-100 mm Hg). With the stethoscope, the pulse rate can be counted for 15 to 30 s. Pressure is released after each measurement. An alternative is for the participant to stop stepping after each stage, taking the HR for a 10-s count 5 s after the stage is completed.

As in most submaximal GXT protocols, HR is plotted against work rate or $\dot{V}O_2$ for each stage, and a line is drawn through the points to the estimated maximal HR. A vertical line is then drawn to the baseline to obtain an estimate of the step rate that would have been achieved if the subject had completed a maximal test. Figure 5.6 shows the results of a step test for a sedentary 55-year-old man before a training program. His estimated maximal step rate was 40 steps $\cdot$ min^{-1}. The $\dot{V}O_2max$, calculated with the formula for stepping in chapter 4, was 7.7 METs or about 27 ml $\cdot$ kg^{-1} $\cdot$ min^{-1}.

Posttest Procedures

When the test is over, the tester should conduct a cool-down phase, monitor test variables, and give posttest instructions. The tester should also organize the test data (see Posttest Protocol on page 91).

8 In Review

A graphic plot of HR responses (>110 beats $\cdot$ min^{-1}) to a GXT on a treadmill, cycle ergometer, or bench step can be used to estimate $\dot{V}O_2max$. A line is drawn through the HR values and is extrapolated to the subject's age-adjusted estimate of maximal HR. A vertical line is drawn to the x-axis to estimate the work rate and $\dot{V}O_2$ the person would have achieved if the test had been a maximal test.

Name: ____________ Age: 55 Estimated HRmax: 165 85% HRmax: 140

Step test protocol
Step height = 16 cm

Ht: ______
Wt: ______
Sex: Male

Step rate	Heart rate
12	100
18	115
24	128
30	142

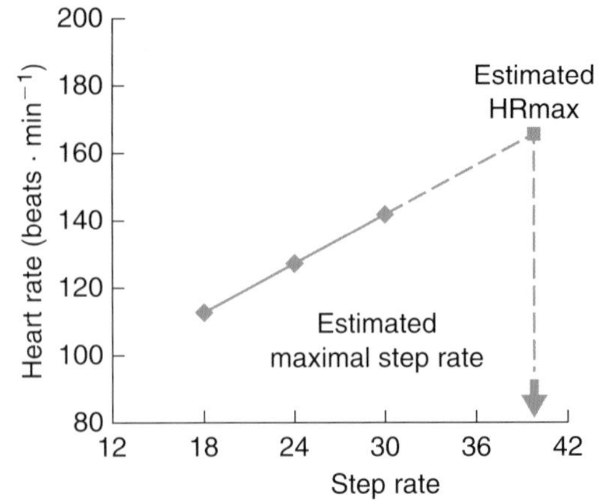

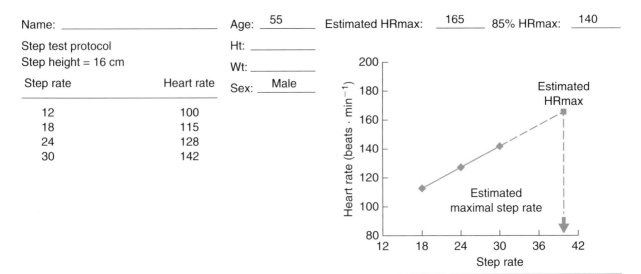

Figure 5.6 Maximal aerobic power estimated by measuring HR response to a submaximal graded exercise step test.

Posttest Protocol

Use a cool-down as programmed per physician and other posttreadmill tests.

Have the individual sit down or lie down depending on posttests (nuclear).

Monitor HR, BP, and ECG immediately and after 1, 2, 4, and 6 min.

Remove cuff and electrodes when double product (HR × SBP) is close to pretest value.

Provide instructions for showering:

Ask subject to wait for about 30 min before showering.

Ask subject to move around in the shower and use warm (not hot) water.

Check for return of person from the shower.

Organize test data and discuss test results with the participant.

Adapted from Howley 1988.

Case Studies

You can check your answers by referring to appendix A.

5.1

You are contacted by a fitness club to review the test it uses to evaluate CRF in middle-age participants. The club requires the participants to perform the 1.5-mile run test during their first exercise session. The club director says he uses this test because so much data exist for it—the test has been used for more than 10 years. What is your reaction?

5.2

You conduct the 1-mile walk test with a 45-year-old male client and record the following information: time = 15 min; HR = 140 beats · min^{-1}; weight = 170 lb. Calculate and evaluate his estimated $\dot{V}O_2$max.

5.3

A 50-year-old male, weighing 180 lb, completes a submaximal GXT on a cycle ergometer, and the following data are obtained:

kgm · min^{-1}	HR
300	100
450	110
600	125
750	140

Estimate the subject's $\dot{V}O_2$max by the extrapolation procedure. Express the value in METs.

5.4

A 30-year-old woman, weighing 120 lb, completes four stages of a submaximal Balke treadmill test (3 miles · hr^{-1}), and the following data are obtained:

% Grade	HR
2.5	96
5	120
7.5	135
10	150

Estimate the subject's $\dot{V}O_2$max by the extrapolation method and express it in ml · kg^{-1} · min^{-1}, L · min^{-1}, and METs.

5.5

A Monark cycle ergometer is calibrated with 0.5-, 1.0-, 1.5-, and 2.0-kg weights, and each of the values is 0.25 kg too high on the scale. What could have caused this?

Appendix

Calibrating Equipment

To **calibrate** is to check the accuracy of a measuring device by comparing it with a known standard and adjusting it to provide an accurate reading. This section explains how to calibrate the equipment used in exercise testing. These are suggestions only and should not be viewed as a substitute for the specific procedures recommended by the equipment manufacturer (23).

Treadmill Speed and Elevation Settings

The treadmill's speed and grade settings must be calibrated because they determine physiological demand and are crucial in estimating cardiorespiratory fitness.

Calibrating Speed

An easy way to calibrate the speed on any treadmill is to measure the length of the belt and count the number of belt revolutions in a certain time period. To calibrate treadmill speed, follow these specific steps (23):

1. Measure the exact length of the belt in meters.
   a. Place a meter stick on the belt surface and mark a starting point.
   b. Advance the belt by hand, marking the belt 1 m at a time until you return to the starting point; record the value for belt length.
2. Place a small piece of tape near the edge of the belt surface.
3. Turn on the treadmill to a given speed by using the speed control.
4. Count 20 revolutions of the belt while tracking time with a stopwatch. Start your watch as the tape first moves past the fixed point, beginning counting with 0.
5. Convert the number of revolutions to revolutions per minute ($rev \cdot min^{-1}$). For example, if the belt made 20 complete revolutions in 35 s, then

$$35\ s / 60\ s \cdot min^{-1} = 0.583\ min$$

So,

$$20\ rev / 0.583\ min = 34.3\ rev \cdot min^{-1}$$

6. Multiply the calculated revolutions per minute (Step 5) times the belt length (Step 1). This will give you the belt speed in meters per minute ($m \cdot min^{-1}$). For example, if the belt length is 5.025 m, then

$$34.3\ rev \cdot min^{-1} \cdot 5.025\ m \cdot rev^{-1} = 72.35\ m \cdot min^{-1}$$

7. To convert meters per minute to miles per hour, divide the answer in Step 6 by 26.8 $(m \cdot min^{-1}) \cdot (miles \cdot hr^{-1})^{-1}$:

$$172.35\ m \cdot min^{-1} / 26.8\ ([m \cdot min^{-1}] \cdot [miles \cdot hr^{-1}]^{-1}) = 6.43\ miles \cdot hr^{-1}$$

8. The value obtained in Step 7 is the actual treadmill speed in miles per hour. If the speed indicator does not agree with this value, adjust the dial to the proper reading. Check the instruction manual for the location of the speed adjustment.
9. Repeat for a number of different speeds to ensure accuracy across the speeds used in test protocols.

Calibrating Elevation

Treadmill manuals describe how to calibrate the grade by using a simple carpenter's level and a square edge. This calibration procedure consists of three steps:

1. Use a carpenter's level to make sure that the treadmill is level, and check the zero setting on the grade meter under these conditions (with the treadmill electronics turned on). If the meter does not read zero, follow instructions to make the adjustment (usually by using the small screw on the face of the dial).

2. Elevate the treadmill so that the percentage-grade dial reads approximately 20%. Measure the exact incline of the treadmill as shown in figure 5.7. When the level's bubble is exactly in the center of the tube, the rise measurement is obtained.

3. Calculate the grade as the rise over the "run" (tangent) and adjust the treadmill meter to read that exact grade. For example, if the rise were 4.5 in. to the run's 22.5 in., the fractional grade would be

$$\text{Grade} = \text{tangent } \phi = \text{rise} / \text{run} = 4.5 \text{ in.} / 22.5 \text{ in.} = 0.20 = 20\%$$

The rise-over-run method is a typical engineering method for calculating grade, giving the tangent of the angle (the opposite side divided by the horizontal distance, as shown in figure 5.7). Although the sine of the angle (opposite side divided by the hypotenuse) provides the most accurate setting of grade, table 5.9 shows that the tangent value is a good approximation of the sine value for grades less than 20%, or 12°. The rise-over-run method can also be used to calibrate steep grades: Obtain the tangent value as described previously and simply look across table 5.9 to obtain the correct sine value to set on the treadmill dial. For example, if the rise-over-run method yielded 0.268, or 26.8% (tangent), the correct setting would be 25.9% (sine). The latter value is set on the grade dial of the treadmill.

9 In Review

Calibrating the treadmill includes checking both the speed and elevation.

Calibrating the Cycle Ergometer

The cycle ergometer must be calibrated routinely to ensure that the work rate is accurate. Altering either the pedal rate or the load on the wheel varies the work rate on the mechanically braked cycle ergometer. Work is equal to force times the distance through which the force acts: W = F × D. The kilopond, defined as the force acting on a mass of 1 kg at the normal acceleration of gravity, is the proper unit for force. However, the kilopond and the kilogram typically are used interchangeably in exercise testing.

On a mechanically braked cycle ergometer, the force (kilograms of weight on the wheel) is moved through a distance (in meters), so work is expressed in kilogram-meters (kgm). Because work is accomplished over some period of time (e.g., minutes), the activity is referred to as a work rate or power output ($kgm \cdot min^{-1}$), not a workload. On the Monark cycle ergometer, a point on the rim of the wheel travels 6 m per pedal revolution, so at 50 $rev \cdot min^{-1}$, the wheel travels 300 $m \cdot min^{-1}$. If a weight of 1 kg were hanging from that wheel, the work rate, or power output, would be 300 $kgm \cdot min^{-1}$. From these simple calculations you can see the importance of maintaining a correct pedal rate during the test—if the subject were pedaling at 60 $rev \cdot min^{-1}$, the work rate would actually be 20% higher (360 vs. 300 $kgm \cdot min^{-1}$) than it appears to be. The force setting (resistance on the wheel) also must be carefully set and checked because it tends to drift as the test progresses. It is crucial that the force (resistance) values on the scale be correct. The following four steps outline the procedures for calibrating the Monark cycle ergometer scale (3) (refer to figure 5.8):

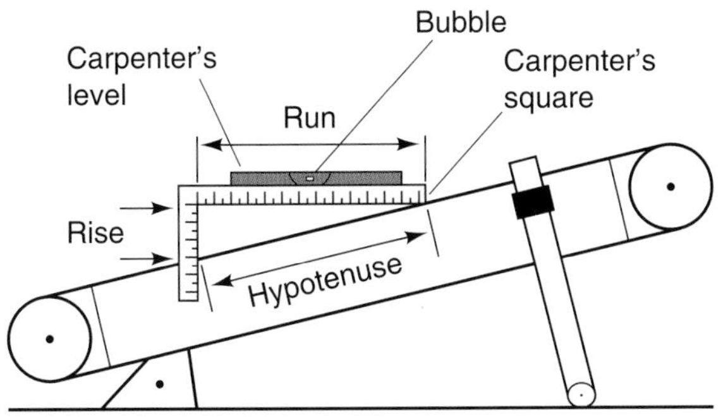

Figure 5.7 Calibrating grade by the tangent method (rise/run) with a carpenter's square and level.

Reprinted from Howley, 1988. The exercise testing laboratory. In *Resource manual for guidelines for exercise testing and prescription.* By permission of Lea & Febiger.

1. Disconnect the "belt" at the spring.

2. Loosen the lock nut and use the adjusting screw on the front of the bike against which the force scale rests so that the vertical mark on the pendulum weight is matched with 0 kp on the weight scale (see figure 5.8*a*). The pendulum must be free-swinging. Lock the adjustment screw with the lock nut. Note: To keep the calibration weights from touching the flywheel, it may be easier to elevate rear of the ergometer (with a 2 × 4 on edge), set the zero as described previously, and proceed to the next step.

3. Suspend a 4.0-kg weight from the spring so that no contact is made with the flywheel, and see if the pendulum moves to the 4.0-kp mark (see figure 5.8*b*). If it doesn't, alter the position or size of the adjusting weight in the pendulum (see figure 5.8*c*). When the lock screw on the back of the pendulum weight is loosened, the adjusting weight can be lowered, raised, or replaced. Check the force scale again and be sure to calibrate the ergometer through the range of values to be used in your tests. Note: If

Table 5.9 Natural Sines and Tangents

Degrees	Sine	% Grade	Tangent	% Grade
0	0.0000	0.0	0.0000	0.0
1	0.0175	1.7	0.075	1.7
2	0.0349	3.5	0.0349	3.5
3	0.0523	5.2	0.0524	5.2
4	0.0698	7.0	0.0699	7.0
5	0.0872	8.7	0.0875	8.7
6	0.1045	10.4	0.1051	10.5
7	0.1219	12.2	0.1228	12.3
8	0.1392	13.9	0.1405	14.0
9	0.1564	15.6	0.1584	15.8
10	0.1736	17.4	0.1763	17.6
11	0.1908	19.1	0.1944	19.4
12	0.2079	20.8	0.2126	21.3
13	0.2250	22.5	0.2309	23.1
14	0.2419	24.2	0.2493	24.9
15	0.2588	25.9	0.2679	26.8
20	0.3420	34.2	0.3640	36.4
25	0.4067	40.7	0.4452	44.5

Reprinted from Howley, 1988, The exercise testing laboratory. In *Resource manual for guidelines for exercise testing and prescription.* By permission of Lea & Febiger.

you used the 2 × 4 to elevate the rear of the ergometer, remove it and reset the zero as described in step 2.

4. Reassemble the cycle ergometer.

10 **In Review**

Calibrating the cycle ergometer involves establishing a true zero, hanging standard weights from the spring, and verifying that they line up with the readings on the scale. Specific steps are listed.

Calibrating the Sphygmomanometer

A **sphygmomanometer** is a BP measurement system composed of an inflatable rubber bladder, an instrument to indicate the applied pressure, an inflation bulb to create pressure, and an adjustable valve to deflate the system. The cuff and the measuring instrument are the most crucial in terms of measurement accuracy. The width of the cuff should be about 20% wider than the diameter of the limb to which it is applied, and when inflated, the bladder should not cause a bulging or displacement. If the bladder is too wide, blood pressure will be underestimated; if too narrow, pressure will be overestimated. Consequently, bladder size (length × width) varies with the type of cuff: child size (21.5 cm × 10 cm), adult size (24 cm × 12.5 cm), and large adult size (33 cm or 42 cm × 15 cm).

The pressure-measuring device, the manometer, can be a mercury or an aneroid type. The mercury type is the standard, and its calibration is easily maintained. The mercury column should rise and fall smoothly, form a clear meniscus, and read zero when the bladder is deflated. If the mercury sticks in the tube, remove the cap and swab out the inside. If it is very dirty, the tube should be removed and cleaned (with detergent, a water rinse, and alcohol for drying). If the mercury column falls below zero, add mercury to bring the meniscus exactly to the zero mark (9, 20, 23). Note: Special care must be taken when handling toxic materials such as mercury; follow your institution's guidelines.

The aneroid gauge uses a metal bellows assembly that expands when pressure is applied, and the expansion moves the pointer on the indicator dial. A spring attached to the pointer moves the pointer

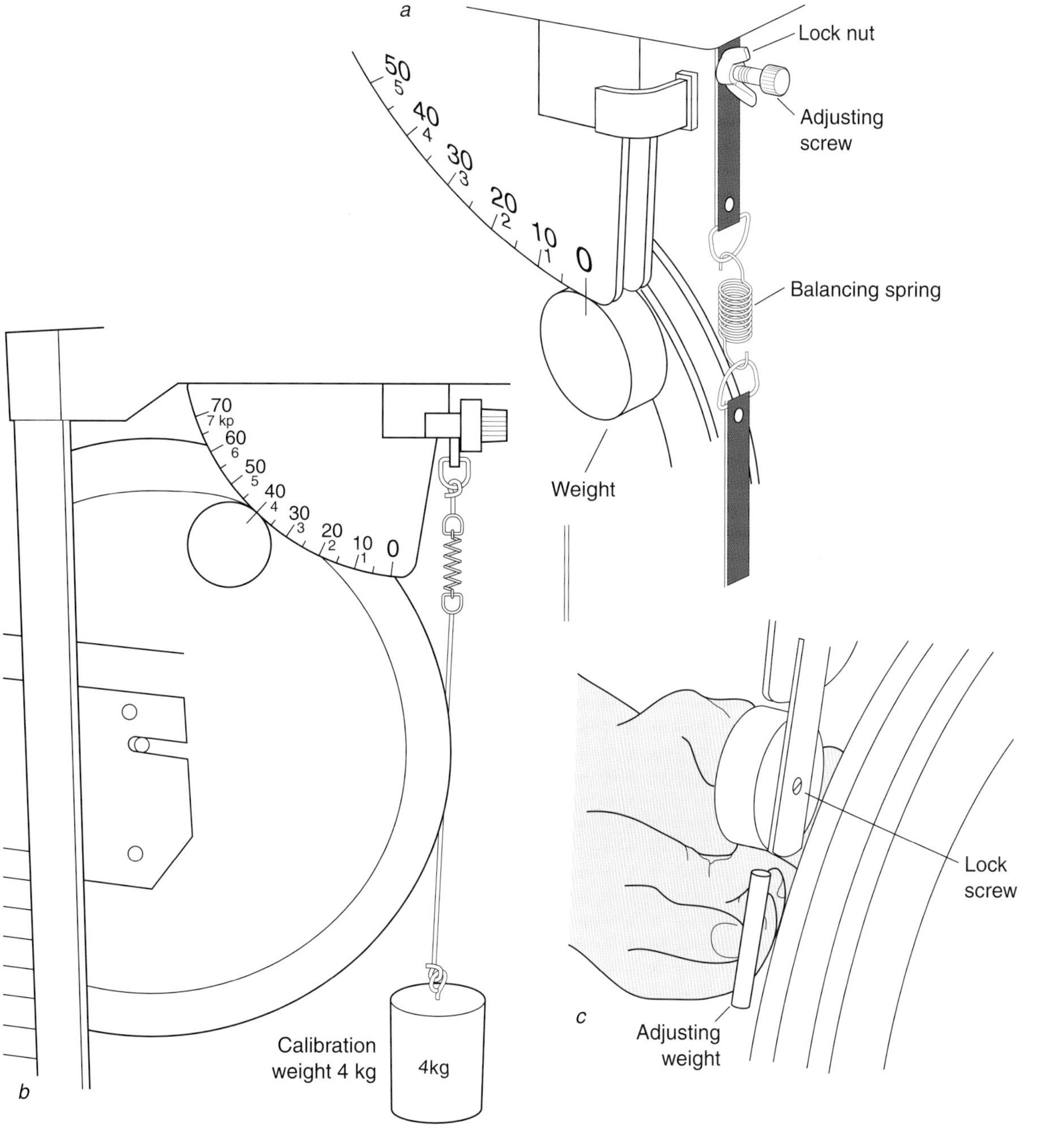

Figure 5.8 Calibrating the Monark cycle ergometer. *(a)* Adjust the pendulum to align with 0; *(b)* suspend a 4.0-kg weight from the spring; and *(c)* adjust the position or size of the weight in the pendulum.

Adapted from Monark Exercise AB.

downscale to zero when the bladder is deflated. This gauge should be calibrated at least once every 6 months at a variety of settings, by using the mercury column just described. A simple Y tube (from the stethoscope) is used to connect the two systems together (see figure 5.9). Readings should be taken with pressure falling to simulate the readings during an actual measurement (23).

11 In Review

It is important to have the correct size cuff when measuring blood pressure. The mercury sphygmomanometer is the standard, and the aneroid gauge should be calibrated against the mercury column every 6 months.

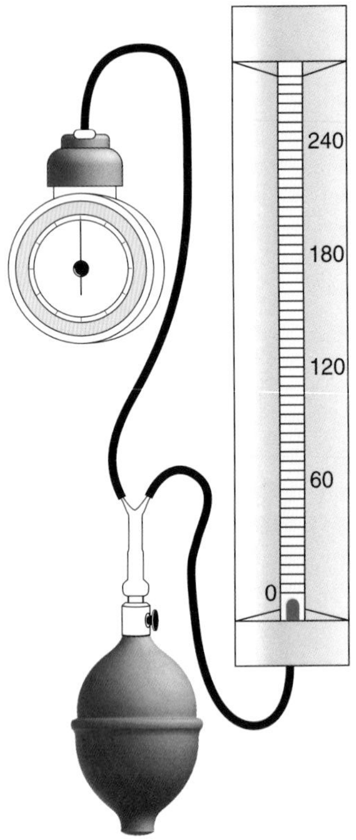

Figure 5.9 Calibrating an aneroid manometer with a mercury manometer.

Reproduced by permission. Human blood pressure determination by sphygmomanometer 1994. Copyright American Heart Association.

Source List

1. American College of Sports Medicine. (2000). *ACSM's guidelines for exercise testing and prescription* (6th ed.). Philadelphia: Lippincott Williams & Wilkins.
2. Åstrand, I. (1960). Aerobic work capacity in men and women with special reference to age. *Acta Physiologica Scandinavica, 49*(Suppl. 169), 1-92.
3. Åstrand, P-O. (1979). *Work tests with the bicycle ergometer.* Varberg, Sweden: Monark-Crescent AB.
4. Åstrand, P-O. (1984). Principles of ergometry and their implications in sport practice. *International Journal of Sports Medicine, 5,* 102-105.
5. Åstrand, P-O., & Rhyming, I. (1954). A nomogram for calculation of aerobic capacity (physical fitness) from pulse rate during submaximal work. *Journal of Applied Physiology, 7,* 218-221.
6. Åstrand, P-O., & Saltin, B. (1961). Maximal oxygen uptake and heart rate in various types of muscular activity. *Journal of Applied Physiology, 16,* 977-981.
7. Balke, B. (1963). A simple field test for assessment of physical fitness. In *Civil Aeromedical Research Institute report* (pp. 63-66). Oklahoma City: Civil Aeromedical Research Institute.
8. Balke, B. (1970). *Advanced exercise procedures for evaluation of the cardiovascular system* (Monograph). Milton, WI: Burdick.
9. Baum, W.A.. (1961). *Sphygmomanometers, principles and precepts.* New York: Baum.
10. Blair, S.N., Kohl, H.W., III, Paffenbarger, R.S., Jr., Clark, D.G., Cooper, K.H., & Gibbons, L.W. (1989). Physical fitness and all-cause mortality. *Journal of the American Medical Association, 262,* 2395-2401.
11. Borg, G. (1998). *Borg's perceived exertion and pain scales.* Champaign, IL: Human Kinetics.
12. Bransford, D.R., & Howley, E.T. (1977). The oxygen cost of running in trained and untrained men and women. *Medicine and Science in Sports, 9,* 41-44.
13. Bruce, R.A. (1972). Multistage treadmill test of submaximal and maximal exercise. In American Heart Association (Ed.), *Exercise testing and training of apparently healthy individuals: A handbook for physicians* (pp. 32-34). New York: American Heart Association.
14. Cooper, K.H. (1977). *The aerobics way.* New York: Bantam Books.
15. Cooper Institute for Aerobics Research (1999). *FITNESSGRAM test administration manual.* Champaign, IL: Human Kinetics.
16. Daniels, J.T. (1985). A physiologist's view of running economy. *Medicine and Science in Sports and Exercise, 17,* 332-338.
17. Daniels, J., Oldridge, N., Nagle, F., & White, B. (1978). Differences and changes in VO_2 among young runners 10-18 years of age. *Medicine and Science in Sports, 10,* 200-203.
18. Ellestad, M. (1994). *Stress testing: Principles and practice.* Philadelphia: Davis.
19. Franks, B.D. (1979). Methodology of the exercise ECG test. In E.K. Chung (Ed.), *Exercise electrocardiography: Practical approach* (pp. 46-61). Baltimore: Williams & Wilkins.
20. Frohlich, E.D., Grim, C., Labarthe, D.R., Maxwell, M.H., Perloff, D., & Weidman, W.H. (1988). Recommendations for human blood-pressure determination by sphygmomanometers. *Circulation, 77,* 501A-514A.
21. Golding, L.A. (2000). *YMCA fitness testing and assessment manual.* Champaign, IL: Human Kinetics.
22. Hagberg, J.M., Mullin, J.P., Giese, M.D., & Spitznagel, E. (1981). Effect of pedaling rate on submaximal exercise responses of competitive cyclists. *Journal of Applied Physiology, 51,* 447-451.
23. Howley, E.T. (1988). The exercise testing laboratory. In S.N. Blair, P. Painter, R.R. Pate, L.K. Smith, & C.B. Taylor (Eds.), *Resource manual for guidelines for exercise testing and prescription* (pp. 406-413). Philadelphia: Lea & Febiger.
24. Kline, G.M., Porcari, J.P., Hintermeister, R., Freedson, P.S., Ward, A., McCarron, R.F., Ross, J., & Rippe, J.M. (1987). Estimation of VO_2max from a 1-mile track walk, gender, age, and body weight. *Medicine and Science in Sports and Exercise, 19,* 253-259.
25. Maritz, J.S., Morrison, J.F., Peter, J., Strydom, N.B., & Wyndham, C.H. (1961). A practical method of estimating an individual's maximal oxygen uptake. *Ergonomics, 4,* 97-122.
26. McArdle, W.D., Katch, F.I., & Pechar, G.S. (1973). Comparison of continuous and discontinuous treadmill and bicycle tests for max VO_2. *Medicine and Science in Sports, 5*(3), 156-160.
27. Montoye, H.J., & Ayen, T. (1986). Body-size adjustment for oxygen requirement in treadmill walking. *Research Quarterly for Exercise and Sport, 57,* 82-84.
28. Montoye, H.J., Ayen, T., Nagle, F., & Howley, E.T. (1986). The oxygen requirement for horizontal and grade walking on a motor-driven treadmill. *Medicine and Science in Sports and Exercise, 17,* 640-645.
29. Naughton, J.P., & Haider, R. (1973). Methods of exercise testing. In J.P. Naughton, H.R. Hellerstein, & L.C. Mohler (Eds.), *Exercise testing and exercise training in coronary heart disease* (pp. 79-91). New York: Academic Press.
30. Oldridge, N.B., Haskell, W.L., & Single, P. (1981). Carotid palpation, coronary heart disease, and exercise rehabilitation. *Medicine and Science in Sports and Exercise, 13,* 6-8.
31. Pollock, M.L., & Wilmore, J.H. (1990). *Exercise in health and disease* (2nd ed.). Philadelphia: Saunders.
32. President's Council on Physical Fitness and Sports. (2002). *President's Challenge Physical Activity and Fitness Award Program.* Washington, DC: Author.
33. Roitman, J.L. (Ed.). (1998). *ACSM's resource manual for guidelines for exercise testing and prescription* (3rd ed.). Philadelphia: Lippincott Williams & Wilkins.
34. Shephard, R.J. (1970). Computer programs for solution of the Åstrand nomogram and the calculation of body surface area. *Journal of Sports Medicine and Physical Fitness, 10,* 206-210.

six

Body Composition

Dixie L. Thompson

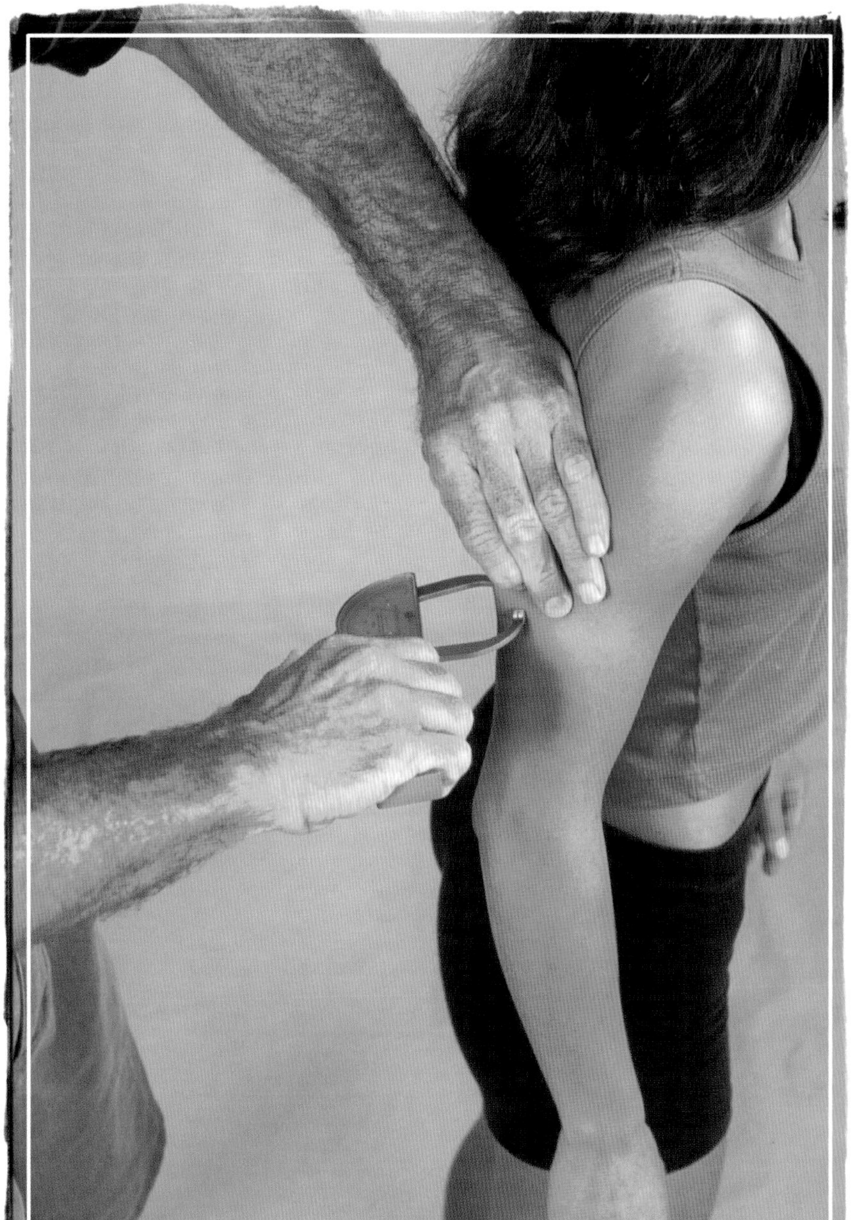

Objectives

The reader will be able to do the following:

1. Discuss the impact of body composition on health and describe the health implications of different types of body fat distribution patterns.
2. Compare and contrast hydrostatic weighing, air displacement plethysmography, bioelectrical impedance analysis, and skinfold measurements as means for estimating body composition.
3. Identify common measurement sites for skinfolds and girths.
4. Calculate and interpret body mass index.
5. Assess body composition using a variety of techniques and describe the advantages and disadvantages of these techniques.

American media is filled with advertisements for programs designed to help people "get in shape." One point of emphasis (many times the primary focus) in these programs is weight loss. An appropriate amount of body fat is an important part of a person's physical fitness. The HFI needs to understand the importance of appropriate amounts of body fat, become aware of the various means for assessing body fat, and become proficient at estimating body fat through skinfolds and girths. As with other aspects of fitness assessment, attention to detail and experience with the techniques used are necessary to become proficient at estimating body fatness. This chapter was written to assist the HFI in acquiring these skills.

Health and Body Composition

Body composition commonly refers to the relative percentages of fat and nonfat tissues in the body. **Fat-free mass** and **percent body fat (%BF)** are typically the most frequently reported values from a body composition assessment. %BF refers to the percentage of the total body weight that is composed of fat: %BF = (fat weight / body weight × 100). Fat-free mass refers to the weight of the nonfat tissues of the body and often is used synonymously with the term **lean body mass**. Table 6.1 lists suggested age-based %BFs (5). Body composition assessment is an important part of a fitness assessment because of the ill effects related to having excessively low or high percentages of body fatness. Various techniques are used to assess body composition, and the HFI should be skilled in their use.

The prevalence of **obesity** and **overweight** among Americans is increasing at an alarming rate. For example, it is estimated that the prevalence of obesity increased by approximately 50% between 1991 and 1998 (18). Another examination found that 63% and 55% of American men and women, respectively, were either overweight or obese (19). Obesity

Table 6.1 Suggested Age-Based Body Fat Percentage Standards for Adults

Men	Recommended range[a]
18-34 years	8-22
35-55 years	10-25
56 years or older	10-25
Women	
18-34 years	20-35
35-55 years	23-38
56 years or older	25-38

[a]Values are body fat percentage.

Adapted from Going and Davis (5).

is a condition in which a person has an excess of **adipose,** or fat, tissue. Obesity may be classified according to either %BF or by the relationship of height and weight (see section on body mass index). Although classification systems vary, a %BF of greater than 38% for females and greater than 25% for males generally is considered in the obese range (5, 15). Overweight is the condition in which a person is above the recommended weight range but is not yet in the obese category (see section on body mass index). Numerous negative health consequences of obesity have been documented including coronary artery disease, hypertension, stroke, type 2 diabetes, increased risk of various cancers, osteoarthritis, degenerative joint disease, abnormal blood lipid profile, and menstrual irregularities (20). Recent estimates attribute approximately 300,000 deaths in the United States each year to obesity (2). Because of the link between obesity and many diseases, it is essential that the HFI provide clients with an accurate assessment of this important fitness component.

When people gain excess fat, genetics determine where the adipose tissue accumulates. Researchers are quite interested in learning how **body fat distribution,** or **fat patterning,** affects health. **Android-type obesity** (i.e., male-pattern obesity, apple shape) is the term used to describe the excessive storage of fat in the trunk and abdominal areas. Excessive fat in the hips and thighs is labeled **gynoid-type obesity** (i.e., female-pattern obesity, pear shape). In terms of negative health consequences, android-type obesity appears to be the most dangerous and is closely linked with cardiovascular disease. The use of waist-to-hip ratios can be a useful tool for differentiating gynoid-type and android-type obesity. Waist circumference also is used to determine when excessive trunk fat is present. Descriptions of how to make these measurements are presented later in this chapter.

Just as too much body fat can be unhealthy, too little body fat also can compromise one's health. Among the many important roles of fat are providing energy, helping with temperature regulation, and cushioning the joints. The minimum body fat level needed to maintain health varies among individuals and is dependent on sex and genetics. The %BF thought to be necessary to allow for good health (i.e., **essential fat**) is 8 to 12% for women and 3 to 5% for men (5). Infertility, depression, impaired temperature regulation, and even death are among the outcomes of excessive weight loss (25). Extreme fat loss results from starvation imposed by internal or external forces. Eating disorders that result in self-starvation are discussed in chapter 11. Because of the important link between health and body composition, an analysis of a client's body fat should be a part of physical fitness assessments.

1 In Review

The prevalence of obesity and overweight is greater than 50% among U.S. adults. Significant health consequences (e.g., cardiovascular disease, type 2 diabetes) may result from obesity. Cardiovascular disease risk is linked more closely with android-type obesity (apple shape) than with gynoid-type obesity (pear shape). Too little body fat also can lead to negative physical outcomes.

Methods for Assessing Body Composition

Numerous techniques have been used successfully in estimating body composition. It is important for the HFI to understand that none of the methods currently used actually *measure* percent body fat. The techniques *estimate* %BF based on the relationship between %BF and other factors that can be accurately measured such as skinfold thicknesses or underwater weight. The only way to truly measure the volume of fat in the body would be to dissect and chemically analyze tissues in the body!

Each of the body composition techniques described in the following sections have inherent advantages and disadvantages. It is important that the HFI understand these so wise decisions can be made when choosing the method for body composition assessment. In many situations encountered by the HFI, ease of measurement, relative accuracy, and cost will be the primary considerations when choosing a technique. In other situations (research or clinical conditions), the accuracy of the measurement may outweigh other considerations.

Hydrostatic Weighing

Hydrostatic (underwater) **weighing** is one of the most common means for estimating body composition in research settings and often is used as the **criterion method** for assessing %BF. A criterion method provides the standard against which other methodologies are compared. In performing this procedure, a person gets into a tank of warm water, submerges him- or herself under the surface of the water, and then exhales fully while technicians record her or his weight (figure 6.1). The submerged weight and body weight (taken on land) are used to calculate %BF.

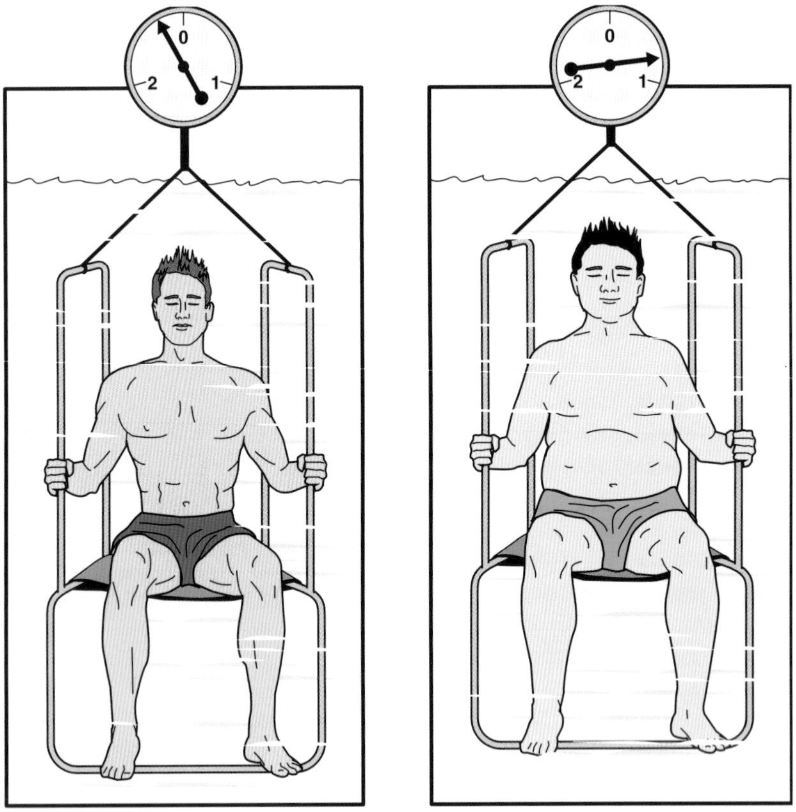

Figure 6.1 Hydrostatic weighing.

Adapted from Pollock and Wilmore 1990.

Hydrostatic weighing is based on Archimedes' principle, which states that a submerged object is "buoyed up" by a force equal to the volume of water it displaces. This buoyant force causes the object to weigh less under water than it does on land. The difference between land weight and underwater weight is used to calculate body volume. Because the density of an object is calculated by dividing weight by volume, body density can be calculated by using the following formula.

$$D_b = \frac{BW}{\frac{(BW - UWW)}{D_{H_2O}} - RV}$$

You will note that in addition to body weight (BW) and underwater weight (UWW), one must determine the density of the water (D_{H_2O}) in the hydrostatic tank and the residual lung volume (RV). Water density is dependent on water temperature and is necessary to convert weight into volume; therefore, accurate measurement of the water temperature is essential. Also, one must correct for the residual lung volume of the person being weighed because any air in the lungs will create an additional buoyant effect that will reduce underwater weight. The oxygen dilution technique described by Wilmore (28) is one of the most frequently used methods for assessing residual lung volume. If residual lung volume must be estimated, the accuracy of hydrostatic weighing is reduced dramatically. Because sex, age, and height are correlated with RV, an estimate of residual lung volume can be obtained by using a formula that incorporates the client's age and height (6). The box on the next page contains formulas for males and females.

Once the body density is calculated, this value must be converted into %BF. To make this conversion, a **two-compartment model** is used. In a two-compartment model, all body tissues are classified as either fat or nonfat. One of the most commonly used equations for this procedure is the Siri (24) equation (%BF = $495/D_b - 450$). In this model, the fat-free portion of the body is composed of all tissues except lipids and is assumed to have a density

Formulas to Calculate Residual Lung Volume From Height and Age (6)

Females:

(0.009 × age in years) + (0.08128 × height in inches) – 3.9 = residual lung volume in liters

Males:

(0.017 × age in years) + (0.06858 × height in inches) – 3.447 = residual lung volume in liters

of 1.1 kg/L. Fat is assumed to have a density of 0.9 kg/L. It has been suggested that the inherent error (caused by variations in hydration or bone density) of this method is 2 to 2.8% in young Caucasian adults (14). The assumption that fat density is 0.9 kg/L appears to hold true for everyone; however, there are situations in which the density of the fat-free body is different from the assumed 1.1 kg/L. For example, if a person's bone density is different from the standard used by Siri, then the assumption that the density of fat-free body equals 1.1 kg/L becomes invalid. Because African-American adults typically have a higher bone density than their Caucasian counterparts, Schutte and colleagues (23) proposed that a different equation be used to calculate %BF for African-American men. A number of equations have been proposed to convert body density into %BF. Some of these are listed in table 6.2. For more equations and information on converting body density into %BF, see the ACSM Guidelines (1) and Heyward and Stolarczyk (8). Researchers sometimes use techniques more advanced than two-compartment models. These techniques are currently impractical for non-research settings (see box on page 102).

Hydrostatic weighing provides an accurate estimation of body composition for most adults, and this technique remains a standard of comparison for various other methods. Major disadvantages to this procedure are the time, expense, and technical expertise required. Also, many individuals are unable to perform this procedure because of their discomfort in being under water.

Following are guidelines that will help ensure accurate assessment of body composition with hydrostatic weighing techniques:

- The participant should not eat within 4 hr of testing.
- The participant should urinate and defecate before testing.
- The participant should wear as little clothing as possible. Remove any trapped air bubbles from clothing before weighing.
- Instruct the participant to exhale completely while submerged. (This will take practice for most individuals.)
- The participant should remain as motionless as possible while submerged to increase accuracy.
- Perform several (5-10) trials to obtain consistent measurements.
- Measure, rather than estimate, residual volume.

Table 6.2 Sample of Equations Used to Convert Body Density Into Body Fat Percentage

Group	Sex	Equation
African American	Male	%BF = $(437/D_b) - 393$
	Female	%BF = $(485/D_b) - 439$
Caucasian	Male	%BF = $(495/D_b) - 450$
	Female	%BF = $(501/D_b) - 457$

Note. %BF = body fat percentage; D_b = body density.

Adapted from Heyward and Stolarczyk (8).

Body Composition Techniques Used in Research Settings

Multicompartment Models

A disadvantage to any two-compartment model of body composition is the number of assumptions that must be made about the composition and density of various body tissues. To avoid this problem, researchers sometimes use models in which combinations of measurements are used to estimate body composition. Although these techniques must still rely on some basic assumptions about the body's "makeup," fewer broad generalizations about the body's component parts are made. Therefore, these multicompartment models provide a more accurate assessment of body composition.

An example of a multicompartment model is Siri's three-compartment model in which the body is divided into fat, water, and solids (protein and mineral) (24). This model requires the measurement of total body density and total body water. Total body water measurements are typically determined through the ingestion of an isotope of hydrogen such as deuterium or tritium. After the ingested isotope spreads through the body's water, a fluid sample (e.g., urine, blood) can be used to calculate total body water. This model is particularly useful in clinical situations when patients have significant alterations in body water. In cases where the bone mineral varies from what is assumed in a two-compartment model (e.g., osteoporotic patient), a technique requiring measurement of bone is needed. Lohman (13) presented a model that divides the body into fat, mineral, and protein and water components. Both body density and bone mineral measurement (usually done with x-ray imaging) are needed for this technique. Sometimes bone and water measurements are added to the body density measurement to provide a four-compartment model (i.e., protein, mineral, fat, and water) of the body (7).

Multicompartment models provide important criterion measures of body composition for researchers. Data from these methodologies are used to develop better field methods for assessing body composition in diverse populations. However, the cost, time, and technical expertise required for this process make it impractical in most nonresearch settings.

Air Displacement Plethysmography

Another technique to determine %BF that uses the concept of density as the ratio of body weight to body volume is **air displacement plethysmography**. In this method, body volume is estimated while the subject sits in a sealed chamber. During testing, a computer-controlled diaphragm moves, changing the volume of the chamber. Pressure changes in the chamber are related to the size of the person being measured. By examining the pressure-volume relationship, the HFI can calculate body volume and therefore body density (4, 17). The two-compartment equations listed in table 6.2 then can be used to convert density into %BF.

The primary advantage of this method compared with hydrostatic weighing is that air displacement plethysmography is quicker and is less anxiety producing for many individuals. Researchers continue to gather data on this device in an attempt to determine if it can be routinely substituted for hydrostatic weighing. The major disadvantage to this method is the cost of the highly technical equipment needed to make the measurements. A major consideration for obtaining accurate measurements with this device is that subjects dress according to manufacturer's specifications (i.e., tight-fitting Lycra swimsuit and swim cap).

Bioelectrical Impedance Analysis

Bioelectrical impedance analysis (BIA) is a simple, quick, noninvasive method that can be used to estimate %BF. This technique is based on the assumption that tissues high in water content will conduct electrical currents with less resistance than those with little water (21). Because adipose tissue contains little water, fat will impede the flow of electrical current.

BIA requires that a small electrical current be sent through the body. This current is undetectable to the person being tested (21). There are several types of commercially available BIA devices. Some place electrodes on the hand and foot, some are hand-held devices, and others, which look much like bathroom scales, have contact points for the bottom of the feet. Whatever the design of the machine, as the introduced current passes through the body, voltage will decrease. This voltage drop (impedance) is used to calculate %BF. Typically, other information such as sex, height, and age are used in conjunction with impedance to predict %BF. BIA has gained wide acceptance in the fitness industry because it is easy, inexpensive, and noninvasive. The accuracy of this technique depends on the type of equipment and equations used; however, a standard error of approximately ±4% commonly is reported (14). In other words, the %BF value from BIA is typically within 4% of that obtained using hydrostatic weighing. A problem with the use of BIA is that the relationship between impedance and %BF varies among populations. This means that the best equation to predict %BF will depend on the person being tested. For more detailed information on choosing an appropriate BIA equation, refer to *Applied Body Composition Assessment* by Heyward and Stolarczyk (8). Furthermore, BIA does not produce accurate results for individuals with amputations, significant muscular atrophy, severe obesity, or diseases that alter the state of hydration. It also has been recommended that people with implanted defibrillators avoid BIA assessment until the safety of BIA with these individuals has been determined (21).

A person's state of hydration can greatly alter BIA results; therefore, it is essential to follow standardized guidelines with this assessment technique (21). Following is a list of guidelines for using BIA.

- Remove oil and lotions from the skin with alcohol before placing electrodes.
- Place electrodes precisely as directed by the manufacturer of the impedance device used. Incorrect electrode placement will greatly reduce the accuracy of the procedure.
- Many of the equations used with BIA require the measurement of height, weight, or both. Height should be measured to the nearest 0.5 cm and weight to the nearest 0.1 kg.
- Any substance that alters the body's hydration state such as alcohol or diuretics should be avoided for at least 48 hr before BIA. (Diuretics being taken under a doctor's direction should not be stopped.)
- Individuals being assessed should avoid eating and should drink only enough to maintain hydration during the 4 hr before assessment.
- Exercise should be avoided for 12 hr preceding BIA.
- Menstrual cycle phase should be noted because of its ability to alter hydration levels.

Page 104 discusses how techniques which produce images of the body (e.g., x-rays) are sometimes used in clinical settings for body composition assessment.

2 In Review

Two-compartment models divide the body into fat and fat-free components. Although the Siri two-compartment model is often used for all adults, other models are available for specific segments of the population. Both hydrostatic weighing and air displacement plethysmography use the concept of a two-compartment model. Bioelectrical impedance analysis is based on the principle that electrical currents will flow easier through more hydrated tissues (muscle) than through less hydrated tissue (fat). Although this technique can be quite useful in body composition screening, steps should be taken to ensure that hydration is normal at the time of testing.

Skinfolds

The measurement of skinfold thickness is one of the most frequently performed tests to estimate body composition. This quick, noninvasive, inexpensive method can, in most cases, provide a fairly accurate assessment of %BF. The fat percentage value obtained by skinfold equations is typically within 4% of the value measured using underwater weighing (14). This methodology is based on the assumption that, as one gains adipose tissue, the increase in skinfold thickness will be proportional to the additional fat weight. Because 50 to 70% of one's adipose tissue is stored subcutaneously, this assumption holds true in most cases.

Because of the widespread use of this type of assessment, the HFI should master the skills involved. Accurate measurement of skinfold thickness requires that several things be done correctly: locating the skinfold site, "pinching" the skinfold away from the underlying tissue, measuring with the caliper, and choosing the proper equation. The following sections address each of these important concerns.

Locating the Skinfold Site

It is critical that the site of the skinfold measurement be accurately determined. To increase the accuracy of the measurement, especially for the inexperienced technician, the site for measurement should

Imaging Techniques in Body Composition Assessment

Dual energy x-ray absorptiometry (DXA) was developed for measuring the density of bones. Although this remains a primary use of this methodology, software has been developed that can estimate %BF from DXA scans. This procedure requires a total-body x-ray with extremely low-dosage energy beams. As the x-ray beams pass through the subject, the density of all parts of the body is determined. Because fat, bone, and nonbone lean tissue have different densities, these three compartments can be identified (12).

Although this technique requires a full-body x-ray, the radiation exposure for the procedure is minimal and is roughly equivalent to 1/50 of the radiation exposure of a chest x-ray. Some claim DXA as the new criterion method for body composition assessment; however, there are still issues unresolved for this technology. For example, differences in DXA software packages may result in varied body fat outcomes. Also, variations in body segment thicknesses tend to alter DXA results (12). Studies investigating the error associated with this technique have reported errors ranging from 1.2 to 4.8% (14). This procedure is relatively quick (approximately 15 min) and has the potential for very accurate results regardless of the age, sex, or race of the individual being tested. The major prohibitive factors for using this procedure are cost and access to the equipment. Because of the radiation exposure involved, DXA equipment is housed in hospitals and/or clinically oriented research centers. At present, DXA methodology is used most frequently as a research tool and in the clinical assessment of body composition.

Magnetic resonance imaging (MRI) and computed tomography (CT) are also imaging techniques that provide important information to clinicians and researchers. One of the common uses of these machines is to determine the amount of fat, particularly deep fat, found in the trunk. Because deep fat (visceral fat) is highly associated with disease, researchers use these techniques to quantify this important fat distribution pattern. CT scans use x-rays to produce images of the fat and nonfat tissues, whereas MRI uses a strong magnetic field for this purpose. The equipment necessary for this type of imaging is very expensive and is found only in clinical settings.

---

be located and then marked with an erasable marker. This will help ensure that the calipers are placed in precisely the correct position each time the skinfold is measured. All skinfold measurements should be taken on the right side of the body unless otherwise specified. Refer to table 6.3 for some of the most commonly used measurement sites. For a more complete description of skinfold site determination, refer to the *Anthropometric Standardization Reference Manual* (16). The HFI should also note that the measurement of skinfolds immediately after exercise may lead to inaccurate results because of fluid volume shifts.

"Pinching" the Skinfold

Once the correct location for the skinfold measurement is determined, the HFI must then gently but firmly pinch and lift the skinfold away from the underlying muscle in order to measure it. The following guidelines describe proper methods for measuring skinfolds:

1. Place the fingers perpendicular to the skinfold approximately 1 cm from the site to be measured.
2. Gently yet firmly pinch the skinfold between the thumb and the first two fingers and lift away from the underlying tissues.
3. Place the jaws of the caliper at the measurement site perpendicular to the skinfold. The jaws of the caliper should be halfway between the bottom and top of the fold. Maintain pinch while taking measurement.
4. Read the measurement on the caliper 1 to 2 s after the jaws come into contact with the skin.
5. Wait at least 15 s before taking a subsequent measurement. To allow time for fold to return to normal, take one measurement at each site, and then repeat measurements. If the second measurement varies by more than 1 to 2 mm, repeat the measurement a third time.

Measuring the skinfolds of obese individuals can be difficult if not impossible. If the jaws of the caliper will not open wide enough to measure the skinfold, use an alternative method for assessing body composition. Girth measurements for predicting %BF (26, 27), body mass index, and waist-to-hip ratio are methods that may be used for obese individuals. These methods are described later in the chapter.

Measuring With the Caliper

Skinfold thickness is measured with a skinfold caliper. A variety of commercially available calipers are available

Table 6.3 Commonly Used Skinfold Site Locations

Skinfold site	Description
Abdominal	Measure vertical fold 2 cm to the right of and level with the umbilicus. Make sure the head of the caliper is not in the umbilicus.
Triceps	Measure the vertical fold over the belly of the triceps muscle. The arm should be relaxed. The specific site is the posterior midline of the upper arm, half the distance between the acromion and olecranon processes.
Chest	The location for this site is half or a third the distance between the anterior axillary line and the nipple for men and women, respectively. The measurement should be a diagonal fold along the natural line of the skin.
Midaxillary	This vertical fold should be taken at the level of the ziphoid process on the midaxillary line.
Subscapular	This site is located 2 cm below the inferior angle of the scapula. The diagonal fold should be measured at a 45° angle.
Suprailiac	This diagonal fold should be measured in line with the natural angle of the iliac crest. The measurement should be taken along the anterior axillary line just above the iliac crest.
Thigh	Measure the vertical fold over the quadriceps muscle on the midline of the thigh. The measurement site is half the distance between the top of the patella and the inguinal crease. Subject's leg should be relaxed.

that vary in price and accuracy. The Lange and Harpenden calipers traditionally have been used most often in research settings because of their precision and reliability; however, other calipers also may be used effectively (3). Obviously, if the calipers that are being used do not measure skinfolds accurately, the estimate of body fat will be compromised. It is advisable to measure with calipers that closely match those used in the development of the equation you are using.

Choosing the Proper Equation

Most skinfold equations were developed by using underwater weighing as the criterion method and actually are designed to estimate body density. To develop skinfold equations, the body density of a large number of people was measured (typically by using hydrostatic weighing), and this value was compared with skinfold thickness through a statistical method called regression analysis. This statistical technique results in the development of an equation that reflects the relationship between skinfolds and body density. By inserting a client's skinfold measurements (and sometimes other information such as age) into these equations, the HFI obtains an estimate of the client's body density. Body density then is converted to %BF by using a two-compartment model equation such as the Siri equation (table 6.2).

Both generalized and population-specific skinfold equations have been developed (10, 14). Generalized equations are designed to estimate body composition in groups of people who vary greatly in age, body composition, and fitness. An advantage of these equations is that they can be used to estimate body composition in most people; however, these equations lose accuracy when testing individuals that are dissimilar to those used to develop the equation. These equations are also typically less accurate for people at either end of the fatness continuum. Population-specific equations are designed to predict body composition in a particular subgroup of the population, such as women runners. The advantage of using population-specific equations is that they tend to have higher accuracy when testing people that fit the physical profile of those in the subgroup of interest.

Because sex influences the areas in which fat is stored, separate skinfold equations for men and women have been developed. The Jackson and Pollock (9) equations for men and the Jackson, Pollock, and Ward (11) equations for women are generalized equations that are used widely. Note that the client's age is used in these equations. This is because the relationship between total body fat and subcutaneous fat changes with age; as one ages, proportionally less fat is stored subcutaneously. Equations from these authors that require the measurement of three or seven sites are listed in the box on page 106. In addition, tables 6.4 and 6.5 provide quick references for estimating body fatness from skinfold thicknesses for men and women, respectively. To use these tables, total the sum of your client's skinfolds (chest, abdominal, and thigh for men; triceps, suprailium, and thigh for women) and locate the corresponding value in the far left column. Then, locate the client's age in the top row. The intersection of the row and column will be the client's estimated %BF.

Equations to Estimate Body Density From Skinfold Thicknesses (9, 10, 11)

Women

3 sites

$$D_b = 1.0994921 - 0.0009929(X1) + 0.0000023(X1)^2 - 0.0001392(X2)$$

3 sites

$$D_b = 1.089733 - 0.0009245(X3) + 0.0000025(X3)^2 - 0.0000979(X2)$$

7 sites

$$D_b = 1.097 - 0.00046971(X4) + 0.00000056(X4)^2 - 0.00012828(X2)$$

X1 = sum of triceps, suprailiac, and thigh skinfolds

X2 = age in years

X3 = sum of triceps, suprailiac, and abdominal skinfolds

X4 = sum of triceps, abdominal, suprailiac, thigh, chest, subscapular, and midaxillary skinfolds

Men

3 sites

$$D_b = 1.10938 - 0.0008267(X1) + 0.0000016(X1)^2 - 0.0002574(X2)$$

3 sites

$$D_b = 1.1125025 - 0.0013125(X3) + 0.0000055(X3)^2 - 0.0002440(X2)$$

7 sites

$$D_b = 1.112 - 0.00043499(X4) + 0.00000055(X4)^2 - 0.00028826(X2)$$

X1 = sum of chest, abdomen, and thigh skinfolds

X2 = age in years

X3 = sum of chest, triceps, and subscapular skinfolds

X4 = sum of triceps, abdominal, suprailiac, thigh, chest, subscapular, and midaxillary skinfolds

Girth Measurements

Several girth measurements (body and limb circumferences) are used as ways to either estimate body composition or describe body proportions. Advantages of making girth measurements are that they provide quick and reliable information about the individual. These measurements are sometimes used in equations to predict body composition and may also be used to track changes in body shape and size during weight loss. The major disadvantage is that they provide little information about the fat and nonfat components of the body. For example, a bodybuilder's thigh can have a larger circumference (yet less fat) than that of an obese individual. A description of several commonly measured girths follows; refer to the *Anthropometric Standardization Reference Manual* (16) for additional circumference sites.

Table 6.4 Percentage Body Fat Estimation for Men From Age and the Sum of Chest, Abdominal, and Thigh Skinfolds

Sum of skinfolds (mm)	Age to the last year: Under 22	23 to 27	28 to 32	33 to 37	38 to 42	43 to 47	48 to 52	53 to 57	Over 57
8-10	1.3	1.8	2.3	2.9	3.4	3.9	4.5	5.0	5.5
11-13	2.2	2.8	3.3	3.9	4.4	4.9	5.5	6.0	6.5
14-16	3.2	3.8	4.3	4.8	5.4	5.9	6.4	7.0	7.5
17-19	4.2	4.7	5.3	5.8	6.3	6.9	7.4	8.0	8.5
20-22	5.1	5.7	6.2	6.8	7.3	7.9	8.4	8.9	9.5
23-25	6.1	6.6	7.2	7.7	8.3	8.8	9.4	9.9	10.5
26-28	7.0	7.6	8.1	8.7	9.2	9.8	10.3	10.9	11.4
29-31	8.0	8.5	9.1	9.6	10.2	10.7	11.3	11.8	12.4
32-34	8.9	9.4	10.0	10.5	11.1	11.6	12.2	12.8	13.3
35-37	9.8	10.4	10.9	11.5	12.0	12.6	13.1	13.7	14.3
38-40	10.7	11.3	11.8	12.4	12.9	13.5	14.1	14.6	15.2
41-43	11.6	12.2	12.7	13.3	13.8	14.4	15.0	15.5	16.1
44-46	12.5	13.1	13.6	14.2	14.7	15.3	15.9	16.4	17.0
47-49	13.4	13.9	14.5	15.1	15.6	16.2	16.8	17.3	17.9
50-52	14.3	14.8	15.4	15.9	16.5	17.1	17.6	18.2	18.8
53-55	15.1	15.7	16.2	16.8	17.4	17.9	18.5	19.1	19.7
56-58	16.0	16.5	17.1	17.7	18.2	18.8	19.4	20.0	20.5
59-61	16.9	17.4	17.9	18.5	19.1	19.7	20.2	20.8	21.4
62-64	17.6	18.2	18.8	19.4	19.9	20.5	21.1	21.7	22.2
65-67	18.5	19.0	19.6	20.2	20.8	21.3	21.9	22.5	23.1
68-70	19.3	19.9	20.4	21.0	21.6	22.2	22.7	23.3	23.9
71-73	20.1	20.7	21.2	21.8	22.4	23.0	23.6	24.1	24.7
74-76	20.9	21.5	22.0	22.6	23.2	23.8	24.4	25.0	25.5
77-79	21.7	22.2	22.8	23.4	24.0	24.6	25.2	25.8	26.3
80-82	22.4	23.0	23.6	24.2	24.8	25.4	25.9	26.5	27.1
83-85	23.2	23.8	24.4	25.0	25.5	26.1	26.7	27.3	27.9
86-88	24.0	24.5	25.1	25.7	26.3	26.9	27.5	28.1	28.7
89-91	24.7	25.3	25.9	26.5	27.1	27.6	28.2	28.8	29.4
92-94	25.4	26.0	26.6	27.2	27.8	28.4	29.0	29.6	30.2
95-97	26.1	26.7	27.3	27.9	28.5	29.1	29.7	30.3	30.9
98-100	26.9	27.4	28.0	28.6	29.2	29.8	30.4	31.0	31.6
101-103	27.5	28.1	28.7	29.3	29.9	30.5	31.1	31.7	32.3
104-106	28.2	28.8	29.4	30.0	30.6	31.2	31.8	32.4	33.0
107-109	28.9	29.5	30.1	30.7	31.3	31.9	32.5	33.1	33.7
110-112	29.6	30.2	30.8	31.4	32.0	32.6	33.2	33.8	34.4
113-115	30.2	30.8	31.4	32.0	32.6	33.2	33.8	34.5	35.1
116-118	30.9	31.5	32.1	32.7	33.3	33.9	34.5	35.1	35.7
119-121	31.5	32.1	32.7	33.3	33.9	34.5	35.1	35.7	36.4
122-124	32.1	32.7	33.3	33.9	34.5	35.1	35.8	36.4	37.0
125-127	32.7	33.3	33.9	34.5	35.1	35.8	36.4	37.0	37.6

Note. Percentage of fat is calculated by the formula of Siri: percent fat = $[(4.95/D_b) - 4.5] \times 100$, where D_b = body density.

Adapted from Pollock, Schmidt, and Jackson (22).

Table 6.5 Percentage Body Fat Estimation for Women From Age and Triceps, Suprailium, and Thigh Skinfolds

Sum of skinfolds (mm)	Age to the last year: Under 22	23 to 27	28 to 32	33 to 37	38 to 42	43 to 47	48 to 52	53 to 57	Over 57
23-25	9.7	9.9	10.2	10.4	10.7	10.9	11.2	11.4	11.7
26-28	11.0	11.2	11.5	11.7	12.0	12.3	12.5	12.7	13.0
29-31	12.3	12.5	12.8	13.0	13.3	13.5	13.8	14.0	14.3
32-34	13.6	13.8	14.0	14.3	14.5	14.8	15.0	15.3	15.5
35-37	14.8	15.0	15.3	15.5	15.8	16.0	16.3	16.5	16.8
38-40	16.0	16.3	16.5	16.7	17.0	17.2	17.5	17.7	18.0
41-43	17.2	17.4	17.7	17.9	18.2	18.4	18.7	18.9	19.2
44-46	18.3	18.6	18.8	19.1	19.3	19.6	19.8	20.1	20.3
47-49	19.5	19.7	20.0	20.2	20.5	20.7	21.0	21.2	21.5
50-52	20.6	20.8	21.1	21.3	21.6	21.8	22.1	22.3	22.6
53-55	21.7	21.9	22.1	22.4	22.6	22.9	23.1	23.4	23.6
56-58	22.7	23.0	23.2	23.4	23.7	23.9	24.2	24.4	24.7
59-61	23.7	24.0	24.2	24.5	24.7	25.0	25.2	25.5	25.7
62-64	24.7	25.0	25.2	25.5	25.7	26.0	26.2	26.4	26.7
65-67	25.7	25.9	26.2	26.4	26.7	26.9	27.2	27.4	27.7
68-70	26.6	26.9	27.1	27.4	27.6	27.9	28.1	28.4	28.6
71-73	27.5	27.8	28.0	28.3	28.5	28.8	29.0	29.3	29.5
74-76	28.4	28.7	28.9	29.2	29.4	29.7	29.9	30.2	30.4
77-79	29.3	29.5	29.8	30.0	30.3	30.5	30.8	31.0	31.3
80-82	30.1	30.4	30.6	30.9	31.1	31.4	31.6	31.9	32.1
83-85	30.9	31.2	31.4	31.7	31.9	32.2	32.4	32.7	32.9
86-88	31.7	32.0	32.2	32.5	32.7	32.9	33.2	33.4	33.7
89-91	32.5	32.7	33.0	33.2	33.5	33.7	33.9	34.2	34.4
92-94	33.2	33.4	33.7	33.9	34.2	34.4	34.7	34.9	35.2
95-97	33.9	34.1	34.4	34.6	34.9	35.1	35.4	35.6	35.9
98-100	34.6	34.8	35.1	35.3	35.5	35.8	36.0	36.3	36.5
101-103	35.3	35.4	35.7	35.9	36.2	36.4	36.7	36.9	37.2
104-106	35.8	36.1	36.3	36.6	36.8	37.1	37.3	37.5	37.8
107-109	36.4	36.7	36.9	37.1	37.4	37.6	37.9	38.1	38.4
110-112	37.0	37.2	37.5	37.7	38.0	38.2	38.5	38.7	38.9
113-115	37.5	37.8	38.1	38.2	38.5	38.7	39.0	39.2	39.5
116-118	38.0	38.3	38.5	38.8	39.0	39.3	39.5	39.7	40.0
119-121	38.5	38.7	39.0	39.2	39.5	39.7	40.0	40.2	40.5
122-124	39.0	39.2	39.4	39.7	39.9	40.2	40.4	40.7	40.9
125-127	39.4	39.6	39.9	40.1	40.4	40.6	40.9	41.1	41.4
128-130	39.8	40.0	40.3	40.5	40.8	41.0	41.3	41.5	41.8

Note. Percentage of fat is calculated by the formula of Siri: percent fat = $[(4.95/D_b) - 4.5] \times 100$, where D_b = body density.

Adapted from Pollock, Schmidt, and Jackson (22).

- Waist—narrowest part of the torso between the ziphoid process and the umbilicus
- Abdomen—circumference of the torso at the level of the umbilicus
- Hips—maximal circumference of the buttocks above the gluteal fold
- Thigh—largest circumference of the right thigh below the gluteal fold

The **waist-to-hip ratio** (WHR) is one of the most used clinical applications of girth measurements. This value is often used to reflect the degree of abdominal, or android-type, obesity. A WHR greater than 0.94 for young men or 0.82 for young women is considered to place the individual at much greater risk for developing negative health consequences as a result of excess abdominal fat (8). Because the relationship between WHR and disease is modified by age, organizations suggest the use of waist circumference as an indicator of disease risk. A waist circumference of greater than 102 cm (40 in.) in men or greater than 88 cm (35 in.) in women is considered to significantly increase the risk of obesity-related disease (1, 20).

When assessing girths, use the following procedures to standardize the measurements:

- Make sure that the measuring tape is horizontal when measuring trunk circumferences and is perpendicular to the long axis of the limb when measuring limbs. Using either a mirror or an assistant will help ensure the tape is placed properly.
- Apply constant pressure to the tape without pinching the skin. Use a tape measure fitted with a handle that indicates the amount of tension exerted.
- When measuring limbs, measure on the right side of the body. Alternately, measure on both sides and record values for right and left.
- Ensure that the person is standing erect, relaxed, and with feet together.
- When measuring girths of the trunk, take the measurement after the person exhales and before he or she begins the next breath.

Body Mass Index

A widely used clinical assessment of the appropriateness of a person's weight is the **body mass index** (BMI), or Quetelet index. This value is calculated by dividing the weight in kilograms by height in meters squared.

BMI is a quick and easy method for determining if one's weight is appropriate for one's height. In the past, height-weight charts were used for this purpose, but BMI is the currently accepted method for interpreting the height-weight relationship. As is the case with girth measurements, BMI does not differentiate between fat and nonfat weight. This is problematic when testing athletic individuals with a large lean mass. For example, a football linebacker who is 6 ft 2 in. and weighs 220 pounds will be considered overweight according to BMI standards (BMI = 28.3 kg/m^2), when in fact he may have a very low %BF. On the other hand, an inactive person with a similar height and weight is probably carrying excess adipose tissue. Even with the limitations of using BMI, for most adults there is a clear correlation between elevated BMI and negative health consequences (19). The recommended BMI range is from 18.5 to 24.9 kg/m^2. Overweight is classified as a BMI of 25 to 29.9 kg/m^2, and a BMI of 30 kg/m^2 or higher is considered obesity (1, 20). In screening situations where body fat estimation is impossible or impractical, BMI can be a useful tool for the HFI to provide feedback to individuals.

Calculating Target Body Weight

As listed in table 6.1, healthy %BF ranges are quite different for females and males and cover a wide range. One of the important tasks of the HFI is helping clients determine an appropriate weight goal. Once an estimate of %BF has been obtained, the HFI can calculate an appropriate target weight. As discussed in chapter 11, setting reasonable goals for weight loss is a major factor in maintaining compliance. To calculate target body weight, one must know body weight, %BF, and the desired level of body fatness (see the box on the next page).

3 In Review

Skinfold measurements can provide a quick and relatively accurate method for estimating body composition; however, care must be taken in making these measurements if the values are to be accurate and reliable. Girth measurements, particularly WHR and waist circumference, can be useful in assessing risk of obesity-related disease. BMI is a useful tool in classifying individuals into overweight and obese categories. The recommended BMI range is from 18.5 to 24.9 kg/m^2. Target body weight can be calculated if current weight and body composition are known.

Calculating Target Body Weight

Fat mass = current body weight × (%BF/100%)

Fat-free mass (FFM) = current body weight – fat mass

$$\text{Target Body Weight} = \frac{\text{FFM}}{1-\left(\frac{\text{Desired \%BF}}{100}\right)}$$

Example: A 40-year-old woman weighs 155 lb and has a body fat percentage of 30%. Her goal is to reach 23% body fat. What is her target weight?

Fat mass = 155 lb × 0.30 = 46.5 lb

FFM = 155 lb – 46.5 lb = 108.5 lb

$$\text{Target Body Weight} = \frac{108.5}{1-\left(\frac{23}{100}\right)} = 140.9 \text{ lb}$$

Case Study

6.1

You are the director of a worksite exercise facility. Mr. Jackson, a 48-year-old man, has joined the exercise program. At his initial evaluation, you make the following measurements:

Height = 5′11"

Weight = 230 lbs

Hip circumference = 43 in

Waist circumference = 36 in

Chest skinfold = 30 mm

Abdomen skinfold = 36 mm

Thigh skinfold = 26 mm

a. Calculate and interpret the following: BMI, WHR, and %BF.

b. Mr. Jackson sets an *initial* %BF goal of 24%. Calculate his target body weight for his goal.

Source List

1. American College of Sports Medicine. (2000). *ACSM's guidelines for exercise testing and prescription* (6th ed.). Philadelphia: Lippincott Williams & Wilkins.
2. Allison, D.B., Fontaine, K.R., Manson, J.E., Stevens, J., & VanItallie, T.B. (1999). Annual deaths attributable to obesity in the United States. *Journal of the American Medical Association, 282*(16), 1530-1538.
3. Cataldo, D., & Heyward, V.H. (2000). Pinch an inch: A comparison of several high-quality and plastic skinfold calipers. *ACSM's Health and Fitness Journal, 4*(3), 12-16.
4. Dempster, P., & Aitkens, S. (1995). A new air displacement method for the determination of human body composition. *Medicine and Science in Sports and Exercise, 27*, 1692-1697.
5. Going, S., & Davis, R. (2001). Body composition. In J.L. Roitman (Ed.), *ACSM's resource manual for guidelines for exercise testing and prescription* (4th ed., pp. 391-400). Baltimore: Lippincott Williams & Wilkins.
6. Goldman, H.I., & Becklake, M.R. (1959). Respiratory function tests. *American Review of Tuberculosis and Pulmonary Disease, 79*, 457-467.
7. Heymsfield, S.B., Lichtman, S.W., Baumgartner, R.N., Wang, J., Kamen, Y., Aliprantis, A., & Pierson, R.N. (1990). Body composition of human: Comparison of two improved four-compartment models that differ in expense, technical complexity, and radiation exposure. *American Journal of Clinical Nutrition, 52*, 52-58.
8. Heyward, V.H., & Stolarczyk, L.M. (1996). *Applied body composition assessment*. Champaign, IL: Human Kinetics.
9. Jackson, A.S., & Pollock, M.L. (1978). Generalized equations for predicting body density of men. *British Journal of Nutrition, 40*, 497-504.
10. Jackson, A.S., & Pollock, M.L. (1985). Practical assessment of body composition. *The Physician and Sportsmedicine, 13*, 76-90.
11. Jackson, A.S., Pollock, M.L., & Ward, A. (1980). Generalized equations for predicting body density in women. *Medicine and Science in Sports and Exercise, 12*, 175-182.
12. Kohrt, W.M. (1995). Body composition by DXA: Tried and true? *Medicine and Science in Sports and Exercise, 27*, 1349-1353.
13. Lohman, T.G. (1986). Applicability of body composition techniques and constants for children and youth. *Exercise and Sport Sciences Reviews, 14*, 325-356.
14. Lohman, T.G. (1992). *Advances in body composition assessment*. Champaign, IL: Human Kinetics.
15. Lohman, T.G., Houtkooper, L., & Going, S.B. (1997). Body fat measurement goes high-tech: Not all are created equal. *ACSM's Health & Fitness Journal, 1*, 30-35.
16. Lohman, T.G., Roche, A.F., & Martorell, R. (1988). *Anthropometric standardization reference manual*. Champaign, IL: Human Kinetics.
17. McCrory, M.A., Gomez, T.D., Bernauer, E.M., & Mole, P.A. (1995). Evaluation of a new air displacement plethysmograph for measuring human body composition. *Medicine and Science in Sports and Exercise, 27*, 1686-1691.
18. Mokdad, A.H., Serdula, M.K., Dietz, W.H., Bowman, B.A., Marks, J.S., & Koplan, J.P. (1999). The spread of the obesity epidemic in the United States, 1991-1998. *Journal of the American Medical Association, 282*(16), 1519-1522.
19. Must, A., Spandano, J., Coakley, E.H., Field, A.E., Colditz, G., & Dietz, W.H. (1999). The disease burden associated with overweight and obesity. *Journal of the American Medical Association, 282*(16), 1523-1529.
20. National Heart, Lung, and Blood Institute. (1998). *Clinical guidelines on the identification, evaluation, and treatment of overweight and obesity in adults* (NIH Publication No. 98-4083). Bethesda, MD: National Institutes of Health, National Heart, Lung, and Blood Institute.
21. National Institutes of Health. (1994). *Bioelectrical impedance analysis in body composition measurement: NIH technology assessment conference statement*. Bethesda, MD: National Institutes of Health.
22. Pollock, M.L., Schmidt, D.H., & Jackson, A.S. (1980). Measurement of cardiorespiratory fitness and body composition in a clinical setting. *Comprehensive Therapy, 6*, 12-27.
23. Schutte, J.E., Townsend, E., Hugg, J., Shoup, R., Malina, R., & Blomqvist, C. (1984). Density of lean body mass is greater in blacks than in whites. *Journal of Applied Physiology: Respiratory, Environmental, and Exercise Physiology, 56*, 1647-1649.
24. Siri, W.E. (1961). Body composition from fluid spaces and density: Analysis of methods. In J. Brozek & A. Henschel (Eds.), *Techniques for measuring body composition* (pp. 223-244). Washington, DC: National Academy of Sciences.
25. Sizer, F., & Whitney, E. (1994). *Hamilton and Whitney's nutrition: Concepts and controversies*. St. Paul: West.
26. Weltman, A., Levine, S., Seip, R.L., & Tran, Z.V. (1988). Accurate assessment of body composition in obese females. *American Journal of Clinical Nutrition, 48*, 1179-1183.
27. Weltman, A., Seip, R.L., & Tran, Z.V. (1987). Practical assessment of body composition in obese males. *Human Biology, 59*, 523-536.
28. Wilmore, J.H. (1969). A simplified method for determination of residual volume. *Journal of Applied Physiology, 27*, 96-100.

seven

Nutrition

Dixie L. Thompson

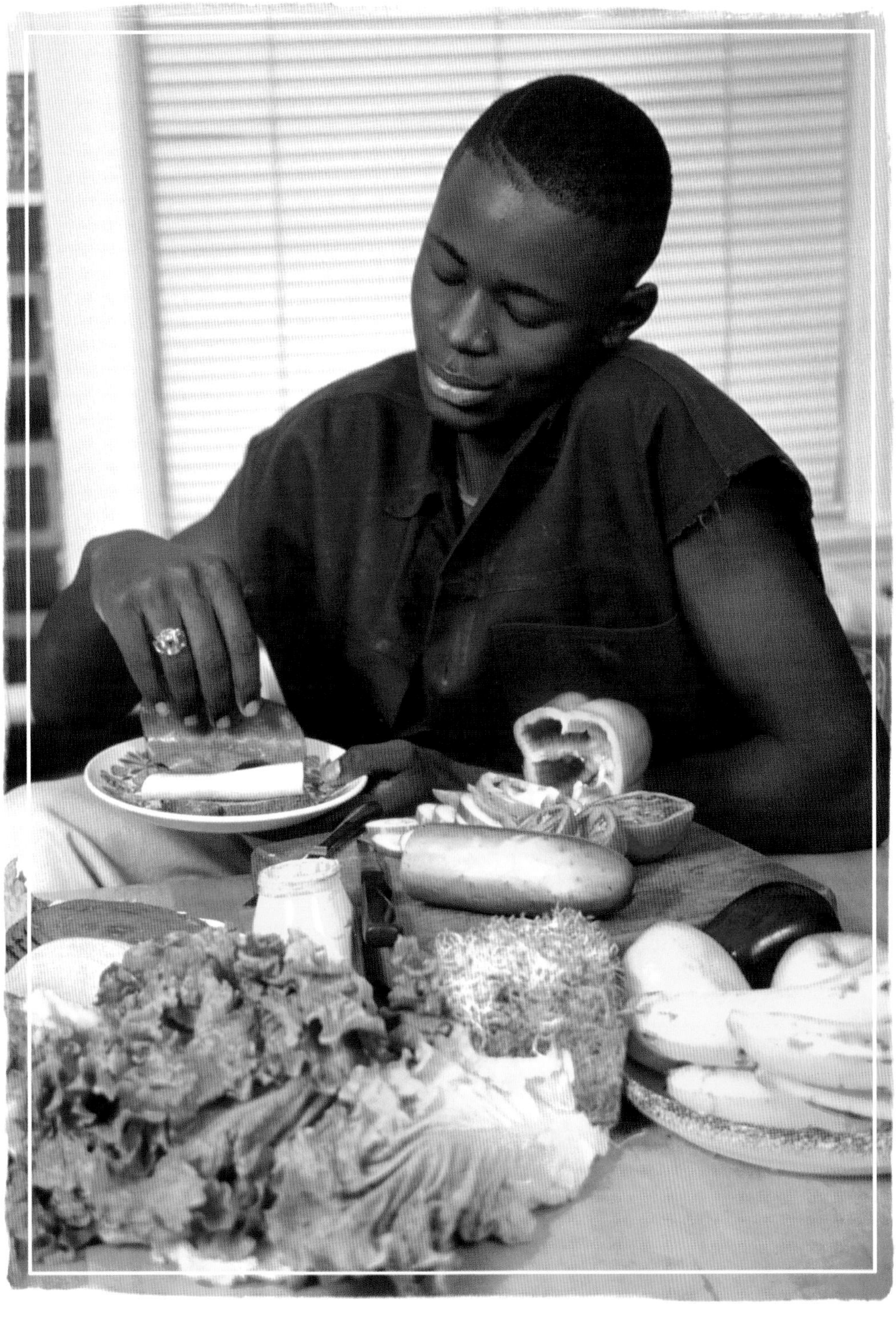

© Cleo Photography

Objectives

The reader will be able to do the following:

1. List the six essential nutrients, describe their role in the proper functioning of the body, and list the recommended percentage of calories from carbohydrates.
2. List the recommended percentage of calories from fats.
3. List the recommended percentage of calories from proteins.
4. Understand the importance of vitamins and minerals, and how to optimize them in the typical diet.
5. Describe assessment of dietary intake for healthy adults.
6. Describe the role of the United States Department of Agriculture (USDA) Food Guide Pyramid and the U.S. Dietary Guidelines in making healthy nutritional choices.
7. Explain the relationship between the blood lipid profile and cardiovascular disease and the role of diet and exercise in modifying blood lipids.
8. Describe appropriate methods for maintaining hydration during exercise.
9. Discuss the protein, vitamin, and mineral needs of a physically active person.
10. Describe an appropriate means for maximizing glycogen storage before competition.
11. List the three components of the female athlete triad.

Good nutrition results from a diet in which foods are eaten in the proper quantities and with the needed distribution of nutrients to maintain good health in the present and in the future. **Malnutrition**, on the other hand, is the outcome of a diet in which there is an underconsumption, overconsumption, or unbalanced consumption of nutrients that leads to disease or an increased susceptibility to disease. Implicit in these definitions is the fact that proper nutrition is essential to good health. A history of poor nutritional choices will eventually lead to health consequences. As will become apparent in this chapter, poor nutritional choices have been linked to chronic conditions including cardiovascular disease and cancer.

The public is bombarded with messages about nutrition, and it is often difficult for the layperson to distinguish good information from bad. The HFI can play an important role in conveying basic nutritional information. It should be emphasized, however, that a registered dietitian is the appropriate health care professional to handle the nutritional counseling of individuals with special needs.

Six Classes of Essential Nutrients

Many substances are necessary for the proper functioning of the body. **Nutrients** are substances that the body requires for the maintenance of health, growth, and repair of tissues. Nutrients can be divided into six classes: carbohydrates, fats, proteins, vitamins, minerals, and water (22).

Carbohydrates

Carbohydrates are nutrients composed of carbon, hydrogen, and oxygen and are essential sources of energy in the body. Carbohydrates can be subdivided into three categories: monosaccharides, di-saccharides, and polysaccharides (22). The monosaccharides and disaccharides are sometimes called simple sugars. Simple sugars provide a significant contribution to the caloric content of foods such as fruit juices, soft drinks, and candy. The most important simple sugar in the human body is **glucose**. The molecular formula for glucose is $C_6H_{12}O_6$. The polysaccharides are commonly referred to as complex carbohydrates or starches. These substances are formed by combining simple sugars. Rice, pasta, and whole grain breads are just a few examples of foods that are high in complex carbohydrates. When carbohydrates are stored in the human body, glucose molecules are joined together to form large molecules called **glycogen**. Glycogen is stored in the liver and skeletal muscle.

Grains, vegetables, and fruits are excellent sources of carbohydrates. It is recommended that at least 55 to 60% of the total number of calories consumed

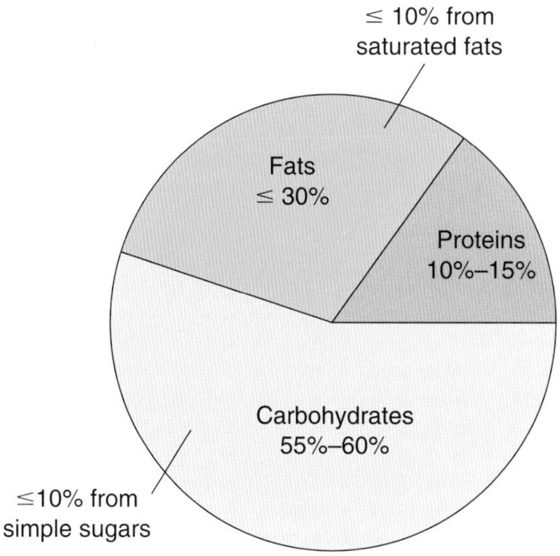

Figure 7.1 Recommended intake of carbohydrates, fats, and proteins.

come from carbohydrates (18) (figure 7.1). It is further recommended that 10% or less of the total calories consumed come from simple sugars. The reason for eating more complex rather than simple carbohydrates is the higher **nutrient density** in complex carbohydrates. Nutrient density refers to amount of essential nutrients in a food in comparison with the calories it contains. For example, a candy bar (simple sugars) has a low nutrient density, whereas a slice of whole grain bread (complex carbohydrates) contains a high nutrient density.

One of the benefits of consuming many foods that are high in complex carbohydrates is that they also typically contain **dietary fiber**. Dietary fiber refers to substances found in plants that cannot be broken down by the human digestive system. Although fiber cannot be digested, it helps prevent cancers of the digestive system, hemorrhoids, and constipation because it helps food move quickly and easily through the digestive system. It is recommended that people consume 20 to 35 g of fiber per day (18). Excellent sources of dietary fiber are grains, vegetables, legumes, and fruit.

As mentioned earlier, carbohydrates are a vital source of energy in the human body. During high-intensity exercise, carbohydrates are the primary fuel source for ATP production. When carbohydrates are broken down in the human body, they yield approximately 4 kcal of energy per gram. This relationship also can be viewed from the food intake perspective. For example, a person who eats 10 g of carbohydrate will have approximately 40 kcal of energy to use or store.

Focus on Glycemic Index

When carbohydrates are ingested, blood glucose rises and subsequently insulin is released from the pancreas. The rapidity with which blood glucose rises after food intake is represented by the **glycemic index**. Foods with a high glycemic index cause a rapid spike in blood glucose, whereas foods with a low glycemic index do not. A number of factors (biochemical composition, preparation method, fiber content) affect glycemic index. Some examples of high glycemic index foods are baked potatoes, white rice, and soft drinks. Lower glycemic index foods include apples, kidney beans, and milk. For more information on the glycemic index of foods, see Walberg-Rankin (25).

Some evidence exists that consuming a diet rich in low glycemic index foods helps fight cardiovascular disease, obesity, and type 2 diabetes (14). Proposed benefits of low glycemic index diets are increased satiety, lower triglycerides, higher HDL-C, and improved insulin sensitivity. Although some evidence exists that health may be improved by eating more lower glycemic index foods, this issue is still under investigation. In fact, recent dietary guidelines from the American Diabetes Association (ADA) do not emphasize the use of glycemic index in making food choices. The ADA stresses attention to the total amount of carbohydrate rather than glycemic index. The ADA suggests that a diet which promotes a healthy weight and is low in fat is preferable for preventing and treating type 2 diabetes and its comorbidities.

1 In Review

The six classes of nutrients are carbohydrates, fats, proteins, vitamins, minerals, and water. The metabolism of 1 g of carbohydrate yields 4 kcal of energy. Carbohydrates should contribute at least 55 to 60% of one's daily calories, with no more than 10% of calories from simple sugars.

Fats

Fats are an essential part of a healthy diet and serve vital functions in the human body. Among the functions performed by fats in the body are temperature regulation, protection of vital organs, distribution of some vitamins, energy production, and formation of component parts of cell membranes (22). Like carbohydrates, fats are composed of carbon, hydrogen, and oxygen; however, their chemical structure is different. **Triglycerides** are the primary storage form of fats in the body. These large molecules are composed of three fatty acid chains connected to a glycerol backbone. The majority of triglycerides are stored in adipose cells (i.e., fat cells). The aerobic metabolism of triglycerides provides much of the energy needed during rest and low-intensity exercise. When metabolized, 1 g of fat yields 9 kcal of energy. **Phospholipids** are another type of fat found in the body. As the name implies, these fats have phosphate groups attached to them. Phospholipids are important constituents of cell membranes. **Cholesterol** is a sterol (a fatty substance in which the carbon, hydrogen, and oxygen atoms are arranged in rings). In addition to the cholesterol we consume in our diet, the body constantly produces cholesterol, which is used in forming cell membranes and making steroidal hormones. Meat and eggs are the major sources of cholesterol in the typical American diet; however, it is recommended that people consume no more than 300 mg of cholesterol per day (24). However, for those attempting to lower blood lipids, limiting cholesterol intake to 200 mg per day is recommended (10). **Lipoproteins** are large molecules that allow fats to travel through the bloodstream. The impact of lipoproteins on cardiovascular health is discussed later in the chapter.

Both animals and plants provide sources of fat. It generally is recommended that no more that 30% of one's total calories be composed of dietary fats (24) (figure 7.1). Saturated fats come primarily from animal sources and are typically solid at room temperature. Plant sources of saturated fats are palm oil, coconut oil, and cocoa butter. The chemical structure of saturated fats contains no double bonds between carbon atoms; in other words, the fat is "saturated" with hydrogen atoms. A high intake of saturated fat is directly related to increased cardiovascular disease. Therefore, one should limit consumption of saturated fats to no more than 10% of total calories (24). Unsaturated fats contain fewer hydrogen atoms because some double bonding between carbon atoms exists. These fats are typically liquid at room temperature. Corn, peanut, canola, and soybean oil are sources of unsaturated fats. Monounsaturated fats (e.g., olive and canola oil) have a single double bond in the fatty acid chain. Polyunsaturated fats (e.g., fish, corn, soybean, and peanut oil) have two or more double bonds between carbon atoms. The impact of various kinds of fats on health risk will be discussed later in the chapter.

2 In Review

No more than 30% of one's daily calories should come from fats, and no more than 10% of calories should come from saturated fats. Cholesterol intake should be limited to 300 mg per day. The breakdown of 1 g of fat yields 9 kcal of energy.

Proteins

Proteins are substances composed of carbon, hydrogen, oxygen, and nitrogen. All proteins are made by combining **amino acids**. Amino acids are molecules composed of an amino group (NH_3), a carboxyl group (COO), a hydrogen atom, a central carbon atom, and a side chain. The difference in the side chains gives unique characteristics to each amino acid. Amino acids can combine in innumerable ways to form proteins, and it is estimated that tens of thousands of different types of proteins exist in the body. The ordering of the amino acids provides the unique structure and function of proteins. The unique chemical properties and structures of proteins allow them to serve many different functions in the body. Some of the most common functions of protein are listed next:

- Carries oxygen (hemoglobin)
- Fights disease (antibodies)
- Catalyzes reactions (enzymes)
- Allows muscle contraction (actin, myosin, and troponin)
- Acts as a connective tissue (collagen)
- Clots blood (prothrombin)
- Acts as a messenger (protein hormones such as growth hormone)

Of the 20 amino acids found in the body, most can be constructed from other substances in the body; however, there are eight **essential amino acids** that must be a part of one's regular diet. Eating a variety of protein-containing foods is typically adequate to meet this need. There are proteins in both meat products and plant products. Animal sources of protein such as meat, milk, and eggs contain the eight essential amino acids. Plant sources of protein such as beans, starchy vegetables, nuts, and grains do not always contain all eight essential amino acids. Because of this, vegetarians must consume a variety of protein-containing foods. Examples of foods that contain complimentary proteins are legumes and grains, vegetables and nuts, and legumes and seeds (8).

It is recommended that proteins make up 10 to 15% of one's daily calories (figure 7.1). This will ensure adequate protein for the growth, maintenance, and repair of cells. The protein requirement for adults generally is met by consuming 0.8 g of protein for each kilogram of body weight (19). As discussed later in this chapter, individuals who are training intensely may have higher protein requirements. In addition, children have higher protein needs to support their continually growing bodies. The recommended protein intake is approximately 2 g/kg for infants, 1.2 g/kg for 1- to 3-year-olds, 1.1 g/kg for 4- to 6-year-olds, 1 g/kg for 7- to 14-year-olds, and 0.9 g/kg for 15- to 18-year-old boys (19).

In addition to the functions of proteins listed previously, these molecules can be metabolized for energy production. The breakdown of 1 g of protein yields approximately 4 kcal of energy to be used by the body. The contribution of protein to resting energy needs or energy needs during exercise is quite small (<5%) in well-nourished individuals. During very long bouts of exercise (>1 hr) or when a person is not well nourished, protein may supply more of the body's energy needs, possibly up to 15%.

3 In Review

Proteins are made of amino acids and serve numerous functions. To ensure that all needed amino acids are available in adequate amounts, people should eat a variety of protein-containing foods each day. The breakdown of 1 g of protein yields 4 kcal of energy.

Vitamins

Vitamins are organic substances that are essential to the normal functioning of the human body. Although vitamins do not contain energy to be used by the body, they are essential in the metabolism of fats, carbohydrates, and proteins. The 13 vitamins are needed for numerous processes including blood clotting, protein synthesis, and bone formation. Because of the critical role vitamins play, it is necessary that they exist in proper quantities in the body. The major functions, important dietary sources, and the recommended intakes of vitamins are listed in table 7.1. There are two major classifications of vitamins: fat-soluble and water-soluble.

The chemical structure of fat-soluble vitamins causes them to be transported and stored with lipids. The four fat-soluble vitamins are A, D, E, and K. Because these vitamins are stored in the body with fats, it is not necessary to continually ingest large amounts of them; however, a small daily intake of each is recommended.

The B vitamins and vitamin C are water-soluble vitamins. Water-soluble vitamins are not stored in large quantities and therefore must be consumed daily. Deficiencies related to water-soluble vitamins such as scurvy (vitamin C deficiency) and beriberi (thiamin deficiency) may appear in a rather short period of time. Overconsumption of either fat-soluble or water-soluble vitamins can lead to toxic effects; however, because fat-soluble vitamins are stored in the body, the potential for overdose with these substances is greater (8).

Focus on Antioxidant Vitamins

During metabolic processes, molecules or fragments of molecules are formed that can damage the body's tissues. These **free radicals** have at least one unpaired electron in their outer shells; thus, they are very chemically reactive. Lipid-rich cell membranes and DNA are highly susceptible to the effects of free radicals, and cell damage can occur when free radicals accumulate. For example, development of atherosclerosis is linked with free radical formation. Fortunately, mechanisms exist to diminish the effects of free radicals. In addition to several enzymes that naturally occur in cells, some vitamins have properties that allow them to react with free radicals. These **antioxidant vitamins** have received a great deal of media attention in the past few years. These substances are hypothesized to counteract the effects of aging and decrease the likelihood of developing cardiovascular disease and cancer. **Beta-carotene** (a precursor of vitamin A), vitamin C, and vitamin E are highly touted antioxidant substances. Several large epidemiological studies are currently underway that may help us understand more about the protective function of these substances. Because of the potential for toxic effects from an overdose of antioxidants, it is wise to avoid overconsumption of these substances (see table 7.1).

Table 7.1 Vitamins: Functions, Sources, and Dietary Reference Intakes

Vitamin	Functions	Sources	Adult RDA[a]		UL[b]
			Men	Women	
Thiamin (B_1)	Functions as part of a coenzyme to aid utilization of energy	Whole grains, nuts, lean pork	1.2 mg	1.1 mg	ND
Riboflavin (B_2)	Involved in energy metabolism as part of a coenzyme	Milk, yogurt, cheese	1.3 mg	1.1 mg	ND
Niacin	Facilitates energy production in cells	Lean meat, fish, poultry, grains	16 mg	14 mg	35 mg
B_6	Absorbs and metabolizes protein; aids in red blood cell formation	Lean meat, vegetables, whole grains	1.3 mg	1.3 mg	100 mg
Pantothenic acid	Aids in metabolism of carbohydrate, fat, and protein	Whole-grain cereals, bread, dark green vegetables	5 mg*	5 mg*	ND
Folic acid	Functions as coenzyme in synthesis of nucleic acids and protein	Green vegetables, beans, whole-wheat products	400 μg	400 μg	1000 μg
B_{12}	Involved in synthesis of nucleic acids, red blood cell formation	Only in animal foods, not plant foods	2.4 μg	2.4 μg	ND
Biotin	Coenzyme in synthesis of fatty acids and glycogen formation	Egg yolk, dark green vegetables	30 μg	30 μg	ND
C	Intracellular maintenance of bone, capillaries, and teeth	Citrus fruits, green peppers, tomatoes	90 mg	75 mg	2000 mg
A	Vision; formation and maintenance of skin and mucous membranes	Carrots, sweet potatoes, margarine, butter, liver	900 μg	700 μg	3000 μg
D	Aids in growth and formation of bones and teeth; promotes calcium absorption	Eggs, tuna, liver, fortified milk	5 μg*	5 μg*	50 μg
E	Protects polyunsaturated fats; prevents cell membrane damage	Vegetable oils, whole-grain cereal and bread, green leafy vegetables	15 mg	15 mg	1000 mg
K	Important in blood clotting	Green leafy vegetables, peas, potatoes	120 μg*	90 μg*	ND

[a]Values are Recommended Daily Allowance (RDA) for adults 19 to 50 years of age, unless marked with an asterisk. The requirements may vary for children, older adults, and pregnant or lactating women. *Values are Adequate Intakes (AI), indicating that sufficient data to set the RDA are unavailable.

[b]Tolerable Upper Intake Levels (UL) for adults 19 to 50 years of age. Intakes above the UL may lead to negative health consequences.

ND = not yet determined.

Adapted from Franks and Howley 1989.

Minerals

Minerals are inorganic elements that serve a variety of functions in the human body. The minerals that appear in the largest quantities (calcium, phosphorus, potassium, sulfur, sodium, chloride, and magnesium) are often called macrominerals or major minerals. Other minerals are also essential to normal functioning of the body, but because they exist in smaller quantities, they are called microminerals, or trace elements. The functions, dietary sources, and recommended intake of minerals are listed in table 7.2.

Calcium is a mineral that often is consumed in inadequate amounts by Americans. Calcium is important in the mineralization of bone, muscle contraction, and transmission of nervous impulses. **Osteoporosis** is a disease characterized by a decrease in the total amount of bone mineral in the body and by a decrease in the strength of the remaining bone. This condition is most common in the elderly but also may exist in younger people who have diets inadequate in calcium, vitamin D, or both. It is estimated that in the United States, osteoporosis results in approximately 1.5 million fractures per year with resultant health care costs of $10 to $15 billion (17). Maximal bone density is achieved during the early adult years, and during older adult years bone density declines in everyone. Those who achieve the highest bone density and maintain adequate intakes of calcium and vitamin D are most protected from the ravages of osteoporosis. The NIH recommendations for calcium intake for Americans are listed in table 7.3 (16). Milk, dark green vegetables, and nuts are excellent sources of calcium. For example, a 30-year-old male should consume 1000 mg of calcium daily. One cup (8 oz) of 1% milk has approximately 300 mg of calcium, which would be almost one third of this daily recommendation.

Iron is another mineral that is often underconsumed by Americans, particularly women and children. In fact, the most prevalent nutrient deficiency in the United States is iron deficiency (8). In addition to being a critical component of hemoglobin and myoglobin, iron is important in immune function, in the formation of brain neurotransmitters, and in the functioning of the electron transport chain (8). The oxygen-carrying properties of hemoglobin depend on the presence of iron. There is a continual turnover of red blood cells in the body, and much of the iron used to form new hemoglobin comes from old red blood cells. However, there is a daily need for iron, and if iron reserves (liver, spleen, bone marrow) and iron intake are inadequate, hemoglobin cannot be formed. The resultant condition is **iron-deficiency anemia**. In this condition, the amount of hemoglobin in red blood cells is reduced, which decreases the capacity of the blood to transport oxygen. The recommended intake of iron for males and postmenopausal women is 8 mg per day (12). For females during the child-bearing years, the recommended intake is 18 mg per day (12). Red meat and eggs are excellent sources of iron. Additionally, spinach, lima and navy beans, and prune juice are excellent vegetarian sources of iron. The consumption of vitamin C with meals increases the body's ability to absorb iron.

Sodium, on the other hand, is a mineral that many Americans overconsume. High sodium intake has been linked with hypertension. It is suggested that adults limit their sodium intake to no more than 2400 mg per day (18, 24). People can substantially reduce their sodium intake by limiting consumption of processed foods and decreasing the amount of salt added to foods when cooking (24).

Water

Water is considered an essential nutrient because of its vital role in the normal functioning of the body. Water contributes approximately 65% to 75% of the total body weight and is essential in creating the environment in which all metabolic processes occur. Water is necessary to regulate temperature and transport substances throughout the body.

It is recommended that each day a person ingest 1 to 1.5 ml of water for each calorie expended (19). For most adults, drinking approximately 2.5 L (10 glasses) of water each day will fulfill this requirement. As discussed later in this chapter, this need is higher for individuals exercising intensely. Water is consumed in both food and beverages. It is suggested that individuals limit their intake of caffeinated beverages because of the diuretic effects of these products.

4 In Review

Vitamins, minerals, and water do not provide energy, but they are essential in many other ways to the healthy functioning of the body. In general, Americans would benefit from limiting sodium consumption (to decrease blood pressure), increasing calcium intake (to improve bone strength), and increasing iron ingestion (to prevent anemia).

Table 7.2 Minerals: Functions, Sources, and Dietary Reference Intakes

Mineral	Functions	Sources	Adult RDA[a]		UL[b]
			Men	Women	
Calcium	Bones, teeth, blood clotting, nerve and muscle function	Milk, sardines, dark green vegetables, nuts	1000 mg*	1000 mg*	2500 mg
Chloride	Nerve and muscle function water balance (with sodium)	Table salt	750 mg	750 mg	ND
Magnesium	Bone growth; nerve, muscle, and enzyme function	Nuts, seafood, whole grains, leafy green vegetables	420 mg	320 mg	350 mg[c]
Phosphorus	Bone, teeth, energy transfer	Meats, poultry, seafood, eggs, milk, beans	700 mg	700 mg	4000 mg
Potassium	Nerve and muscle function	Fresh vegetables, bananas, citrus fruits, milk, meats, fish	2000 mg	2000 mg	ND
Sodium	Nerve and muscle function, water balance	Table salt	500 mg	500 mg	ND
Chromium	Glucose metabolism	Meats, liver, whole grains, dried beans	35 µg*	25 µg*	ND
Copper	Enzyme function, energy production	Meats, seafood, nuts, grains	900 µg	900 µg	10,000 µg
Fluoride	Bone and teeth growth	Drinking water, fish, milk	4 mg	3 mg	10 mg
Iodine	Thyroid hormone formation	Iodized salt, seafood	150 µg	150 µg	1100 µg
Iron	O_2 transport in red blood cells; enzyme function	Red meat, liver, eggs, beans, leafy vegetables, shellfish	8 mg	18 mg	45 mg
Manganese	Enzyme function	Whole grains, nuts, fruits, vegetables	2.3 mg*	1.8 mg*	11 mg
Molybdenum	Energy metabolism in cells	Whole grains, organ meats, peas, beans	45 µg	45 µg	2000 µg
Selenium	Works with vitamin E	Meat, fish, whole grains, eggs	55 µg	55 µg	400 µg
Zinc	Part of enzymes, growth	Meat, shellfish, yeast, whole grains	11 mg	8 mg	40 mg

[a]Values are Recommended Daily Allowance (RDA) for adults 19 to 50 years of age, unless marked with an asterisk. The requirements may vary for children, older adults, and pregnant or lactating women. *Values are Adequate Intakes (AI), indicating that sufficient data to set the RDA are unavailable.

[b]Tolerable Upper Intake Levels (UL) for adults 19 to 50 years of age. Intakes above the UL may lead to negative health consequences.

[c]This refers to pharmacological agents only, and not amounts contained in food and water. No evidence of ill effects from ingestion of naturally occurring amounts in food and water.

ND = not yet determined.

Adapted from Franks and Howley 1989.

Table 7.3 Guidelines for Calcium Intake

Age	Recommended intake (mg/day)
0–6 months	400
6–12 months	600
1–5 years	800
6–10 years	800–1200
11–24 years	1200–1500
Women 25–50 years	1000
Pregnant or lactating women	1200–1500
Postmenopausal on estrogen	1000
Postmenopausal without estrogen	1500
Men 25–65 years	1000
All people >65 years	1500

Note. Up to 2000 mg/day appears safe in most individuals.
Data from NIH Consensus Statement on Optimal Calcium Intake (16).

Assessing Dietary Intake

Examining a person's dietary habits allows the HFI to make suggestions about how to better meet nutritional and weight loss / weight maintenance goals. This information can be gathered through the use of a food diary in which the client records everything that is consumed. These records typically are kept for 3 or 7 days and usually are adequate to provide a general idea of a person's nutritional habits. If a 3-day food diary is kept, it is important that one of the days be a weekend day because many people eat differently on weekends than on weekdays (13). Once the records are compiled, a number of software packages can be used to analyze the diet. Although food diaries provide important information, there are problems with this practice (26):

- People tend to underreport what they eat.
- People do not keep records specific enough to provide quality information.
- People often temporarily change how they eat when they are required to record their food intake.

The HFI can take steps to minimize these problems. First, make sure that the client understands the importance of completely and honestly recording what is eaten. Emphasize to the client that the accuracy and usefulness of the feedback depend on the information he or she provides and that the client is not going to be criticized or judged for what he or she has eaten. Additionally, the HFI should provide the client with models or descriptions of portion sizes. For more information on serving sizes, see the USDA's Home and Garden Bulletin 252 (23). Providing explicit instructions about how to complete the food diary will allow the client to provide a more useful and accurate record. Additionally, the food diary should be user friendly and include cues to elicit complete responses. A sample food diary and instructions are provided on form 7.1.

As indicated earlier, the HFI can provide general nutrition information to the public. Clients with special metabolic needs such as diabetes mellitus should be referred to a registered dietitian. Comparing dietary intake to **Dietary Reference Intake** (DRI) can be particularly informative (11). The DRI is a set of values for nutrients, separated by age and sex, which includes the **Recommended Dietary Allowance** (RDA, amount found to be adequate for approximately 97% of the population) or the **Adequate Intake** (AI, amount considered adequate although insufficient data exist to establish RDA) and **Tolerable Upper Intake Levels** (UL, highest intake believed to pose no health risk). For the typical client, the following special areas of emphasis should be included in a nutritional profile:

- Total calories
- Percentage of calories from fats, carbohydrates, and protein
- Amount of saturated fat and cholesterol
- Sodium intake
- Iron intake
- Calcium intake
- Fiber

It is also important to examine the food diary for emotional and / or social cues to eating behaviors. For example, some people eat when depressed or only eat when alone. This type of information can be quite helpful in making behavior changes needed for weight loss and weight maintenance. More information on this topic is covered in chapter 11.

5 In Review

Food diaries can be used to assess dietary practices. The client must provide detailed information for the dietary assessment to be accurate.

form **7.1**

Sample Food Log

Instructions

1. Record everything you eat. This should include foods and beverages eaten at meals and snacks.
2. Record carefullly how the food was prepared. Be as descriptive as possible (e.g., fried in corn oil, broiled in 1 T of margarine).
3. Be sure to indicate the amount of food eaten. Use typical household measures when possible (t = teaspoon; T = tablespoon; c = cup; oz = ounce).
4. Provide brand names and labels for packaged foods.
5. For composite foods such as sandwiches, casseroles, and soups, indicate the ingredients contained in the food. For example, a turkey sandwich might be described as 2 slices of whole wheat bread, 1 oz of baked turkey breast without skin, 1 slice of tomato, 2 leaves of iceberg lettuce, 1 T light mayonnaise.
6. Indicate where and with whom you were when you ate. Also describe your feelings at the time—were you worried, content, lonely, stressed? (Be honest with yourself.)
7. Carry this form with you so that you can write down foods as they are eaten. Do not wait until the end of the day to record your food intake.

Food/Drink	**Description** (e.g., amount, cooking method, brand name)	**Location** (e.g., place, people, alone)	**Feelings** (e.g., hunger, anger, joy)	**Time**

From Edward T. Howley and B. Don Franks, 2003, *Health Fitness Instructor's Handbook*, 4th ed. (Champaign, IL: Human Kinetics).

Recommendations for Dietary Intake

Many different plans have been suggested to guide food intake. The USDA has suggested using the **food guide pyramid** as a guide to eating (24). The food guide pyramid is reproduced in figure 7.2, along with a quantification of serving sizes. This plan separates foods into six categories:

- Bread, cereal, rice, and pasta group (6-11 servings)
- Fruit group (2-4 servings)
- Vegetable group (3-5 servings)
- Milk, yogurt, and cheese group (2-3 servings)
- Meat, poultry, fish, dry beans, eggs, and nuts group (2-3 servings)
- Fats, oils, and sweets (use sparingly)

This helpful guide to eating provides a suggested number of servings for each group. It is important to note that there is a recommended range of servings for each group. The low end of the range should be used by a person who is smaller or less active, and a person who is very active or large should consume the higher number of servings. In addition to using the food guide pyramid to guide nutritional choices, the USDA makes other general nutritional recommendations:

- Eat a variety of foods.
- Engage in regular physical activity.
- Achieve and maintain a healthy weight.
- Choose a diet with plenty of grain products, vegetables, and fruits.
- Choose a diet low in saturated fat and cholesterol.
- Choose a diet moderate in sugars.
- Choose a diet moderate in salt and sodium.
- Drink alcoholic beverages in moderation, if at all.

The entire USDA Dietary Guidelines for Americans (24) can be accessed via the Internet from the

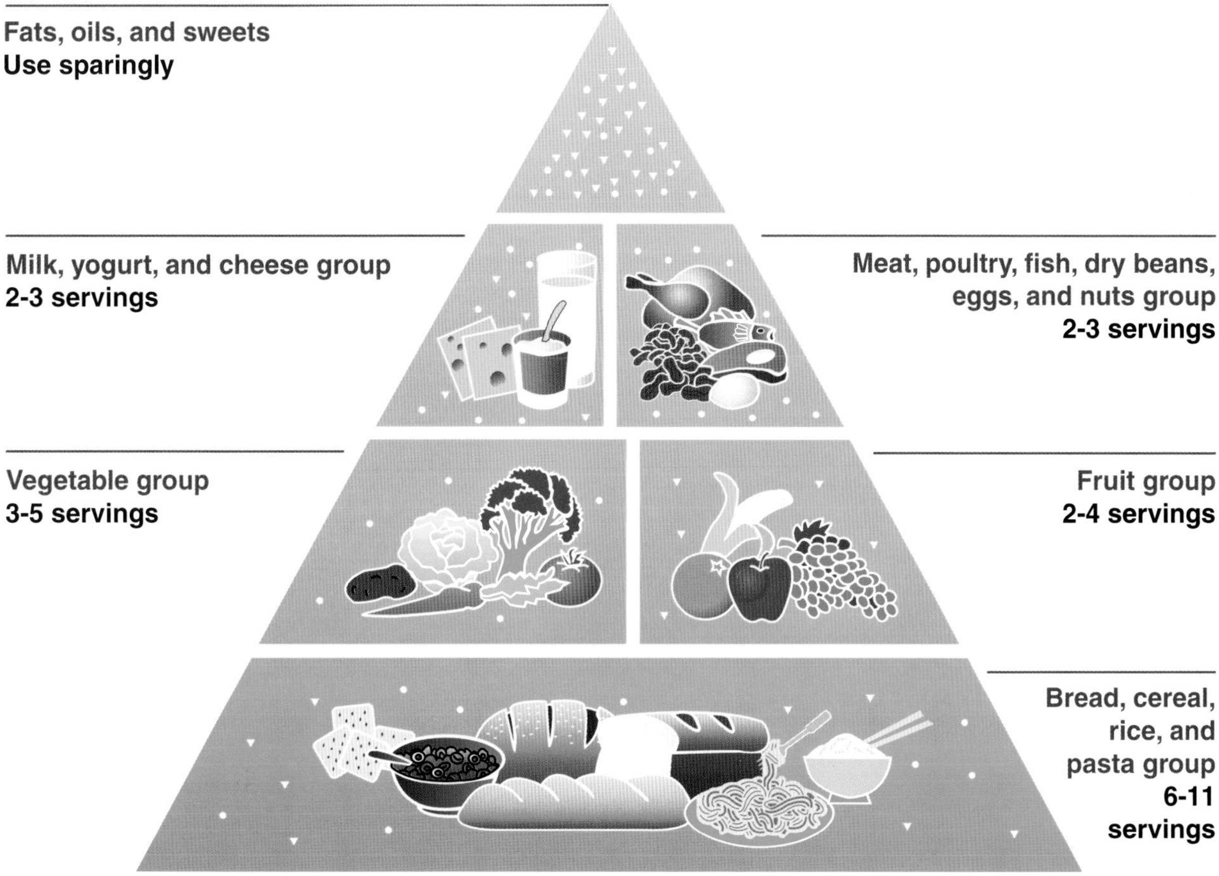

Figure 7.2 The food guide pyramid.

usda.gov Web site. These guidelines can be used in an attempt to meet the RDAs (11, 19). The RDAs, developed by the National Research Council of the National Academy of Sciences, suggest levels that appear to be adequate to meet the nutritional needs of practically all healthy people. The RDAs were determined by estimating the average need for the nutrient and then increasing the value by 2 standard deviations. Ultimately, these recommendations are adequate for more than 97% of the population. The recommendations are divided into age and sex categories to allow more specificity. For nutrients about which less is known, an estimated AI is suggested. As mentioned previously, new guidelines also establish ULs for some nutrients. These ULs can be used to help prevent overdose. The Dietary Reference Intake (RDAs, AIs, and ULs) for various nutrients can be found on the Web site for National Academy Press (15).

The Food and Drug Administration publishes recommended **Daily Values (DV)** to be used in food labeling. The DVs were developed in an attempt to inform the public about the nutritional content of the foods they buy. All foods must have labels containing information about the total calories, fat (including saturated fat), cholesterol, sodium, carbohydrates (including dietary fiber), protein, and various vitamins and minerals. The nutritional labels also contain the percentage of the recommended DVs provided by the food. For example, the suggested DV for cholesterol is 300 mg; therefore, if a food contains 15 mg of cholesterol, it will constitute 5% of the recommended daily intake of cholesterol. Additional information on DVs can be found in the *Dietary Guidelines for Americans* (24).

6 In Review

The Food Guide Pyramid provides information about the amount and types of food that should be consumed daily. The RDAs, AIs, and ULs provide specific information about needed nutrient intake. DVs allow consumers to evaluate the nutritional content of foods.

Diet, Exercise, and the Blood Lipid Profile

Cardiovascular disease is the leading cause of death in the United States. One of the primary risk factors for development of cardiovascular disease is a poor blood lipid profile. Both diet and exercise can have positive effects on this very important risk factor.

Lipoproteins and Risk of Cardiovascular Disease

Because lipids are hydrophobic (i.e., not water soluble), they need to bind with some other substance to be transported in the blood. Lipoproteins are macromolecules composed of cholesterol, triglycerides, protein, and phospholipids. Classifications for these molecules are based on their size and makeup. The two classes of lipoproteins most closely linked with cardiovascular disease are low-density lipoproteins (LDL) and high-density lipoproteins (HDL). LDL transports cholesterol and triglycerides from the liver to be used in various cellular processes. HDL retrieves cholesterol from the body's cells and returns it to the liver to be metabolized.

Elevated levels of total cholesterol (the sum of all forms of cholesterol) and low-density lipoprotein cholesterol (LDL-C) are linked with the development of atherosclerotic plaque in the arteries. Increased levels of high-density lipoprotein cholesterol (HDL-C) help prevent the atherosclerotic process. According to the 2001 National Cholesterol Education Program (NCEP) guidelines, total cholesterol levels below 200 mg/dL and LDL-C values below 100 mg/dL are desirable (10). This recommendation is the same as previous guidelines for total cholesterol but establishes a more stringent value for LDL-C (100 compared with 130 mg/dL). Total cholesterol of 240 mg/dL or higher and LDL-C of 160 mg/dL or higher are considered high and are associated with greater risk of cardiovascular disease (10) (see table 7.4). In addition, HDL-C below 40 mg/dL is considered too low and HDL-C 60 mg/dL or higher is considered ideal (10). This lower limit for HDL-C is also more stringent than in previous years (40 compared with 35 mg/dL).

Effects of Diet and Exercise on the Blood Lipid Profile

Consuming a diet low in saturated fat and cholesterol, losing weight, and participating in regular aerobic exercise all have been linked to positive changes in the blood lipid profile. The 2001 NCEP guidelines (10) suggest that individuals follow a therapeutic lifestyle changes (TLC) diet to improve the blood lipid profile. The TLC diet supersedes the NCEP Step I and Step II diets previously recommended. The TLC diet includes the following dietary practices:

Table 7.4 Cholesterol Classification Categories Recommended by the Expert Panel on Detection, Evaluation, and Treatment of High Blood Cholesterol in Adults (10)

Total cholesterol	
<200	Desirable
200–239	Borderline high
≥240	High
LDL cholesterol	
<100	Optimal
100–129	Near or above optimal
130–159	Borderline high
160–189	High
≥190	Very high
HDL cholesterol	
<40	Low
≥60	High

Note. Values are mg/dl.

- Limiting total fat intake to 25% to 35% of calories (Note: If at the higher end of the range, care should be taken to ensure that most fats are monounsaturated.)
- Limiting saturated fat intake to 7%, polyunsaturated fat to 10%, and monounsaturated fat to 20% of calories
- Limiting cholesterol intake to <200 mg/day
- Limiting intake of **trans fats**

Focus on Trans Fats

Recent attention has been focused on the health risk of **trans fatty acids** (i.e., trans fats). Although small amounts of trans fats are found in animal products, the majority of these hydrogenated fats are found in processed foods produced by using fats from plants. The hydrogenation process causes a chemical transformation that changes the orientation of hydrogen atoms in the fat. This hardens the liquid oil and leads to a more stable product that is better suited for cooking. Consequently, many processed foods (e.g., cookies, chips, doughnuts, french fries) are prepared with trans fats. On food labels, items high in trans fats will have partially hydrogenated vegetable oils as a primary ingredient. The problem with trans fats is that they can be as harmful to the blood lipid profile as saturated fats. Trans fats elevate LDL-C and lower HDL-C. Therefore, trans fats should be avoided to improve the lipid profile.

The intake of some fats, such as omega-3 fatty acids, appears to benefit health. Omega-3 fatty acids are found in canola oil as well as fish such as salmon and tuna. Omega-3 fatty acids are polyunsaturated fats that get their name from the site of the first double bond in the fatty acid chain. American diets are typically low in omega-3 fatty acids and higher in omega-6 fatty acids (e.g., peanut, corn, and soybean oil). Bringing the intake of these two types of fats into better balance appears to improve the lipoprotein profile and lower the risk of cardiovascular disease (20).

People who engage in regular aerobic exercise and maintain a healthy weight typically have a better blood lipid profile than their sedentary counterparts. It is difficult to ascertain which of these changes are attributable to the exercise and which are related to a healthy body weight. It appears that the primary blood lipid changes attributable to aerobic exercise are increases in HDL-C and decreases in blood levels of triglycerides (9). Weight loss has been linked with lower total cholesterol, LDL-C, and triglycerides as well as higher HDL-C.

7 In Review

Elevated total cholesterol and LDL-C and depressed HDL-C are risk factors for development of cardiovascular disease. Aerobic exercise, weight loss, and low intake of saturated fat, trans fat, and cholesterol are effective means of improving the blood lipid profile.

Nutrition for Physically Active Individuals

As discussed previously, nutrition plays an important role in health. Proper nutrition is also essential for optimal performance during physical activity. The ACSM, ADA, and the Dietitians of Canada released a joint position statement in 2000 that addresses the needs of physically active adults (4). The HFI should be familiar with these guidelines to provide basic nutritional advice to clients who exercise regularly.

Hydration Before, During, and After Exercise

Sweating is the body's primary mechanism for heat dissipation during exercise. The amount of sweat lost during exercise depends on the environmental heat and humidity, the type and intensity of exercise, and individual characteristics. Dehydration reduces the body's capacity for sweating and can impair performance by decreasing strength, endurance, and coordination. In addition, dehydration increases the risk of heat cramps, heat exhaustion, and heat stroke (see chapter 25).

A person should consume 14 to 20 oz (400-600 ml) of water 2 hr before an endurance exercise bout (1, 4, 7) and then drink an additional 7 to 10 oz (200-300 ml) 10 to 20 min before beginning exercise (7). Fluid replacement during exercise is essential in activities that last an hour or longer, especially if they take place in hot, humid environments. During exercise one should drink approximately 150 to 350 ml (6-12 oz) of water every 15 to 20 min (4). Water that is slightly chilled (5-10° C) is suggested for increasing palatability and absorption (1).

In activities where large amounts of sweat are lost, it is important that the fluid is fully replaced. Weighing before and after these types of activities is recommended. One should drink approximately 16 to 24 oz (475-700 ml) of water for each pound of weight lost (4). If on subsequent days the weight has not returned to normal, additional water should be consumed before beginning exercise. For reviews of the hydration needs of athletes, refer to the position stands of the National Athletic Trainers' Association (7) and the ACSM (1).

8 In Review

Adequate hydration is essential to performance. Water should be consumed before, during, and after extended bouts of exercise.

Protein Intake for Athletes

It has been reported that athletes who are training intensely may benefit from increasing their protein intake above the level recommended for a sedentary person (i.e., 0.8 g/kg). An athlete training intensively in primarily endurance activities may benefit from consuming 1.2 to 1.4 g of protein per kilogram of body weight (4). For athletes engaging in high-intensity, high-volume strength and resistance training, a protein intake of up to 1.6 to 1.7 g/kg may be needed (4). To this point, most of the studies in this area have focused on male athletes, so little is known about the protein needs of women athletes (4).

The additional protein requirements of athletes should be met through food choices, not supplements. There is an upper limit to the rate at which muscle can be accrued; therefore, excessive protein intake (i.e., above the recommendations) does not enhance performance or increase muscle mass (4). Because of the higher caloric intake of intensively training athletes, a diet with the normal distribution of macronutrients (i.e., 55-60% carbohydrates, ≤30% fats, and 10-15% protein) typically contains adequate amounts of protein so that additional purposeful increases in protein intake are usually not necessary (4, 27).

Another issue that sometimes arises is the adequacy of protein intake for vegetarian athletes. Because plant proteins are not digested as well as animal proteins, it is suggested that athletes following a strict vegetarian diet consume 1.3 to 1.8 g of protein per kilogram of body weight (4).

Ergogenic Aids

The search for nutritional and pharmacological agents that improve performance has led to the marketing of numerous products touted as **ergogenic aids**. Some of these products (e.g., bee pollen, brewer's yeast) provide no physiological advantage. Other products such as caffeine may improve performance in some instances (27) and have been regulated by various sporting agencies such as the International Olympic Committee. Some ergogenic aids must be strictly avoided, such as anabolic steroids, because of severe and sometimes fatal side effects (21). The ACSM has released a number of "Current Comments" on potential ergogenic aids.

Vitamins and minerals are often consumed by athletes in amounts higher than the RDA in an attempt to improve performance. There is no evidence that this costly practice enhances performance; however, if an athlete's diet provides inadequate amounts of any nutrient, health and performance could suffer (27). The two minerals that often need to be increased in the diet are iron and calcium (6). The most common mineral deficiency among athletes is iron deficiency (27). For athletes with anemia, increased iron consumption is advised and in many cases will improve performance (27). For female athletes with menstrual cycle irregularities, calcium supplementation often is prescribed to promote bone health. See chapter 21 for more information on this topic.

Focus on Creatine Supplementation

Creatine phosphate, a high-energy compound found in skeletal muscle, is an important source of energy during bursts of high-intensity exercise. Creatine supplementation is used by athletes to increase amounts of creatine phosphate in muscle in an effort to enhance high-intensity exercise performance. Studies demonstrate that creatine supplementation does improve high-intensity exercise performance, particularly repeated bouts of high-intensity cycling, under laboratory conditions. Less is known about the impact on performance under competitive conditions. Creatine supplementation also is associated with weight gain (~1 kg) as a result of water retention. It is unclear if this extra weight could impede, rather than enhance, performance in weight-bearing activities such as sprinting. There are some reports of muscle cramping and gastrointestinal distress with creatine use. No studies have examined the side effects of long-term creatine use. For more information on creatine supplementation, refer to the ACSM *Current Comments* by Kraemer and Volek (3) and the review by Williams (27).

9 In Review

The typical protein RDA for adults of 0.8 g/kg appears inadequate for athletes. People who are training intensely should consume 1 to 1.5 g of protein per kilogram of body weight. Ergogenic aids are pharmacological or nutritional agents thought to improve athletic performance. Although a few of these products may enhance performance, there are many highly touted products with unproven results. In healthy, well-nourished athletes, extra vitamins and minerals (i.e., above the RDAs) do not improve performance.

Carbohydrate Loading and Intake During Exercise

Adequate intake of carbohydrates is necessary for optimal athletic performance in endurance events. Glucose is the major source of energy during exercise; when blood glucose levels decline, the ability to continue exercise is limited. A physically active person should routinely consume a diet in which 60 to 65% of the calories are carbohydrates. For an athlete who trains heavily on consecutive days or who engages in frequent exhaustive exercise bouts, a diet providing 6 to 10 g of carbohydrate per kilogram of body weight is recommended (4).

Carbohydrate loading is a practice used to maximize glycogen storage before competition. This practice is most beneficial for athletes who compete in events requiring continuous activity lasting longer than an hour, such as marathon running. The ADA recommends the following practices to enhance glycogen storage (5):

- Consume a diet in which 65 to 70% of the total calories are carbohydrates.
- Decrease the duration of exercise bouts during the week before competition.
- Rest completely on the day before competition.

During events that involve continuous vigorous activity for 60 min or more, it is beneficial to consume easily absorbed carbohydrates during the exercise. The ACSM recommends that solutions containing 4 to 8% carbohydrates (glucose, sucrose, or starch) are best to balance the need for blood glucose maintenance and fluid replacement. The solution should be consumed in small to moderate amounts (150-350 ml) every 15 to 20 min (1).

Female Athlete Triad

The **female athlete triad** is a condition characterized by the presence of disordered eating, amenorrhea, and osteoporosis (2). As discussed in chapter 21, disordered eating is more common in female athletes than in the general population. It is thought that the pressure to succeed and the drive to be thin lead many female athletes to begin unhealthy eating practices such as severe caloric restriction (anorexia), purging of food after eating (bulimia), and compulsive overexercising. These unhealthy patterns interfere with normal hormone secretion and eventually can lead to irregular menses (**oligomenorrhea**) or a lack of menses altogether (**amenorrhea**). Because estrogen is essential in maintaining strong bones in women, the low estrogen levels observed in athletes with menstrual cycle irregularities can lead to a loss of bone. The weakening of the bones makes the athlete more susceptible to stress fractures and can lead to an early and severe onset of osteoporosis.

The HFI should encourage all physically active people to consume adequate calories and nutrients to support their energy expenditure. Active females who begin to miss menstrual periods should be referred to a physician to evaluate the need for hormonal therapy or calcium supplementation. Some signs of disordered eating are listed in chapter 11. Athletes who exhibit these signs should be referred to a nutritionist, a psychologist, or both, who is qualified to counsel a person with eating disorders.

10 **In Review**

Adequate glycogen is necessary for optimal performance. Carbohydrate loading is beneficial for extended exercise bouts. Glucose intake during exercise can be beneficial if vigorous exercise lasts 60 min or more.

11 **In Review**

The female athlete triad (disordered eating, amenorrhea, and osteoporosis) can lead to serious health consequences. Athletes who exhibit signs of an eating disorder should be referred to a qualified nutritionist, psychologist, or both.

Research Insight

The Institute of Medicine recently released new dietary recommendations. Although most are congruent with those recommendations found in this chapter, here are some highlights from the new report.

- Acceptable Macronutrient Distribution Ranges (AMDR) for healthy diets were established, suggesting that 20 to 35% of calories come from fats, 45 to 65% from carbohydrates, and 10 to 35% from protein.
- The AI for total fiber was established at 38 g per day for men and 25 g per day for women.
- The RDA for carbohydrate intake was set at 130 g per day. This establishes a lower level that ensures adequate glucose for functioning of the central nervous system.
- Adequate Intakes (AI) were established for some fatty acids.

At the time of this writing, this text (Dietary Reference Intakes for Energy, Carbohydrate, Fiber, Fat, Fatty Acids, Cholesterol, Protein, and Amino Acids) was not available in hard copy. The information can be accessed on the Internet World Wide Web from the National Academies Press at www.nap.edu.

Case Study

You can check your answers by referring to appendix A.

7.01

A male college basketball player (weight = 190 lb) with a daily caloric intake of 3500 kcal is considering additional protein supplements. He currently consumes approximately 15% of his calories from protein. Is his protein intake adequate? Would you recommend that he increase his protein intake?

Source List

1. American College of Sports Medicine. (1996). Position stand on exercise and fluid replacement. *Medicine and Science in Sports and Exercise, 28,* i-vii.
2. American College of Sports Medicine. (1997). Position stand on the female athlete triad. *Medicine and Science in Sports and Exercise, 29*(5), i-ix.
3. American College of Sports Medicine. (1998). Current comment from the American College of Sports Medicine : Creatine Supplemenation. [Online] Available: acsm.org/pdf/CREATINE3.pdf [July 10, 2002].
4. American College of Sports Medicine, American Dietetic Association, & Dietitians of Canada. (2000). Nutrition and athletic performance. *Medicine and Science in Sports and Exercise, 32*(12), 2130-2145.
5. American Dietetic Association & Canadian Dietetic Association. (1993). Position of the American Dietetic Association and the Canadian Dietetic Association: Nutrition for physical fitness and athletic performance for adults. *Journal of the American Dietetic Association, 93,* 691-696.
6. Berning, J.R. (1995). Nutritional concerns of recreational endurance athletes with an emphasis on swimming. In C.G.R. Jackson (Ed.), *Nutrition for the recreational athlete* (pp. 55-68). Boca Raton, FL: CRC Press.
7. Casa, D.J., Armstrong, L.E., Hillman, S.K., Montain, S.J., Reiff, R.V., Rich, B.S.E., Roberts, W.O., & Stone, J.A. (2000). National Athletic Trainers' Association position statement: Fluid replacement for athletes. *Journal of Athletic Training, 35*(2), 212-224.
8. Driskell, J.A. (2000). *Sports nutrition.* Boca Raton, FL: CRC Press.
9. Durstine, J.L., & Haskell, W.L. (1994). Effects of exercise training on plasma lipids and lipoproteins. *Exercise and Sport Sciences Reviews, 22,* 477-521.
10. Expert Panel on Detection, Evaluation, and Treatment of High Blood Cholesterol in Adults. (2001). Executive Summary of the Third Report of the National Cholesterol Education Program (NCEP) Expert Panel on Detection, Evaluation, and Treatment of High Blood Cholesterol in Adults (Adult Treatment Panel III). *Journal of the American Medical Association, 285*(19), 2486-2497.
11. Food and Nutrition Board, Institute of Medicine. (2001). *Dietary reference intakes: Applications in dietary assessment.* Washington, DC: National Academic Press.
12. Food and Nutrition Board, Institute of Medicine. (2001). *Dietary reference intakes for vitamin A, vitamin K, arsenic, boron, chromium, copper, iodine, iron, manganese, molybdenum, nickel, silicon, vanadium, and zinc.* Washington, DC: National Academy Press.
13. Gibson, R.S. (1993). *Nutritional assessment: A laboratory manual.* New York: Oxford University Press.
14. Morris, K.L., & Zemel, M.B. (1999). Glycemic index, cardiovascular disease, and obesity. *Nutrition Reviews, 57*(9), 273-276.
15. National Academy Press. (2002). Food and nutrition. [Online] Available: books.nap.edu/v3/makepage.phtml ?val1=subject&vak2=fn [July 10, 2002].
16. National Institutes of Health. (1994). *Optimal calcium intake: NIH Consensus Development Conference statement.* Bethesda, MD: Author.
17. National Institutes of Health. (2000). *Osteoporosis prevention, diagnosis, and therapy: NIH Consensus Development Conference statement.* Bethesda, MD: Author.
18. National Research Council, Committee on Diet and Health. (1989). *Diet and health: Implications for reducing chronic disease risk.* Washington, DC: National Academy Press.
19. National Research Council, Food and Nutrition Board. (1989). *Recommended dietary allowances* (10th ed.). Washington, DC: National Academy Press.
20. Poindexter, S., St. Clair, L., & Wheeler, K. (2001). Diet and chronic disease. In J.L. Roitman (Ed.), *ACSM's resource manual for guidelines for exercise testing and prescription* (4th ed., pp. 34-40). Philadelphia: Lippincott Williams & Wilkins.
21. Ruud, J.S., & Wolinsky, I. (1995). Nutritional concerns of recreational strength athletes. In C.G.R. Jackson (Ed.), *Nutrition for the recreational athlete* (pp. 55-68). Boca Raton, FL: CRC Press.
22. Sizer, F., & Whitney, E. (1994). *Hamilton and Whitney's nutrition: Concepts and controversies.* St. Paul: West.
23. United States Department of Agriculture and the Center for Nutrition Policy. (1996). The food guide pyramid (Home and Garden Bulletin 252). Washington, DC: Author.
24. United States Department of Agriculture & United States Department of Health and Human Services. (2000). *Nutrition and your health: Dietary guidelines for Americans* (Home and Garden Bulletin No. 232). Washington, DC: Author.
25. Walberg-Rankin, J. (1997). Glycemic index and exercise metabolism. *Gatorade Sports Science Institute: Sports Science Exchange, 10*(1), 1-7.
26. Westerterp, K.R. (2000). The assessment of energy and nutrient intake in humans. In C. Bouchard (Ed.), *Physical activity and obesity* (pp. 133-149). Champaign, IL: Human Kinetics.
27. Williams, M.H. (1998). Nutritional ergogenics and sports performance. *PCPFS Physical Activity and Fitness Research Digest, 3*(2), 1-14.

eight

Assessment of Muscular Fitness

Kyle J. McInnis and Avery Faigenbaum

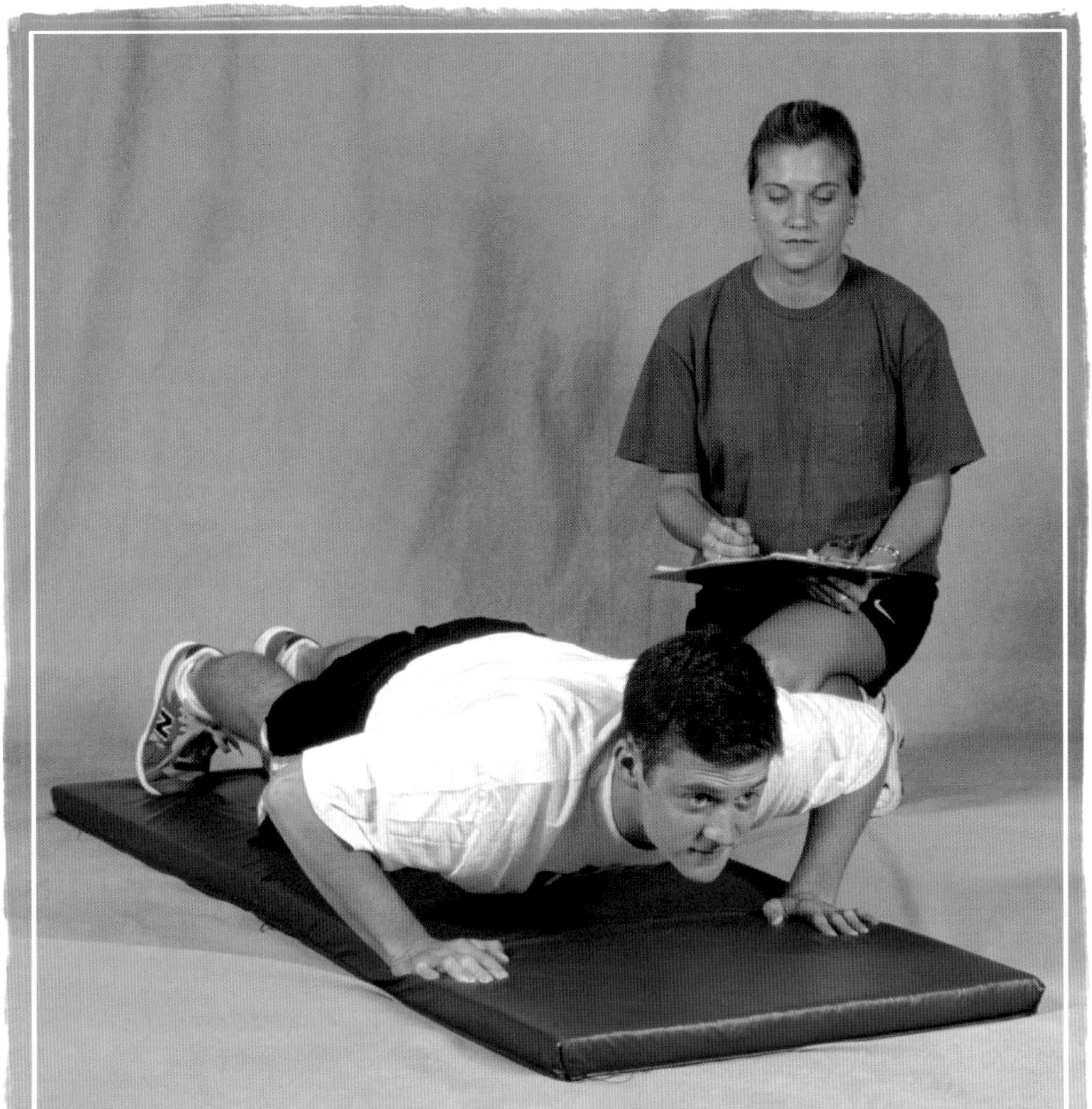

Objectives

The reader will be able to do the following:

1. Discuss precautions to enhance participant safety during muscular fitness assessments.
2. Describe methods of assessing muscular strength and endurance, including the 1 repetition maximum (1RM) and 10 repetition maximum (10RM) tests, push-up test, abdominal curl-up test, and YMCA bench press test.
3. Describe how to interpret the results from various muscular strength and endurance tests in relation to health and fitness.
4. Discuss indications for muscular fitness testing in older adults.
5. Describe how to assess muscular strength/endurance in older adults by using the 30-s chair stand test and single-arm curl test.
6. Describe the benefits, safety, and precautions for assessing muscular fitness in coronary prone clients.

The term **muscular fitness** has been used to describe the integrated status of **muscular strength** (maximal force a muscle can generate at a given velocity) and **muscular endurance** (ability of a muscle to make repeated contractions or to resist muscular fatigue) (4, 16, 21). Muscular fitness is important in both promoting and maintaining health and enhancing athletic performance (3) (see box on page 131). Accordingly, the American College of Sports Medicine (ACSM) includes muscular fitness in its position stand on the recommended quantity and quality of exercise to achieve and maintain fitness in healthy adults (3). In general, the ACSM recommends that resistance training of a moderate to high intensity, sufficient to develop and maintain muscle mass, become an integral part of fitness programs (see chapter 12). This chapter describes tests commonly used in the health/fitness setting to assess muscular strength and endurance. Particular emphasis is given to strength tests that can be performed safely in the fitness setting, especially those that do not require specialized equipment or sophisticated procedures. The assessment of muscular fitness and functional capabilities in older adults and in persons with coronary heart disease and high blood pressure (hypertension) is also described.

Preliminary Considerations

Muscular fitness often is assessed by the number of repetitions a person is capable of performing using a given weight. This may be viewed as representing a continuum with "strength" at one end of the assessment scale and "endurance" at the other (figure 8.1) (4). In general, tests allowing few repetitions of a task measure muscular strength, whereas those that require high numbers of repetitions measure muscular endurance. Performing fitness tests to assess muscular strength/endurance before commencing exercise training or as part of a fitness screening evaluation can provide valuable information on a client's baseline fitness level. For example, test results can be compared with established standards and can help identify weaknesses in certain muscle groups or muscle imbalances that could be targeted in exercise training programs. The infor-mation obtained during baseline muscular fitness assessments also can serve as a basis for designing individualized exercise training programs. An equally useful application of fitness testing is to show a client's progressive improvements over time as a result of the training program and thus provide beneficial feedback that promotes long-term exercise adherence.

Factors such as those listed next are important in promoting safe muscular fitness tests that yield valid and reproducible results.

- Preparticipation evaluation—All participants who undergo fitness testing should first complete a medical history questionnaire to identify individuals who may pose a cardiovascular or orthopedic risk during testing and training. The ACSM's procedures for administering an appropriate health appraisal and subsequent risk stratification and medical evaluation have been described in detail in this textbook (see chapter 3) and elsewhere (4).

Components of Muscular Fitness Related to Promoting or Maintaining Good Health, Fitness, and Athletic Performance (3)

Health Aspects of Muscular Fitness

- Preservation or enhancement of fat-free mass and resting metabolic rate
- Preservation or enhancement of bone mass with aging
- Improved glucose tolerance and insulin sensitivity
- Reduced HR and BP response while lifting any submaximal load (which reduces myocardial oxygen demand during activities requiring muscular force)
- Lowered risk of musculoskeletal injury, including low back pain
- Improved ability to carry out activities of daily living in older age
- Improved balance and decreased risk of falls in older age
- Improved self-esteem

Athletic Performance Aspects of Muscular Fitness

- Enhanced muscular strength and muscular endurance
- Enhanced speed, power, agility, and balance
- Reduced risk for musculoskeletal injuries
- Improved body composition for various events or activities
- Improved confidence for performing certain athletic events and activities involving high levels of muscular fitness
- Enhanced performance in most athletic activities

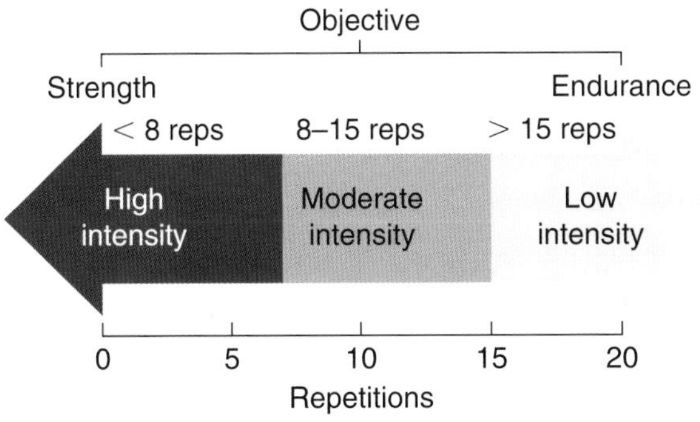

Figure 8.1 Classification of resistance exercise intensity for training and assessment. Weight loads allowing few reps (e.g., <15) test for muscular strength, and weight loads that can be repeatedly lifted (e.g., ≥15 reps) assess muscular endurance.

Adapted with permission from the ACSM (4).

- Familiarization—To obtain a reliable test score that can be used to track physiological adaptations over time, individuals should become familiar with the testing equipment and protocol by participating in one or more practice sessions with qualified instruction.

- Warm-up—A 5- to 10-min general warm-up including brief cardiovascular exercise, light stretching, and several light repetitions of the specific testing exercise should proceed muscular fitness testing. This increases muscle temperature and localized blood flow and promotes appropriate cardiovascular responses to exercise (3).

- Specificity—Muscle strength and muscular endurance are specific to the muscle or muscle group, the type of muscular action (static or dynamic; concentric or eccentric), the speed of muscular action (slow or fast), and the joint angle being tested (16, 21). Accordingly, muscular fitness tests should involve similar characteristics as used during the training program.

- Safety—Safety measures related to the testing equipment, testing environment, proper instruction, and the use of spotters should be reviewed.

- Interpretation of results—The availability of health criteria or population-specific norms should be considered when you choose a test, particularly when it is desirable to classify an individual's test data, such as when performing tests as part of a fitness screening evaluation. However, availability of norms is less of a concern when the test is used primarily to detect improvements in an individual's muscular fitness over time, where the absolute strength values (e.g., kilograms lifted) or relative scores (e.g., kilograms lifted per kilogram of body weight) can be compared during repeated testing.

1 In Review

Muscular strength is best assessed by using resistance that requires maximum or near-maximum tension with few repetitions, whereas muscular endurance is assessed by using lighter resistance with a greater number of repetitions. In either case, muscular fitness can be assessed safely in the health/fitness setting and provides important information for individualized exercise prescription. An ideal application of these tests is to evaluate changes in muscular fitness over time.

Muscular Strength

Muscular strength refers to the maximal force that can be generated by a specific muscle or muscle group. **Isometric** or **static strength** (constant muscle length during muscle activation) can be measured conveniently with a variety of devices, including cable tensiometers and handgrip dynamometers, which measure strength at one specific point in the range of motion. These tests and devices occasionally are used in research and academic settings but are not used routinely by most health/fitness practitioners. Thus, the procedures for these tests are described in detail elsewhere (5, 16). **Isokinetic testing** involves the assessment of maximal muscle tension throughout a range of joint motion at a constant angular velocity (e.g., 60°/s). Isokinetic testing devices measure peak rotational force or torque, and data are obtained with specialized equipment that allows the tester to control the speed of rotation (degrees per second) around various joints (e.g., knee, hip, shoulder, elbow). Although the data collected from isokinetic strength assessments may be useful to health/fitness professionals, the necessary computerized equipment is expensive and therefore is limited almost entirely to rehabilitation and research settings. Consequently, isokinetic strength evaluations may not be a practical consideration for most health/fitness practitioners.

The most common type of strength assessment performed by fitness professionals is **dynamic testing**, which involves movement of the body (e.g., a push-up) or an external load (e.g., bench press). Dynamic strength testing is typically inexpensive because it does not require sophisticated or specialized equipment. Moreover, dynamic assessments can be performed with different types of equipment, such as free weights (barbells and dumbbells) or weight-stack machines, and can be used to test any major muscle or muscle group through a variety of different exercises. Examples of exercises typically used for dynamic strength testing in fitness centers include the bench press, lat pull-down, and leg press.

Repetition Maximum Testing

The "gold standard" of dynamic strength testing is the **1 repetition maximum (1RM)**, the heaviest weight that can be lifted only once using good form. Peak force development in such tests commonly is referred to as the **maximum voluntary contraction (MVC)**. In general, 1RM tests are good indicators of strength and can be performed safely in the health/fitness setting with qualified supervision, for example, by fitness professionals who are familiar with, and adhere to, current guidelines of exercise leadership such as those described here and previously by the ACSM (3). Multiple RM tests that involve 8 to 12 repetitions can also be used to safely and effectively assess strength in adults who are apparently healthy or have controlled disease conditions (26). Moreover, when the purpose of testing is to define an initial training load, a multiple RM testing procedure is beneficial because it minimizes the potential error compared with extrapolating the exercise intensity as a percentage of a 1RM. For example, determining the maximum weight load a person can lift 10 times during testing also can be used to identify an appropriate weight load for this number of repetitions performed during training. The procedures used to assess 1RM are shown on the next page and can be modified to test any given number of repetitions (e.g., 10RM).

Interpretation of Results

For meaningful comparative strength assessments in men and women of different body mass, it is best to express strength with a ratio of weight lifted during a single or multiple RM test relative to one's own body weight. The following procedures describe how to determine a strength ratio from a 10RM test (21):

Procedures for Performing 1RM Testing

1. The subject performs a light warm-up of 5 to 10 repetitions at 40 to 60% of perceived maximum (e.g., light-to-moderate exertion).
2. After a 1-min rest with light stretching, the subject performs 3 to 5 repetitions at 60 to 80% of perceived maximum (e.g., moderate-to-hard exertion).
3. The subject attempts a 1RM lift. If the lift is successful, a rest period of 3 to 5 min is provided. The goal is to find the 1RM within 3 to 5 maximal efforts.The process of increasing the weight up to a true 1RM can be improved by familiarization sessions that allow approximation of the 1RM.This process is continued until a failed attempt occurs.
4. The 1RM is reported as the weight of the last successfully completed lift.

Adapted from Kraemer and Fry (21).

1. Determine the heaviest weight load the client can perform for 10 good repetitions (10RM weight load).
2. Convert the 10RM weight load to a 1RM estimation by dividing the weight load by 0.75.
3. Divide the 1RM estimated weight load by the client's body weight to obtain the strength ratio.

For example, a client who weighs 140 lb and completes 10 leg presses with 120 lb would have an estimated 1RM of 160 lb (120 lb divided by 0.75). Her leg press weight ratio would be 1.14 (160 divided by 140).

Normative Data

Normative strength scores such as lower or upper body strength ratios for different age and sex categories have been published in the ACSM's *Guidelines for Exercise Testing and Prescription* (4). However, normative data to date have been derived from a relatively homogeneous sample of subjects (mostly middle to upper class Caucasians) using only certain types of resistance training equipment, which limits interpretation of test scores. For example, because equipment design can vary significantly from one manufacturer to another and because of inherent differences in using free weights versus machines weights, strength scores can vary widely by testing equipment used. Thus, comparison of individual client scores should be limited to tests performed with the type of equipment used to generate the norms. Future research is needed to provide additional norms for different types of resistance-training equipment as well as norms on diverse races/ethnicities and age groups.

Serial Comparisons

Often, the primary purpose of performing muscular fitness tests is to evaluate changes in strength over the course of a fitness program. Periodic muscle fitness testing is particularly appealing because it eliminates the need to compare individual data with that provided in normative tables, as described previously. The frequency of follow-up testing will depend on the quality and quantity of exercise training by the client as well as the client's desire and staff availability. When multiple tests are performed, appropriate feedback to the client should include percentage improvement of strength or endurance (i.e., by dividing original pretraining score by posttraining score and multiplying by 100) and recommendations for improving or maintaining muscular fitness based on the client's individualized goals.

Muscular Endurance

Muscular endurance, also called local muscle endurance, is the ability of a muscle group to execute repeated contractions over a period of time sufficient to cause muscular fatigue or to maintain a specific percentage of the maximum voluntary contraction for a prolonged period of time (4). Devices (e.g., free weights or machines) for measuring strength also can be used to assess muscular endurance. In addition, simple field tests such as an abdominal curl-up (crunch) test (10, 12) or the maximum number of push-ups that can be performed without rest (8) can be used to evaluate the endurance of the abdominal or upper body muscles, respectively. These field tests can be used either independently or in combination with other methods of strength or endurance assessment such as

RM testing. One indication for tests such as the abdominal curl-up or push-up is to screen for muscle weaknesses related to various health indicators. For example, there are sufficient scientific data to suggest that poor abdominal strength/endurance is an important predisposing factor for muscular low back pain and that the curl-up test can help identify individuals with abdominal strength/endurance weakness that may contribute to this condition (4, 19). Moreover, the muscles of the upper body, such as those activated in the push-up test, are used in many daily activities such as raking or gardening, carrying luggage, or painting. Thus, these tests provide a practical mechanism of evaluating a client's muscular fitness and provide useful feedback to the client about how muscular conditioning, or deconditioning, affects performance of many common activities.

Push-Up and Curl-Up Tests

The procedures used to perform the push-up and curl-up tests as described by the ACSM are presented on the next page and shown in figures 8.2 and 8.3 (push-up test) and 8.4 (curl-up test). The purpose of the push-up test is to evaluate muscular endurance of the upper body, including the triceps, anterior deltoid, and pectoral muscles. Men typically use the standard push-up position with only the hands and toes in contact with the floor and women typically use the modified push-up position from the knees. However, either position of the push-up test may be used for men or women, based on client's strength, but this limits interpretation to normative data.

The purpose of the bent-knee curl-up test is to evaluate abdominal muscle endurance. Full sit-up tests are unsatisfactory because hip flexor involvement during the sit-up motion has the potential to harm the low back (see chapter 9). Even though modifications to the traditional sit-up have been instituted, including a bent-knee position, stress to the low back is still present during the motion. Consequently, the bent-knee curl-up test recently was modified to reduce the potential for low back injury and to better assess abdominal muscle function (10).

Both the push-up and curl-up tests are relatively simple, inexpensive methods for assessing muscular endurance and can be used for both men and women of various ages. Results of the full push-up test for men and partial push-up test for women and curl-up tests for men and women can be compared with the standards in tables 8.1 and 8.2, respectively. As with RM testing, the push-up and curl-up tests can be performed serially to reliably assess changes in muscular endurance after training. Finally, for very deconditioned individuals, especially those who are overweight or obese, these tests may be very difficult to perform. In such cases, poor results obtained during testing may discourage individuals from exercise participation. Thus, for each participant, the HFI must carefully consider whether these tests are appropriate and likely to yield useful information.

YMCA Bench Press Test

Alternatives to the push-up and curl-up test to assess muscular endurance also exist. The HFI can adapt resistance training equipment to measure muscular endurance by selecting an appropriate submaximal level of resistance and measuring the number of repetitions or the duration of static contraction before fatigue. For example, the YMCA bench press test involves performing standardized repetitions at a rate of 30 lifts/min to test muscular endurance of the upper body (15). Men are tested using an 80-lb barbell and women using a 35-lb barbell, and subjects are scored by the number of successful repetitions completed. The main disadvantage of the test is that it uses a fixed weight, which places lighter clients at a disadvantage or may represent a weight that is too heavy for deconditioned or older clients to lift repeatedly. On the other hand, the load may be too light for very fit individuals, leading the individual to perform significantly more repetitions than typically used during training. Despite these limitations, this test can be used independently or in combination with other tests in the overall assessment of muscular fitness. The procedures for this test are summarized next, and norms are shown in table 8.3:

1. Use a 35-lb (straight) barbell for women or an 80-lb (straight) barbell for men. A spotter should be present during the test.
2. Set a metronome to 60 beats $\cdot$ min^{-1}.
3. The test begins with the bar in the down position touching the chest, with the elbows flexed and hands shoulder-width apart.
4. A repetition is counted when the elbows are fully extended. After each extension, the participant should lower the bar to touch the chest.
5. Up or down movements should be in time to the 60 beats $\cdot$ min^{-1} rhythm, which should be 30 lifts per minute.
6. Count the total number of repetitions completed in good form.

Push-Up and Curl-Up (Crunch) Test Procedures for for Measurement of Muscular Endurance

Push-Up

1. Explain the purpose of the test to the client (e.g., to determine how many push-ups can be completed to reflect upper body muscular strength and endurance).
2. Inform clients of proper breathing technique—to exhale with the effort (when pushing away from the floor).
3. The push-up test usually is administered with male subjects in the standard "up" position with hands shoulder-width apart, back straight, and head up, using the toes as the pivotal point. For female subjects, the modified "knee push-up" position usually is used, with legs together, lower leg in contact with mat, ankles plantar flexed, back straight, hands shoulder-width apart, and head up. (Note: Some males will need to use the modified position, and some females can use the full body position as described in this chapter).
4. The subject must lower the body until the chin touches the mat or until chest touches the fist of examiner. The stomach should not touch the mat.
5. For both men and women, the subject's back must be straight at all times and the subject must push up to a straight arm position.
6. Demonstrate the test and allow clients to practice if desired.
7. Remind the client that a brief rest is allowed only in the up position.
8. Begin the test when the client is ready, and count the total number of push-ups the client completes before reaching the point of exhaustion.
9. The client's score is the total number of push-ups performed.

Curl-Up (Crunch)

1. Explain the purpose of the test to the client (e.g., to determine how many curl-ups can be completed to reflect abdominal muscular strength and endurance).
2. Explain proper breathing technique—to exhale with the effort (when curling up from the floor).
3. The individual assumes a supine position on a mat with the knees at 90°. The arms are at the side, with fingers touching a piece of masking tape. A second piece of masking tape is placed 8 cm (for those who are ≥ 45 years) or 12 cm (for those who are < 45 years) beyond the first.*
4. A metronome is set to 40 beats · min^{-1}, and the individual does slow, controlled curl-ups to lift the shoulder blades off the mat (the trunk makes a 30° angle with the mat) in time with the metronome (20 curl-ups/min). The low back should be flattened before curling up.
5. Demonstrate the test and allow clients to practice if desired.
6. The individual performs as many curl-ups as possible without pausing up to a maximum of 75.**

Note. Descriptions of procedures are adapted from the ACSM (4).

*Alternatives include (a) holding the hands across the chest and counting when the trunk reaches a 30° position or (b) placing the hands on the thighs and curling up until the hands reach the kneecaps. Elevation of the trunk to 30° is the important aspect of the movement.

**An alternative includes doing as many curl-ups as possible in 1 min.

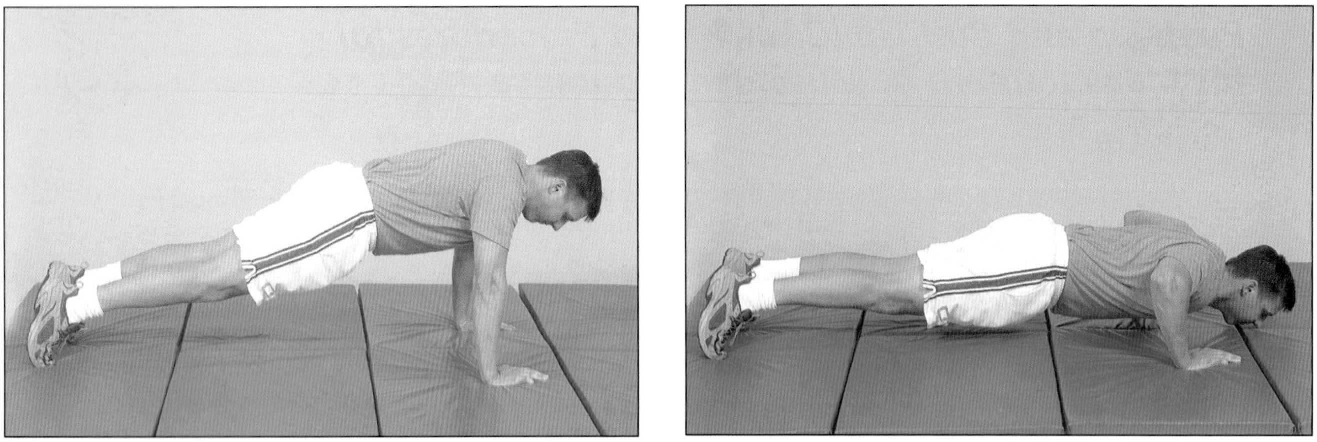

Figure 8.2 Proper form for the starting position (*a*) and finishing position (*b*) of the standard push-up test, as described by the ACSM (4).

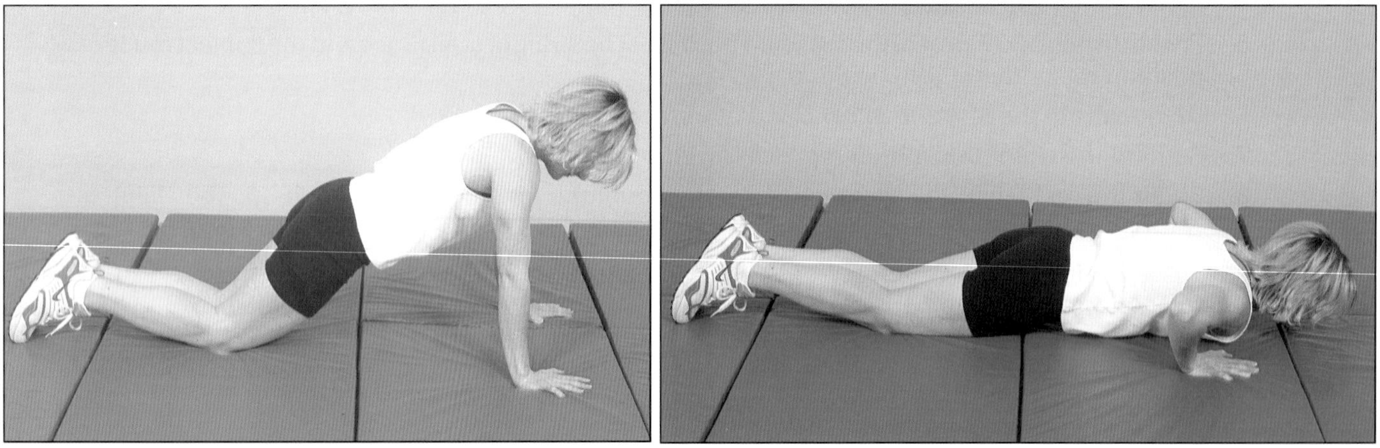

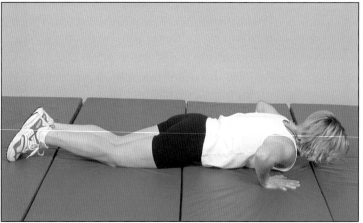

Figure 8.3 Proper form for the starting position (*a*) and finishing position (*b*) of the modified push-up test, as described by the ACSM (4).

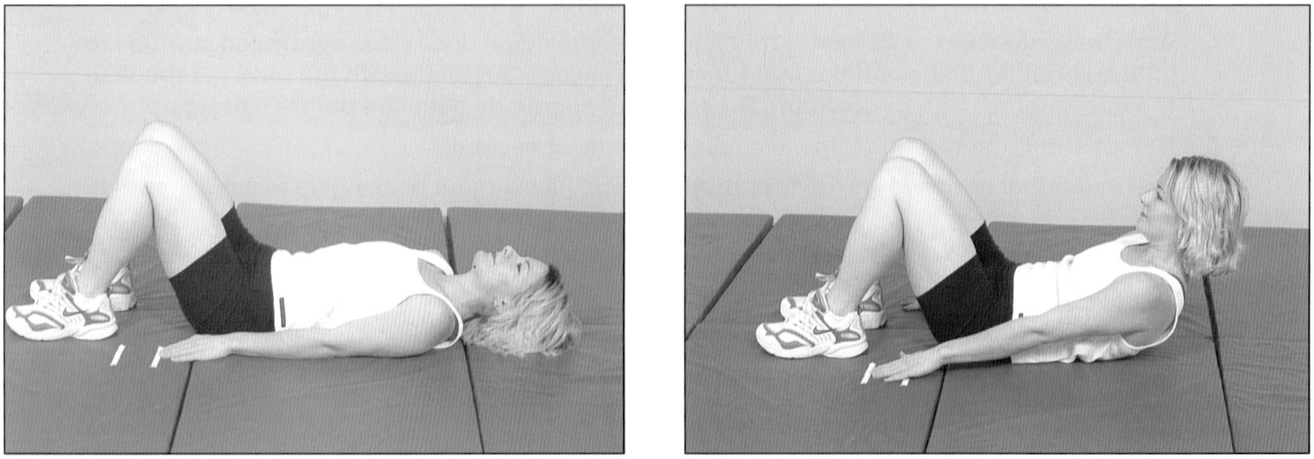

Figure 8.4 Proper form for the starting position (*a*) and finishing position (*b*) of the abdominal curl-up test as described by the ACSM (4).

Table 8.1 Push-Up Norms for Men and Women by Age Groups Using Number Completed

Age (years)	(15–19) M	(15–19) F	(20–29) M	(20–29) F	(30–39) M	(30–39) F	(40–49) M	(40–49) F	(50–59) M	(50–59) F	(60–69) M	(60–69) F
Excellent	>39	>33	>36	>30	>30	>27	>22	>24	>21	>21	>18	>17
Above average	29–38	25–32	29–35	21–29	22–29	20–26	17–21	15–23	13–20	11–20	11–17	12–16
Average	23–28	18–24	22–28	15–20	17–21	13–19	13–16	11–14	10–12	7–10	8–10	5–11
Below average	18–22	12–17	17–21	10–14	12–16	8–12	10–12	5–10	7–9	2–6	5–7	1–4
Poor	<17	<11	<16	<9	<11	<7	<9	<4	<6	<1	<4	<1

Note. The Canadian Standardized Test of Fitness was developed by and is reproduced with permission of the Government of Canada, Fitness and Amateur Sport (8).

Source: *CSTF operation manual,* (3rd ed.). Ottawa: Government of Canada, Fitness and Amateur Sport, 1986.

Table 8.2 Curl-Up Norms by Age Group Using Number Completed

	Men			Women		
	<35 yr	35–44 yr	45 yr	<35 yr	35–44 yr	45 yr
Excellent	60	50	40	50	40	30
Good	45	40	25	40	30	15
Marginal	30	25	15	25	15	10
Needs work	15	10	5	10	6	4

Source: Faulkner et al. (12).

Table 8.3a YMCA Bench Press Norms for Number of Repetitions Completed for Men Using 80 lb

	Age (years)					
Fitness	16–25	26–35	36–45	46–55	56–65	65+
Excellent	>37	>33	>29	>23	>21	>17
Good	29–37	26–33	23–29	19–23	14–21	10–17
Above average	24–28	22–25	19–22	14–18	10–13	8–9
Average	21–23	18–21	15–18	10–13	7–9	5–7
Below average	15–20	13–17	11–14	7–9	4–6	3–4
Poor	9–14	6–12	6–10	3–6	1–3	1–2
Very poor	<9	<6	<6	<3	<1	0

Source: Adapted from Golding et al. (15), *The Y's way to physical fitness* (3rd ed.).

Table 8.3b YMCA Bench Press Norms for Number of Repetitions Completed for Women Using 35 lb

	Age (years)					
Fitness	18–25	26–35	36–45	46–55	56–65	65+
Excellent	>35	>32	>27	>25	>21	>17
Good	27–35	24–32	21–27	19–25	16–21	12–17
Above average	22–26	19–23	6–20	13–18	11–15	9–11
Average	17–21	15–18	12–15	10–12	8–10	5–8
Below average	13–16	11–14	9–11	6–9	4–7	2–4
Poor	7–12	4–10	3–8	2–5	1–3	0–1
Very poor	<7	<4	<3	<2	0	0

Source: Adapted from Golding et al. (15), *The Y's way to physical fitness,* (3rd ed.).

2 In Review

The most common type of muscle fitness assessment in the fitness setting is dynamic strength testing with a single or multiple repetition maximum protocol. Although lack of adequate normative data often limits the evaluation of individual test data, such tests are valuable as a means of tracking strength and endurance improvement. Field tests such as the push-up and abdominal curl-up tests provide a practical approach for evaluating muscular fitness, either as stand-alone procedures or as adjuncts to other types of muscular fitness evaluations.

Special Considerations: Older Adults

The number of older adults in the United States is expected to increase exponentially over the next several decades. For instance, in 1990 there were 31.2 million U.S. adults (13%) who were age 65 years or older, but this number is expected to more than double to 70.3 million (20%) by the year 2030 (24). Because people are living longer, it is becoming increasingly more important to find ways to extend active, healthy lifestyles and reduce physical frailty in later years (2, 22). Assessing muscular strength and endurance and other aspects of physical fitness in older adults can reveal physical weaknesses and yield important information used to design exercise programs that improve strength before serious functional limitations occur.

The Senior Fitness Test

Rikli and Jones (28) have developed a functional fitness test battery—The Senior Fitness Test (SFT)—for older adults in response to a need for improved assessment tools for this population. The test was designed to assess the key physiological parameters (e.g., strength, endurance, agility, and balance) needed to perform common everyday physical activities that are often difficult in later years. One aspect of the SFT is the 30-s chair stand test (see Research Insight.) This test, as well as others of the SFT, meets scientific standards for reliability and validity, is simple and easy to administer in the field setting, and has accompanying performance norms for older men and women ages 60 to 94 based on a study of more than 7000 older Americans (27). This test has been shown to correlate well with other strength tests such as the 1RM. The SFT can be used by the HFI to safely and effectively assess muscular strength/endurance in most older adults.

Research Insight

Measuring lower body strength is critical in evaluating the functional performance of older adults. Jones, Rikli, and Beam's 1999 study (20) was designed to assess the test-retest reliability and validity of a 30-s chair stand as a measure of lower body strength in adults over the age of 60 years. Seventy-six community-dwelling older adults (mean age = 70.5 years) volunteered to participate in the study, which involved performing two 30-s chair stand tests and two maximum leg press tests, each conducted on separate days 2 to 5 days apart. Test-retest interclass correlations of .84 for men and .92 for women, together with a nonsignificant change in scores for Day 1 testing to Day 2, indicate that the 30-s chair stand has good stability reliability. A moderately high correlation between chair stand performance and maximum weight-adjusted leg press performance for both men and women ($r = .78$ and .71, respectively) supports the criterion related to validity of the chair stand as a measure of lower body strength. Construct (or discriminant) validity of the chair stand was demonstrated by the test's ability to detect differences between various age and physical activity level groups. As expected, chair stand performance decreased significantly across age groups in decades—from the 60s to the 70s to the 80s ($p < .01$)—and was significantly lower for low active participants than for high active participants ($p < .0001$). It was concluded that the 30-s chair stand provides a reliable and valid indicator of lower body strength in generally active, community-dwelling older adults.

Assessing Muscular Fitness With the SFT

Before testing, all participants should warm up and follow other preliminary procedures as described previously. In addition, for both the chair stand and arm curl test, the following instruction is recommended as a standardization procedure for administering tests on all clients:

"Do the best you can on each test item but never push yourself to a point of overexertion or beyond what you think is safe for you."

The 30-s Chair Stand Test

The 30-s chair stand test, selected to reflect lower body strength, involves counting the number of times within 30 s that an individual can rise to a full stand from a seated position, without pushing off with the arms (figure 8.5). Studies have shown that chair stand performance, a common method of assessing lower body strength in older adults, correlates well with major criterion indicators of lower body strength (e.g., Cybex II knee extensor and knee flexor strength and other functional measures), stair-climbing ability, walking speed, and risk of falling (6) and has been found to detect normal age-related declines in strength (9). Furthermore, the chair stand has been found to be safe and sensitive in detecting the effects of physical training in older adults (17, 23). Table 8.4 summarizes the normal range of scores of participants ages 60 to 94. The normal range is defined as the middle 50% of the population tested for each age group, with the lower limits being equivalent to the 25th percentile rank and the upper limits equivalent to the 75th percentile rank within each 5-year age group.

The Single-Arm Curl Test

Upper body function, including arm strength and endurance, is important in executing many normal everyday activities such as household chores, carrying groceries, lifting a suitcase, and picking up grandchildren (24). The 30-s arm curl test, a measure of upper body strength / endurance, involves determining the number of times a dumbbell (5 lb for women, 8 lb for men) can be curled through a full range of motion in 30 s. The prescribed arm position protocol includes holding the weight in a handshake grip at full extension (to the side of the chair) and then supinating during flexion so that the palm of the hand faces the biceps at full flexion (figure 8.6). Results of studies indicate that the 30-s arm curl is a good predictor of both biceps strength and overall upper body strength (27). It is important to consider that most participants, including those

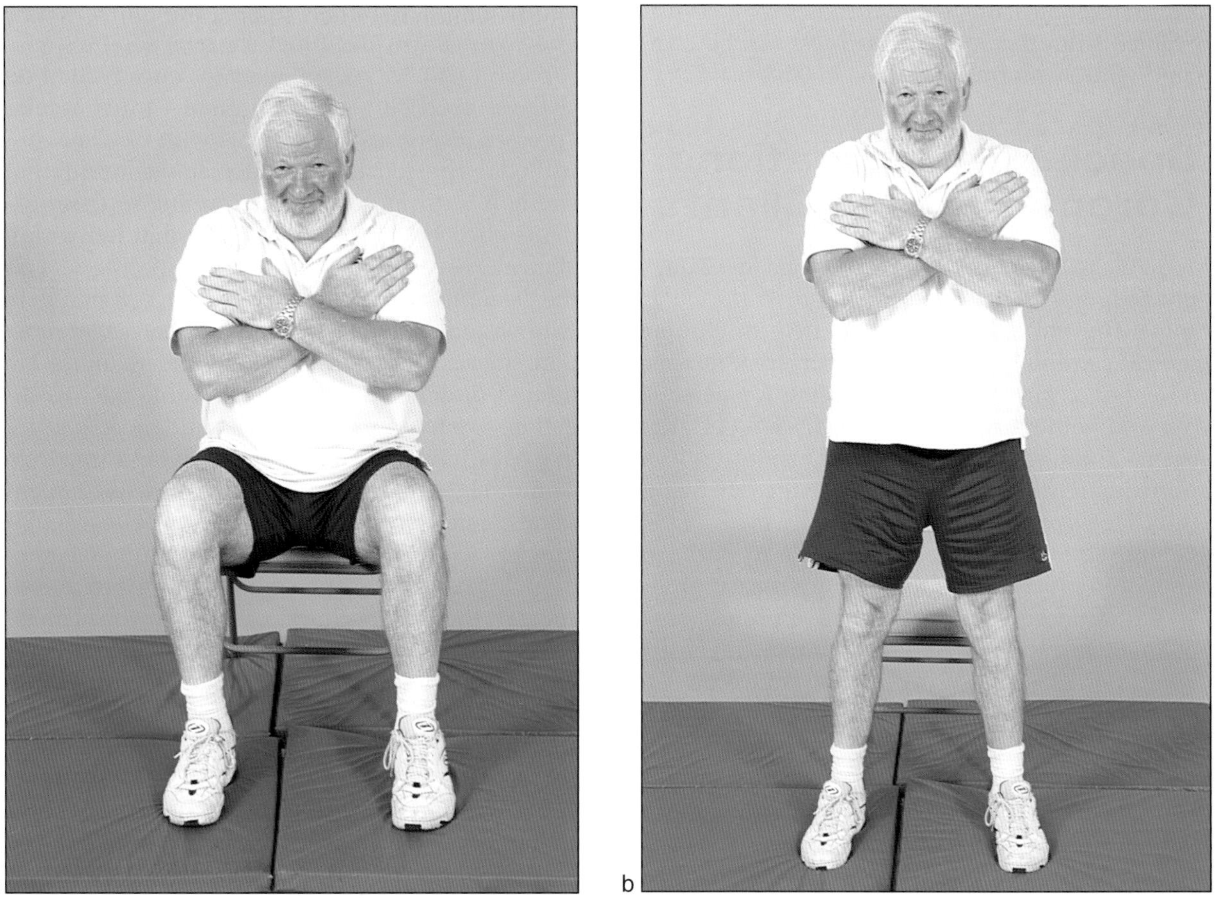

a b

Figure 8.5 Procedures for administering the 30-s chair stand test (28).

Table 8.4 Normal Range of Scores on the 30-s Chair Stand and 30-s Arm Curl Tests for Older Adults

	Age (years)						
	60–64	**65–69**	**70–74**	**75–79**	**80–84**	**85–89**	**90–94**
Chair stand (no. of stands)							
Women	12–17	11–16	10–15	10–15	9–14	8–13	4–11
Men	14–19	12–18	12–17	11–17	10–15	8–14	7–12
Arm curl (no. of reps)							
Women	13–19	12–18	12–17	11–17	10–16	10–15	8–13
Men	16–22	15–21	14–21	13–19	13–19	11–17	10–17

Note. "Normal" is defined as the middle 50% of the population. Participants scoring above or below these ranges would be considered "above normal" or "below normal" for their age.

Adapted by permission from R.E. Rikli and C.J. Jones 2001.

with arthritis, were able to perform the arm curl test without much discomfort and were less bothered performing the arm curl test described here than the maximum-grip strength protocol commonly used as a strength measure in other studies (27). Results obtained from the 30-s arm curl test can be compared with the norms presented in table 8.4.

Special Considerations: Coronary Prone Clients

Moderate resistance training performed just 2 days per week has been shown to improve muscular fitness, prevent and manage a variety of chronic medical conditions, modify coronary risk factors, and enhance psychosocial well-being for persons with and without cardiovascular disease (14). Resistance training could benefit the majority of the approximately 13.5 million people in the U.S. living with CHD, because many cardiac patients lack the physical strength and self-confidence to perform common daily activities that require muscular effort (26). Consequently, authoritative professional health organizations including the American Heart Association (26), ACSM (4), and the American Association of Cardiovascular and Pulmonary Rehabilitation (1) support the inclusion of resistance training as an adjunct to endurance-type exercise in their current recommendations and guidelines on exercise for individuals with cardiovascular disease. Resistance training is also recommended in the evidence-based report clinical practice guidelines on cardiac rehabilitation (29).

Both moderate- to high-intensity (e.g., 40-80% 1RM) resistance testing and training can be performed safely by cardiac patients deemed "low risk" (e.g., those with absence of angina or serious ventricular arrhythmias during normal activities, good left ventricular function, and good exercise capacity) (26). Moreover, despite concerns that resistance exercise elicits abnormal cardiovascular "pressor responses" in patients with CHD or controlled hypertension, studies have found that strength tests and resistance training in these patients elicit HR and BP responses that fall within clinically acceptable limits (11, 25). Specific data on the benefits and safety of resistance training in women and patients with poor left ventricular function, such as those with congestive heart failure, are limited, and these areas require additional investigation. Contemporary exercise guidelines suggest that patients with uncontrolled hypertension (>160/90 mm Hg), unstable angina pectoris, uncompensated congestive heart failure, poor left ventricular function (ejection fraction < 30%), abnormal hemodynamic responses during a clinical exercise test, severe orthopedic limitations, or uncontrolled metabolic diseases (e.g. uncontrolled diabetes or thyroid disease) should be excluded from strength testing and or training until their clinical status improves or stabilizes and until they receive appropriate medical clearance (26).

As with graded exercise testing, the risk of a serious cardiac event during strength testing can be minimized by proper preparticipation screening and close supervision by HFIs. During exercise testing of patients with known or suspected CHD or

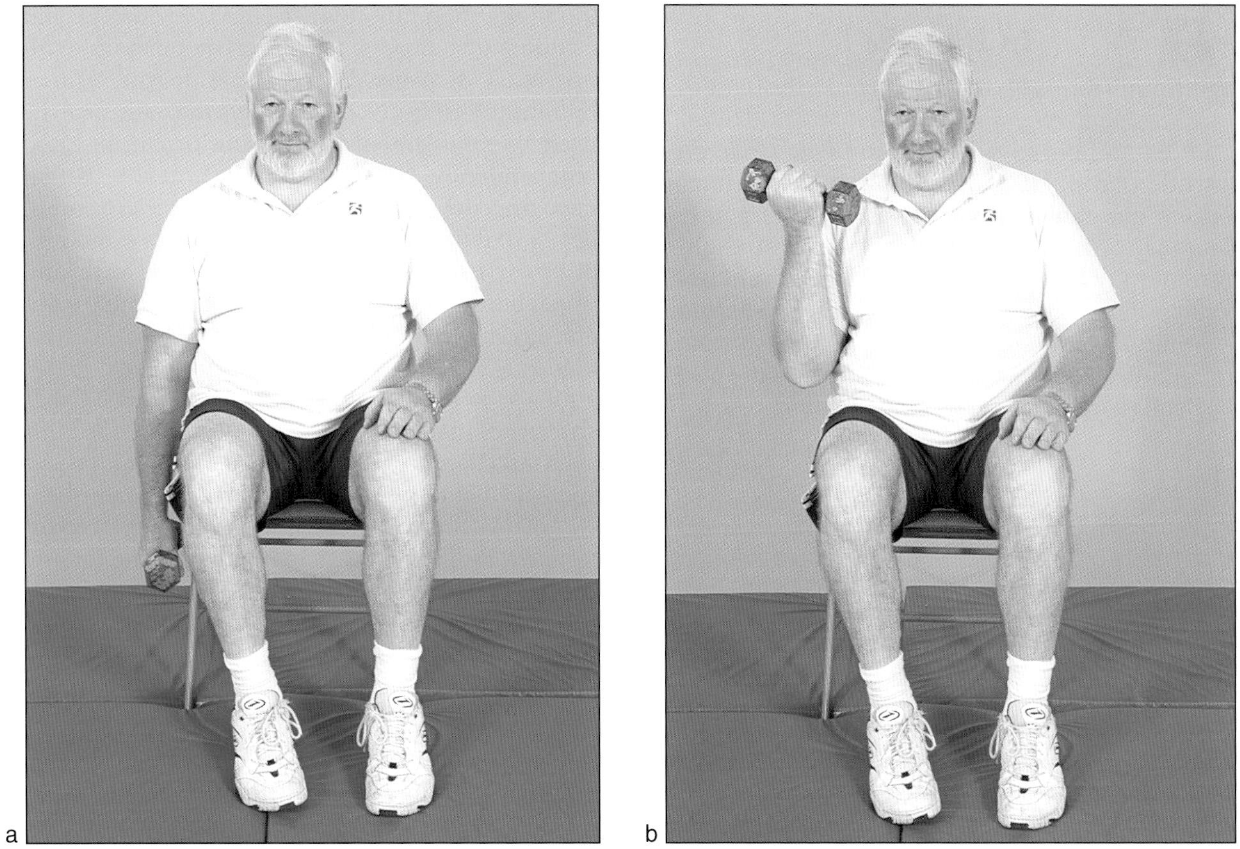

Figure 8.6 Procedures for administering the 30-s arm curl test (28).

hypertension, the HFI should do preliminary work to establish appropriate weight loads and instruct the participant on proper lifting techniques. This should include demonstrating proper ROM and speed of movement for each exercise as well as correct breathing patterns to avoid the Valsalva maneuver. The monitoring of resting and recovery BPs (e.g., every 1-3 min) and identification and evaluation of abnormal signs and symptoms should be considered standard protocol during the initial evaluation of the cardiovascular response during testing. Exaggerated BP responses, clinical signs or symptoms of CHD, or any other abnormal findings as previously described by the ACSM that occur during resistance testing or training should be considered indications for the HFI to terminate the activity until further evaluation by a qualified healthcare provider (4). Because BP measured immediately postexercise tends to underestimate values during contractions, the HFI should act conservatively when evaluating the cardiovascular responses to testing in this population (13, 18).

Studies thus far have shown no adverse hemodynamic responses in low-risk cardiac patients who perform 1RM or multiple RM testing for upper and lower body exercises (11, 13). Moreover, there is no scientific evidence suggesting that 1RM testing is "riskier" than 10RM testing for low-risk cardiac patients. However, multiple repetition testing (e.g., 5RM or 10RM) is a more conservative and, therefore, sensible approach to testing clients with a history of cardiovascular disease. Regardless of the number of repetitions used during testing, the initial resistance or weight should be set at a moderate level that allows the participant to achieve the proper repetition range at a "somewhat hard" level (e.g., 13-15 on the original Borg perceived exertion scale; see chapter 5) (7). Furthermore, the procedures previously described in this chapter for strength assessment can be applied safely to clients with a history of known or occult CHD who are clinically stable and those with controlled hypertension. Careful screening and astute monitoring of abnormal signs or symptoms, such as angina, by the HFI are paramount to minimizing any potential risks while simultaneously maximizing the benefits of resistance training for persons with and without cardiovascular disease.

3 In Review

Although strength tests were once thought to evoke unsafe physiological responses in older adults and persons with high BP or CHD, an accumulating body of scientific evidence supports the conclusion that such tests are safe and can provide useful information for strength training prescription in these and other special populations. Proper screening and astute monitoring of clients with controlled chronic conditions are warranted to promote safe and effective muscular fitness evaluations.

Conclusions

Numerous tests exist to assess muscular fitness in apparently healthy adults and in those with controlled chronic medical conditions. Assessment options vary from tests that rely on sophisticated and expensive laboratory equipment (e.g., isokinetic tests) to others that are inexpensive and quite simple to administer. Tests that determine the single RM (i.e., 1RM) or a multiple RM (e.g., 10RM) by using either free weights or weight machines provide a practical, valid, and reliable means of gathering muscular fitness outcome data for both determining pretraining muscular strength/endurance and evaluating changes over time. The push-up, curl-up, and YMCA bench press tests provide further options to assess muscular fitness that either can be used to complement RM testing or can be used independently. Newer muscular fitness tests that have been developed and validated in a large number of older adults (e.g., the 30-s chair stand and bicep curl test) provide a valid measure of lower and upper body strength. Such tests are extremely valuable given their association with functional performance in the rapidly increasing number of older adults who participate in fitness programs. Other special populations commonly encountered by HFIs such as clients with known or overt CHD and controlled hypertension can share in the same benefits of muscle fitness testing as their healthier counterparts. Proper preparticipation screening for any contraindications to exercise participation and careful monitoring are needed to promote safe exercise participation.

Case Study

Answers to 1 and 2 can be found in the tables and figures presented in this chapter. See details in the chapter for 3.

8.1

A middle-age female who recently joined your health/fitness facility would like to participate in an initial fitness assessment and receive advice about beginning an overall fitness program. She has not participated in a structured exercise program for several years, although she reports that she leads an active lifestyle that often includes accumulating moderate amounts of daily physical activity. Her preparticipation health history questionnaire reveals that she is without signs, symptoms, or diagnosis of any cardiovascular, metabolic, or musculoskeletal diseases or conditions. Using a classmate to play the role of this client, practice the procedures presented in this chapter as described in the following three directives:

1. Explain, demonstrate, and perform the procedures for one muscle strength test for the upper body and one for the lower body.
2. Explain, demonstrate, and perform the procedures for a muscular endurance test used to evaluate the abdominal muscles and one for the upper body.
3. Explain the results of the tests performed in 1 and 2 to your client. Where appropriate, give specific reference to her level of muscular fitness and implications for subsequent training.

Source List

1. American Association of Cardiovascular and Pulmonary Rehabilitation. (1999). *Guidelines for cardiac rehabilitation and secondary prevention programs* (3rd ed.). Champaign, IL: Human Kinetics.
2. American College of Sports Medicine. (1998). ACSM position stand on exercise and physical activity for older adults. *Medicine and Science in Sports and Exercise, 30,* 992-1008.
3. American College of Sports Medicine. (1998). ACSM position stand. The recommended quantity and quality of exercise for developing and maintaining cardiorespiratory and muscular fitness, and flexibility in healthy adults. *Medicine and Science in Sports and Exercise, 30,* 875-991.
4. American College of Sports Medicine. (2000). *ACSM's guidelines for exercise testing and prescription* (6th ed.). Baltimore: Lippincott Williams & Wilkins.
5. Bohannon, R.W. (1990). Muscle strength testing with hand-held dynamometers. In L.R. Amundsen (Ed.), *Muscle strength testing. Instrumented and non-instrumented systems* (pp. 69-112). New York: Churchill Livingstone.
6. Bohannon, R.W. (1995). Sit to stand test for measuring performance of lower extremity muscles. *Perceptual and Motor Skills, 80,* 163-166.
7. Borg, G. (1982). Psychophysical bases of perceived exertion. *Medicine and Science in Sports and Exercise, 14,* 377-381.
8. *Canadian Standardized Test of Fitness Operations Manual* (3rd ed.). (1986). Ottawa: Government of Canada, Fitness and Amateur Sport.
9. Csuka, M., & McCarty, D.J. (1985). Simple method for measurement of lower extremity muscle strength. *Journal of the American Medical Association, 78,* 77-81.
10. Diener, M.H., Golding, L.A., & Diener, D. (1995). Validity and reliability of a one-minute half sit-up test of abdominal muscle strength and endurance. *Sports Medicine Training and Rehabilitation, 6,* 105-119.
11. Faigenbaum, A., Skrinar, G., Cesare, W., Kraemer, W., & Thomas, H. (1990). Physiologic and symptomatic responses of cardiac patients to resistance exercise. *Archives of Physical Medicine and Rehabilitation, 71,* 395-398.
12. Faulkner, R.A., Springings, E.S., McQuarrie, A., Bell, R.D. (1989). A partial curl-up protocol for adults based on an analysis of two procedures. *Canadian Journal of Sports Science, 14,* 135-141.
13. Featherstone, J.F., Holly, R., & Amsterdam, E. (1993). Physiologic responses to weight lifting in coronary artery disease. *American Journal of Cardiology, 71,* 287-292.
14. Fletcher, G.F., Balady, G., Froelicher, V.F., Hartley, L.H., Haskell, W.L., & Pollock, M.L. (1995). Exercise standards: A statement for healthcare professionals from the American Heart Association. *Circulation, 91,* 580-615.
15. Golding, L.A., Myers, C.R., & Sinning, W.E. (1989). *The Y's way to physical fitness* (3rd ed.). Champaign, IL: Human Kinetics.
16. Graves, J.E., Pollock, M.L., & Bryant, C.X. (2001). Assessment of muscular strength and endurance. In Roitman, J.L. (Ed.), *ACSM's resource manual for guidelines for exercise testing and prescription* (4th ed., pp. 376-380). Baltimore: Williams & Wilkins.
17. Guralnik, J.M., Simosick, E.M., Ferrucci, L., Glynn, R.J., Berkman, L.F., Blazer, D.G., Scherr, P.A., & Wallace, R.B. (1994). A short physical performance battery assessing lower extremity function: Association with self reported disability and prediction of mortality and nursing home admission. *Journal of Gerontology, 49,* M85-M94.
18. Haslam, K.A., McCartney, S.N., McKelvie, R.S., & MacDougall, J.D. (1988). Direct measurements of arterial blood pressure during formal weightlifting in cardiac patients. *Journal of Cardiopulmonary Rehabilitation, 8,* 213-225.
19. Jackson, A.W., Morrow, J.R., Brill, P.A., Kohl, H.W. (1998). Relations of sit-up and sit-and-reach to low back pain in adults. *Journal of Orthopaedic and Sports Physical Therapy, 27,* 22-26.
20. Jones, C.J., Rikli, R.E., & Beam, B.C. (1999). A 30-s chair-stand test as a measure of lower body strength in community-residing older adults. *Research Quarterly for Exercise and Sports, 70,* 113-119.
21. Kraemer, W., & Fry, A. (1995). Strength testing development and evaluation of methodology. In P.J. Maud & C. Foster (Eds.), *Physiological assessments of human fitness* (pp. 115-138). Champaign, IL: Human Kinetics.
22. Lawrence, R., & Jette, A.M. (1996). Disentangling the disablement process. *Journals of Gerontology. Series B, Psychological Sciences and Social Sciences, 51b,* 5173-5182.
23. McMurdo, M., & Rennie, L. (1993). A controlled trial of exercise by residents of old people's homes. *Age and Aging, 22,* 11-15.
24. *Older Americans 2000: Key indicators of well-being.* Hyattsville, MD: Federal Interagency Forum on Aging Related Statistics.
25. Pollock, M., & Evans, W. (1999). Resistance training for health and disease. *Medicine and Science in Sports and Exercise, 31,* 10-11.
26. Pollock, M.L., Franklin, B.A., Balady, G.J., Bernard, L., Chaitman, M.D., Fleg, J.L., Fletcher, B., Limacher, M., Pina, I.L., Stein, R.A., Williams, M., & Bazzarre, T. (2000). Resistance exercise in individuals with and without cardiovascular disease benefits, rationale, safety, and prescription. *Circulation, 101,* 828-833.
27. Rikli, R.E., & Jones, C.J. (1999). Development and validation of a functional fitness test for community residing older adults. *Journal of Aging and Physical Activity, 7,* 129-161.
28. Rikli, R.E., & Jones, C.J. (2001). *Senior fitness test manual.* Champaign, IL: Human Kinetics.
29. Wenger, N.K., Froelicher, E.S., Smith, L.K., Ades, P.A., Berra, K., Blumenthal, J.A., Cerro, C.M., Dattilo, A.M., Davis, D., DeBusk, R.F., Drozda, J.P., Fletcher, B.J., Franklin, B.A., Gaston, H., Greenland, P., McBride, P.E., McGregor, C.G.A., Oldridge, N.B., Piscarella, J.C., & Rogers, F.J. (1995). *Cardiac rehabilitation as secondary prevention. Clinical practice guideline* (AHCPR publication no. 96-0672). Rockville, MD: U.S. Department of Health and Human Services, Public Health Service, Agency for Health Care Policy and Research and the National Heart, Lung, and Blood Institute.

nine

Flexibility and Low Back Function

Wendell Liemohn

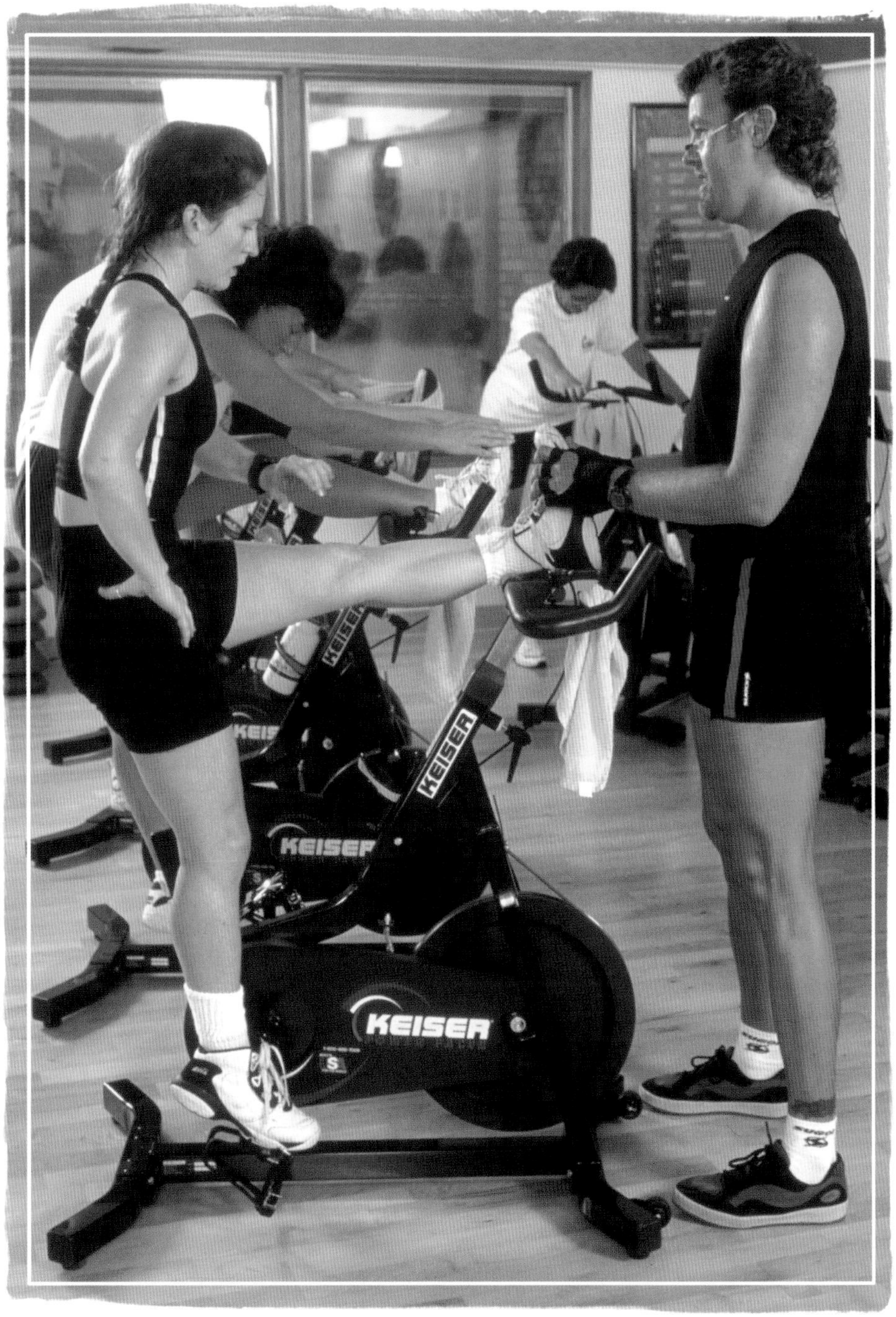

Objectives

The reader will be able to do the following:

1. Describe the relationship between flexibility/ROM and low back function.
2. List five factors that can affect the degree of an individual's flexibility/ROM.
3. Describe the amount of flexion that can occur between the rib cage and the sacrum and state a general rule to follow in performing lumbar extension exercises.
4. Explain why having good ROM at the hip joint is important to having a healthy back.
5. Describe the pluses and minuses of the sit-and-reach test.

Flexibility relates to the ability to bend without breaking; the related word *flexion* is the act of bending or being bent. In applied anatomy, flexion is used to denote a bending movement in the sagittal plane as two body segments are moved in approximation to each other (see chapter 27). If you were to bend over and touch your toes from the standing position, you would be demonstrating flexion at both iliofemoral (hip) joints and limited flexion in the lower intervertebral joints of the spine.[1] When you returned to the standing position, the movement would be called extension; further movement of the trunk backward beyond your normal standing posture would be called hyperextension (see chapter 27). What is somewhat ironic is that individuals may be called flexible if they can show an extreme amount of mobility in either forward bending (i.e., flexion) or backward bending (i.e., hyperextension) because both movements meet the criteria for the definition of flexion. In part because there is potential confusion in describing an individual's ability to hyperextend as being indicative of flexibility, *range of motion* (ROM) frequently is used in place of flexibility. The terms flexibility and ROM, however, often are interchanged.

Having functional ROM at all joints of the musculoskeletal system is desirable to ensure efficient body movement; this is one reason why flexibility is a key component of physical fitness. Although some individuals might be considered to have very good ROM because they performed well in a flexibility test, flexibility is considered a joint-specific characteristic. In other words, having good trunk flexion ROM does not guarantee having good trunk extension ROM. Moreover, sometimes ROM might be related to one's genotype (i.e., heredity related). In other cases, ROM might be related more to the activities in which one participates. For example, many years of ballet or gymnastics training would be expected to make an individual more flexible than someone of the same age, the same sex, and a comparable genotype who did not participate in such training.

If the body is viewed as a kinetic chain, any asymmetrical tightness or looseness in the joints of the lower extremities could affect the spine. When low back function is considered, good ROM usually is considered desirable too. Once a low back problem occurs, increasing ROM can reduce both the severity of the problem and the amount of time it takes to recover and return to work. However, it is also possible that too much mobility can contribute to instability; an example of this could occur if there were damage to a disc and the supporting ligaments of this motion segment.

1 In Review

Flexibility and ROM are joint specific. Having good ROM can decrease chances of having a low back problem. Once a low back problem has occurred, increasing ROM is a goal in most therapeutic exercise programs. However, in some cases a damaged motion segment may enable too much ROM and cause instability.

Factors Affecting ROM

Many different factors can affect ROM. Although age, sex, and genotype may be good predictors, there are always exceptions.

[1]The greatest amount of intervertebral movement occurs between the fifth lumbar vertebra (L5) and the fused sacrum (which begins with S1); this is referred to as the lumbosacral joint. The intervertebral joint between L4 and L5 also permits a substantial portion of the movement in the lower portion of the spine; however, the amount of movement permitted between L1 and L4 is nominal.

Effect of Age and Sex on ROM

The amount of ROM one has depends on several demographic variables. For example, ROM typically decreases in adulthood; however, it is unknown how much of this diminution in ROM is attributable to aging per se or to the reduction in physical activity related to aging. Sex is another consideration; although females are generally considered to be more flexible than males, the opposite has been found to be true in flexion/extension movements of the spine.

Nature/Nurture Considerations

Marked increases in ROM may be achieved by some individuals who participate in good flexibility training programs; however, one's genotype imposes limitations. Some people have relatively poor flexibility; no matter how hard they train, their flexibility will improve nominally. Although an individual with great flexibility may devote a considerable amount of time to stretching exercises, one's genotype is important too. Moreover, some research suggests that improvements in ROM may relate more to the ability to tolerate pain than to actual changes in connective tissue length (14, 16).

Postural Considerations

If individuals did not use their full ROM at a joint, tendinous tissue would compensate by shortening. It then would become very difficult to make some of the movements used by many in activities of daily living. For example, a person sitting at a computer terminal for many hours each day without adequate postural support might develop a greater thoracic curve (e.g., a dorsal kyphosis) and round shoulders (see figure 9.1). If habitual postures such as this are maintained excessively, tendinous tissue that previously permitted a wide degree of movement would shorten and impede movement.

Effects of Disease Processes on ROM

The process of disease can have a significant negative impact on a person's ROM. The disease processes of arthritis and osteoporosis and their effect on ROM are discussed next.

Arthritis

Arthritis can have a debilitating effect on ROM because it affects articular cartilage. Articular cartilage,

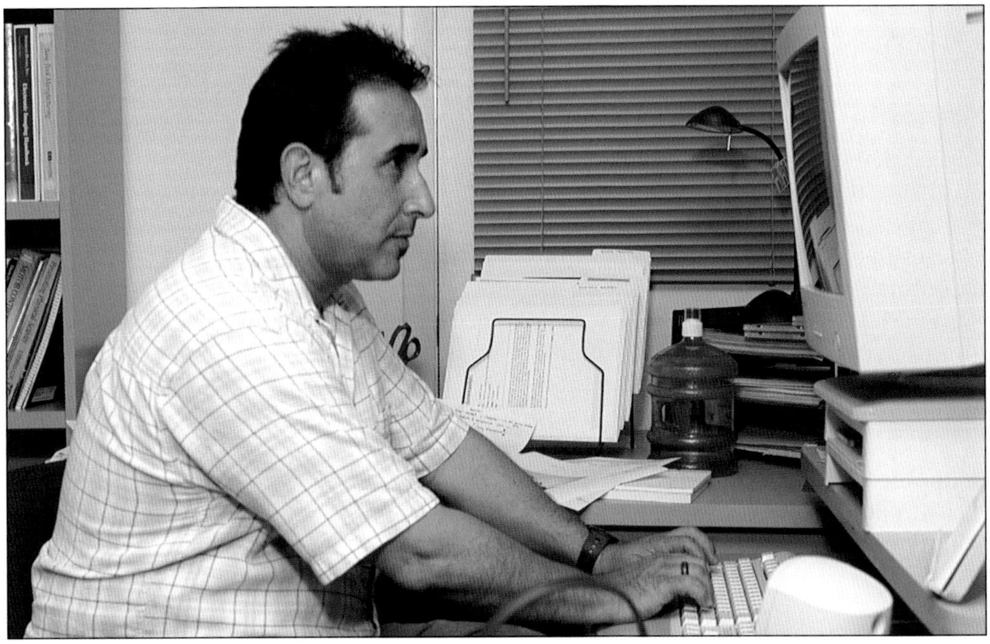

Figure 9.1 Connective tissue structures (e.g., ligaments and tendons) adapt to habitual poor sitting posture by lengthening in response to stress and thus shorten in the absence of stress. Eventually, if no attempt is made to remove these stresses and/or develop counterbalancing ones, poor sitting postures can transfer to poor standing postures.

also called hyaline cartilage, is **avascular** (i.e., it does not have a blood supply); because of this, its healing capability is not good. Thus, if one or more joints have injury or disease, the body's compensatory adaptations may work for a while but often become deficient as the individual ages. Because articular cartilage does not repair itself well, fibrocartilage and / or bony spicules are often the replacement tissues, which further diminishes joint movement. Two of the more common types of arthritis are **rheumatoid arthritis** and **osteoarthritis**. Rheumatoid arthritis affects females more than males and can occur anytime in life but most often between the ages of 25 and 60. It appears to be an autoimmune disease in some cases, but the exact cause is unknown; it can affect a few joints (pauciarticular) or many joints (polyarticular). Osteoarthritis is much more prevalent and accounts for 90 to 95% of arthritis cases. It can be considered a disease of aging, because after age 70 about 85% of the population may be affected. Its cause is usually some injury or mechanical derangement; however, in some cases the cause is unknown.

Lack of mobility attributable to arthritis often is seen in joints such as the fingers or the knee; however, arthritis also can decrease mobility in the spine if the site is a facet joint (see figure 9.2). Because articular cartilage is avascular, it depends on the diffusion of nutrients from tissue fluid; further deterioration can result from lack of movement. Thus, it is desirable for the individual with arthritis to maintain as much ROM as possible.

Osteoporosis

Osteoporosis is characterized by a loss in bone mineral density or bone mass. Although it is a problem seen particularly in women after menopause, it can also affect men and may be genetically influenced. Common osteoporotic sites include the hip, wrist, and vertebrae; a common characteristic of these sites is that cancellous bone predominates (see chapter 27). In the spine, osteoporosis can cause an actual buckling and compression of vertebrae; a person afflicted with this condition may show extreme curves in the spine as well as loss of ROM. Fortunately, cancellous bone can become denser through weight-bearing activities such as weight training.

2 In Review

Factors that relate to one's ROM are age, sex, heredity, posture, and disease. If joint ROM is not used, it will be lost; although declines in ROM relate to increased age, some declines in ROM are related to a decline in physical activity. ROM relates to both nature and nurture; one's genotype as well as the type of activities in which one participates can affect ROM. Habitual poor posture also can decrease ROM. Arthritis is a disease of joints and thus tends to reduce joint ROM. Osteoporosis can reduce spine ROM because of its destructive effect on vertebrae.

ROM and Low Back Function

Spinal carriage is functionally integrated with most movements because many movements emanate from the spine. A strong argument also has been made that the spine and its associated tissues are the primary engine of locomotion in our species (5).

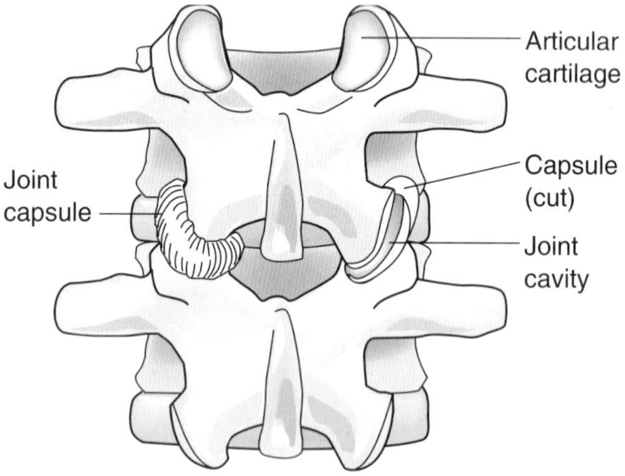

Figure 9.2 Posterior junctions between two vertebrae often are referred to as facet joints. Facet joints are synovial joints and have articular cartilage; if articular cartilage is damaged, arthritis can occur.

Acceptance of this view demands an appreciation of the importance of maintaining good spinal mobility.

Spine ROM

ROM deficiencies in the spine and its supporting structures have been viewed as prognostic indicators of low back pain (1, 19). ROM by itself, however, is not as good a predictor of impending low back problems (2). In other words, although ROM can be a causal factor in some cases of low back pain, more often two or more variables are jointly responsible for the problem. Moreover, individuals with chronic low back pain often receive therapeutic stretching regimens to improve trunk and hip-joint ROM (see chapter 13).

A very important concept is that the flexion movement between the rib cage and the sacrum is, in essence, a straightening of one's "normal" **lumbar lordotic curve** (figure 9.3). Although there may be a progressive decline in spinal mobility in all planes with aging, McKenzie (17) contended that there is a greater decline in extension movement because this movement is used less as a person ages. Unfortunately, extension of the spine is an issue often ignored or misinterpreted in exercise programs (see chapter 13). Although ballistic extension movements of the spine (and ballistic rotation movements) are totally inappropriate, slow and controlled extension movements to maintain ROM and strengthen the erector spinae are appropriate for inclusion in exercise programs. Nevertheless, if active back extension is done, one should not exceed the upper limit of one's normal lumbar lordosis as seen in standing (20).

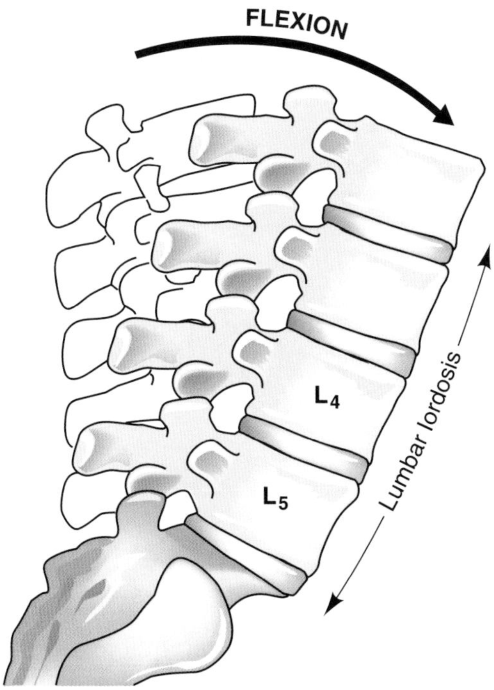

Figure 9.3 In forward movement of the trunk, lumbar flexion per se does not occur. What some may view as lumbar flexion is in essence a removal of the lordotic curve.

An extreme lateral curvature is called **scoliosis**; the HFI can use the Adam's test to get a better perception of the presence or absence of scoliosis in a client (figure 9.4). Although many causes have been identified for scoliosis, usually the cause is unknown. It is not surprising that leg-length discrepancy leading to a lateral tilt of the pelvis is associated with scoliosis and low back pain; however, the evidence that scoliosis causes low back pain is not conclusive. Dependent on the degree of scoliosis seen, a person with this condition may present with a different posturing of the rib cage when performing abdominal strengthening exercises because of the spinal rotation that scoliosis may cause.

Iliofemoral-Joint ROM

The muscles crossing the hip joint sometimes are viewed as "guy wires" bracing the pelvis (see figure 9.5); if any of these guy wires are too tight, the trunk musculature, regardless of how well it is developed, may have difficulty controlling pelvic position. Because the sacral portion of the pelvis is the foundation for the 24 vertebrae stacked on it, pelvic positioning plays an important role in the integrity of the spine. For example, tightness in the hip flexors such as the iliopsoas will produce an anterior or forward pelvic tilt; tightness in the hip extensors such as the hamstrings will produce a backward or posterior pelvic tilt (see figure 9.5). Thus, if either of these muscle groups is tight, the ability of the abdominal muscles to control pelvic positioning will be adversely affected. Individuals who cannot control their pelvic positioning with their abdominal muscles are vulnerable to having low back pain; this is one of the reasons why good ROM at the iliofemoral joint is important.

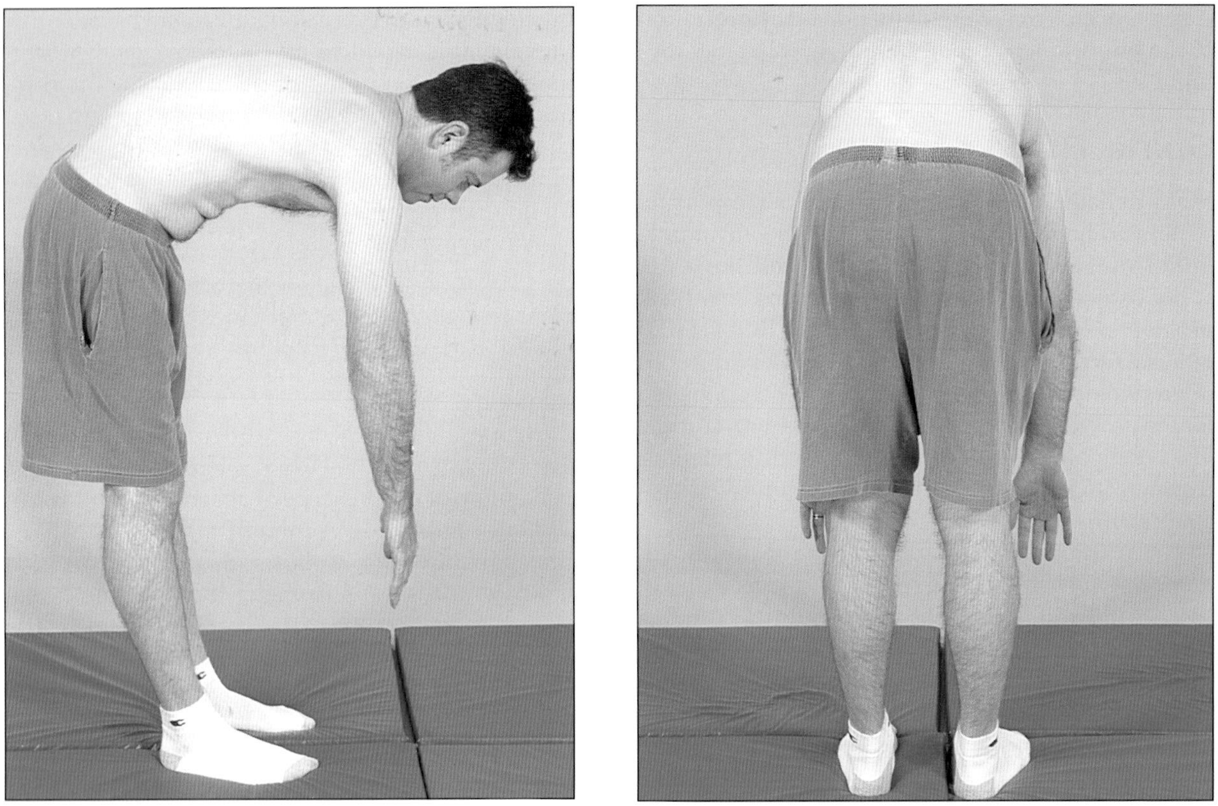

Figure 9.4 Adam's test. Viewing the spinous processes as the subject is standing does not always reveal scoliotic curves even if present. However, it is much easier to see a scoliotic curve after the subject bends forward at the waist.

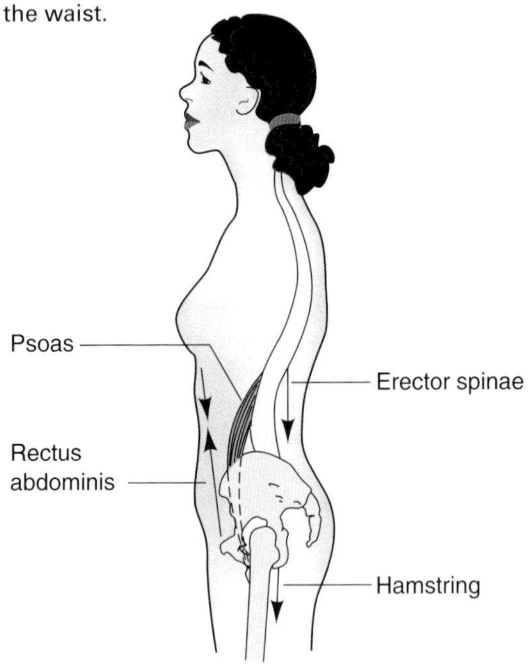

Figure 9.5 The muscles crossing the hip joint can be viewed as guy wires. If, for example, the hamstring guy wires are too tight, the rectus abdominis will have difficulty in controlling pelvic positioning. Inability to control pelvic positioning with the abdominal musculature makes one vulnerable to low back problems.

It is also possible that tightness may be caused by factors other than the muscles that are active in movement at the hip joint. For example, tightness in the iliotibial (I-T) band can limit adduction of the thigh. Tightness in the piriformis muscle can limit movement in the transverse plane; this is a little more complex because it can limit outward or inward rotation of the femur dependent on the hip-thigh angle (22).

3 In Review

Spine flexion between the rib cage and the sacrum is limited to the straightening of one's normal lordotic curve. Although maintenance of spine extension ROM is important, ballistic back extension movements should be avoided and back extension should not exceed the exerciser's normal lumbar lordosis. I-T band and piriformis tightness also can have a deleterious effect on the biomechanics of the iliofemoral joint.

Measuring Spine and Hip-Joint ROM

Some of the techniques used to measure ROM as it relates to low back function are specific to the spine or to the hip joint; other techniques purport to measure spine and hip-joint ROM concurrently. Because some of these techniques warrant more discussion than others, some techniques are discussed here and others are shown in this chapter's appendix.

Trunk-Extension ROM

In Imrie and Barbuto's (8) test for back extension, the back musculature is not actively used; it is considered a passive test of back ROM because the hyperextension movement in the spine is the result of arm and shoulder muscle contraction (see appendix). An active test of spine-extension ROM called the trunk lift was developed by the Cooper Institute for Aerobics Research (4). It is an active test because muscles of the spine (i.e., erector spinae and multifidus) are responsible for hyperextending the spine (see appendix). Because both trunk-extensor muscle strength and ROM contribute to performance on the trunk lift test and only ROM contributes to performance on the passive test, we used multiple regression analyses to further study performance on these tests by university students. Somewhat to our surprise we found that the two tests in essence measure the same construct (12).

Hip-Joint ROM

The Thomas test (see appendix) typically is used to measure tightness in the hip flexors. Two of the more popular tests used to measure tightness in the hip extensors include the relatively new active knee-extension test (see appendix) and the often used passive straight-leg raise test (see appendix). In some instances it may be desirable to check for tightness in the I-T bands and in the piriformis muscles (these tests are illustrated in the appendix).

4 In Review

Good ROM at the hip joint is important for good biomechanics of the spine. Although hip-flexor tightness is not seen as often as hip-extensor tightness, both are important factors in maintaining a healthy spine. Tightness in the muscles crossing the hip joint may make an individual susceptible to low back problems.

Combined Tests of Trunk and Hip-Joint Flexion ROM

The fingertips-to-floor and the sit-and-reach tests have often been used under the pretense that they measure flexibility in the low back as well as at the hip joint. It has been shown conclusively, however, that although both can be used as measures of hip-joint flexibility (e.g., hamstring length), in their conventional use neither test is an effective measure of low back ROM (15). Because the sit-and-reach is used more as a field test than the fingertips-to-floor test, it is examined here in greater detail. Most of the following comments apply to its use either as an exercise or as a test.

Using the sit-and-reach test as an exercise has been questioned clinically. For example, if the hamstrings are tight and one performs the sitting stretch ballistically, the structures of the spine may be obligated to absorb these stresses; over time these repetitive motions may have a serious consequence on low back function. Moreover, it has also been shown that even if the sit-and-reach is done slowly, the static postures resulting during the stretching phase can place high compressive forces on the intervertebral discs (18). Cailliet (3) cautioned that this exercise might damage ligaments of the spine, particularly if the participant's hamstrings are tight.

To reduce the stress on the spine incumbent in the sit-and-reach, Cailliet (3) recommended what he called a "protective hamstring stretch" (see the appendix to this chapter). In this exercise, the hamstrings of each leg are stretched alternately while the nonstretched limb is bent at the knee joint with its foot flat on the floor next to the contralateral knee. Cailliet contended that lumbosacral stress is less in his hamstring stretch than in the more typical sit-and-reach with both legs extended; if this is true, the same reasoning would warrant administering the sit-and-reach test with only one leg extended. However, we examined lumbosacral movement in university students tested with both legs extended as well as with just one leg extended and found that less flexion movement (which would imply less stress) was not seen in Cailliet's version of the sit-and-reach (13). Nevertheless, Cailliet's protective hamstring stretch has other factors in its favor (e.g., permits checking for symmetry) and is deemed to be a safer activity for the spine than the sit-and-reach with both legs extended.

The sit-and-reach has also been questioned because it does not allow for proportional differences between arm, trunk, and leg length. In response to the latter, Hopkins and Hoeger (6) developed a protocol that purportedly would control for some of this variance (see appendix to this chapter for description). More recent research of others suggests that their limb length adjustment did not improve validity (7).

We noted that performance on the sit-and-reach was significantly better with the ankle of the tested leg in passive plantar flexion as opposed to the fixed dorsiflexion posture usually required when the test is administered (11). Our research suggests that factors such as tightness in the connective tissue structures located behind the knee and tension on the **sciatic nerve** can affect performance on the sit-and-reach. (We used a sit-and-reach box that restrained only the heel of the tested leg and permitted the foot to plantar flex into the box.) Most recently, Hui and Yuen (7) reported on a test that also permits plantar flexion of the foot of the tested leg and that does not require a sit-and-reach box. Although their test appears to have some advantages to the sit-and-reach tests previously discussed (see appendix for description), the trunk posturing that this protocol permits might be problematic for some individuals who have disc disease.

Even though the sit-and-reach activity has medical contraindications and a host of factors can affect its performance, it can still be of value as a field test provided that test users are aware of these shortcomings. Following are suggestions that can make the sit-and-reach a better test:

- It is argued that the number of centimeters reached is not the most valid indicator of performance. The test administrator is better advised to examine the quality of the movement of the individual being tested. Quality points to look for include the angle of the sacrum (see figure 9.6) and the "smoothness" of the spinal curve. These relatively simple determinations can be used to make the sit-and-reach a measure of low back mobility as well as a measure of hamstring length. These and other quality points are delineated in figure 9.6.
- It is recommended that the sit-and-reach be administered with only one leg extended. Although this technique doubles the number of measurements required, the tester will be able to evaluate symmetry.
- If a sit-and-reach box is used to make measurements, it is recommended that it be altered to permit passive plantar flexion at the ankle joint. This may be done by converting the standard sit-and-reach box by simply replacing the vertical surface under the cantilever extension with a 4-cm rod; this permits plantar flexion into the box but restrains the heel. This adjustment is not necessary if the protocol of Hui and Yuen (7) is followed.

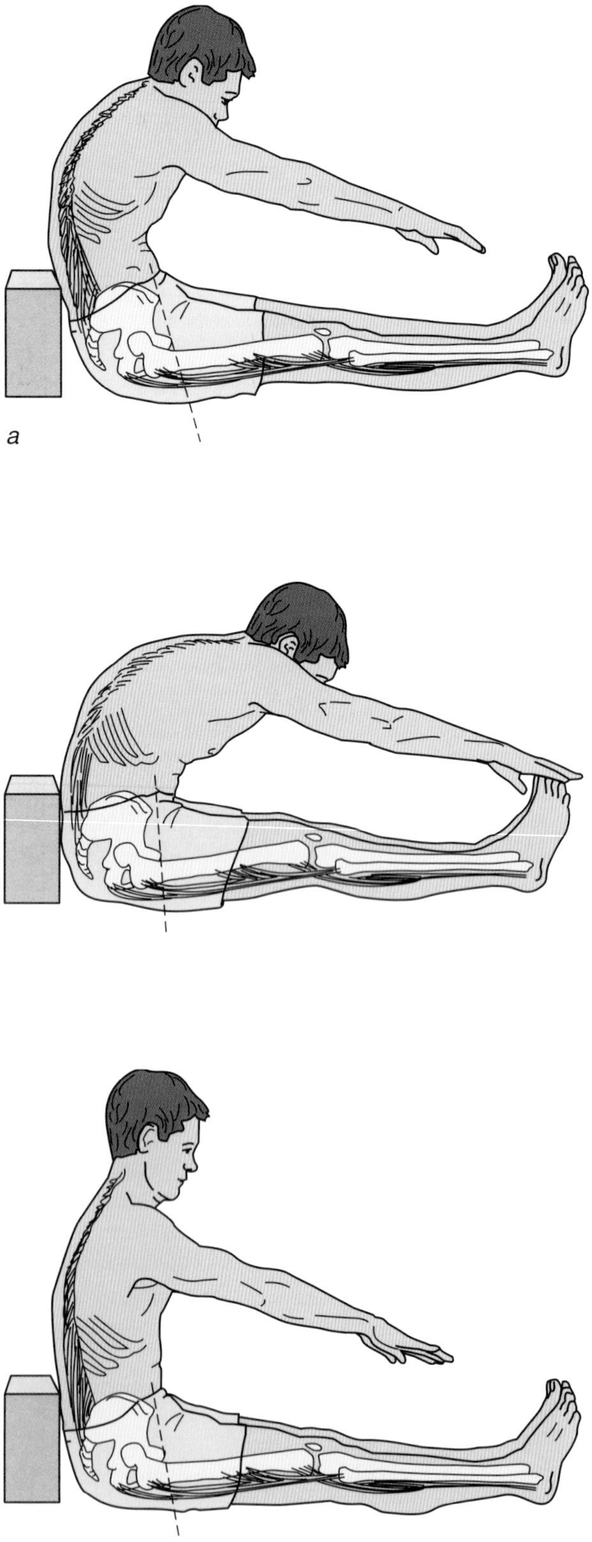

a

c

Figure 9.6 Sit-and-reach test. Quality points to look for: (*a*) tight hamstrings (note tilt of pelvis), tight low back and stretched upper back; (*b*) normal length of hamstrings and low back; (*c*) tight hamstrings (note tilt of pelvis), tight low back.

If you are interested in other tests that are designed specifically to measure spine ROM, two suggestions are offered; however, both require the ability to locate bony landmarks on the pelvis and spine. Keeley et al. (9) described a test protocol for a double inclinometer technique that is used in clinical settings; although inclinometers are expensive (approximately $100 each), they are more versatile than the less expensive goniometer. Williams et al. (21) described a modification of the Schober technique that is used to measure spine ROM; although a tape measure is the only equipment required, this test is used primarily in clinical settings in part because the location of bony landmarks requires the removal of clothing.

5 In Review

If a person with tight hamstrings practices the sit-and-reach maneuver with both legs extended, the soft tissue structures of the spine can be damaged. In administering the sit-and-reach test, the HFI should consider the quality of the movement; it can be more important than the number of centimeters reached.

Case Studies

You can check your answers by referring to appendix A.

9.1

After learning that one of the individuals participating in your physical fitness program was told that his hamstrings were tight, you administer the sit-and-reach test to get some baseline data on his tightness. Somewhat to your surprise you find that he can reach beyond the plane of his toes. What quality factors (i.e., something other than centimeters reached) in his sit-and-reach performance might you further examine to explain this disparity? What other hamstring length test might you administer?

9.2

Another individual's record indicates that she has very tight hip flexors based on an administration of the Thomas test. However, when you administer the Thomas test, you do not find evidence of hip-flexor tightness. Assume that this individual has done nothing to increase her ROM and that you are confident that you administered the Thomas test correctly. Explain how the prior administrator of the test might have erred.

Appendix

Tests for Measuring ROM As It Relates to Low-Back Function

Spine ROM

Passive-Back ROM Test

While keeping the anterior part of the pelvis (i.e., anterior superior iliac spines) in contact with the floor, the subject elevates the torso with arm and shoulder muscles; the muscles of the back are not used in this movement. The score is the perpendicular distance from the suprasternal notch to the floor; from a geometric perspective it should be easy for individuals with longer trunks to have better scores. Scoring: 30 cm (12 in.) or more is excellent, 20 cm (8 in.) or more is good, and 10 cm (4 in.) or more is fair.

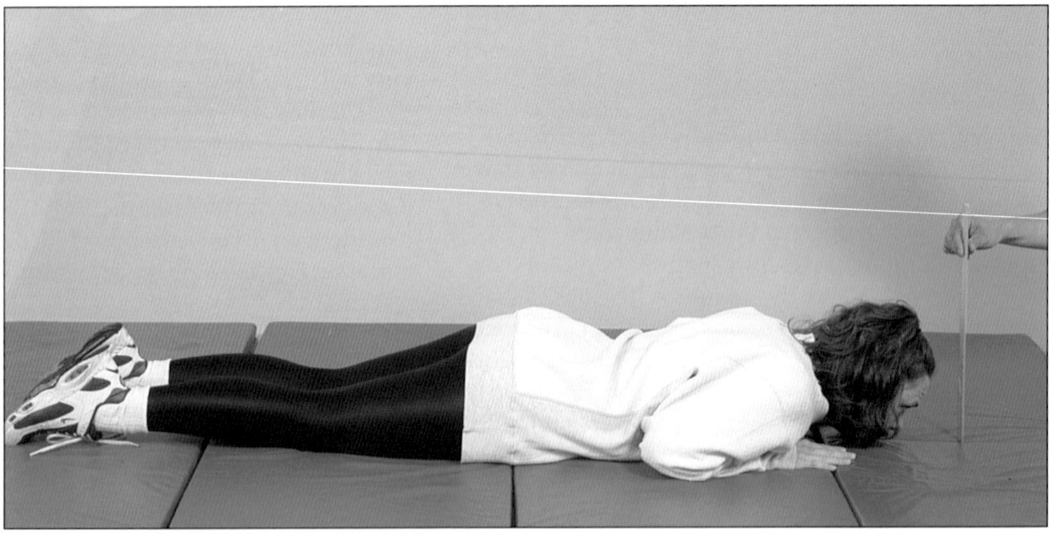

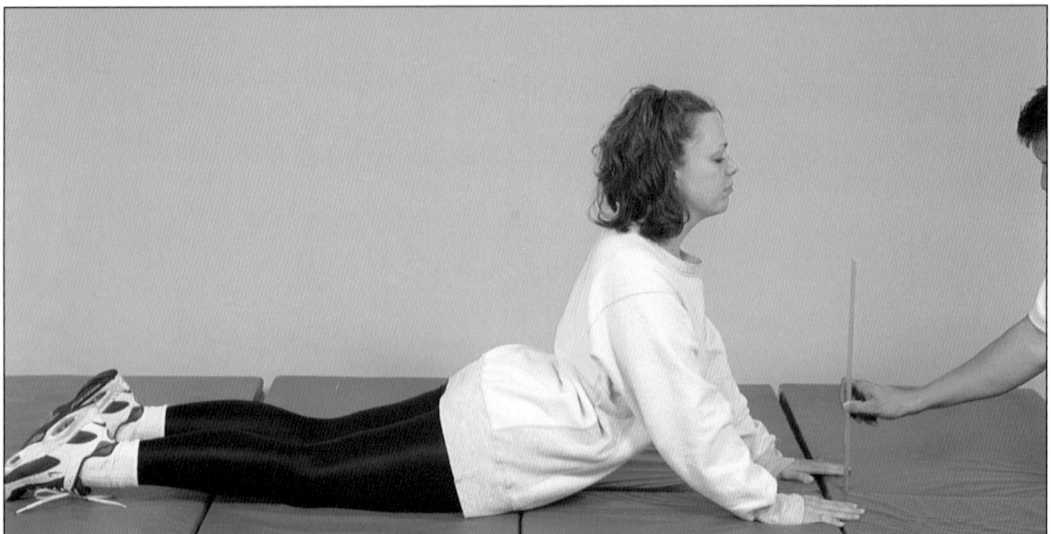

Active Back ROM/Strength Test

In this test, the individual slowly lifts the torso by contracting the erector spinae and multifidus muscle groups until the chin is a maximum of 30 cm (12 in.) from the mat. This item is from the *Cooper Institute for Aerobics Research* (4); although norms were not presented, most individuals tested should be able to raise the chin at least 15 cm (6 in.). (From a geometric perspective, it should be easier for individuals with longer trunks to have better scores; you should consider this factor when administering this test.)

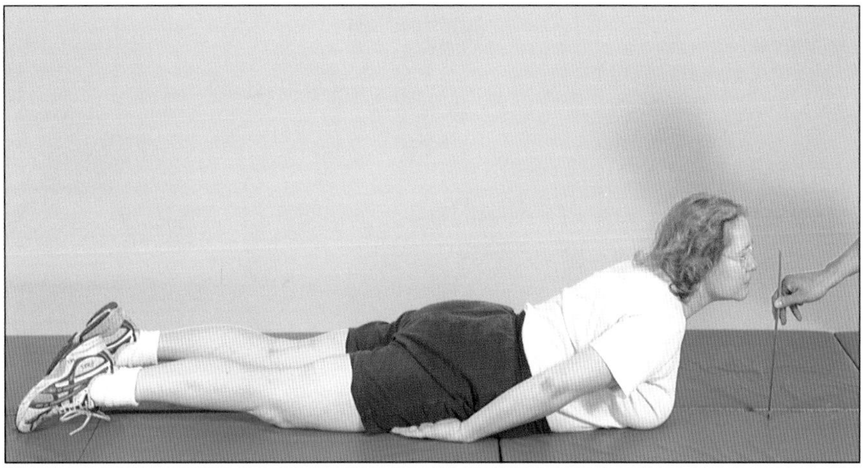

Hip-Joint ROM

Thomas Test

The individual being tested pulls the contralateral leg toward his or her chest until the low back touches the testing surface. The test is successful if the thigh of the straight leg remains in contact with table or floor. If it does not, the degree of elevation indicates the tightness of the hip flexors. The tester must ensure that there is not too much posterior rotation of the pelvis. Some subjects may be able to posteriorly rotate the pelvis beyond the point where the low back touches the testing surface and this could suggest a false positive (i.e., with too much posterior rotation of the pelvis, anyone's hip flexors might look tight).

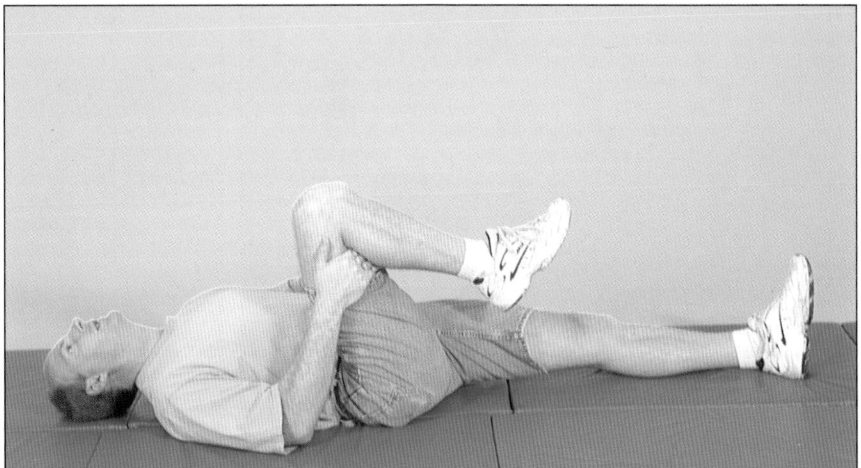

Ober's Test (I-T band tightness)

The pelvis is in the neutral position with the hips stacked. The score is the number of finger breadths that the medial femoral condyle remains elevated from the testing surface (22). This test can be helpful in determining the effect of exercise programming on I-T band tightness, a problem seen in "runner's knee" (also referred to as patellofemoral syndrome or chondromalacia patella).

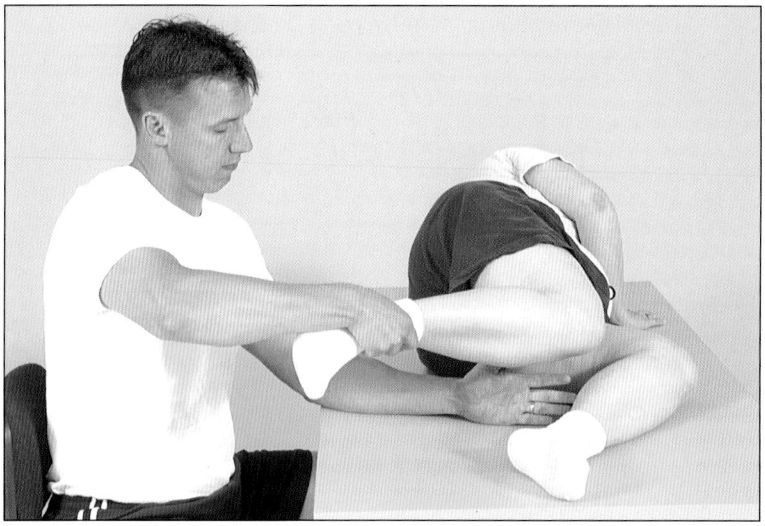

Piriformis ROM

The examination of piriformis ROM is difficult and thus should be done only by those with appropriate experience. It includes (a) assessment below 90° of hip flexion (in this position it is an external rotator and abductor) and (b) assessment above 90° of hip flexion (in this position it is an internal rotator and adductor) (22). This test can be helpful in determining the effect of exercise programming on piriformis tightness.

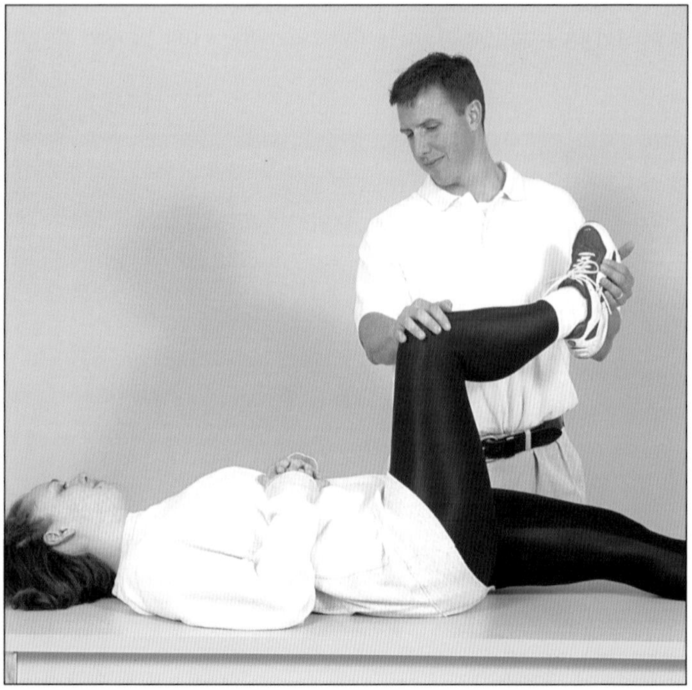

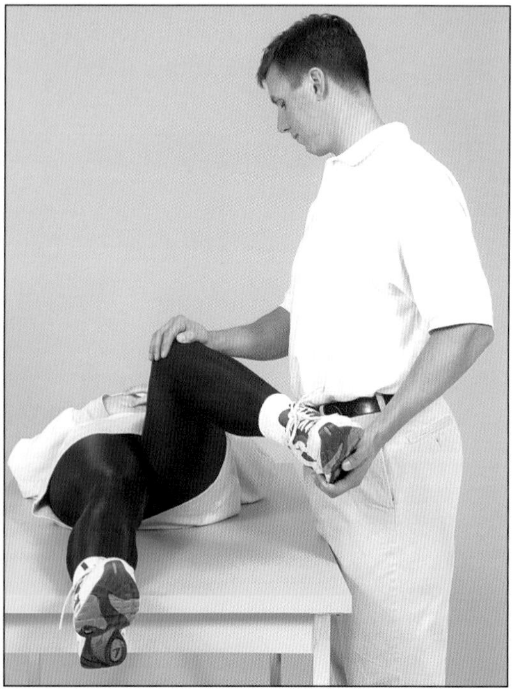

Passive Straight Leg Raise Test

In the straight leg raise test recommended, the pelvis is first posteriorly rotated until the low back is snug against the table; one leg is then raised by the tester while ensuring that the other one remains extended and flat on the testing surface. ROM in flexion can be determined with a goniometer placed on its axis on the greater trochanter or an inclinometer placed just below the tibial tubercle. A minimum of 80° is desirable on the passive straight leg raise; however, most therapists would like to see 90°. If large numbers of subjects are being tested, a protractor-type device can be contrived to speed up the testing process; however, the measurement will not be as precise. (Although the Leighton Flexometer can be used for measuring ROM of the extremities in a test such as this one, its use was not seen in the literature reviewed.)

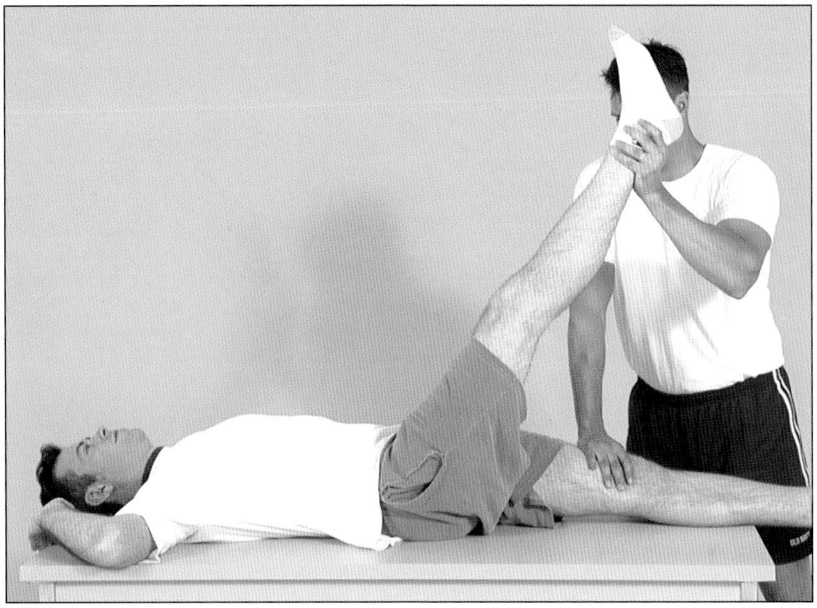

Active Knee-Extension (AKE) Test (Also Called the 90/90 Test)

In this test, the thigh of one leg is raised perpendicular (i.e., 90° to the floor) with the lower 90° to the thigh (the tester will have to hold it in this position). The subject then actively extends the lower leg. A zero score indicates that the leg was moved 90° (i.e., perpendicular to the table and in line with the thigh); a score of 10 indicates that the leg was moved 80°. A score of 5 to 15 is desirable. Many therapists like this test because the individual being tested controls the amount of movement. (Some therapists determine passing ROM using the 90/90 starting position.)

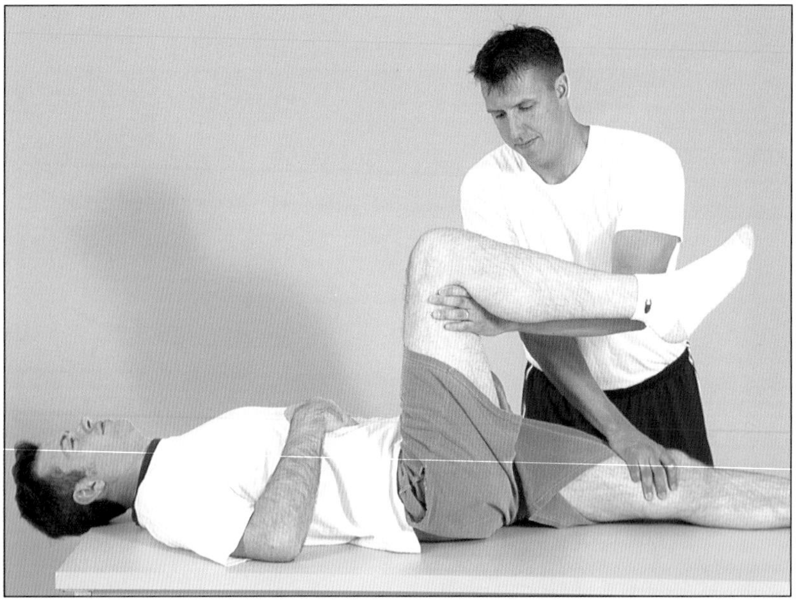

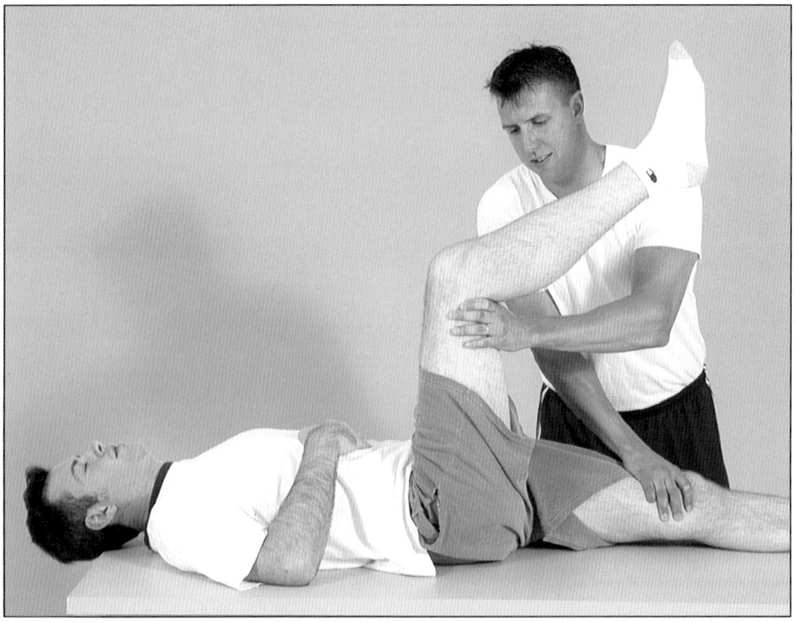

Combined Tests of Trunk and Hip-Joint Flexion

Cailliet Protective Hamstring Stretch

As the participant flexes the hip and knee of the contralateral leg, the attendant posterior rotation of the pelvis decreases the turning moment of inertia of the torso; this is one reason why some believe that this exercise / test is safer than the bilateral sit-and-reach activity (3).

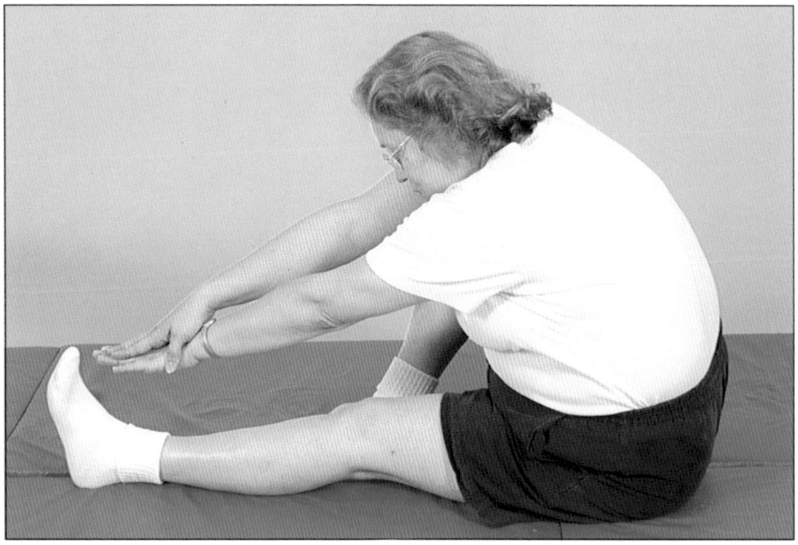

Hopkins and Hoeger Sit-and-Reach

A reach score is first determined with the back against the wall; this score then is subtracted from the maximum reach score (6). Recent research has questioned its validity in adjusting for arm- and leg-length discrepancy.

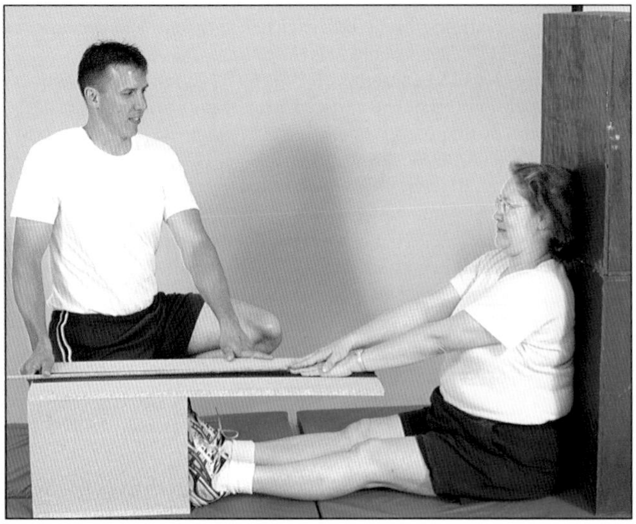

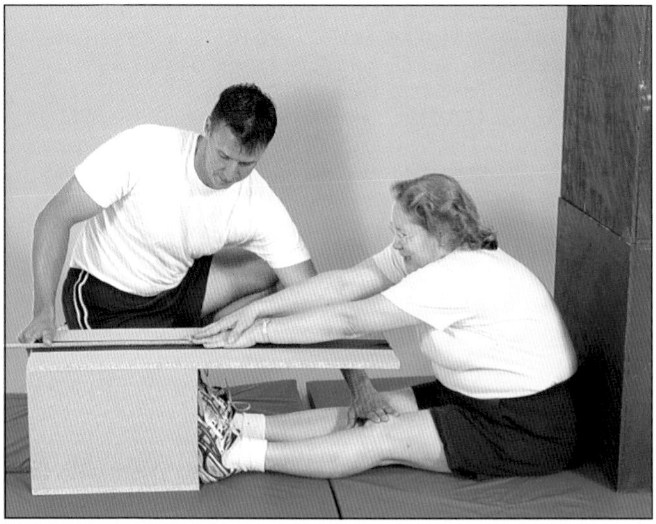

Modified Back-Saver Sit-and-Reach

The only equipment required for this test is a meter rule and a bench. Because the ankle is permitted to passively plantar flex, connective tissue tightness behind the knee, as well as other factors such as sciatic nerve tension, does not affect performance (7).

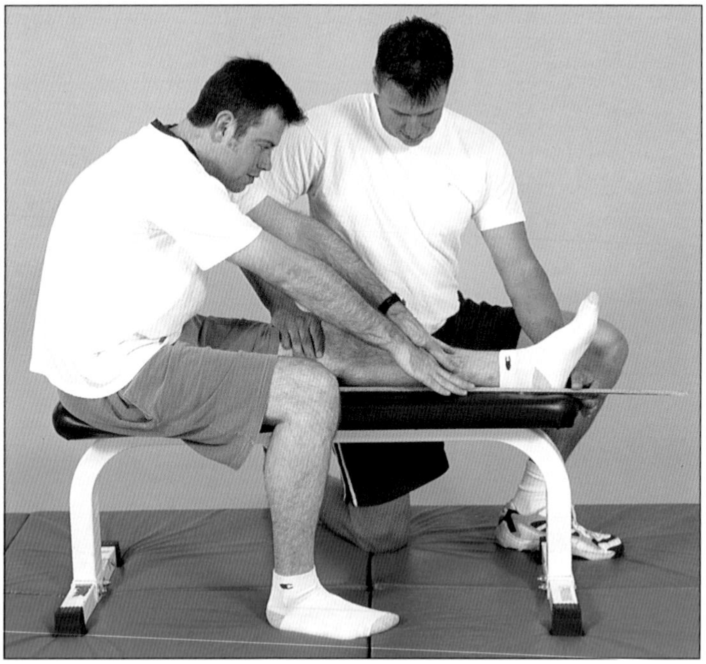

Source List

1. Biering-Sorensen, F. (1984). Physical measurements as risk indicators for low-back trouble over a one-year period. *Spine, 9*(2), 106-119.
2. Cady, L.D., Bischoff, D.P., O'Connell, E.R., Thomas, P.C., Allan, J.H. (1979). Strength and fitness and subsequent back injuries in firefighters. *Journal of Occupational Medicine, 21*(4), 269-272.
3. Cailliet, R. (1988). *Low back pain syndrome*. Philadelphia: Davis.
4. Cooper Institute for Aerobics Research. (1992). *The Prudential FITNESSGRAM*. Dallas: Author.
5. Gracovetsky, S. (1988). *The spinal engine*. New York: Springer-Verlag.
6. Hopkins, D.R., & Hoeger, W.W.K. (1992). A comparison of the sit-and-reach test and the modified sit-and-reach test in the measurement of flexibility for males. *Journal of Applied Sport Science Research, 6*, 7-10.
7. Hui, S.S., & Yuen, P.Y. (2000). Validity of the modified back-saver sit-and-reach test: A comparison with other protocols. *Medicine and Science in Sports and Exercise, 32*(9), 1655-1659.
8. Imrie, D., & Barbuto, L. (1988). *The back power program*. Toronto: Stoddart.
9. Keeley, J., Mayer, T.G., Cox, R., Gatchel, R., Smith, J., Mooney, V. (1986). Quantification of lumbar function. Part 5: Reliability of range-of-motion measures in the sagittal plane and an in vivo torso rotation measurement technique. *Spine, 11*, 31-35.
10. Kendall, F.P., McCreary, E.K., Provance, P.G. (1993). *Muscles: testing and function* (4th ed.). Baltimore: Williams & Wilkins.
11. Liemohn, W., Martin, S.B., Pariser, G. (1997). The effect of ankle posture on sit-and-reach test performance in young adults. *Journal of Strength and Conditioning Research, 11*, 239-241.
12. Liemohn, W., Miller, M., Haydu, T., Ostravski, S., Miles, S., Riggs, S. (2000). An examination of a passive and an active back extension range of motion (ROM) tests. *Medicine and Science in Sports and Exercise, 32*(5), S307.
13. Liemohn, W., Sharpe, G.L., Wasserman, J.F. (1994). Lumbosacral movement in the sit-and-reach and in Cailliet's protective-hamstring stretch. *Spine, 19*, 2127-2130.
14. Magnusson, S.P., Simonsen, E.B., Aagaard, P., Gleim, G.W., McHugh, M.P., Kjaer, M. (1995). Viscoelastic response to repeated static stretching in the human hamstring muscle. *Scandinavian Journal of Medicine and Science in Sports, 5*, 342-347.
15. Martin, S.B., Jackson, A.W., Morrow, J.R., Liemohn, W. (1998). The rationale for the sit and reach test revisited. *Measurement in Physical Education and Exercise Science, 2*(2), 85-92.
16. McHugh, M.P., Kremenic, I.J., Fox, M.B., Gleim, G.W. (1998). The role of mechanical and neural restraints to joint range of motion during passive stretch. *Medicine and Science in Sports and Exercise, 30*(6), 928-932.
17. McKenzie, R. (1981). *The lumbar spine—Mechanical diagnosis and therapy*. Waikanae, New Zealand: Spinal Publications.
18. Nachemson, A. (1975). Towards a better understanding of low-back pain: A review of the mechanics of the lumbar disc. *Rheumatology Rehabilitation, 14*, 129-143.
19. Pope, M.H., Bevins, T., Wilder, D.G., Frymoyer, J.W. (1985). The relationship between anthropometric, postural, muscular, and mobility characteristics of males ages 18-55. *Spine, 10*, 644-648.
20. Saal, J.S., & Saal, J.A. (1991). Strength training and flexibility. In A.H. White & R. Anderson (Eds.), *Conservative care of low back pain* (pp. 65-77). Baltimore: Williams & Wilkins.
21. Williams, R., Binkley, J., Bloch, R., Goldsmith, C.H., Minuk, T. (1993). Reliability of the modified-modified Schober and double inclinometer methods for measuring lumbar flexion and extension. *Physical Therapy, 73*, 26-37.
22. Zuhosky, J.P., & Young, J.L. (2001). Functional physical assessment for low back injuries in the athlete. In W. Liemohn (Ed.), *Exercise prescription and the back* (pp. 67-88). New York: McGraw-Hill Medical.

part three

Exercise Prescription for Health and Fitness

In **part III** we provide guidelines and recommendations for exercise programming for each of the fitness components: cardiorespiratory fitness **(chapter 10)**, weight management **(chapter 11)**, muscular strength and endurance **(chapter 12)**, and flexibility and low-back function **(chapter 13)**. We describe the importance of exercise leadership with examples of a variety of activities in **chapter 14**. **Part IV** includes modifications recommended for individuals with special characteristics or conditions. These recommendations are based on two exercise training principles. The degree to which a tissue such as bone, skeletal muscle, or cardiac muscle functions depends on the activity to which it is exposed. This statement summarizes the two major principles underlying training programs: overload and specificity.

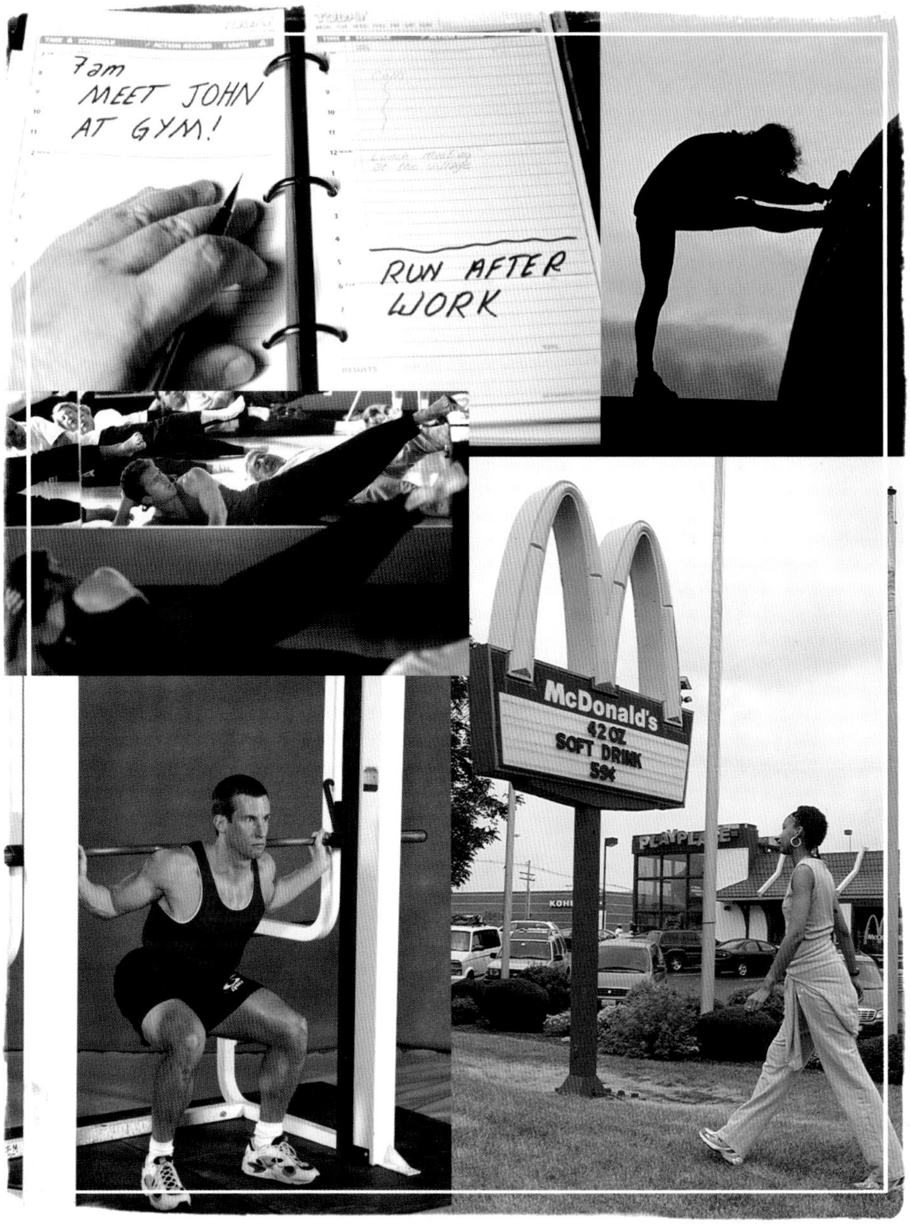
7am
MEET JOHN
AT GYM!
RUN AFTER
WORK
McDonald's
42 OZ
SOFT DRINK
59¢

The principle of **overload** describes a dynamic characteristic of living creatures: Use increases functional capacity. If a tissue or organ system is required to work against a load to which it is not accustomed, it becomes stronger instead of wearing out and becoming weaker. The slang for this principle is "use it or lose it." The corollary of the overload principle is the principle of **reversibility**, which indicates that physiological gains are lost when the load against which a tissue or organ system is working is reduced. The variables that contribute to an overload in an exercise program include the intensity, duration, and frequency of the exercise. As we will see, it is the combination of these elements that results in a sufficient amount of total work, or energy expenditure, to cause an increase in the functional capacity of the cardiorespiratory (CR) systems.

The principle of **specificity** states that the training effects derived from an exercise program are specific to the exercise done and the muscles involved. For example, a person who runs as a primary form of exercise shows little change in the arm muscles. The person who exercises at a low intensity that recruits only slow-twitch muscle fibers will have little or no training effect in the fast-twitch fibers in the same muscle groups. If muscle fibers are not used they cannot adapt, and, consequently, they will not become "trained." The type of adaptation that occurs as a result of training is specific to the type of training taking place (e.g., endurance vs. heavy resistive strength training). Running causes an increase in the number of capillaries and mitochondria in the muscle fibers involved in the exercise and make them more resistant to fatigue. Strength training causes a hypertrophy of the muscles involved, due to an increase in the amount of contractile proteins, actin and myosin, in the muscle.

In summary:

- Tissues adapt to the load to which they are exposed
- To increase the functional capacity of a tissue, it must be *overloaded* (i.e., subjected to a load to which it is not accustomed).
- The type of adaptation is *specific* to the muscle fibers involved and the type of exercise.
- Endurance exercise increases mitochondria and capillary number
- Strength training increases contractile protein and size of the muscle.

ten

Exercise Prescription for Cardiorespiratory Fitness

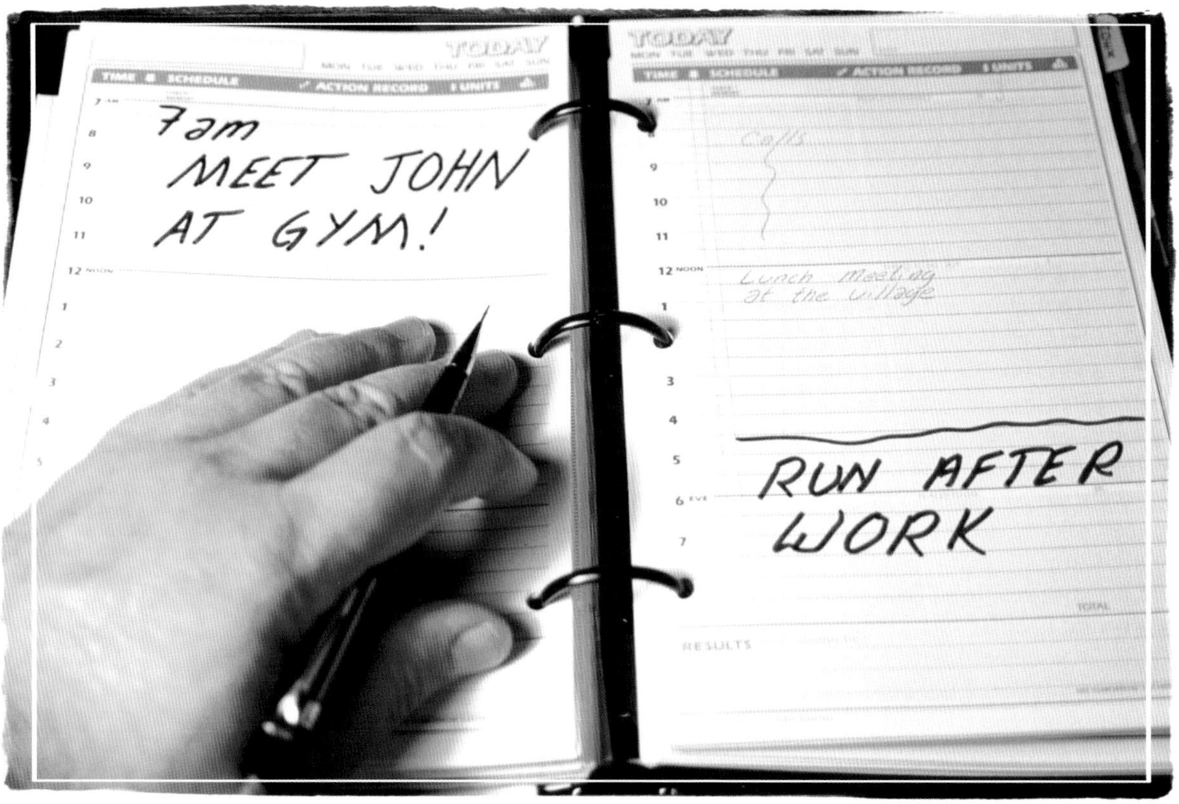

© Will Funk

Objectives

The reader will be able to do the following:

1. Characterize the "dose" of exercise in an exercise prescription and identify means by which a health-related effect might occur.
2. Describe the public health recommendation for physical activity.
3. Explain the concepts of overload and specificity as they relate to training programs, and describe general guidelines related to cardiorespiratory fitness programs, including those related to warm-up and cool-down.
4. Develop an exercise prescription for correct exercise intensity, duration, and frequency to achieve and maintain cardiorespiratory fitness goals.
5. Express exercise intensity in terms of energy production, HR, and RPE.
6. Contrast the approaches used for developing exercise prescriptions for the general public, the fit population, and people whose complete GXT results are available; describe the differences between a supervised and an unsupervised program.
7. Describe the effects of temperature and humidity, altitude, and pollution on the exercise prescription.

In the introductory chapters to this text we indicated the importance of physical activity and physical fitness for health. In fact, the *Surgeon General's Report on Physical Activity and Health* (58) concluded that physical inactivity is a major risk factor for cardiovascular, respiratory, and metabolic diseases. Of more than 450 health objectives for the nation, *Healthy People 2010* (59) selected physical activity as one of the top 10 health indicators. A recent symposium on dose-response issues concerning physical activity and health concluded that regular physical activity is associated with a reduction in all-cause mortality, fatal and nonfatal total cardiovascular disease (CVD), and CHD. Physical activity also was linked to a reduction in the incidence of obesity and type 2 diabetes and an improvement in metabolic control in individuals with type 2 diabetes (12, 36). This chapter deals with the important question of how much activity is needed to bring about the desired effects, with a focus on cardiorespiratory fitness (CRF).

Prescribing Exercise

There is a close parallel between the HFI wishing to know the proper **dose** of exercise needed to bring about a desired **effect** (response) and the physician's need to know the type and quantity of a drug needed to cure a disease. We recognize that there is a difference between what is needed to cure a headache and what is needed to cure tuberculosis. In concert with that, there is no question that the dose of physical activity necessary to achieve a high level of performance is different from that required to improve a health-related outcome (e.g., lowered BP, reduced risk of coronary heart disease). Similarities can be drawn between the dose-response relationship for medications and that for exercise in figure 10.1 (16).

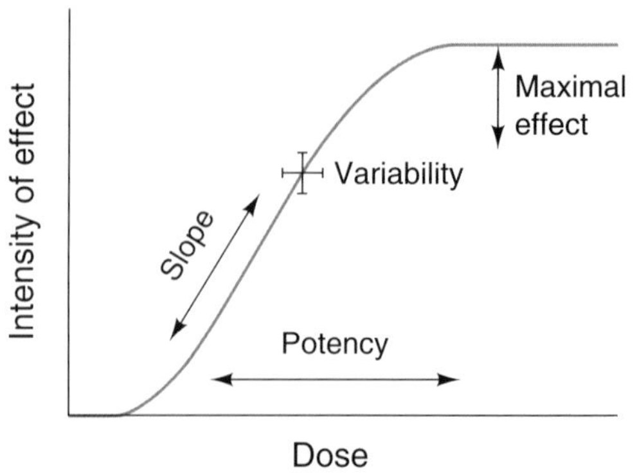

Figure 10.1 Representative log dose-effect curve illustrating its four characterizing parameters.

Reprinted from Goodman and Gilman 1975.

• Potency: The potency of a drug is a relatively unimportant characteristic in that it makes little difference whether the effective dose is 1 mg or 100 mg as long as it can be administered in an appropriate dosage (16). Applied to exercise prescriptions, walking 4 miles at a moderate pace is as effective in expending calories as running 2 miles.

• Slope: The slope of the curve describes how much of an effect comes from a change in dose (16). Some physiological measures such as HR and lactate responses to a fixed exercise task change quickly (in days) for a dose of exercise, whereas some health-related effects (e.g., changes in serum cholesterol) are realized only after many months of exercise.

• Maximal effect: The maximal effect (efficacy) of a drug varies with the type of drug. For example, morphine can relieve pain of all intensities, whereas aspirin is effective against only mild to moderate pain (16). Similarly, strenuous exercise can increase $\dot{V}O_2$max and modify risk factors, whereas light to moderate exercise can change risk factors with only a minimal impact on $\dot{V}O_2$max.

• Variability: The effect of a drug varies between individuals and within individuals depending on the circumstances. The point where the slop changes in figure 10.1 indicates the variability in the dose required to bring about a particular effect and the variability in the effect associated with a given dose (16). For example, gains in $\dot{V}O_2$max attributable to endurance training show considerable variation, even when the initial $\dot{V}O_2$max value is controlled for (10).

• Side effect: A last point worth mentioning is that no drug produces a single effect (16). The effects might include adverse (side) effects that limit the usefulness of the drug. For exercise, the side effects might include an increased risk of injury.

Unlike most drugs, which people stop taking when a disease is cured, there is a need to engage in some form of physical activity throughout life to experience the health-related and fitness effects.

The exercise dose is usually is characterized by the intensity, frequency, duration, and type of activity; we discuss each of these in detail later in this chapter. However, in contrast to what we know about the role of each of these variables in improving $\dot{V}O_2$max, little is known about the minimum or optimal quantities of each variable related to achieving health outcomes (24). In the recent symposium on dose-response issues related to physical activity and health, it was concluded that there was strong evidence of an inverse and generally linear relationship between physical activity and the rates of all-cause mortality, total CVD, CHD incidence and mortality, and the incidence of type 2 diabetes. On the other hand, it was more difficult to determine a dose-response relationship for other health outcomes (12, 36). The following Research Insight provides more information.

Research Insight

Although physical activity is known to have a favorable impact on many health-related problems, there has been some question as to whether evidence exists to support a dose-response relationship. To address this issue, scientists examined both the quality and the quantity of evidence linking physical activity to a wide variety of health-related problems. The results of their deliberations were published in a special supplement of *Medicine and Science in Sports and Exercise* (12). The consensus statement (36) from that meeting found that more activity was associated with lower rates of the following:

- All-cause mortality
- Total cardiovascular disease
- Incidence of CHD and mortality
- Incidence of type 2 diabetes
- Total fat
- Colon and breast cancer
- Osteoporosis

More (of certain types) activity may cause problems:

- Low back pain
- Osteoarthritis

Although physical activity is important to prevent or treat the following health problems, the symposium found no evidence of a dose-response for physical activity in the following health problems:

- Blood pressure
- Stroke
- Glucose control in type 2 diabetes
- Blood lipids
- Abdominal and visceral fat
- Depression
- Anxiety
- Independent living in older adults

Cause and Effect

The response (effect) generated by a particular dose of exercise can include changes in $\dot{V}O_2$max, resting BP, insulin sensitivity, body weight (percentage body fat), and depression. However, as Haskell (23, 24) pointed out, we may have to reexamine our understanding of cause and effect when we study how a dose of physical activity is related to the responses of physical fitness and health. Physical activity could bring about favorable changes by improving

- fitness (especially cardiovascular fitness) and thereby improving health,
- fitness and health simultaneously and separately,
- fitness but not a specific health outcome, or
- some specific health outcome but not fitness.

It has become clear that improvements in a variety of health-related concerns are not dependent on an increase in $\dot{V}O_2$max; this distinction is important to mention at the beginning of this chapter, which concerns itself with appropriate ways to improve $\dot{V}O_2$max.

1 In Review

An exercise dose reflects the interaction of the intensity, frequency, duration, and type of exercise. The cause of the health-related response may be related to an improvement in $\dot{V}O_2$max or may act through some other mechanism, making health-related outcomes and gains in $\dot{V}O_2$max independent of each other.

Short- and Long-Term Responses to Exercise

Haskell indicated that in addition to understanding the cause-and-effect connection between physical activity and specific outcomes, we need to distinguish between short-term (acute) and long-term (training) responses (22, 25). The patterns of responses in the days and weeks after the initiation of a dose of exercise can vary substantially, depending on the variable being measured:

- Acute responses—Responses occur with one or several exercise bouts but do not improve further.
- Rapid responses—Benefits occur early and plateau.
- Linear responses—Gains are made continuously over time.
- Delayed responses—Responses occur only after weeks of training.

The need for such distinctions can be seen in figure 10.2 (34), which shows proposed dose-response relationships between physical activity, defined as minutes of exercise per week at 60 to 70% of maximal work capacity, and a variety of physiological responses:

- BP and insulin sensitivity are most responsive to exercise.
- Changes in $\dot{V}O_2$max and resting HR are intermediate.
- Serum lipid changes such as increases in HDL are delayed.

The dose-response relationship of exercise to positive physiological responses has important implications when exercise is used alone or in concert with medication to control disease; we discuss this further in chapter 24.

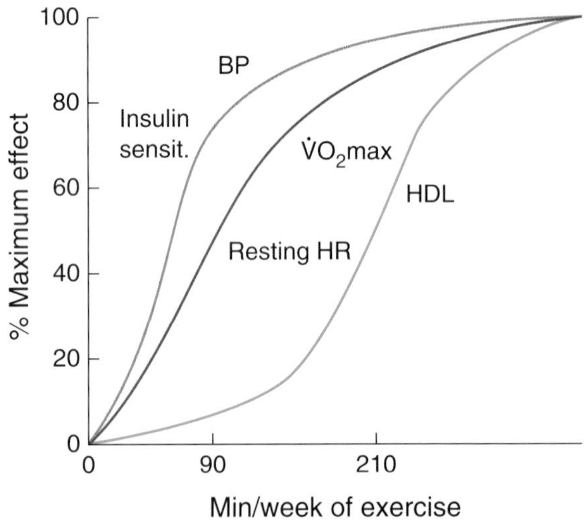

Figure 10.2 Proposed dose-response relationships between amount of exercise performed per week at 60 to 70% maximum work capacity and changes in BP and insulin sensitivity (curve to the left side), which appear most sensitive to exercise; maximum oxygen consumption ($\dot{V}O_2$max) and resting HR, which are parameters of physical fitness (middle curve); and lipid changes, such as HDL (right-hand curve).

Reprinted from G.L. Jennings et al. 1991.

Public Health Recommendations for Physical Activity

It should be no surprise, given the previous discussion, that it is difficult to provide a single exercise prescription that addresses all issues related to prevention and treatment of various diseases. Despite this, there has been a great need to provide a general exercise recommendation to improve the health status of all adults in the United States. The ACSM and the CDC responded to this need by publishing guidelines for physical activity (42): Every U.S. adult should accumulate 30 min or more of moderate-intensity (3-6 METs) physical activity on most, preferably all, days of the week.

These guidelines were based on a comprehensive review of the literature dealing with health-related aspects of physical activity; the dose-response curve in figure 10.3 summarizes the findings. By having the most sedentary group (Group A) move up just one level of physical activity shown in figure 10.3, the greatest gains in health-related benefits can be realized. These physical activity recommendations were based on the finding that caloric expenditure and total time of physical activity are associated with reduced cardiovascular disease and mortality. Furthermore, doing the activity in intermittent bouts (e.g., 10 min) is an alternative way of meeting the 30-min goal (42, 59).

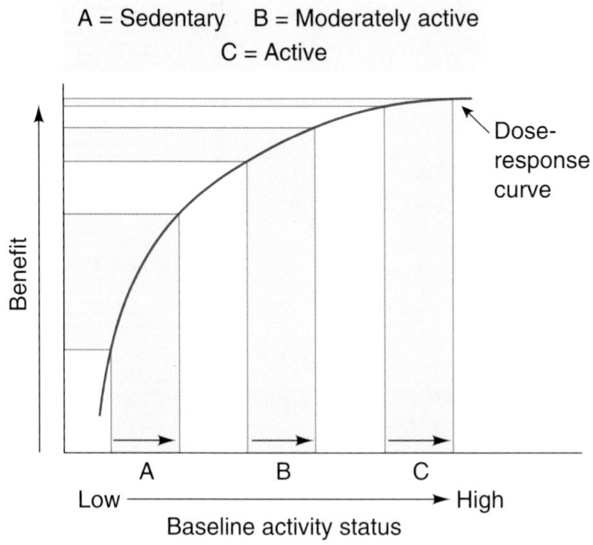

Figure 10.3 The dose-response curve represents the best estimate of the relationship between physical activity (dose) and health benefit (response). The lower the baseline physical activity status, the greater will be the health benefit associated with a given increase in physical activity (arrows A, B, and C).

Reprinted from Pate et al. 1995.

2 In Review

The basis for the public health physical activity recommendations is that the health-related benefits of physical activity may be more related to the total number of calories expended than to the intensity level of the exercise. The focus of this exercise prescription aimed at sedentary individuals is for moderate activity to be done most, if not all, days of the week for a total of 30 min per day.

The preceding physical activity recommendations are appropriate for individuals taking the first step from being sedentary to becoming active. However, individuals who expend more than 2000 kcal per week, or who possess a high $\dot{V}O_2$max, show the lowest death rate from all causes (5, 41). Consequently, there are benefits to be gained not only when a sedentary person becomes active but also as a moderately active person engages in more vigorous exercise that increases functional capacity ($\dot{V}O_2$max). The purpose of this chapter is to lead you through the steps involved in developing an exercise prescription to improve CRF in apparently healthy individuals.

General Guidelines for CRF Programs

To apply the principles of overload and specificity (see Introduction to part III) to CRF, activities that overload the heart and respiratory systems need to be used in exercise programs. Activities that use the large-muscle groups contracting in a rhythmic and continuous manner are effective in overloading the cardiorespiratory systems. Activities involving a small-muscle mass and weight training exercises are less appropriate because they tend to generate very high cardiovascular loads relative to energy expenditure (see chapter 28). Activities that improve CRF are high in caloric cost and therefore help to achieve a relative leanness goal. How do you get someone started?

Screen Participants

If the person has not already done so, have him or her fill out one of the health status forms. Chapter 3 provides guidelines for who should and should not seek medical clearance before exercising.

Encourage Regular Participation

Exercise must become a valuable part of a person's lifestyle. It is not something that can be done sporadically, nor will doing it for only a few months or years build up a fitness reserve. Dramatic gains accomplished through fitness activities are lost quickly with inactivity (see chapter 28). Only people who continue activity as a way of life enjoy its long-term benefits (remember the principle of reversibility).

Provide Different Types of Activities

A fitness program starts with easily quantified activities, such as walking or cycling, so that the proper exercise intensity can be achieved. After a minimum level of fitness is achieved, a variety of activities are included in the program. Chapter 14 outlines three phases of activities: (a) work up to walking briskly for 4 miles per workout; (b) gradually begin jogging, and work up to jogging continuously for 3 miles; and (c) introduce a variety of activities, including exercise to music.

Program for Progression

Given the importance of helping sedentary people become active, the emphasis in any health-related fitness program that includes such individuals should be to start slowly and, when in doubt, do too little rather than too much. Participants should begin at work levels that can be easily completed and should be encouraged to gradually increase the amount of work they can do during a workout. For example, a sedentary participant who is interested in jogging as a goal should begin a training program by walking a distance that she or he can complete without feeling fatigued or sore. With time, the participant will be able to walk a greater distance at a faster pace without discomfort. After this person can walk 4 miles briskly without stopping, she or he can gradually work up to jogging 3 miles continuously per workout. For the participant who is ready to begin jogging, you might introduce the interval-type workout (walking / jogging / walking / jogging). As individuals adapt to the interval workouts, they will be able to gradually increase the amount of jogging while decreasing the distance walked (see the walking and jogging programs in chapter 14).

Adhere to Format for a Fitness Workout

The main body of the fitness workout consists of dynamic large-muscle group activities at an intensity high enough and a duration long enough to accomplish enough total work to specifically overload the cardiorespiratory systems. Stretching and light endurance activities are included before the workout (warm-up) and after the workout (cool-down) for safety and to improve low back function.

There are physiological, psychological, and safety reasons for including warm-up and cool-down. In general, the warm-up and cool-down should consist of the following:

- Activities similar to the activities done in the main body of the workout but done at a lower intensity (e.g., walking, jogging, or cycling below THR)
- Stretching exercises for the muscles involved in the activity as well as those in the midtrunk area
- Muscular endurance exercises, especially for the muscles in the abdominal region

These activities help participants ease into and out of a workout and promote a healthy low back. If a workout is going to be shorter than usual, the reduction in time should take place in the main body of the workout, so that 5 to 10 min are retained for the warm-up and cool-down portions.

Conduct Periodic CRF Tests

Routine health-related physical fitness testing to determine a participant's progress can be motivational and may help alter programs that are not achieving desired results. The HFI can help by setting realistic goals for the next testing session when discussing test results. A general rule would be a 10% improvement in 3 months in the test scores that need to change. Once the person has reached a desirable level, the goal is to maintain that level.

3 In Review

People interested in a fitness program should be screened for risk factors and encouraged to participate regularly. The program should provide different types of activities that use large muscle groups and overload the heart and respiratory systems, and the individual should start slowly and progress gradually to higher levels of work. The workout should have a warm-up and a cool-down period, including stretching and muscular endurance exercises for the midtrunk areas. Periodic CRF tests can be used to alter the exercise prescription.

Formulating the Exercise Prescription

The CRF training effect depends on the degree to which the systems are overloaded, that is, the intensity, duration, and frequency of training. Intensity generally is expressed as a percentage of some maximal physiological response, typically, oxygen uptake (%$\dot{V}O_2$max) or HR (%HRmax), or derivatives of these—oxygen uptake reserve ($\dot{V}O_2$R) or HR reserve (HRR). These are described in detail in the next section. The interaction of intensity (low to high), duration (short to long), and frequency (seldom to often) should result in an energy expenditure (total work) of 150 to 400 kcal per day. The lower end of this range is a little over the 1000 kcal / week recommended for health benefits for previously sedentary individuals (3).

Intensity

How hard does a person have to work to provide sufficient overload for the cardiovascular and respiratory systems to increase CRF? To answer this question, we must first define and describe the different expressions of exercise intensity and show how they relate to each other.

- Percentage of maximal oxygen uptake (%$\dot{V}O_2$max). Across a broad range of CRF levels, many physiological responses are normalized (i.e., made similar between individuals) when the intensity of exercise is expressed as a percentage of $\dot{V}O_2$max (%$\dot{V}O_2$max). A person who is working at 24.5 ml · kg^{-1} · min^{-1} and has a $\dot{V}O_2$max of 35 ml · kg^{-1} · min^{-1} is working at 70% $\dot{V}O_2$max. This approach has been used extensively in the development of exercise guidelines, as seen in the *ACSM's Guidelines for Exercise Testing and Prescription* and its position stands. However, in the most recent updates of both of these documents, the relative intensity is expressed as the percentage of oxygen uptake reserve (%$\dot{V}O_2$R) (2, 3).
- Percentage of oxygen uptake reserve (%$\dot{V}O_2$R). $\dot{V}O_2$R is calculated by subtracting one MET (3.5 ml · kg^{-1} · min^{-1}) from the subject's $\dot{V}O_2$max. The %$\dot{V}O_2$R is a percentage of the difference between resting $\dot{V}O_2$ and $\dot{V}O_2$max and is calculated by subtracting 1 MET from the exercise oxygen uptake, dividing by the subject's $\dot{V}O_2$R, and multiplying by 100%. For example, an individual with a $\dot{V}O_2$max of 35 ml · kg^{-1} · min^{-1} who is exercising at 24.5 ml · kg^{-1} · min^{-1} would be at 67% $\dot{V}O_2$R: (24.5 – 3.5) / (35 – 3.5) × 100%. The %$\dot{V}O_2$R is equal to the HR response when it is expressed as a percentage of the HRR (55, 56).
- Percentage of HRR (%HRR). The HRR is calculated by subtracting resting HR from maximal HR. The %HRR is a percentage of the difference between resting and maximal HR and is calculated by subtracting resting HR from the exercise HR, dividing by the HRR, and multiplying by 100%. An individual exercising at 160 beats · min^{-1} who has a maximal HR of 200 beats · min^{-1} and a resting HR of 60 beats · min^{-1} is working at 71% of the HRR: (160 – 60) / (200 – 60) × 100%. Prior to the most recent ACSM position stand, the %HRR was believed to be closely linked to the %$\dot{V}O_2$max on a one-to-one basis, that is, 70% HRR = 70% $\dot{V}O_2$max. Swain et al. (55, 56) pointed out that although this is the case when vigorous exercise is done by fit individuals, it is not the case for low intensities of exercise, especially when performed by those with low fitness levels. For example, a 3 MET activity for someone with a 5 MET maximal aerobic power is 60% $\dot{V}O_2$max but only 50% of $\dot{V}O_2$R: 2 METs / (5 METs – 1 MET) × 100%. An advantage of expressing exercise intensity as %HHR is that the %$\dot{V}O_2$R is numerically identical to the %HRR across the fitness continuum.
- Percentage of maximal HR (%HRmax). Because of the linear relationship between HR (above ~110 beats · min^{-1}) and $\dot{V}O_2$ during dynamic exercise, investigators and clinicians have long used a simple percentage of maximal HR (%HRmax) as an estimate the %$\dot{V}O_2$max in setting exercise intensity. An advantage of this method of expressing exercise intensity is that it is easier to teach than the %HRR.
- Rating of perceived exertion (RPE). The RPE is not viewed as a substitute for prescribing exercise intensity by HR, but once the relationship between the HR and RPE has been established, RPE can be used in its place (2). However, the RPE may not consistently translate to the same intensity for different modes of exercise, so one should not expect an exact matching of the RPE to a %HRmax or %HRR (3).

Table 10.1 shows the categories of exercise intensity as described in the 1998 ACSM position stand, with %$\dot{V}O_2$R and %HRR used to set the standard for the other expressions of exercise intensity (2). These are shown on the left side of the table with intensities ranging from very light to maximal.

The RPE values are based on Borg's 6 to 20 RPE scale (6). The values in table 10.1 for %HRmax and %$\dot{V}O_2$max have been updated to reflect more accurately the relationship between them and %$\dot{V}O_2$R (%HRR) (32). Furthermore, Table 10.1 provides the absolute exercise intensities (in METs) for each of the intensity classifications for four groups that vary in $\dot{V}O_2$max. As you can see, by looking across

Table 10.1 Classification of Physical Activity Intensity

	Endurance-type Activity										
	Relative Intensity			Intensity (METs and %$\dot{V}O_2$max) in Healthy Adults Differing in $\dot{V}O_2$							
Intensity	%$\dot{V}O_2$R %HRR	%HR_{max} [y]	RPE‡	$\dot{V}O_2$max=12 METs		$\dot{V}O_2$max=10 METs		$\dot{V}O_2$max=8 METs		$\dot{V}O_2$max=5 METs	
				METs	%$\dot{V}O_2$max**	METs	%$\dot{V}O_2$max	METs	%$\dot{V}O_2$max	METs	%$\dot{V}O_2$max
Very light	<20	<50	<10	<3.2	<27	<2.8	<28	<2.4	<30	<1.8	<36
Light	20-39	50-63	10-11	3.2-5.3	27-44	2.8-4.5	28-45	2.4-3.7	30-47	1.8-2.5	36-51
Moderate	40-59	64-76	12-13	5.4-7.5	45-62	4.6-6.3	46-63	3.8-5.1	48-64	2.6-3.3	52-67
Hard	60-84	77-93	14-16	7.6-10.2	63-85	6.4-8.6	64-86	5.2-6.9	65-86	3.4-4.3	68-87
Very hard	≥85	≥94	17-19	≥10.3	≥86	≥8.7	≥87	≥7.0	≥87	≥4.4	≥88
Maximal	100	100	20	12	100	10	100	8	100	5	100

Modified from Table 1 of ACSM position stand (ACSM 1998) by Howley (2001).

*%$\dot{V}O_2$R – percent of oxygen uptake reserve; %HRR – percent of heart rate reserve.

[Y]%HRmax = 0.7305 (%$\dot{V}O_2$max) + 29.95 (Londeree and Ames 1976); values based on 10-MET group

[1]Borg Rating of Perceived Exertion 6-20 scale (Borg 1998)

**$\dot{V}O_2$max = [(100%-%$\dot{V}O_2$R) METmax^{-1}] + %$\dot{V}O_2$R (Personal communication, David Swain, 2000)

the table from the 12 MET to the 5 MET column, the difference between %$\dot{V}O_2$max and %$\dot{V}O_2$R is larger as $\dot{V}O_2$max becomes smaller, with the difference more obvious for the "very light" to "moderate" range of exercise intensities. For those with $\dot{V}O_2$max values of 10 METs, there is little practical difference between %$\dot{V}O_2$R and %$\dot{V}O_2$max values. The MET values listed for each fitness level equal the stated %$\dot{V}O_2$max and %$\dot{V}O_2$R values. The %$\dot{V}O_2$R can be converted to %$\dot{V}O_2$max by using the following equation (D.P. Swain, personal communication, 2000):

$$\%\dot{V}O_2max = [(100\% - \%\dot{V}O_2R)\,METmax^{-1}] + \%\dot{V}O_2R.$$

The %HRmax values listed in Table 10.1 were derived from an equation by Londeree and Ames (37).

$$\%HRmax = 0.7305\,(\%\dot{V}O_2max) + 29.95.$$

This equation is similar to those of Swain et al. (54) and Hellerstein and Franklin (27). There was little difference in the %HRmax values across the four fitness groups for each of the intensity classifications, so the %$\dot{V}O_2$max values for the 10-MET fitness group were used to provide the %HRmax values for table 10.1.

Table 10.1 allows the HFI to classify data on exercise intensity in a consistent manner, whether expressed in oxygen uptake (METs), HR, or RPE. From a practical standpoint, for those with average CRF levels and who work at moderate to hard intensities of exercise, there is little practical difference between %$\dot{V}O_2$max and %$\dot{V}O_2$R.

The 1998 ACSM position stand recommended a range of exercise intensities of 40 or 50% to 85% of $\dot{V}O_2$R (%HRR) to achieve CRF goals. However, the position stand also indicated that the lower end of this continuum of intensities (i.e., 40-49% $\dot{V}O_2$R) was appropriate for those who were quite unfit (2). That is consistent with the needs for this group to focus on moderate exercise that can be carried out long enough to achieve health-related benefits and perhaps gains in CRF. Consequently, for the average sedentary individual, the appropriate range of exercise intensities to achieve CRF goals is 50 to 85% of $\dot{V}O_2$R (HRR). As you can see in table 10.1, for an individual with a CRF of 10 METs, there is, at most, a 6% difference between the values for %$\dot{V}O_2$max and %$\dot{V}O_2$R (% HHR) for moderate to very hard exercise intensities. If a person's CRF were only 8 METs, the value for %$\dot{V}O_2$max would be 2% $\dot{V}O_2$max higher compared with 10 METs. For that reason we will use %$\dot{V}O_2$max and %$\dot{V}O_2$R interchangeably, except where special attention is warranted. The following Research Insight provides more information on oxygen uptake reserve.

Research Insight

Traditionally, the intensity of the exercise prescription was based on a percentage of one's maximal oxygen uptake, expressed in ml · kg^{-1} · min^{-1} or in METs. Estimates of the percentage of $\dot{V}O_2$max were derived from the percentage of maximal HR or percentage of HRR. The 1998 ACSM position statement (2) recommended that a percentage of oxygen uptake reserve ($\dot{V}O_2$R) be used. The oxygen uptake reserve uses the same principle as the HRR; that is, the resting oxygen intake is taken into account. Thus, to determine the exercise intensity of 60% $\dot{V}O_2$R in an individual with a $\dot{V}O_2$max of 40 ml · kg^{-1} · min^{-1}, the following calculation would be made:

$$\dot{V}O_2R = \dot{V}O_2max - resting\ \dot{V}O_2$$

In this example, 40 – 3.5 ml · kg^{-1} · min^{-1} = 36.5 ml · kg^{-1} · min^{-1}

60% of 36.5 ml · kg^{-1} · min^{-1} = 21.9 ml · kg^{-1} · min^{-1}

This number is added to the resting oxygen uptake

$$\dot{V}O_2 = 21.9 + 3.5 = 25.4\ ml \cdot kg^{-1} \cdot min^{-1}$$

As Table 10.2 shows, using $\dot{V}O_2$R results in the person working at a slightly higher target $\dot{V}O_2$ (ml · kg^{-1} · min^{-1}) than simply taking the percentage of one's $\dot{V}O_2$max without regard to the resting level. In the preceding example, the individual would be working at 25.4 ml · kg^{-1} · min^{-1} for 60% of $\dot{V}O_2$R, whereas it would be 24 ml · kg^{-1} · min^{-1} for the direct percentage of $\dot{V}O_2$max. The difference between % $\dot{V}O_2$R and % $\dot{V}O_2$max is greater at lower intensity levels and for individuals with lower $\dot{V}O_2$max levels.

To recap, it generally is believed that the intensity threshold for a training effect is at the low end of the intensity continuum for those who are sedentary and at the high end of the scale for those who are fit (3). For older, deconditioned adults, 40 to 60% $\dot{V}O_2$max is a good place to start, and for those who are physically active and at the high end of the fitness scale, intensities >80% $\dot{V}O_2$max are appropriate. However, for most people who are cleared to participate in a structured exercise program, 60 to 80% $\dot{V}O_2$max seems to be the optimum range of exercise intensities. Figure 10.4 shows that exercise at the high end of the scale has been associated with

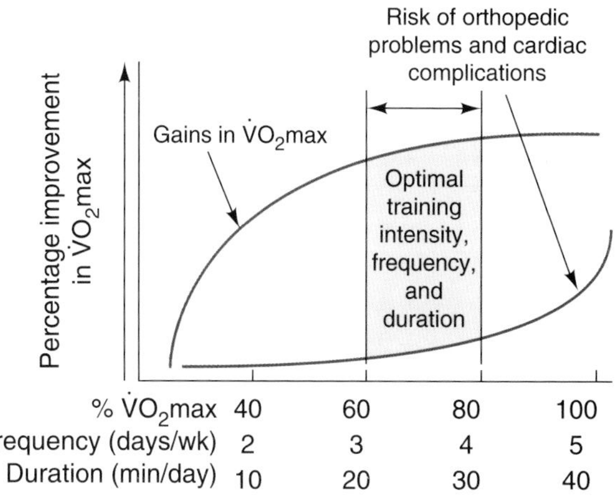

Figure 10.4 Effects of increasing the frequency, duration, and intensity of exercise on the increase in $\dot{V}O_2$max in a training program. This figure demonstrates the increasing risk of orthopedic problems attributable to exercise sessions that are too long or conducted too many times per week. The probability of cardiac complications increases with exercise intensity beyond that recommended for improvements in cardiorespiratory fitness.

From Powers and Howley 1997. Drawing based on Dehn and Mullins 1977, and Hellerstein and Franklin 1984.

Table 10.2 Differences in $\dot{V}O_2$ When Training Intensities Are Expressed As %$\dot{V}O_2$R Versus %$\dot{V}O_2$max for Individuals With Different $\dot{V}O_2$max Values

	$\dot{V}O_2$max					
	20 ml · kg^{-1} · min^{-1}		40 ml · kg^{-1} · min^{-1} Target $\dot{V}O_2$ (ml · kg^{-1} · min^{-1})		60 ml · kg^{-1} · min^{-1}	
Percent	%$\dot{V}O_2$max	%$\dot{V}O_2$R	%$\dot{V}O_2$max	%$\dot{V}O_2$R	%$\dot{V}O_2$max	%$\dot{V}O_2$R
40	8	10.1	16	18.1	24	26.1
50	10	11.75	20	21.75	30	31.75
60	12	13.4	24	25.4	36	37.4
70	14	15.05	28	29.05	42	43.05
80	16	16.7	32	32.7	48	48.7

more cardiac complications (9, 27). Exercise intensity must be balanced against the duration so that the person can exercise long enough to expend 150 to 400 kcal per day, consistent with achieving CRF and body composition goals. If the exercise intensity is too high, the person may not be able to exercise long enough to achieve the total work goal.

Duration

How many minutes of exercise should a person do per session? Figure 10.4 shows that improvements in $\dot{V}O_2$max increase with the **duration** of the exercise session. However, the optimum duration of an exercise session depends on the intensity. The total work accomplished in a session is the most important variable determining CRF gains, once the minimal intensity **threshold** is achieved (3). If the goal were to accomplish 300 kcal of total work in an exercise session in which the individual is working at 10 kcal $\cdot$ min^{-1} (2 L of oxygen per min), the duration of the session would have to be 30 min. If the person were working at half that intensity, 5 kcal $\cdot$ min^{-1}, the duration would have to be twice as long. Thirty minutes of exercise can be taken as one 30-min session, two 15-min sessions, or three 10-min sessions. Figure 10.4 also shows that when the duration of hard exercise (75% $\dot{V}O_2$max) exceeds 30 min, the risk of orthopedic injury increases (43).

Frequency

Why recommend that someone do 3 to 5 workouts per week, if 2 would suffice? Figure 10.4 shows that gains in CRF increase with the frequency of exercise but begin to level off at 4 days per week. People who start a fitness program should plan to exercise 3 or 4 times per week. The long recommended work-a-day-then-rest-a-day routine has been validated on the basis of improvements in CRF, low incidence of injuries, and achievement of weight loss goals. Although exercising for fewer than 3 days per week can improve CRF, the participant would have to exercise at a higher intensity, and weight loss goals may be difficult to achieve (43). Exercising for more than 4 days per week for previously sedentary people seems to be too much and results in more dropouts and injuries and less psychological adjustment to the exercise (9, 43).

4 In Review

CRF is improved with exercise intensities of 40 to 85% $\dot{V}O_2R$. The intensity threshold for a training effect is lower (40-60% $\dot{V}O_2R$) for those who are sedentary and higher (>80% $\dot{V}O_2R$) for those who are physically active and possess high levels of CRF. The optimal training intensity for the average individual is approximately 60 to 80% $\dot{V}O_2R$. The duration of an exercise session should balance the exercise intensity to result in an energy expenditure of 150 to 400 kcal per day (minimum of 1000 kcal per week). The optimum frequency of training, based on improvements in CRF and a low risk of injuries, is 3 to 4 times per week for exercise intensities rated "hard."

Determining Intensity

How is exercise intensity set for a particular individual? Direct and indirect methods to determine appropriate exercise intensity are reviewed in this section, with a focus on the typically sedentary individual. The approach would be the same for those with very low or very high levels of physical activity and CRF but would use different intensity guidelines.

Metabolic Load

The most direct way to determine the appropriate exercise intensity is to use a percentage of the measured maximal oxygen consumption. Remember, the optimum range of exercise intensities associated with improvements in CRF in typically sedentary individuals is 60 to 80% $\dot{V}O_2$max. The advantage of measuring oxygen consumption to determine exercise intensity is that the method is based on the criterion test for CRF—maximal oxygen consumption. The major disadvantages are the expense and difficulty of measuring oxygen consumption for each individual and trying to suit specific fitness activities to meet the specific metabolic demand for each person.

QUESTION: A 75-kg man completes a maximal GXT, and his $\dot{V}O_2max$ is 3.0 $L \cdot min^{-1}$. This is equal to 15 $kcal \cdot min^{-1}$ (5 $kcal \cdot L^{-1} \times 3\ L \cdot min^{-1}$), 40 $ml \cdot kg^{-1} \cdot min^{-1}$, and 11.4 METs. At what exercise intensities should he work to be at 60 to 80% $\dot{V}O_2max$?

1. 60% of 3.0 $L \cdot min^{-1}$ = 1.8 $L \cdot min^{-1}$;
   80% of 3.0 $L \cdot min^{-1}$ = 2.4 $L \cdot min^{-1}$.
2. 60% of 15 $kcal \cdot min^{-1}$ = 9 $kcal \cdot min^{-1}$;
   80% of 15 $kcal \cdot min^{-1}$ = 12 $kcal \cdot min^{-1}$.
3. 60% of 40 $ml \cdot kg^{-1} \cdot min^{-1}$ = 24 $ml \cdot kg^{-1} \cdot min^{-1}$;
   80% of 40 $ml \cdot kg^{-1} \cdot min^{-1}$ = 32 $ml \cdot kg^{-1} \cdot min^{-1}$.
4. 60% of 11.4 METs = 6.8 METs;
   80% of 11.4 METs = 9.1 METs.

Answer:

He should use activities that require the following:

1.8 to 2.4 $L \cdot min^{-1}$
9 to 12 $kcal \cdot min^{-1}$
24 to 32 $ml \cdot kg^{-1} \cdot min^{-1}$
6.8 to 9.1 METs

$\dot{V}O_2R$—Using the preceding data, we find that 60 to 60% of $\dot{V}O_2R$ = 60% × (40 $ml \cdot kg^{-1} \cdot min^{-1}$ – 3.5 $ml \cdot kg^{-1} \cdot min^{-1}$) + 3.5

$$\text{Target } \dot{V}O_2 = 0.6 \times (36.5\ ml \cdot kg^{-1} \cdot min^{-1}) + 3.5\ ml \cdot kg^{-1} \cdot min^{-1}$$

$$\text{Target } \dot{V}O_2 = 21.9 + 3.5 = 25.4\ ml \cdot kg^{-1} \cdot min^{-1} = 7.3\ \text{METs (i.e., } 25.4/3.5)$$

$$80\% \times (40\ ml \cdot kg^{-1} \cdot min^{-1} - 3.5\ ml \cdot kg^{-1} \cdot min^{-1}) + 3.5$$

$$\text{Target } \dot{V}O_2 = 0.8 \times (36.5\ ml \cdot kg^{-1} \cdot min^{-1}) + 3.5\ ml \cdot kg^{-1} \cdot min^{-1}$$

$$\text{Target } \dot{V}O_2 = 29.2 + 3.5 = 32.7\ ml \cdot kg^{-1} \cdot min^{-1} = 9.3\ \text{METs (i.e., } 32.7/3.5)$$

Answer:

He should use activities that require the following:

25.4 to 32.7 $ml \cdot kg^{-1} \cdot min^{-1}$

7.3 to 9.3 METs

When these values are known, appropriate activities can be selected from tables listing the energy costs of various activities (see appendix C for these tables). However, this is a very cumbersome method for prescribing exercise. Prescribing on the basis of the caloric cost of the activity does not take into consideration the effect that environmental (e.g., heat, humidity, altitude, cold, pollution), dietary (e.g., adequate hydration), and other variables have on a person's response to some absolute exercise intensity. The participant's ability to complete a workout will depend on her or his physiological responses and the perception of effort associated with the activity, rather than the metabolic cost of the activity itself. Fortunately, by using specific HR values that are approximately equal to 60 to 80% $\dot{V}O_2max$, you can formulate an exercise prescription that takes many of these factors into consideration. These HR values are called the **target heart rate (THR)** range. How is the THR range determined?

THR: Direct Method

As described in chapters 5 and 28, HR increases linearly with the metabolic load. In the direct method for determining THR, HR is monitored at each stage of a maximal GXT. HR is then plotted on a graph against the $\dot{V}O_2$ (or MET) equivalents of each stage of the test. The HFI determines the THR range by taking appropriate percentages of $\dot{V}O_2max$ (%$\dot{V}O_2max$) at which the person should train and finds what the HR responses were at those points. Figure 10.5 shows this method being used for a subject with a functional capacity of 10.5 METs. Work rates of 60 to 80% of maximal METs demanded HR responses of 132 to 156 $beats \cdot min^{-1}$, respectively. The HR values become the intensity guide for the subject and represent the THR range (2).

THR: Indirect Methods

In contrast to the direct method, which requires the participant to complete a maximal GXT, two indirect methods have been developed to estimate an appropriate THR.

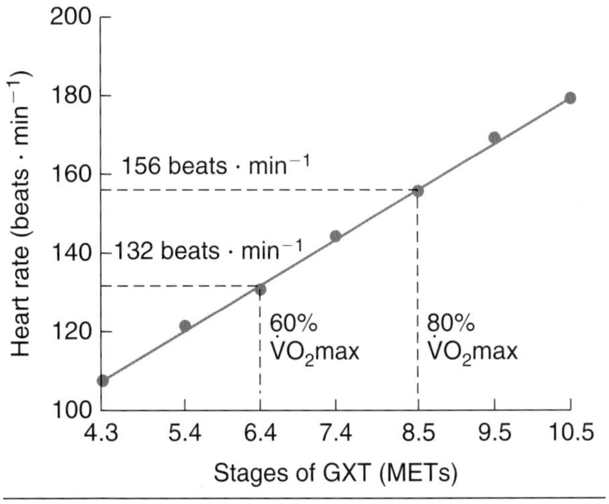

Figure 10.5 Direct method of determining the THR zone when maximal aerobic power (functional capacity) is measured during a GXT.

HRR Method

The HRR is the difference between resting and maximal HR. For a maximal HR of 200 beats · min^{-1} and a resting HR of 60 beats · min^{-1}, the HRR is 140 beats · min^{-1}. As shown in figure 10.6, the percentage of the HRR is equal to the percentage of $\dot{V}O_2R$ across the range of exercise intensities (55, 56). For those with average to high levels of CRF, the HRR is approximately equal to the $\%\dot{V}O_2max$.

The HRR method of determining the THR range, made popular by Karvonen, requires a few simple calculations (35):

1. Subtract the resting HR from the maximal HR to obtain the HRR.
2. Calculate 60% and 80% of the HRR.
3. Add each value to the resting HR to obtain the THR range.

QUESTION: A 40-year-old male participant has a measured maximal HR of 175 beats · min^{-1} and a resting HR of 75 beats · min^{-1}. What is his THR range, calculated by the Karvonen (HRR) method?

Answer:

1. HRR = 175 beats · min^{-1} – 75 beats · min^{-1} = 100 beats · min^{-1}
2. 60% of 100 beats · min^{-1} = 60 beats · min^{-1}
3. 80% of 100 beats · min^{-1} = 80 beats · min^{-1}

60 beats · min^{-1} + 75 beats · min^{-1} = 135 beats · min^{-1} for 60% $\dot{V}O_2max$

80 beats · min^{-1} + 75 beats · min^{-1} = 155 beats · min^{-1} for 80% $\dot{V}O_2max$

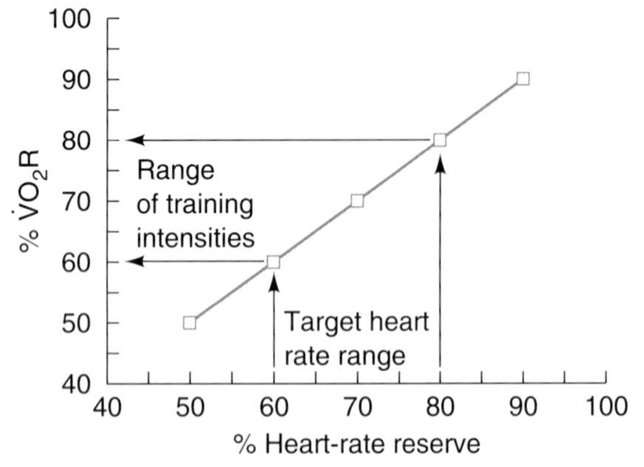

Figure 10.6 Relationship of percentage HRR and percentage of oxygen uptake reserve ($\%\dot{V}O_2R$).

Based on Swain 1997, 1998.

The advantages of this procedure for determining exercise intensity are that the recommended THR is always between the person's resting and maximal HRs, and the %HRR is equal to the $\%\dot{V}O_2R$ across the entire range of CRF levels. Although the resting HR is variable and can be influenced by factors such as caffeine, lack of sleep, dehydration, emotional state, and training, this does not introduce serious errors into the calculation of the THR by the Karvonen method (21). Consider the following example:

QUESTION: The 40-year-old subject mentioned previously participates in an endurance training program, and his resting HR decreases by 10 beats · min^{-1}. Because maximal HR (175 beats · min^{-1}) is not affected by training, what happens to his THR range?

Answer:

1. The HRR now equals 175 beats · min^{-1} – 65 beats · min^{-1} = 110 beats · min^{-1}
2. 60% of 110 beats · min^{-1} = 66 beats · min^{-1} + 65 beats · min^{-1} = 131 beats · min^{-1}
3. 80% of 110 beats · min^{-1} = 88 beats · min^{-1} + 65 beats · min^{-1} = 153 beats · min^{-1}

Consequently, the change in resting HR had only a minimal effect on the THR range.

Percentage of Maximal HR Method

Another method of determining THR range is to use a fixed percentage of the maximal HR (%HRmax). The advantage of this method is its simplicity and the fact that it has been validated across many populations (27, 38, 54). Figure 10.7 shows the relationship between %HRmax and $\%\dot{V}O_2max$.

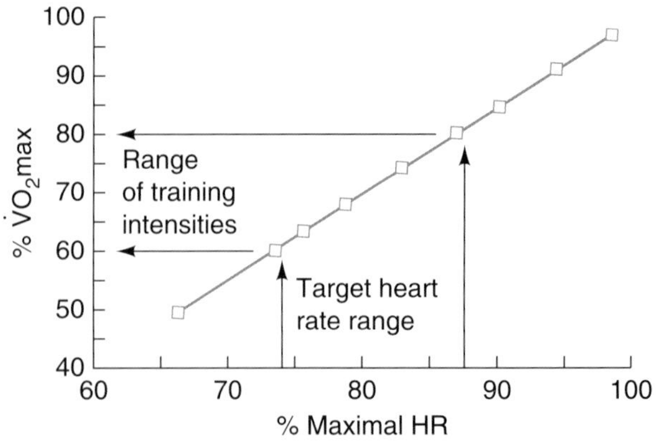

Figure 10.7 Relationship of percentage of maximal HR and percentage of maximal aerobic power ($\dot{V}O_2max$).

Data from Londeree and Ames 1976.

It is clear that %HRmax and %$\dot{V}O_2$max are linearly related, and the %HRmax can be used to estimate the metabolic load in training programs. The usual guideline to estimate reasonable exercise intensity for the typically sedentary individual is 70 to 85% HRmax. However, this THR range is equal to approximately 55 to 75% $\dot{V}O_2$max, respectively, and represents a slightly more conservative intensity prescription than that generated by the HRR method when 60 to 80% of the HRR is used. The range of 75 to 90% HRmax is more similar to 60 to 80% $\dot{V}O_2$max and HRR; the following example shows how to use the %HRmax method of calculating the THR range.

QUESTION: How can I calculate a THR range if I don't know what the resting HR is? Use the data from the 40-year-old subject mentioned previously who had a measured maximal HR of 175 beats · min^{-1}.

Answer:

Take 75% and 90% of that value:

75% of 175 beats · min^{-1} = 131 beats · min^{-1}

90% of 175 beats · min^{-1} = 158 beats · min^{-1}

These values are similar to those calculated by using the %HRR method described earlier. Table 10.3 shows the relationship between %$\dot{V}O_2$max and %HRmax across the range of exercise intensities from 50 to 85% $\dot{V}O_2$max. This table can be used to simplify the process of making specific exercise intensity recommendations by using the %HRmax method.

Threshold

As mentioned earlier, the intensity of exercise that provides an adequate stimulus for cardiorespiratory improvement varies with activity level and age and spans the range of 40 to 85% $\dot{V}O_2$R and $\dot{V}O_2$max. However, for most of the population, the optimal intensity threshold is in the following ranges:

- 60 to 80% of $\dot{V}O_2$max, HRR, and $\dot{V}O_2$R
- 75 to 90% of HRmax

As we mentioned at the beginning of this section, the threshold is toward the lower part of the range (50-60% $\dot{V}O_2$R) for older, sedentary populations and toward the upper part of the range (>80% $\dot{V}O_2$R) for younger, more fit populations. The middle of the range (70% $\dot{V}O_2$R, 70% $\dot{V}O_2$max, or 80% HRmax) is an average training intensity and is appropriate for the typical apparently healthy person who wishes to be involved in a regular fitness program. Participating in activities at these intensities places a reasonable load on the cardiorespiratory systems to constitute an overload, resulting in an adaptation over time.

Table 10.3 Relationship of %HRmax and %$\dot{V}O_2$max

%$\dot{V}O_2$max	%HRmax
50	66
55	70
60	74
65	77
70	81
75	85
80	88
85	92

From Londeree and Ames 1976.

HRmax

The indirect methods for determining exercise intensity use HRmax. It is recommended that the HRmax be measured directly (by maximal GXT) when possible. If it cannot be measured, then any estimation must consider the effect of age on HRmax. Previously, HRmax had been estimated with the formula, HRmax = 220 − age. However, a recent study pointed out that this formula results in an underestimation of HRmax for older individuals (see the Research Insight below).

Research Insight

In a recent study, Tanaka, Monahan, and Seals (57) evaluated the validity of the classic "220 – age" formula to estimate HRmax. They analyzed 351 published studies and cross-validated these findings with a well-controlled laboratory study. They found almost identical results for both approaches: HRmax = 208 – 0.7 × age. This new formula yields HRmax values that are 6 beats · min^{-1} lower for 20-year-olds and 6 beats · min^{-1} higher for 60-year-olds. Although the new formula yields better estimates of HRmax on average, the investigators emphasize the fact that the estimated HRmax for a given individual is still associated with a standard deviation of 10 beats · min^{-1}.

Any estimate of HRmax is a potential source of error for both the HRR and the %HRmax methods of calculating a THR. For example, given that 1 SD of this estimate of HRmax is about 10 beats · min^{-1}, a 45-year-old person's true HRmax may be anywhere between 145 and 205 beats · min^{-1} (±3 SD) rather than the estimated 175. However, 68% (±1 SD) of the population would be between 165 and 185 beats · min^{-1}. If the HRmax is known (e.g., from a GXT), the HFI should use this measured HRmax to determine THR rather than using the estimate with its potential error (38). This is another reason for using caution when relying solely on the THR range as an indicator of exercise intensity. Error potential exists both in the estimate of HRmax and in the equations in which various percentages of HRmax are used to predict %$\dot{V}O_2$max. The intensity levels should only be considered guidelines (see Research Insight).

Research Insight

The two indirect HR methods for estimating exercise intensity provide guidelines to use in an exercise program, and small differences between methods are not important. Both approaches must be used as guidelines because, as for any prediction equation, an error is involved in the estimate provided by the equation. For example, 2 SDs of the estimate of %$\dot{V}O_2$max determined from HR equal ±11.4% $\dot{V}O_2$max (37). Therefore, for 95% of participants, when we use %HRR or %HRmax to predict a work intensity that is 60% $\dot{V}O_2$max, the true intensity is somewhere between 48.6% and 71.4% $\dot{V}O_2$max! This is why these calculated THR values should be used as guidelines in helping individuals increase or maintain CRF. The HFI or personal fitness trainer needs other indicators of exercise intensity to compensate for some of the inherent variability in the THR prescription (see later in this chapter).

Use of THR

The concept of an intensity threshold provides the basis for the importance of regular fitness workouts. Low-intensity activity around the house, yard, and office should be encouraged, but specific workouts above the intensity threshold are necessary to achieve optimum CRF results. At the other extreme, a person who pushes him- or herself near maximum does not have a fitness advantage because similar results can be obtained at a lower intensity that is above the threshold.

The THR can be used as an intensity guide for large muscle group, continuous, whole-body types of activities such as walking, running, swimming, rowing, cycling, skiing, and dancing. However, the same training results may not occur from activities using small muscle groups or resistance exercises because these exercises elevate the HR much higher for the same metabolic load.

People who are less active and have more risk factors should use the lower part of the THR range. More active people with fewer risk factors should use the upper part of the THR range. The THR can be divided by 6 to provide the desired 10-s THR. If the person's HRmax is unknown, the estimated THR for 10 s, by age and activity level, can be found in table 10.4. People can learn to exercise at their THRs by walking or jogging for several minutes and then stopping and immediately taking a 10-s HR. If the person's HR is not within the target range, then the individual should adjust the intensity (by going slower or faster to try to get within the THR range) for a few minutes and take another 10-s count. Using the THR to set exercise intensity has many advantages:

- It has a built-in individualized progression (i.e., as a person increases fitness, harder work has to be done to achieve the THR).
- It takes into account environmental conditions (e.g., a person decreases the intensity while working in very hot temperatures).
- It is easily determined, learned, and monitored.

Table 10.4 Estimated 10-s Target Heart Rate for People Whose Maximal Heart Rate Is Unknown

Population	Intensity %$\dot{V}O_2$max	Age (years) 20	30	40	50	60	70	80
Inactive	50	22	21	20	18	17	16	15
with several	55	23	22	21	19	18	17	16
risk factors								
Normal activity	60	24	23	22	20	19	18	17
with few	65	25	24	23	21	20	19	18
risk factors	70	26	25	24	22	21	20	18
	75	28	26	25	24	22	21	19
	80	29	28	26	25	23	22	20
Very active	85	30	29	27	26	24	23	21
with low risk	90	31	30	28	27	25	24	22

These recommendations are appropriate for most people, but individuals differ in terms of the threshold needed for a training effect, the rate of adaptation to the training, and how exercise feels to them. The HFI must use subjective judgment, based on observations of the person exercising, to determine whether the intensity should be higher or lower. If the work is so easy that the person experiences little or no increase in ventilation and is able to do the work without effort, then the intensity should be increased. At the other extreme, if a person shows signs of doing very hard work and is still unable to reach THR, then a lower intensity should be chosen. In this case, the top part of the THR range might be above the person's true HRmax because the 220 – age formula provides only a rough estimate of the true value. The HFI should not rely on the THR as the only method of judging whether the participant is exercising at the correct intensity. Attention should be paid to other signs and symptoms of overexertion; Borg's RPE might be useful in this regard (see box below).

RPE

The Borg RPE scale that is used to indicate the subjective sensation of effort experienced by the subject during a GXT (see chapter 5) can be used in prescribing exercise for the apparently healthy individual (6). Exercise perceived as just below "somewhat hard" to just above "hard," a rating of 12 to 16 on the original RPE scale, approximates 40/50 to 85% of $\dot{V}O_2R$ or 60/65 to 90% of HRmax (2, 3). With the RPE, if the HRmax is not known and the THR range is perceived as too low or too high, an RPE rating can provide an estimate of the overall effort experienced by the individual; the exercise intensity can then be adjusted accordingly. Furthermore, as a participant becomes accustomed to the physical sensations experienced when exercising at the THR range, there will be less need for frequent pulse rate measurements.

5 In Review

The exercise intensity for a CRF training effect can be described in a variety of ways: 40/50 to 85% $\dot{V}O_2R$ (HRR), 60/65 to 90% HRmax, and 12 to 16 on the original RPE scale.

Exercise Recommendations for the Untested Masses

Certain general recommendations can be made for any person wanting to begin a fitness program. Although the HFI might wish to have each individual go through a complete testing protocol before beginning exercise, that simply is not realistic. In addition, people without known health problems who follow the general guidelines mentioned before can begin to exercise at low risk. In fact, continuing not to exercise places a person at a higher risk for CHD than if he or she begins a modest

When "Moderate-Intensity" Exercise May Be "Hard"

The ACSM and CDC have recommended that every U.S. adult accumulate 30 min or more of moderate-intensity (3-6 METs) physical activity on most, preferably all, days of the week. It is important for the HFI to recognize that the range of 3 to 6 METs, while being moderate exercise for some, may be hard exercise for others. Figure 10.8 shows the relative intensity for a fixed exercise to vary considerably across the range of $\dot{V}O_2max$ values (32). Consequently, some individuals with low $\dot{V}O_2max$ values would function in the intensity range consistent with achieving gains in $\dot{V}O_2max$, whereas those with higher CRF values would not. This example emphasizes the need to consider the THR range and the RPE when following recommendations that specify absolute exercise intensities (e.g., METs).

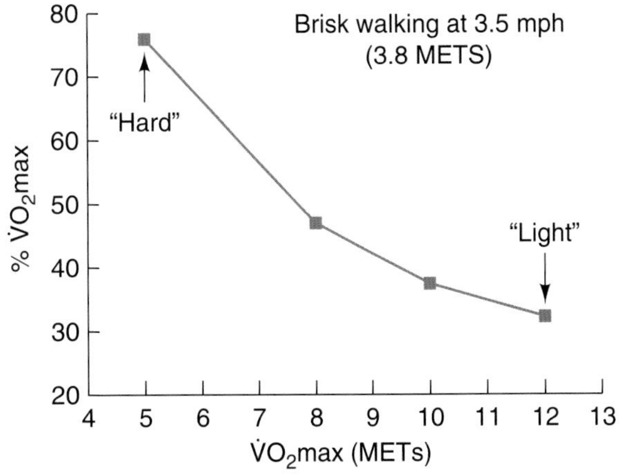

Figure 10.8 Changes in the relative intensity of exercise (% $\dot{V}O_2max$) when the same absolute intensity of exercise is performed by groups differing in $\dot{V}O_2max$ (METs).

From Howley 2001.

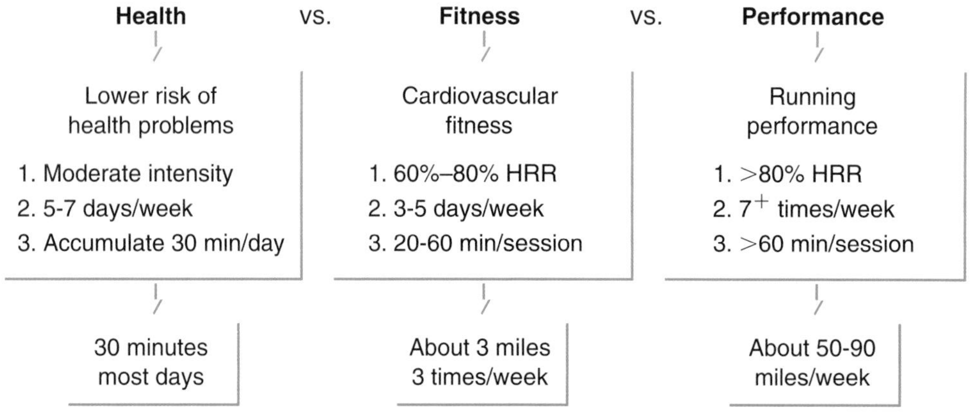

Figure 10.9 Contrasting recommendations for achieving health, fitness, and performance goals.

exercise program. Figure 10.9 summarizes the recommendations for achieving health, fitness, and performance goals.

Exercise Programming for the Fit Population

Exercise recommendations written for people who possess reasonably high levels of fitness tend to be associated with less risk, and these participants require less supervision. In fact, people in this group may focus on performance, in contrast to health and fitness, as the primary goal. A wide variety of programs, activities, races, and competitions are available to address the needs of this group.

The THR range will be calculated as described before, but very fit individuals will work at the top part of the range (>85% of $\dot{V}O_2$max or >90% of HRmax). As was mentioned earlier, a less fit person can start working out at the low end of the range and still experience a training effect. The more fit individual needs to work at the top end of the range to maintain a high level of fitness.

Training for competition demands more than the training intensity needed for CRF. Individuals who do interval-type training programs have peak HRs close to maximum during the intervals. The recovery period between the intervals should include some work at a lower intensity (near 40-50% $\dot{V}O_2$max) to help metabolize the lactate produced during the interval (11) and to reduce the chance of cardiovascular complications that can occur when a person comes to a complete rest at the end of a strenuous exercise bout (44).

For people who participate in sports that are intermittent in nature but that still require high levels of aerobic fitness for success, a running/jogging program is a good way to maintain general conditioning when not participating in the primary sport. However, given the specificity of training, there is no substitute for the real activity when conditioning for a sport.

As figure 10.9 shows, people interested in performance who work at the top end of the THR range, who exercise 5 to 7 or more times per week, and who exercise for longer than 60 min each exercise session are doing much more than the person interested in fitness, and it should be no surprise that they tend to experience more injuries. When this is coupled with the inherent risks associated with competitive activities, it is clear that alternative activities should be planned that can be done when participation in the primary activity is not possible. This reduces the chance of becoming detrained when injuries do occur.

Exercise Prescriptions Using Complete GXT Results

In the previous sections, the exercise recommendation was made on the basis of little or no specific information about the person involved. In many adult fitness programs, potential participants have had a general medical exam or a maximal GXT with appropriate monitoring of the HR, BP, and possibly ECG responses. Unfortunately, this information sometimes is not used in designing the exercise program; instead, the measured HRmax is used in the THR formulas and the rest of the data are ignored. This section outlines the steps that should be followed when the HFI is involved in making the exercise recommendation based on information about the person's functional capacity and the cardiovascular responses to graded exercise. The HFI is not directly involved in the clinical evaluation of a GXT, but an understanding of the steps and the procedures used to make clinical judgments clearly enhances communication between the HFI and the program director, exercise specialist, and physician. The following information on using GXTs for exercise prescription and programming (see box below) was written with this intent.

Program Selection

Exercise program options include exercising alone, in small groups, in fitness clubs, and in clinically oriented settings. The HFI must consider a variety of factors before recommending participation in a supervised or unsupervised program.

Supervised Program

The risk factors, the response to the GXT, the health and activity history, and personal preference influence the type of program in which an individual should participate. Generally, the higher the risk, the more important it is that the person participate in a supervised program. People at high risk for CHD and those who have diseases such as diabetes, hypertension, asthma, and CHD should be encouraged to participate under supervision, at least at the beginning of an exercise program. The personnel in the supervised program are trained to provide the necessary instruction in the appropriate activities, to help monitor the participant's response to the activity, and to administer appropriate first aid or emergency care.

Supervised programs run the gambit from those conducted within a hospital for patients with CHD and other diseases to programs conducted in fitness clubs for people at low risk for CHD. In general, as a person moves along the continuum from inpatient to outpatient, less formal monitoring is required. In addition, the background and training of the personnel tend to vary. The exercise programs aimed at maintaining the fitness level of the CHD patients who went through a hospital-based program have

Using GXTs for Exercise Prescription and Programming

Steps in GXT Analysis for Exercise Prescription

1. Analyze the person's history and list the known risk factors for CHD; also, identify those factors that might have a direct bearing on the exercise program, such as orthopedic problems, previous physical activity, and current interests.
2. Determine if the functional capacity is a true maximum or if it is sign or symptom limited. Express the functional capacity in METs, and record the highest HR and RPE achieved without significant signs or symptoms.
3. If ECG was monitored, itemize the person's ECG changes as indicated by the physician.
4. Examine the HR and BP responses to see if they are normal.
5. List the symptoms reported at each stage.
6. List the reasons why the test was stopped (e.g., ECG changes, falling SBP, dizziness).

Steps in Designing an Exercise Program on the Basis of a GXT

1. Based on the overall response to the GXT, decide to either refer for additional medical care or initiate an exercise program.
2. Identify the THR range and approximate MET intensities of selected activities needed to be within that THR range.
3. Specify the frequency and duration of activity needed to meet the goals of increased CRF and weight loss.
4. Recommend that the person (a) participate in either a supervised or an unsupervised program, (b) be monitored or unmonitored, and (c) do group or individual activities.
5. Select a variety of activities at the appropriate MET level that allow the person to achieve THR. Consider environmental factors, medication, and any physical limitations of the participant when making this recommendation.

medical personnel and emergency equipment appropriate for the population being served. Supervised fitness programs for the apparently healthy have an HFI who can focus more on the appropriate exercise, diet, and other lifestyle behaviors needed to improve health.

The supervised program offers a socially supportive environment for individuals to become and stay active. This is important, given the difficulty of changing lifestyle behaviors. The group program allows for more variety in the types of activities to be used (e.g., group games) and reduces the chance of boredom. To be effective in the long run, the program leader should try to wean the participants from the group in a way that encourages them to maintain their activity patterns when they are no longer in the program.

Unsupervised Program

Despite the risks just described, the vast majority of people at risk for or already having CHD participate in unsupervised exercise programs. Reasons for this include the limited number of supervised programs, the level of interest of the participant and physician in such programs, and the financial resources required to conduct such programs.

Participation in an unsupervised exercise program requires clear communication of correct information from the HFI or physician about how to begin and maintain the exercise program. The emphasis in beginning an unsupervised exercise program is on low intensity (e.g., 40-50% $\dot{V}O_2R$, ~50% $\dot{V}O_2max$, or ~65% HRmax), because the threshold for a training effect is lower in deconditioned people. The goal is to increase the duration of the activity, with exercise frequency approaching every day. This reduces the chance of muscular, skeletal, or cardiovascular problems caused by the exercise intensity and increases muscle function with the expenditure of a relatively large number of calories. In addition, the regularity of the exercise program encourages a positive habit. The outcome of such programs results in the individual being able to conduct her or his daily affairs with more comfort and sets the stage for people who would like to exercise at higher levels.

In an unsupervised exercise program, the person should be provided explicit information about the intensity (THR), duration, and frequency of exercise so that no doubt remains about what should be done. For example, the exercise recommendation might read, "Walk 1 mile in 30 min each day for 2 weeks. Monitor and record your heart rate." The person must be told how to take the pulse rate and be encouraged to follow through on the recording.

Updating the Exercise Program

During participation in an endurance training program, an individual's capacity for work increases. The best sign of this is that the "regular" exercise is no longer sufficient to reach THR; clearly the person is adapting to the exercise. Taking the HR during a regular activity session provides a sound basis for upgrading the intensity or duration of the exercise session.

The exercise program, including the THR, should be updated periodically. The need to update is greater for those with a lower initial level of fitness and a greater number of risk factors. An individual who has a low functional capacity because of heart disease, orthopedic limitations, or chronic inactivity (which might include prolonged bed rest) has difficulty reaching a true maximum on a first treadmill test. Furthermore, she or he experiences the greatest improvements in the shortest period of time in a fitness program. This individual benefits from frequent retesting because the test allows progress (or the lack thereof) to be monitored, and it may give new information that influences the exercise prescription. If the person has had a change in medication that influences the HR response to exercise, the exercise program must be reevaluated.

For people who reach a true maximum in the first test, actual THR will change little during a fitness program because the HRmax is affected very little by regular endurance exercise. However, these people still benefit from a regular evaluation of the overall exercise program, given that their activity interests may change or they may develop orthopedic problems that did not exist before. The reevaluation allows the HFI to probe for information that may enable her or him to refer the person for treatment at a time when treatment will do the most good. Such contact increases the chance that the person will stay involved in an activity program—which is the most important factor in maintaining aerobic fitness.

6 In Review

Exercise recommendations for the general public emphasize low intensity and regular participation; see the public health physical activity recommendations described earlier. Exercise performed at 60 to 80% $\dot{V}O_2R$, for 20 to 40 min, 3 or 4 times per week increases and maintains CRF. Exercise recommendations for very fit individuals emphasize the top end of the training intensity (>80% $\dot{V}O_2R$) and frequent (almost daily) participation. The potential for injury is greater for such performance-driven workouts. For those who undergo a comprehensive, diagnostic GXT with ECG monitoring, all test results are used to select an optimal and safe exercise prescription. Participants with multiple risk factors for CHD and those with existing diseases would benefit from participation in a supervised program. However, most of such individuals will participate in an unsupervised program, necessitating clear communication about the exercise prescription and safety concerns.

Environmental Concerns

THR is used to indicate the proper exercise intensity in health-related fitness programs. However, environmental factors such as heat, humidity, pollution, and altitude can cause HR and the perception of effort to increase during an exercise session. This could shorten the exercise session and reduce participant's chance of expending sufficient calories and experiencing a training effect. Fortunately, by decreasing the exercise intensity we can "control" these environmental problems to provide a safe and effective exercise prescription. The purpose of this section is to discuss the effects that different environmental factors have on the exercise prescription and what we can do about them.

Environmental Heat and Humidity

Chapter 28 describes the increases in body temperature that occur with exercise, the heat-loss mechanisms called into play, and the benefits of becoming acclimatized to the heat. Our core temperature (37° C, or 98.6° F) is within a few degrees of a value that could lead to death by heat injury. As described in chapter 25, however, to prevent a progression from the least to the most serious heat injury, individuals should recognize and attend to a series of stages from heat cramps to heat stroke. Although treatment of these problems is important, prevention is a better approach.

Each of the following factors influences susceptibility to heat injury and can alter the HR and metabolic responses to exercise:

- Fitness—Fit people have a lower risk of heat injury (15), can tolerate more work in the heat (13), and acclimatize to heat faster (8).
- Acclimatization—Seven to 14 days of exercise in the heat increases our capacity to sweat, initiates sweating at a lower body temperature, and reduces salt loss. Body temperature and HR responses are lower during exercise, and the chance of salt depletion is reduced (3, 8).
- Hydration—Inadequate hydration reduces sweat rate and increases the chance of heat injury (8, 50, 51). Generally, during exercise the focus should be on replacing water, not salt or carbohydrate stores.
- Environmental temperature—Exercising in temperatures greater than skin temperatures results in a heat gain by convection and radiation. Evaporation of sweat must compensate if body temperature is to remain at a safe level.
- Clothing—As much skin surface as possible should be exposed to encourage evaporation, although the skin should be protected from too much exposure to the sun with sunblock. Materials should be chosen that will "wick" sweat to the surface for evaporation; materials impermeable to water will increase the risk of heat injury and should be avoided.
- Humidity (water vapor pressure)—Evaporation of sweat is dependent on the water vapor pressure gradient between skin and environment. In warm and hot environments, the relative humidity is a good index of the water vapor pressure, with a lower relative humidity facilitating the evaporation of sweat.
- Metabolic rate—During times of high heat and humidity, decreasing the exercise intensity decreases the heat load, as well as the strain on the physiological systems that must deal with it.
- Wind—Wind places more air molecules into contact with the skin and can influence heat loss in two ways: If there is a temperature gradient for heat loss between the skin and the air, wind will increase the rate of heat loss by convection. In a similar manner, wind increases the rate of evaporation, assuming the air can accept moisture.

Recommendations for Fitness

The members of a fitness program should be educated about all of the heat-related factors just mentioned. The HFI might suggest the following:

- Learning about heat-illness symptoms (e.g., cramps, lightheadedness) and how to deal with them (see chapter 25)
- Exercising in the cooler parts of the day to avoid heat gain from the sun or from building or road surfaces heated by the sun
- Gradually increasing exposure to high heat and humidity to safely acclimatize over a period of 7 to 14 days
- Drinking water before, during, and after exercise and weighing in each day to monitor hydration
- Wearing only shorts and a tank top to expose as much skin as possible, but being careful to use a sunblock to reduce the chance of skin cancer
- Taking HR measurements several times during the activity and reducing exercise intensity to stay in the THR zone

The last recommendation, regarding THR, is most important. HR is a sensitive indicator of dehydration, environmental heat load, and acclimatization. Variation in any of these factors will modify the HR response to any fixed submaximal exercise. It is therefore important for fitness participants to monitor HR regularly and slow down to stay within the THR zone. The RPE also can be used in circumstances of extreme heat to provide an index of the overall physiological strain that the participant is experiencing.

Implications for Performance

Any athlete performing in an environment that is not conducive to heat loss is at an increased risk of heat injury. This has been a major problem for football, where clothing and equipment prevent heat loss, but the increased number of people participating in 10K races, marathons, and triathlons has shifted our focus of attention (18, 33). In the latter cases, the athlete has a very high metabolic rate while exercising in direct exposure to the sun. In response to this problem and on the basis of sound research, the ACSM developed its position stand on thermal injuries (both heat and cold) during distance running (1). The elements in this position stand are consistent with the information presented earlier in the chapter.

Environmental Heat Stress

The preceding discussion mentioned high temperature and relative humidity as factors increasing the risk of heat injuries. To quantify the overall heat stress associated with any environment, a **wet-bulb globe temperature (WBGT)** guide has been developed (1). This overall heat stress index is composed of the following measurements:

- **Dry-bulb temperature** (T_{db})—Ordinary measure of air temperature taken in the shade
- **Black-globe temperature** (T_g)—Measure of the radiant heat load in direct sunlight; temperature is measured inside a 15-cm diameter copper globe painted flat black
- **Wet-bulb temperature** (T_{wb})—Measurement of air temperature with a thermometer whose mercury bulb is covered with a wet cotton wick, which makes it sensitive to the relative humidity (water vapor pressure) and provides an index of the ability to evaporate sweat

The formula used to calculate the WBGT temperature shows the importance of the wet-bulb temperature, being 70% (0.7) of the WBGT index, in determining heat stress (1). This is related to the role the wet-bulb temperature plays in estimating the ability to evaporate sweat, the most important heat-loss mechanism in most situations. The formula is as follows:

$$\text{WBGT} = 0.7\ T_{wb} + 0.2\ T_g + 0.1\ T_{db}$$

The risk of heat illness (**hyperthermia**) attributable to environmental stress while wearing shorts, socks, shoes, and T-shirt is rated on the following scale:

Very high risk: WBGT exceeds 28° C (82° F)
High risk: WBGT = 23 to 28° C (73-82° F)
Moderate risk: WBGT = 18 to 23° C (65-73° F)
Low risk: WBGT less than 18° C (less than 65° F)

The risk of **hypothermia** while wearing shorts, socks, shoes, and T-shirt also must be considered in distance running. A WBGT index of less than 10° C (less than 50° F) is associated with an increased risk of hypothermia, especially in wet and windy conditions.

Table 10.5 provides an estimate of the WBGT using just air temperature and relative humidity. Because this table does not include radiant heat load (globe temperature), 4° F should be added to the estimated WBGT if exercise is conducted in direct sunlight (4).

Table 10.5 Estimate of Wet-Bulb Globe Temperature (WBGT) (°F) From Air Temperature and Relative Humidity (RH%)

RH%	WBGT (°F) 60	65	70	75	80	85	90	95	100	105	110
90	60	64	69	74	79	85	90	95	100	105	110
80	59	63	68	72	77	82	88	93	99	105	110
70	58	62	66	71	76	80	85	90	96	102	108
60	57	60	66	69	73	78	83	87	93	98	103
50	55	59	63	67	71	75	80	84	89	94	99
40	54	58	62	65	69	73	77	82	88	90	95
30	53	57	60	64	67	71	76	79	83	87	91
20	52	55	58	62	65	69	72	76	79	83	87
10	51	54	57	60	63	68	69	73	76	79	82

Note. For inside or outside, WBGT can be estimated from air temperature at the time and place of exercise. Relative humidity is very sensitive to air temperature. If the exercise occurs in direct sunlight, add 4° F to the estimated WBGT.

Exercise and Cold Exposure

Exercising in the cold can create problems if certain precautions are not taken. As mentioned previously, a WBGT of 10° C (50° F) or less is associated with hypothermia. Hypothermia is a decrease in body temperature that occurs when heat loss exceeds heat production. In cold air, there is a larger gradient for convective heat loss from the skin; cold air also is "dry" (has a low water vapor pressure) and facilitates the evaporation of moisture from the skin to further cool the body. The combined effects can be deadly, as shown in Pugh's report of three deaths during a walking competition in very cold temperatures over a 45-mile distance (46).

Factors related to hypothermia include environmental factors, such as temperature, water vapor pressure, wind, and whether air or water are involved; insulating factors, such as clothing and subcutaneous fat; and the capacity for sustained energy production. Each of these factors is discussed in the following paragraphs.

Environmental Factors

Conduction, convection, and radiation depend on a temperature gradient between the skin and the environment; the larger the gradient, the greater the rate of heat loss. What surprises many is that the environmental temperature does not have to be below freezing to cause hypothermia. Other environmental factors interact with temperature to create the dangerous condition by facilitating heat loss: namely, wind and water.

Windchill Index

The rate of heat loss at any given temperature is influenced directly by wind speed. Wind increases the number of cold air molecules coming into contact with the skin, increasing the rate of heat loss. The **windchill index** indicates the temperature equivalent (under calm air conditions) for any combination of temperature and wind speed (see figure 10.10) This allows the HFI to properly gauge the cold stress associated with a variety of wind velocities and temperatures. Keep in mind that for activities such as running, riding, or cross-country skiing into the wind, the speed of the activity must be added to the wind speed to evaluate the full impact of the windchill. For example, cycling at 20 miles · hr^{-1} into calm air at 0° F has a windchill value of –22° F! However, wind is not the only factor that can increase the rate of heat loss at any given temperature.

Water

Heat is lost 25 times faster in water compared with air of the same temperature. Unlike air, water offers little or no insulation where the skin meets the water, so heat is lost rapidly from the body. Movement in cold water increases heat loss from the arms and legs (29), so it is better to stay as still as possible in long-term "unplanned" immersions or wear a wetsuit for anticipated activities in cold water.

Insulating Factors

The rate at which heat is lost from the body is related inversely to the insulation between the body and the environment. The insulating quality is related to

Temperature (°F)

Wind (mph) / Calm	40	35	30	25	20	15	10	5	0	−5	−10	−15	−20	−25	−30	−35	−40	−45
5	36	31	25	19	13	7	1	−5	−11	−16	−22	−28	−34	−40	−46	−52	−57	−63
10	34	27	21	15	9	3	−4	−10	−16	−22	−28	−35	−41	−47	−53	−59	−66	−72
15	32	25	19	13	6	0	−7	−13	−19	−26	−32	−39	−45	−51	−58	−64	−71	−77
20	30	24	17	11	4	−2	−9	−15	−22	−29	−35	−42	−48	−55	−61	−68	−74	−81
25	29	23	16	9	3	−4	−11	−17	−24	−31	−37	−44	−51	−58	−64	−71	−78	−84
30	28	22	15	8	1	−5	−12	−19	−26	−33	−39	−46	−53	−60	−67	−73	−80	−87
35	28	21	14	7	0	−7	−14	−21	−27	−34	−41	−48	−55	−62	−69	−76	−82	−89
40	27	20	13	6	−1	−8	−15	−22	−29	−36	−43	−50	−57	−64	−71	−78	−84	−91
45	26	19	12	5	−2	−9	−16	−23	−30	−37	−44	−51	−58	−65	−72	−79	−86	−93
50	26	19	12	4	−3	−10	−17	−24	−31	−38	−45	−52	−60	−67	−74	−81	−88	−95
55	25	18	11	4	−3	−11	−18	−25	−32	−39	−46	−54	−61	−68	−75	−82	−89	−97
60	25	17	10	3	−4	−11	−19	−26	−33	−40	−48	−55	−62	−69	−76	−84	−91	−98
Frostbite occurs in:							30 minutes		10 minutes		5 minutes							

Wind chill (°F) = $35.74 + 0.6215T - 35.75(V^{0.16}) + 0.4275T(V^{0.16})$

T = Air temperature (°F) V = Wind speed (mph)

Figure 10.10 Windchill index.

the thickness of subcutaneous fat, the ability of clothing to trap air, and whether the clothing is wet or dry.

Body Fat

Subcutaneous fat thickness is an excellent indicator of total body insulation per unit surface area through which heat is lost (26). For example, in one report a fat man was able to swim for 7 hr in 16° C water with no change in body temperature, but a thin man had to leave the water in 30 min with a core temperature of 34.5° C (47). For this reason, long-distance swimmers tend to have more body fat than short-course swimmers; the higher body fatness provides more buoyancy, requiring less energy to swim at any set speed (28).

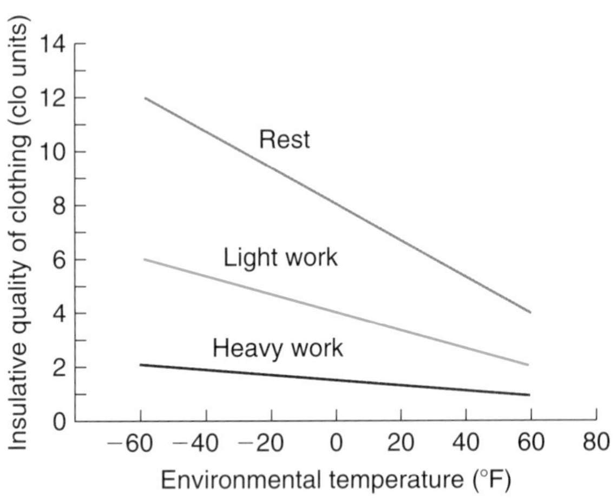

Figure 10.11 As work intensity increases, less insulation is needed to maintain core temperature.

Data from Burton & Edholm 1955.

Clothing

Clothing can extend our natural subcutaneous fat insulation, allowing us to endure very cold environments. The insulation quality of clothing is given in "clo" units, where 1 clo unit is the insulation needed at rest (1 MET) to maintain core temperature when the environment is 21° C (70° F), the relative humidity is 50%, and the air movement is 6 miles · hr^{-1} (7). As the air temperature falls, clothing with a higher clo value must be worn to maintain core temperature because the gradient between skin and environment is increasing. Figure 10.11 shows the insulation needed at different energy expenditures across a broad range of environmental temperatures, from −60 to +80° F (7). It is clear that as energy production increases, insulation must decrease to maintain core temperature. When clothing is worn in layers, insulation can be removed as needed to maintain core temperature. By following these steps, the sweat rate will be reduced and the clothing will retain more of its insulating value. If the clothing becomes wet, the insulating quality decreases because the water can now conduct heat away from the body about 25 times better than air (29). A primary goal, then, is to avoid wetness caused by either sweat or weather. This problem is exacerbated by the cold environment's very dry air, which causes a greater evaporation of moisture. When this problem of cold, dry air and wet clothing is coupled with windy conditions, the risk is even greater. The wind not only provides for greater convective heat loss, as described in the windchill section, but it also accelerates evaporation (19).

Energy Production

Energy production can modify the amount of insulation needed to maintain core temperature and prevent hypothermia (see figure 10.11). When thin (less than 16.8% fat) male subjects were immersed in cold water, the drop in body temperature that occurred at rest was prevented when they did exercise at an energy expenditure of about 8.5 kcal · min^{-1} (39, 40).

Table 10.6 shows the progression of signs and symptoms of hypothermia that occur as body temperature decreases (53). It is important to deal with these problems "on site" rather than wait until the person can be taken to an emergency room. According to Sharkey (52), one should do the following:

- Get the person out of the cold, wind, and rain.
- Remove all wet clothing.
- Provide warm drinks, dry clothing, and a warm dry sleeping bag for a mildly impaired person.
- Keep the person awake; if semiconscious, undress the person and put him or her into a sleeping bag with another person.
- Find a heat source, such as a campfire.

Effect of Air Pollution

Air pollution includes a variety of gases and particulates that are products of the combustion of fossil fuels. The smog that results when these pollutants are highly concentrated can have detrimental effects on health and performance. The gases can affect performance by decreasing the capacity to transport oxygen, increasing airway resistance, and altering the perception of effort required when the eyes burn and the chest hurts.

Physiological responses to these pollutants are related to the amount, or "dose," received. Several major factors determine the dose:

- Concentration of the pollutant
- Duration of the exposure to the pollutant
- Volume of air inhaled

Table 10.6 Clinical Symptoms of Hypothermia

Core temperature (°C)	Symptoms and signs
37	Feeling of cold; skin cooling; decreased social interaction
36	Goose pimples
35	Shivering; muscle tension; fatigue
34.5	Deep cold Numbness Loss of coordination Stumbling Dysarthria Muscle rigidity
32	Disorientation Decreased visual acuity
31–30	Semicoma—coma
28	Ventricular fibrillation and cardiovascular death

Reprinted from Hart and Sutton 1987.

The volume of air inhaled is clearly large during exercise, and this is one reason why physical activity should be curtailed during times of peak pollution levels (14). The following discussion focuses on the major air pollutants: ozone, sulfur dioxide, and carbon monoxide.

Ozone

The **ozone** in the air we breathe is generated by the reaction between ultraviolet (UV) light and emissions from internal combustion engines. There is evidence that a single 2-hr exposure to a high ozone concentration, 0.75 parts per million (PPM), decreases $\dot{V}O_2max$; furthermore, recent studies show that a 6- to 12-hr exposure to a concentration of only 0.12 PPM (the U.S. air-quality standard) decreases lung function and increases respiratory symptoms. Interestingly, people can adapt to ozone exposure, showing diminished responses to subsequent exposures during the "ozone season." Concern about long-term lung health suggests, however, that it would be prudent to avoid heavy exercise during the time of day when ozone and other pollutants are elevated (14).

Sulfur Dioxide

Sulfur dioxide (SO_2) is produced by smelters, refineries, and electrical utilities that use fossil fuel for energy generation. SO_2 does not affect lung function in normal individuals, but it causes bronchoconstriction in asthmatics—a response influenced by the temperature and humidity of the inspired air. Nose breathing is encouraged to "scrub" the SO_2, and drugs like cromolyn sodium and β-agonists can partially block the asthmatic's response to SO_2 (14).

Carbon Monoxide

Carbon monoxide (CO) is derived from the burning of fossil fuel, coal, oil, gasoline, and wood, as well as from cigarette smoke. CO can bind to hemoglobin (HbCO) and decrease the capacity for oxygen transport. The CO concentration in blood is generally less than 1% in nonsmokers but may be as high as 10% in smokers (49). As mentioned in chapter 28, beyond an HbCO concentration of 4.3% there is a 1% reduction in $\dot{V}O_2max$ for each 1% increase in the HbCO concentration. In contrast, when one exercises at about 40% $\dot{V}O_2max$, the HbCO concentration can be as high as 15% before endurance is affected. The cardiovascular system simply has a greater capacity to respond with a larger cardiac output when the oxygen concentration of the blood is reduced during submaximal work (30, 48, 49). This, of course, requires a higher HR for the same work task, and a participant needs to reduce the intensity of exercise during exposure to CO to stay in the THR range. Because it takes about 2 to 4 hr to remove half the CO from the blood once the exposure has been removed, CO can have a lasting effect on performance (14). Unfortunately, it is difficult to predict what the actual CO concentration will be in any given environment. Because we must consider the previous exposure to the pollutant, as well as the length of time and rate of ventilation associated with the current exposure, the following guidelines are provided for exercising in an area with air pollution (49):

- Reduce exposure to the pollutant before exercise because the physiological effects are time and dose dependent.
- Stay away from areas where one might receive a "bolus" dose of CO: smoking areas, high traffic areas, and urban environments.
- Do not schedule activities during the times when pollutants are at their highest levels because of traffic: 7 to 10 A.M. and 4 to 7 P.M.

Effect of Altitude

An increase in altitude decreases the partial pressure of oxygen and reduces the amount of oxygen bound to hemoglobin. As a result, the volume of oxygen carried in each liter of blood decreases. As mentioned in chapter 4, maximal aerobic power steadily decreases with increasing altitude, so that by 2300 m (7500 ft) the value is only 88% of that measured at sea level. This means that an activity that demanded 88% of $\dot{V}O_2max$ at sea level now requires 100% of the "new" $\dot{V}O_2max$.

More than maximal aerobic power is affected by altitude exposure. Any submaximal work rate is going to demand a higher HR at altitude compared with sea level (shown in figure 10.12). The reason is quite simple. Because each liter of blood has less oxygen at altitude, more blood is required to deliver the same quantity of oxygen to the tissues. Consequently, the HR response is elevated at any given submaximal work rate. To stay within the THR range, a person must decrease the intensity of the exercise when at altitude. As with exercise in high heat and humidity, monitoring the THR allows the exerciser to modify the intensity of the activity relative to any additional environmental demand (31).

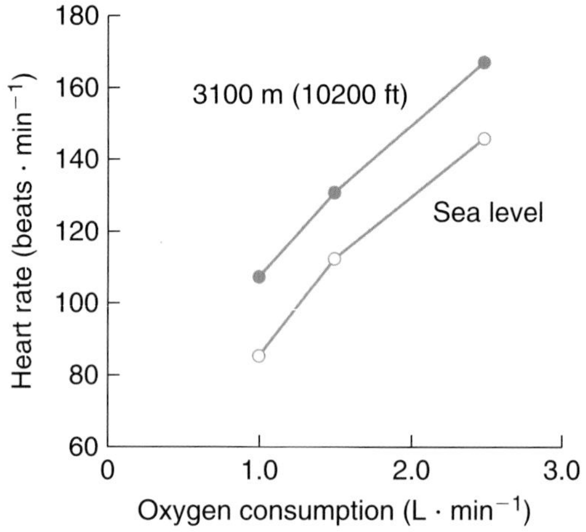

Figure 10.12 The effect of altitude on the HR response to submaximal exercise.

Based on data of R. Grover et al. 1967.

7 In Review

In conditions of high heat and humidity, the exerciser should decrease the work rate to stay in the THR zone. Exercisers should acclimatize to heat over 7 to 14 days to reduce the risk of heat injury. Advise participants to drink water before, during, and after exercise, and exercise in the early morning to reduce environmental heat load. When exercising in cold weather, participants should wear clothing in layers and remove layers to minimize sweating and stay dry. Participants should avoid exercising at times and in places in which air pollution is a problem. When exercising at altitude, participants should decrease work intensity to stay in the THR zone.

Case Studies

In the following case studies you are given general information about an individual, data on risk factors, and the results of an exercise test. Analyze each case, delineate the risk factors, and react to the person's responses to the test (whether normal or not). Then, on the basis of your analysis, make some recommendations for the individual relative to an exercise program and risk-factor reduction program. You can check your answers in appendix A.

10.1

Paul is a Caucasian male, 36 years of age, 88 kg, and 178 cm tall, and he has 28% body fat. Blood chemistry values indicate that his total cholesterol is 270 mg/dl and HDL cholesterol is 38 mg/dl. His mother died of a heart attack at the age of 63, and his father had a heart attack at the age of 68. He is sedentary and has engaged in no endurance training program since college. The following are the results of a maximal GXT conducted by his physician.

Test: Balke, 3 mi · hr^{-1}; 2.5% per 2 min

Grade %	METs	SBP mm Hg	DBP mm Hg	HR beats/min	ECG	Symptoms
	Rest	126	88	70	normal	—
2.5	4.3	142	86	142	normal	—
5	5.4	148	88	150	normal	—
7.5	6.4	162	86	160	normal	—
10	7.4	174	84	168	normal	—
12.5	8.5	186	84	176	normal	—
15	9.5	194	84	190	normal	calf tight
17.5	10.5	198	84	198	normal	fatigue

10.2

Mary is a 38-year-old Hispanic-American female, 170 cm tall, and 61.4 kg, and she has 30% body fat. Blood chemistry values indicate a total cholesterol of 188 mg/dl and an HDL-C of 59 mg/dl. Her resting blood pressure is 124/80. Family history indicates that her father suffered a nonfatal heart attack at the age of 67. She has smoked one pack of cigarettes per day for the past 13 years, and her lifestyle is sedentary. The following is the result of her submaximal cycle ergometer test.

Test: YMCA cycle test

Work rate (kpm · min^{-1})	HR (min 2)	HR (min 3)
150	118	120
300	134	136

Note: Pedal rate = 50 rev · min^{-1}; predicted HRmax = 182 beats · min^{-1}; seat height = 6; and 85% HRmax = 155 beats · min^{-1}

Source List

1. American College of Sports Medicine. (1996). Heat and cold illnesses during distance running. *Medicine and Science in Sports and Exercise, 28,* i-x.
2. American College of Sports Medicine. (1998). The recommended quantity and quality of exercise for developing and maintaining cardiorespiratory and muscular fitness, and flexibility in healthy adults. *Medicine and Science of Sports and Exercise, 30*(6), 975-991.
3. American College of Sports Medicine. (2000). *ACSM's guidelines for exercise testing and prescription* (6th ed.). Philadelphia: Lippincott Williams & Wilkins.
4. Bernard, T.E. (2001). Environmental considerations: heat and cold. In J.L. Roitman (Ed.), *ACSM's resource manual for guidelines for exercise testing and prescription* (4th ed., pp. 209-216). Baltimore: Lippincott Williams & Wilkins.
5. Blair, S.N., Kohl, H.W., III, Paffenbarger, R.S., Jr., Clark, D.G., Cooper, K.H., & Gibbons, L.W. (1989). Physical fitness and all-cause mortality. *Journal of the American Medical Association, 262,* 2395-2401.
6. Borg, G. (1998). *Borg's perceived exertion and pain scales.* Champaign, IL: Human Kinetics.
7. Burton, A.C., & Edholm, O.G. (1955). *Man in a cold environment.* London: Edward Arnold.
8. Buskirk, E.R., & Bass, D.E. (1974). Climate and exercise. In W.R. Johnson & E.R. Buskirk (Eds.), *Science and medicine of exercise and sport* (pp. 190-205). New York: Harper & Row.
9. Dehn, M.M., & Mullins, C.B. (1977). Physiologic effects and importance of exercise in patients with coronary artery disease. *Cardiovascular Medicine, 2,* 365.
10. Dionne, F.T., Turcotte, L., Thibault, M-C., Boulay, M.R., Skinner, J.S., & Bouchard, C. (1991). Mitochondrial DNA sequence polymorphism, $\dot{V}O_2$max, and response to endurance training. *Medicine and Science in Sports and Exercise, 23,* 177-185.
11. Dodd, S., Powers, S.K., Callender, T., & Brooks, E. (1984). Blood lactate disappearance at various intensities of recovery exercise. *Journal of Applied Physiology, 57,* 1462-1465.
12. Dose-response issues concerning physical activity and health: An evidence-based symposium (Supplement). (2001). *Medicine and Science in Sports and Exercise, 33*(6).

13. Drinkwater, B.L., Denton, J.E., Kupprat, I.C., Talag, T.S., & Horvath, S.M. (1976). Aerobic power as a factor in women's response to work within hot environments. *Journal of Applied Physiology, 41,* 815-821.
14. Folinsbee, L.J. (1990). Discussion: Exercise and the environment. In C. Bouchard, R.J. Shephard, T. Stephens, J.R. Sutton, & B.D. McPherson (Eds.), *Exercise, fitness, and health* (pp. 179-183). Champaign, IL: Human Kinetics.
15. Gisolfi, G.V., & Cohen, J. (1979). Relationships among training, heat acclimation, and heat tolerance in men and women: The controversy revisited. *Medicine and Science in Sports and Exercise, 11,* 56-59.
16. Goodman, L.S., & Gilman, A. (Eds.). (1975). *The pharmacological basis of therapeutics.* New York: Macmillan.
17. Grover, R., Reeves, J., Grover, E., & Leathers, J. (1967). Muscular exercise in young men native to 3,100 m altitude. *Journal of Applied Physiology, 22,* 555-564.
18. Hanson, P.G., & Zimmerman, S.W. (1979). Exertional heatstroke in novice runners. *Journal of the American Medical Association, 242,* 154-157.
19. Hardy, J.D., & Bard, P. (1974). Body temperature regulation. In V.B. Mountcastle (Ed.), *Medical physiology* (Vol. 2, 13th ed., pp. 1305-1342). St. Louis: Mosby.
20. Hart, L.E., & Sutton, J.R. (1987). Environmental considerations for exercise. *Cardiology Clinics, 5,* 245-258.
21. Haskell, W.L. (1978). Design and implementation of cardiac conditioning programs. In N.K. Wenger & H.K. Hellerstein (Eds.), *Rehabilitation of the coronary patient* (pp. 203-241). New York: Wiley.
22. Haskell, W.L. (1984). The influence of exercise on the concentrations of triglyceride and cholesterol in human plasma. *Exercise and Sport Sciences Reviews, 12,* 205-244.
23. Haskell, W.L. (1985). Physical activity and health: Need to define the required stimulus. *American Journal of Cardiology, 55,* 4D-9D.
24. Haskell, W.L. (1994). Dose-response issues from a biological perspective. In C. Bouchard, R.J. Shephard, & T. Stevens (Eds.), *Physical activity, fitness, and health* (pp. 1030-1039). Champaign, IL: Human Kinetics.
25. Haskell, W.L. (2001). What to look for in assessing responsiveness to exercise in a health context. *Medicine and Science in Sports and Exercise, 33,* S454-S458.
26. Hayward, M.G., & Keatinge, W.R. (1981). Roles of subcutaneous fat and thermoregulatory reflexes in determining ability to stabilize body temperature in water. *Journal of Physiology* (London), *320,* 229-251.
27. Hellerstein, H.K., & Franklin, B.A. (1984). Exercise testing and prescription. In N.K. Wenger & H.K. Hellerstein (Eds.), *Rehabilitation of the coronary patient* (2nd ed., pp. 197-284). New York: Wiley.
28. Holmer, I. (1979). Physiology of swimming man. *Exercise and Sport Sciences Reviews, 7,* 87-123.
29. Horvath, S.M. (1981). Exercise in a cold environment. *Exercise and Sport Sciences Reviews, 9,* 221-263.
30. Horvath, S.M., Raven, P.R., Dahms, T.E., & Gray, D.J. (1975). Maximal aerobic capacity of different levels of carboxyhemoglobin. *Journal of Applied Physiology, 38,* 300-303.
31. Howley, E.T. (1980). Effect of altitude on physical performance. In G.A. Stull & T.K. Cureton (Eds.), *Encyclopedia of physical education, fitness, and sports: Training, environment, nutrition, and fitness* (pp. 177-187). Salt Lake City: Brighton.
32. Howley, E.T. (2001). Type of activity: resistance, aerobic and leisure versus occupational physical activity. *Medicine and Science in Sports and Exercise, 33,* S364-S369.
33. Hughson, R.L., Green, H.J., Houston, M.E., Thompson, J.A., MacLean, D.R., & Sutton, J.R. (1980). Heat injuries in Canadian mass-participation runs. *Canadian Medical Association Journal, 122,* 1141-1144.
34. Jennings, G.L., Deakin, G., Korner, P., Meredith, I., Kingwell, B., & Nelson, L. (1991). What is the dose-response relationship between exercise training and blood pressure? *Annals of Medicine, 23,* 313-318.
35. Karvonen, M.J., Kentala, E., & Mustala, O. (1957). The effects of training heart rate: A longitudinal study. *Annales Medicinae Experimentalis et Biologiae Fenniae, 35,* 307-315.
36. Kesaniemi, Y.A., Danforth, E., Jr., Jensen, M.D., Kopelman, P.G., Lefebvre, P., & Reeder, B.A. (2001). Dose-response issues concerning physical activity and health: An evidence-based symposium. *Medicine and Science in Sports and Exercise, 33,* S351-S358.
37. Londeree, B.R., & Ames, S.A. (1976). Trend analysis of the % VO_2max-HR regression. *Medicine and Science in Sports, 8,* 122-125.
38. Londeree, B.R., & Moeschberger, M.L. (1982). Effect of age and other factors on maximal heart rate. *Research Quarterly for Exercise and Sport, 53,* 297-304.
39. McArdle, W.D., Magel, J.R., Gergley, T.J., Spina, R.J., & Toner, M.M. (1984). Thermal adjustment to cold-water exposure in resting men and women. *Journal of Physiology: Respiratory, Environmental and Exercise Physiology, 56,* 1565-1571.
40. McArdle, W.D., Magel, J.R., Spina, R.J., Gergley, T.J., & Toner, M.M. (1984). Thermal adjustments to cold-water exposure in exercising men and women. *Journal of Applied Physiology, 56,* 1572-1577.
41. Paffenbarger, R.S., Hyde, R.T., & Wing, A.L. (1986). Physical activity, all-cause mortality, and longevity of college alumni. *New England Journal of Medicine, 314,* 605-613.
42. Pate, R.R., Pratt, M., Blair, S.N., Haskell, W.L., Marcera, C.A., & Bouchard, C. (1995). Physical activity and public health: A recommendation from the Centers for Disease Control and Prevention and the American College of Sports Medicine. *Journal of the American Medical Association, 273,* 402-407.
43. Pollock, M.L., Gettman, L.R., Mileses, C.A., Bah, M.D., Durstine, J.L., & Johnson, R.B. (1977). Effects of frequency and duration of training on attrition and incidence of injury. *Medicine and Science in Sports, 9,* 31-36.
44. Pollock, M.L., & Wilmore, J.H. (1990). *Exercise in health and disease* (2nd ed.). Philadelphia: Saunders.
45. Powers, S.K., & Howley, E.T. (1997). *Exercise physiology.* Madison, WI: Brown & Benchmark.
46. Pugh, L.G.C. (1964). Deaths from exposure in Four Inns Walking Competition, March 14-15, 1964. *Lancet, 1,* 1210-1212.
47. Pugh, L.G.C., & Edholm, O.G. (1955). The physiology of Channel swimmers. *Lancet, 2,* 761-768.
48. Raven, P.B. (1980). Effects of air pollution on physical performance. In G.A. Stull & T.K. Cureton (Ed.), *Encyclopedia of physical education: Physical fitness, training, environment and nutrition related to performance* (Vol. 2, pp. 201-216). Salt Lake City: Brighton.
49. Raven, P.B., Drinkwater, B.L., Ruhling, R.O., Bolduan, N., Taguchi, S., Gliner, J., & Horvath, S.M. (1974). Effect of carbon monoxide and peroxyacetyl nitrate on man's maximal aerobic capacity. *Journal of Applied Physiology, 36,* 288-293.
50. Sawka, M.N., Francesconi, R.P., Young, A.J., & Pandolf, K.B. (1984). Influence of hydration level and body fluids on exercise performance in the heat. *Journal of the American Medical Association, 252*(9), 1165-1169.
51. Sawka, M.N., Young, A.J., Francesconi, R.P., Muza, S.R., & Pandolf, K.B. (1985). Thermoregulatory and blood responses during exercise at graded hypohydration levels. *Journal of Applied Physiology, 59,* 1394-1401.
52. Sharkey, B.J. (1990). *Physiology of fitness* (3rd ed.). Champaign, IL: Human Kinetics.
53. Sutton, J.R. (1990). Exercise and the environment. In C. Bouchard, R.J. Shephard, T. Stephens, J.R. Sutton, & B.D. McPherson (Eds.), *Exercise, fitness, and health* (pp. 165-178). Champaign, IL: Human Kinetics.
54. Swain, D.P., Abernathy, K.S., Smith, C.S., Lee, S.J., & Bunn, S.A. (1994). Target heart rates for the development of cardiorespiratory fitness. *Medicine and Science in Sports and Exercise, 26,* 112-116.
55. Swain, D.P., & Leutholtz, B.C. (1997). Heart rate reserve is equivalent to %VO_2Reserve, not to %VO_2max. *Medicine and Science in Sports and Exercise, 29,* 410-414.
56. Swain, D.P., Leutholtz, B.C., King, M.E., Haas, L.A., & Branch, J.D. (1998). Relationship between % heart rate reserve and % VO_2reserve in treadmill exercise. *Medicine and Science in Sports and Exercise, 30,* 318-321.
57. Tanaka, H., Monahan, K.D., & Seals, D.R. (2001). Age-predicted maximal heart rate revisited. *Journal of the American College of Cardiology, 37,* 153-156.
58. United States Department of Health and Human Services. (1996). *Surgeon General's report on physical activity and health.* Washington, DC: Author.
59. United States Department of Health and Human Services. (2000). *Healthy people 2010: National health promotion and disease prevention objectives.* Washington, DC: Author.

eleven

Exercise Prescription for Weight Management

Dixie L. Thompson

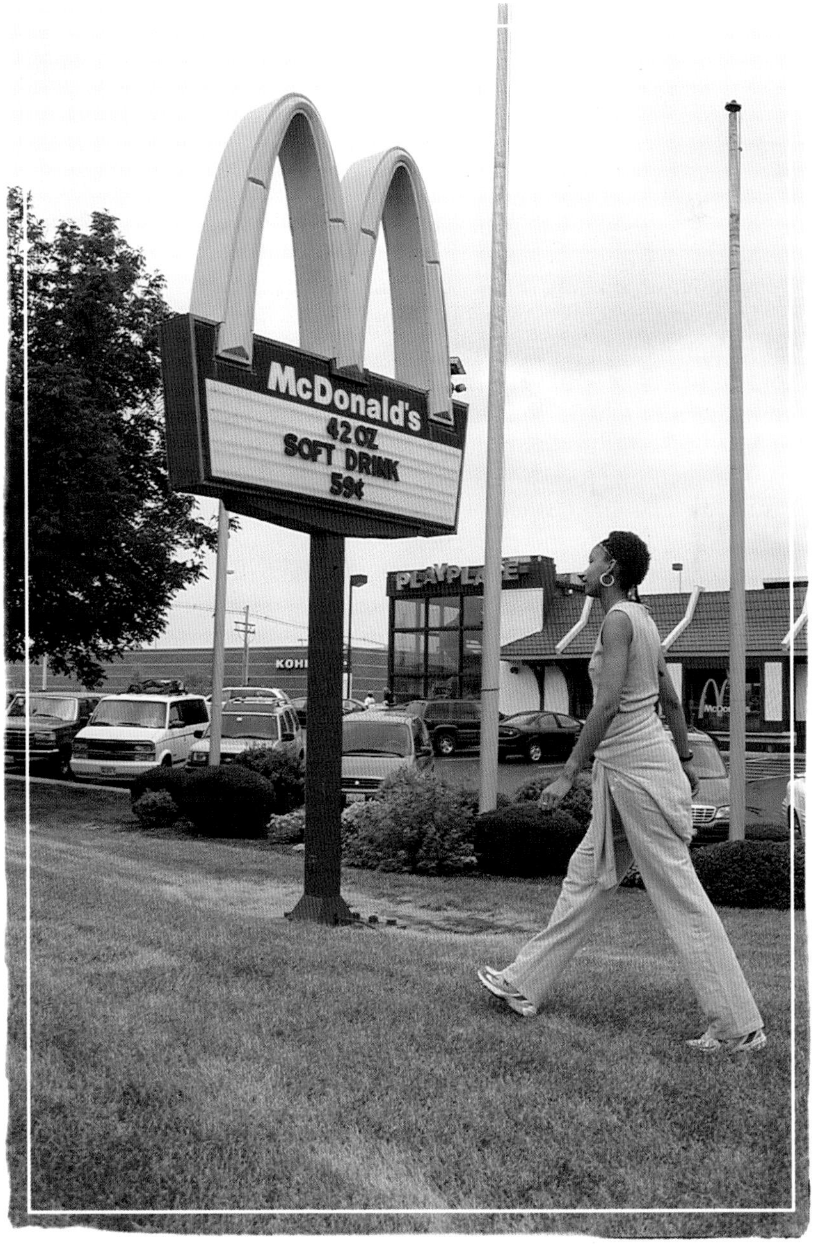

Objectives

The reader will be able to do the following:

1. Identify factors that contribute to obesity.
2. Describe the role that energy balance plays in weight loss and weight maintenance.
3. Provide guidelines for caloric intake to facilitate appropriate weight loss, discuss the role of exercise in weight loss and weight maintenance, and prescribe safe and effective exercise programs for weight management.
4. Describe appropriate behavioral change strategies for modifying and/or maintaining body composition.
5. State the efficacy of quick-fix weight loss methods.
6. Recognize signs of eating disorders.
7. Provide healthy guidelines for gaining weight.

Billions of dollars are spent each year on weight loss. The weight loss industry provides a broad spectrum of goods and services, including over-the-counter and prescription drugs, motivational and educational books, and weight loss clinics. Weight loss groups have sprung up in many environments, ranging from schools to health clinics to churches. Despite this multi-billion dollar industry, Americans are getting fatter. More than 50% of American adults are classified as either overweight or obese (21). Unfortunately, this same negative trend is occurring among U.S. children (9). Although the fight against obesity is lost by many Americans, some manage to maintain a healthy weight throughout their lives, and many successfully lose excess weight. The lessons from these groups of people provide a roadmap for successful weight maintenance (11, 31).

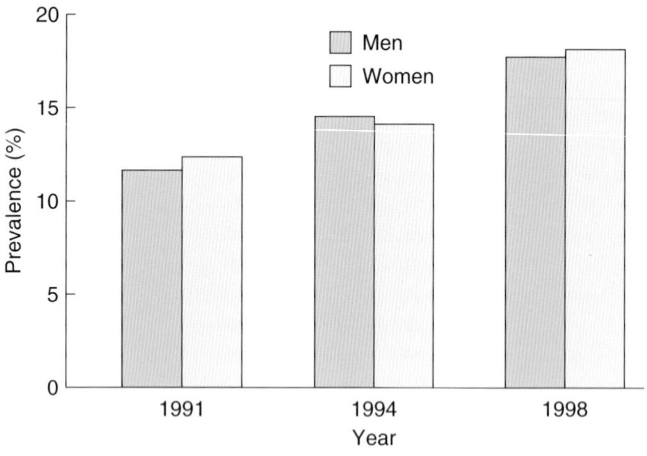

Figure 11.1 Prevalence of obesity among American adults.

Adapted from Mokdad et al. (18).

Increasing Prevalence of Obesity in the United States

There was an approximately 50% increase in the prevalence of obesity (BMI ≥ 30 kg/m^2) during the 1990s (18). Figure 11.1 shows this increasing prevalence of obesity from 1991 to 1998 for both men and women. Some segments of the population are experiencing an even more rapid increase in obesity prevalence. For example, the prevalence of obesity rose by 69.9% among adults ages 18 to 29 years, and obesity rates climbed by 80% for Hispanics during this same time period. Because of the rapid changes in obesity prevalence, this trend does not appear to be causally linked to genetics. As discussed later, lifestyle changes seem to be the major culprits.

It is common for adults to accumulate additional adipose tissue as they age. This gradual accumulation of fat is sometimes called **creeping obesity**. Part of this change in body composition is attributable to a natural loss of muscle caused by aging. A decreasing metabolic rate, a more sedentary lifestyle, and a lack of adjustment in eating patterns, however, appear to be the most important factors contributing to increased body fat (6). Although some fat accumulation is acceptable (see chapter 6, table 6.1), when BMI climbs to obese levels one can expect negative health consequences to follow (21, 22).

1 In Review

Although billions of dollars are spent each year in weight loss attempts, the prevalence of obesity in America is increasing. People tend to accumulate fat as they age, but creeping obesity is not healthy. A change in eating and exercise habits is needed to prevent obesity.

Etiology of Obesity

The cause of obesity cannot be described simply, because many factors contribute to its development. Ultimately, **positive caloric balance** (i.e., taking in more calories than are expended) leads to obesity. It is clear, however, that factors contributing to obesity can be discussed under two broad categories: genetics and lifestyle.

Genetics

Evidence exists that inheritance contributes to the development of obesity (11, 25). In evaluating the impact of genetics on the development of obesity, researchers have attempted to differentiate among factors that are truly genetic and sociocultural factors that are passed down through the generations. Bouchard and colleagues (5) estimated that approximately 25% of the variance in body fat percentage is attributable to genetics. Interestingly, these authors found that inheritance has a larger effect on total fat and deep deposits of adipose tissue than on subcutaneous fat. Additional evidence on the importance of genetics in the transmission of obesity comes from data demonstrating that the BMI of adopted children is more similar to their biological parents than that of their adoptive parents (26). The recent discoveries of genes linked with obesity provide additional evidence that genetics is important in determining the likelihood of obesity.

A negative consequence of our growing knowledge of the genetic link to obesity is that people from families where many are overweight may become discouraged and believe there is nothing to be done about their weight status. Although genetics can be an important contributor to the development of obesity, the primary reason that an individual becomes obese is related to lifestyle. It is important that the HFI emphasize to clients that genetics may predispose one to obesity, but one still can significantly affect her or his body weight.

Lifestyle

The choices that one makes about caloric expenditure and caloric intake have a predominant impact on the development of obesity. The number of calories consumed, the types of foods eaten, and the amount of daily activity all affect one's weight. If more calories are consumed than are expended, the positive caloric balance will result in weight (fat) gain. To lose fat weight, a **negative caloric balance** must be established. This can be achieved by decreasing caloric intake, increasing caloric expenditure, or both.

Food Intake

When excess calories (particularly fat calories) are consumed, the energy is stored as fat. From an evolutionary standpoint, this is a positive adaptation to variations in food availability. In other words, fat accumulation occurs during times of plenty, and this stored energy is used when food supplies are low. In populations that have a constant abundance of high caloric density food, this mechanism often results in excessive fat accumulation.

Health professionals sometimes question whether obese individuals typically consume more calories than their average weight counterparts. Dietary recall studies provide little clear information about this issue because people tend to underreport dietary intake and overestimate physical activity (17). Some research suggests that obese subjects particularly underreport consumption of high-fat and snack-type foods (29). Highly advanced research procedures in which people ingest isotopes of oxygen and hydrogen (doubly labeled water) indicate that overweight individuals expend and consume more calories than normal weight persons (28). The higher energy expenditure is caused by the metabolic cost of supporting the excess body weight. The reasons for consumption of extra calories are not well defined.

Types of Food Eaten and Obesity

When fat is consumed, it is stored as fat more readily than are either protein or carbohydrates. From a theoretical perspective, the low thermic effect of fat (i.e., the energy needed to digest, absorb, transport, and store fat), the ease with which fat is stored as adipose tissue, and the high-caloric density of high-fat foods make fat a likely culprit in the development of obesity.

Several studies indicate that obese and overweight individuals tend to consume a higher percentage of calories from fat than normal weight individuals (29). It appears that the availability of foods high in fat and simple sugars puts individuals at higher risk for development of obesity. In cultures where the majority of calories consumed are complex carbohydrates, the rates of obesity are lower than in the United States.

Daily Energy Expenditure

Data demonstrate a relationship between low physical activity and the development of obesity (30). It is less clear, however, whether low physical activity leads to obesity or if obesity causes people to reduce their activity levels. The role of regular exercise in weight loss is complex and has been reviewed by several authors (10, 22, 24). Certainly an increase in physical activity can play an important role in creating a negative caloric balance. Additionally, some studies have supported the role of exercise in the maintenance of fat-free mass and metabolic rate during periods of weight loss. Although studies sometimes differ in their findings of the short-term effects of exercise on weight loss, the long-term positive consequences of physical activity on weight maintenance are more clear. Exercise appears to be one of the strongest predictors of long-term weight maintenance (16, 30, 31). Additionally, regular physical activity attenuates the age-related weight gain typically observed in populations (8).

2 In Review

Both genetics and lifestyle factors contribute to the development of obesity. Caloric intake, food choices, and daily physical activity are all aspects of lifestyle that affect fat accumulation. A positive caloric balance results in weight gain; a negative caloric balance results in weight loss.

Maintaining a Healthy Weight

Numerous methods can be used to maintain a healthy weight or to lose weight when necessary. The HFI should encourage clients to choose weight maintenance or weight loss techniques that are effective yet pose little threat to overall health. The following sections outline practices that can be implemented safely for the majority of adults.

Assessing Daily Caloric Need

Whether planning individualized weight loss or weight maintenance programs, it is helpful to know the number of calories the client needs to sustain his or her current body weight. This can be done by estimating **daily caloric need**. Daily caloric need represents the number of calories a person needs to sustain current body weight, assuming that activity levels remain constant. The daily caloric need comprises the resting metabolic rate, the thermic effect of food, and the calories used in daily activities (figure 11.2).

Resting metabolic rate (RMR) is the number of calories expended to maintain the body during resting conditions. For most individuals, RMR represents 60 to 70% of the daily caloric need. RMR generally is measured by indirect calorimetry. For people who engage in regular, vigorous exercise, the RMR may account for a smaller proportion of daily caloric need. To accurately measure RMR, the assessment should occur when the client has not eaten for several hours, has not exercised vigorously for the past 12 hr, and has been in a resting,

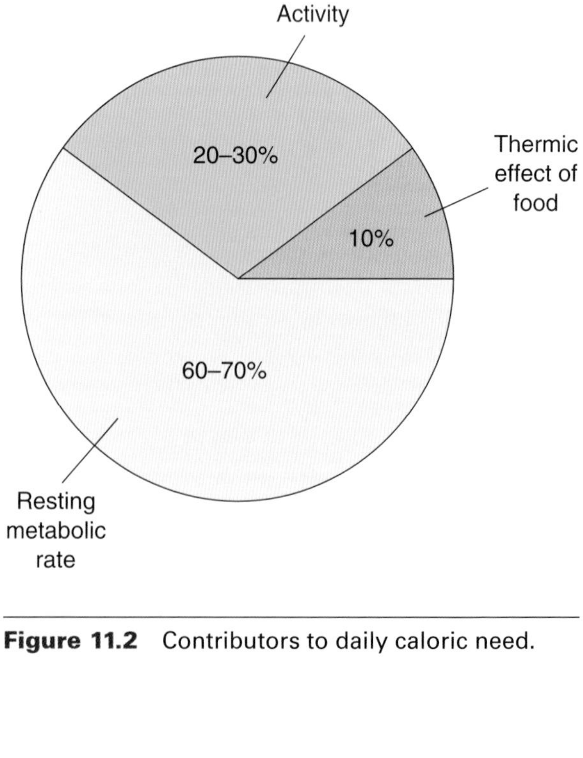

Figure 11.2 Contributors to daily caloric need.

reclined position for 30 min (19). Because of the cost of indirect calorimetry systems and the strict control needed to obtain accurate results, measuring RMR is not always practical; therefore, a number of equations have been developed to predict RMR. These RMR equations are based on the following principles:

- RMR is proportional to body size.
- RMR decreases with age.
- Muscle is more metabolically active than fat.

The larger the body size, the more calories needed to sustain it. This relationship is reflected in all RMR equations. In addition to body size, age, significantly affects RMR. As a person ages, his or her RMR decreases, meaning that a person's daily caloric need will decrease with age. Children typically have higher metabolic rates than adults of any age. RMR remains relatively stable during the early adult years; however, it begins to decline rather substantially after age 45. The effects of age and body size on RMR are reflected in the equations in the following box. Notice that these estimates of RMR use separate equations for males and females. This is because many males have more fat-free mass than females, and fat-free mass requires more energy to sustain it than does fat tissue.

If the HFI knows the fat-free mass of a client, the following equation can be used to predict RMR (7). There is no need for separate equations when fat-free mass is known, because a gram of muscle has the same metabolic need whether it is housed in a male or a female body.

$$\text{RMR (kcal/day)} = 370 + (21.6 \times \text{fat-free mass in kg})$$

When attempting to determine daily caloric need, the HFI also must estimate the calories burned in physical activity. This assessment must contain information about work and leisure-time activity. Although there are numerous ways to gather information about daily activity, one method typically used is to have the client complete an activity log in which he or she records work and leisure activity. Once the activity pattern is established, the information in chapter 4 about the caloric cost of various activities can be used to estimate the energy burned in activity. This would be especially important if working with an individual who trains extensively. Alternately, one can estimate daily caloric need by using the methods outlined in the box on page 194.

The smallest part of the daily caloric need is the **thermic effect of food**. This is the energy needed to digest, absorb, transport, and store the food that is eaten. Although this value may vary slightly depending on the types of food eaten, the thermic effect of food typically accounts for 10% of the daily caloric need (20).

Changing Lifestyle to Promote a Healthy Weight

Although each individual must assess which areas of her or his lifestyle most contribute to excessive weight accumulation, some common steps that would benefit the majority of people who are attempting to lose weight include the following:

- Reduce total calories.
- Reduce fat intake.
- Increase physical activity.
- Change eating behaviors.

As previously mentioned, a negative caloric balance must be established for weight loss to occur. The number of calories consumed while attempting to lose weight should be determined by the client's health, caloric need, and ultimate weight loss goals.

Equations for Estimating Resting Metabolic Rate (12)

MALES:

$$\text{RMR} = 66 + (5 \times \text{height}) + (13.8 \times \text{weight}) - (6.8 \times \text{age})$$

FEMALES:

$$\text{RMR} = 655 + (1.8 \times \text{height}) + (9.6 \times \text{weight}) - (4.7 \times \text{age})$$

RMR expressed in kilocalories per day
height expressed in centimeters
weight expressed in kilograms
age expressed in years

Guidelines for Estimating Daily Caloric Need (12)

Once resting metabolic rate (RMR) has been assessed, use the following criteria for estimating daily caloric need. The calculated value will be a rough estimate of the calories needed to sustain current body weight.

- For a person confined to bed rest, multiply by 1.2.
- For those who are sedentary both in work and leisure time, multiply by 1.3.
- For those who lead a somewhat active life, multiply by 1.4.
- For those who are very active, multiply by 1.5.

EXAMPLE:

Calculate the daily caloric need of a 50-year-old male office worker. He is six feet tall and weighs 215 lb. He walks 2 miles briskly 3 times per week but otherwise is rather inactive.

6 ft × 12 in./ft = 72 in.

72 in. × 2.54 cm/in. = 182.9 cm

215 lb ÷ 2.2 lb/kg = 97.7 kg

1. Calculate RMR (as described previously).

   RMR = 66 + (5 × height) + (13.8 × weight) − (6.8 × age)

   RMR = 66 + (5 × 182.9) + (13.8 × 97.7) − (6.8 × 50)

   RMR = 1989 kcal per day

2. Add calories expended in activity. For a moderately active individual or one who engages in low to moderate activity 3 days per week, multiply RMR by 1.4.

   Daily caloric need = RMR × 1.4

   Daily caloric need = 1989 × 1.4 = 2785 kcal/day

The ACSM recommends that weekly weight loss goals should not exceed 1 kg (about 2.2 lb) per week (1). A general guideline is to establish a caloric deficit of 3500 to 7000 kcal per week (500-1000 kcal/day), which, theoretically, will result in a 1- to 2-lb loss of fat each week (1 lb of fat = 3500 kcal).

Most healthy adults who need to lose weight can institute a low-calorie diet (LCD) consisting of 800 to 1500 kcal/day without major adverse consequences. However, it is not recommended that people institute a very low-calorie diet (VLCD) in which caloric intake is reduced below 800 kcal/day (22). Based on evidence from weight loss studies, VLCDs may result in greater initial weight loss, but the success measured at 1 year is no better that seen with LCDs (22). The ACSM recommends a daily caloric intake of no fewer than 1200 kcal/day (1). This is a general recommendation, and those with special needs (e.g., athletes, the elderly, people with metabolic disorders) may require a different caloric intake. With any caloric restriction, the potential negative side effects of decreases in RMR and fat-free mass can be expected. These negative side effects will be greater in those who establish large daily caloric deficits (22).

Exercise Prescription for Weight Management

The ACSM recommends a combined approach of exercise and moderate caloric restriction for those attempting weight loss (1, 2). Although debate continues over the precise contribution of exercise to weight management, this recommended combination appears to be most effective in maintaining lean mass and avoiding excessive decreases in RMR. It is clear from existing data that engaging in regular aerobic activity is common for those who are successful in maintaining weight loss (31). Studies also show that regular exercise is important in helping prevent weight gain (8, 14). From a theoretical perspective, the addition of exercise to one's everyday life can significantly alter one's weight. For example, expending just 100 kcal per day beyond daily caloric need for a year creates a caloric deficit of 36,500 kcal. Expending 300 to 500 kcal per day in physical activity is a reasonable goal for weight management for most healthy adults (1). The intensity and mode of activity seem less important than ensuring that the exercise is a routine part of one's daily life. The addition of resistance activity to regular aerobic activity may be particularly helpful in maintaining lean mass with aging.

In addition to the physical benefits of regular physical activity, psychological variables have also been reported to improve with exercise. Improvements in self-esteem and self-efficacy are commonly reported outcomes of engaging in regular exercise. The empowerment that comes from becoming more fit can add to the resolve to live a healthy lifestyle and maintain a healthy weight.

3 In Review

Daily caloric need is determined by the RMR, the thermic effect of food, and activity levels. Some common steps from which many people who are attempting to lose weight could benefit are reducing total calories, decreasing fat intake, increasing physical activity, and changing eating behaviors. The exercise prescription for weight management should involve regular aerobic activity that burns 300 to 500 kcal per day. When weight reduction is needed, weight loss goals of 1 to 2 lb per week can be safely initiated by most healthy adults.

Behavior Modification Techniques for Weight Loss and Maintenance

The majority of attempts to lose weight and maintain weight loss are unsuccessful. Behavior modification (changes in lifestyle habits and patterns) is an important component of successful weight loss and weight maintenance programs (22). For additional information on behavior modification, see chapter 22.

When people are committed to changing eating and activity patterns, a number of strategies can be used to improve the chances of long-term success. During the initial phase of weight loss (the "action stage"—see chapter 22), implementing these strategies requires a great deal of effort and there is a significant chance of failure (relapse). After 6 months or more of using these strategies (the "maintenance stage"—see chapter 22), changes in diet and lifestyle become a more natural part of one's routine. Some strategies shown to be effective for losing weight and maintaining weight loss are listed in the following box. Not every client will respond well to the same techniques. Each situation should be considered separately, and an individualized weight loss or weight maintenance plan should be developed for each client.

Record Keeping

Before implementing a weight loss / weight maintenance program, it is wise to obtain information about the current eating patterns. This is most easily done through the use of an eating diary or food log. A sample food log and instructions are provided in chapter 7. Remember, it is important to gather information about the types and quantities of food eaten as well as the social and emotional circumstances surrounding eating.

Careful record keeping helps accomplish several objectives. First, food logs document the problem areas of food intake. Many individuals are unaware of the number of total calories or the amount of fat that they consume daily. Another important purpose of eating diaries is to document the social/

Strategies for Success in Weight Loss or Weight Maintenance

- Keeping records
- Planning meals and snacks
- Soliciting support
- Setting behavioral as well as outcome-oriented goals
- Developing a reward system
- Avoiding self-defeating behaviors
- Combining moderate caloric restriction with aerobic exercise
- Developing healthy eating patterns
- Committing to lifelong maintenance

emotional cues to eating. After a period of record keeping, individuals begin to recognize the factors, other than hunger, that lead to eating (e.g., socializing with friends, watching television, feeling stressed). To combat these cues to eating and, in many cases, overeating, the social and emotional situations one is in when one eats must be recognized and strategies developed to overcome them. A third major purpose of keeping eating records is to make eating a cognitive process. For many people eating is a habit, and their automatic choices about how much and what to eat are made without conscious consideration. As discussed next, appropriate planning of meals and snacks is an important component of a successful weight loss plan.

Planning Meals and Snacks

Weight loss does not occur by accident; it takes a concerted effort. Purchasing appropriate foods and planning meals is imperative for successful weight loss or weight maintenance. One of the most helpful practices in controlling food intake is avoiding the purchase of high-fat/high-caloric-density food. Substituting low-calorie and/or low-fat foods for high-calorie and/or high-fat foods also can substantially affect weight loss. For example, substituting 1% milk for whole milk represents a decrease of approximately 50 kcal per cup. If a person drinks 2 cups of milk per day, this will reduce caloric intake by 36,500 kcal in 1 year!

Meal planning is also essential. In households where the adults work outside of the home, there is little time for meal preparation. Buying breakfast foods that are quick to prepare, nutritious, and relatively low in calories (e.g., fresh fruit, bagels, low-fat yogurt, whole grain cereals) helps provide a morning meal to offset hunger and provide important nutrients. Because many Americans are not at home for the noon meal, food choices often depend on the restaurants that are convenient, affordable, and quick. This leads many to visit fast-food restaurants. Although many of these restaurant chains have added lower fat items to their menus, the majority of fast-food items are high in both fat and calories. It has been shown that individuals who choose to eat fast foods are less successful at maintaining weight loss than those who avoid these food choices (12). Planning ahead might allow some individuals to carry their lunch to work and ensure that a variety of healthy, low-fat, low-calorie food choices are available for this important meal. The evening meal represents a significant percentage of the daily caloric intake of many Americans. It is not uncommon for individuals who may have limited their food intake during the day to overindulge at night. The effort to cook a meal often results in people choosing to eat at restaurants or purchase packaged meals that tend to be high in fat and calories. The effort necessary for cooking nutritious nightly meals can be reduced by the following:

- Cook and store meals ahead of time.
- Find a variety of quick and easy to prepare low-calorie meals.
- Purchase food items ahead of time to avoid unnecessary shopping.
- Keep a variety of fresh vegetables on hand to serve.

It is also important to consider what types of foods are available for snacks. Although avoiding food between meals may be ideal for many, there are times when food is needed between meals. Foods that provide nutrients and are also low calorie are the best choices (e.g., fresh fruit, raw vegetables, low-fat yogurt).

Establishing a Support System

A number of studies have shown the benefit of having a support system when trying to lose weight (22). It is important to understand, however, that the source of the support will vary depending on the client. The support system may be a friend, spouse, significant other, parent, coworker, therapist, or support group. No matter what the source of the support, the HFI should encourage clients in a weight loss or weight maintenance program to seek out individuals to encourage them in their efforts.

Many people are encouraged by the support of other people who also are attempting to lose weight. Many commercial weight loss centers provide support groups. These groups serve several functions: They provide a group to whom participants are accountable, a setting in which helpful hints and success stories can be shared, and a nonthreatening environment where all of the participants are chasing the same objective. For some people, the reasons for overeating are emotional and deeply rooted. In these cases, the guidance provided by a trained therapist may be needed.

Committing to Behavioral As Well As Outcome-Oriented Goals

It is important for clients to develop goals that encourage healthy eating practices. Goal setting is important to help individuals remain focused on weight loss or weight maintenance. Goal setting should take place in a mutual exchange between the HFI and the client. The HFI's role is to provide information about healthy weight loss or management practices; the client is responsible for identifying the behavioral goals to which she or he is willing to commit.

Typically, weight loss is an outcome-oriented goal (i.e., the end result is the measure of success). Weight loss goals should be reasonable for the client involved and should follow the guidelines listed previously. In contrast to outcome goals, behavioral goals focus on the process of weight loss, not the final outcome. Behavioral goals can be used to help make behavior and lifestyle changes that will affect weight loss or weight maintenance. Among the areas that might be targeted by these goals are altering eating patterns, making wise food choices, and increasing daily energy expenditure. An example of a behavioral goal that might be implemented is, "I will walk the stairs to my office daily rather than riding the elevator." More specific information on goal setting can be found in chapter 22.

Designing a Reward System

A part of human nature is the desire to be rewarded for accomplishing goals. When you are designing a weight loss or weight maintenance program, it is wise to provide motivation by planning a way to reward success. As with goal setting, it is vital that the client be involved in developing the rewards that will be used. One rule that the HFI should encourage, however, is to avoid using food as a reward. It is important to establish a reward program that will recognize the achievement of both outcome-oriented and behavioral goals. This is important because the attainment of an outcome goal may take a substantial amount of time, longer than it may take to change certain behaviors. Also, there will be times when a person's weight will plateau, and it is important that behavioral goals be rewarded during these times. Examples of rewards that might be used are listed next.

- Purchasing new clothes
- Purchasing hobby items (e.g., books, compact discs, tools)
- Taking a trip
- Attending special events (movies, music and dance concerts, lectures)

Avoiding Self-Defeating Behaviors

For all of us, there are situations that increase the likelihood we will overeat. It is important when trying to lose weight to acknowledge these situations and institute measures to minimize the chance of falling victim to these self-defeating behaviors. For example, a person who tends to snack on high-calorie foods late at night might avoid purchasing such foods and also implement a behavioral objective of not eating after 7:00 P.M. A person who loves pizza but tends to overindulge when going out to a restaurant might make pizza at home using low-fat ingredients and vegetables as toppings.

It is important to remember that we are all human. There are special times (birthdays, holiday dinners) when people will want to eat foods that are not a part of their weight management plan. The HFI should explain to clients that there will be times when they will not meet all their behavioral objectives. A crucial factor for weight management clients to keep in mind is that a lapse in eating (or activity) should not mean an end to the weight management plan. The HFI should encourage individuals to immediately return to their healthy eating and exercise plan after the lapse. The HFI might help reduce some of the guilty feelings by helping the client view the lapse not as a failure but as an opportunity to renew his or her commitment to the weight loss or weight maintenance process.

Combining Moderate Caloric Restriction With Aerobic Exercise

Regular exercise has been shown to be an important facet of successful weight loss and weight maintenance programs. As mentioned previously, the ACSM (1, 2) and NIH (22) support the use of exercise for weight loss and weight maintenance. The majority of weight loss studies that compare diet with diet plus exercise show that the combined approach leads to greater weight loss (22). Regular aerobic activity expending 300 to 500 kcal each day is recommended for individuals attempting to lose or maintain weight (1). See previous comments in this chapter and also in chapter 18 for more information on exercise prescription for weight loss or weight maintenance.

Changing Unhealthy Eating Patterns

Specific eating patterns have been linked with excessive weight gain (6). Being aware of these behaviors and implementing plans to avoid them increases the likelihood that weight management will be successful. These four changes in eating patterns are recommended:

- Slow down.
- Make wise substitutions.
- Keep variety in your diet.
- Eat smaller and fewer portions.

It is common for people to eat rapidly and then begin to feel uncomfortably full several minutes after they are finished eating. When food is eaten rapidly, inadequate time is allowed for the satiety mechanisms to help curb hunger. This results in people eating more than necessary before they realize that they are no longer hungry. Some ways that can help people slow their eating are to put down the eating utensil between bites, pause at least 30 s between bites, and chew food completely and swallow before taking another bite (6).

As mentioned previously, the substitution of foods that contain less fat and calories for foods that are high in fat and calories can significantly reduce caloric intake. For example, if a person eats a roasted chicken breast without the skin instead of a fried chicken breast with the skin, approximately 160 kcal will be saved. It is important to remember that the wise consumer looks closely at both the total calories in a food as well as the calories that are contributed by fat. Not only will reducing fat intake help with weight control, but it also will help improve the blood lipid profile.

One problem that people face when trying to manage weight is "diet burnout." It is not uncommon to find people on "diets" who consume only certain foods. To help avoid becoming bored and frustrated with one's diet, it is important to consume a variety of healthy, low-calorie, and tasty foods. This objective is linked to the planning process that was described previously. Maintaining variety in the diet not only helps avoid boredom but also provides nutritional balance.

When one is attempting to lose weight, one of the most helpful changes is to decrease the portion size as well as the number of portions consumed. Many people are in the habit of completely filling their plates and eating everything that is on the plate. Additionally, one of the ways that Americans demonstrate to their host or hostess that the food is being enjoyed is by eating extra portions. Taking smaller portions of foods as well as avoiding "seconds" will contribute significantly to caloric restriction.

Committing to Lifelong Maintenance

Weight loss is only a temporary condition unless a plan is in place to maintain the loss. In examining the variables that predict success in maintaining weight loss, Lavery and Loewy (16) concluded, "There are no quick-fix, easy solutions to obesity. The solution is the harsh realization of the need for permanent lifestyle changes to maintain a desired weight status." The HFI should help clients understand the need to commit to long-term lifestyle changes rather than focus solely on short-term weight loss goals. It is encouraging, however, to learn that longer term maintenance of weight loss is much more likely once people have been able to keep weight off for 2 to 5 years (31).

4 In Review

Some strategies leading to successful weight management are keeping records, planning meals and snacks, developing a support system, designing a reward system, committing to both outcome-oriented and behavioral goals, avoiding self-defeating behaviors, combining moderate caloric restriction with aerobic exercise, changing unhealthy eating patterns, and committing to lifelong weight maintenance.

Gimmicks and Gadgets for Weight Loss

Over the years numerous devices have been marketed for weight loss. The majority of these devices are ineffective, and, unfortunately, some are potentially harmful.

Saunas and sweatsuits have, at times, been recommended to help weight loss by burning off or melting away fat. This is a false claim. These devices may induce short-term (i.e., a number of hours) loss of weight by dehydration. These devices do not burn fat but can cause people to sweat profusely. Overuse of saunas and sweatsuits potentially can lead to severe dehydration. Furthermore, the increase in core temperature that is caused by these devices could be harmful to fetuses during the first trimester of pregnancy.

Other devices such as vibrating belts, body wraps, and electrical stimulators have been used in an attempt to lose weight. Although these devices may not be harmful, they do not lead to weight loss. The money spent on these useless devices would be better spent on proven techniques. Additionally, if one puts faith and effort into these unproven techniques, one may delay making lifestyle changes that could lead to long-term weight changes.

A widely held myth is that exercise emphasizing a particular body part will cause that area to lose fat quicker than the rest of the body. This false theory is called **spot reduction**. Curl-ups are commonly used exercises that people perform in an attempt to decrease their waistlines. Although curl-ups are terrific exercises for increasing the muscular strength and endurance of the abdominal muscles, they are not very effective for burning fat. As a person establishes a caloric deficit through regular aerobic exercise, fat loss will occur all over the body, not just the parts where he or she would like to see the decrease.

Programs that advertise rapid, large weight losses are typically deceptive. The rapid weight losses seen at the beginning of such a "diet" are primarily the result of reductions in water weight. It is also important to understand that dietary plans that establish extremely large caloric deficits will substantially reduce RMR and lean body mass and do not establish healthy, lifelong eating habits. As stated earlier, diets consisting of less than 800 kcal per day are not recommended (22). The following box provides useful information about these fad diets.

Focus on Fad Diets

Dietary plans that promise incredible results can be found easily on book shelves, in media ads, and on the Internet. Many people are looking for quick, easy ways to lose weight, and entrepreneurs are eager to supply them. No one description will summarize all fad diets. Many focus on eating one food or food group, whereas others emphasize avoiding certain foods. Most of these plans are low in calories and will result in weight loss (at least according to anecdotal evidence!). However, there are problems. The majority of these diets do not emphasize a balanced diet with an adequate supply of essential nutrients. Over time, these nutritional deficiencies can lead to serious health consequences. Because of the potential for negative health consequences of fad diets, the AHA has "declared war" on fad diets. Another problem with these diets is that they do not lead to lifestyle changes that result in permanent weight loss. Many people follow these diets for a short period of time and then regain their excess weight when they return to their previous pattern of overconsuming calories. These diets typically are focused on food rather than behavior change (increasing physical activity, using food substitution). For more information on making healthy diet choices, see the Web sites of the American Dietetic Association (3) and National Institute of Diabetes and Digestive and Kidney Diseases (23).

5 In Review

A number of "quick fixes" for weight loss are marketed, but these products are at best ineffective and at worst potentially dangerous.

Disordered Eating Patterns

There are conditions in which a person's eating pattern has a negative impact on his or her health. **Eating disorders** are clinically diagnosed conditions in which the unhealthy eating patterns may lead to severe declines in health and even to death. **Anorexia nervosa, bulimia nervosa,** and **binge eating disorder** are three of the eating disorders recognized by the American Psychiatric Association (APA) (4). **Disordered eating** refers to subclinical, unhealthy eating patterns that are often the precursors of eating disorders.

In America, anorexia nervosa and bulimia nervosa occur at a rate of 0.5 to 1% and 2 to 4%, respectively (15). No single mechanism has been identified as the primary cause of disordered eating or eating disorders. It appears that genetic/biological, psychological, and sociocultural factors may predispose one to these conditions. The groups in the American population in which these conditions are most common are young women from middle and high socioeconomic environments and female athletes in sports that emphasize extreme leanness. It is hypothesized that the social pressure to be thin as well as discomfort with sexual development contribute to unhealthy eating patterns in young women. For female athletes, unfortunately, the pressure to perform in some sports is linked with extremely low body weights. For example, it has been reported that more than 60% of female gymnasts exhibit some type of disordered eating pattern (15).

Anorexia nervosa is an eating disorder in which a preoccupation with body weight leads to self-starvation. People with anorexia nervosa typically view themselves as overweight even when their weight is substantially below normal. The APA lists the following criteria for diagnosis of anorexia nervosa (4):

- Purposefully maintaining weight at less than 85% of expected weight for age and height
- Extreme fear of gaining weight and/or fat
- Unhealthy body image in which the person views her- or himself as overweight even when underweight; often associated with a severe intertwining of body image and self-esteem and/or a disregard for the seriousness of maintaining an extremely low body weight
- Absence of at least three consecutive menstrual cycles in postmenarchal women

Bulimia nervosa is characterized by consuming large amounts of food followed by periods of food purging (4). Misuse of laxatives, self-induced vomiting, and excessive exercise are among the methods that may be used to purge. To meet the diagnostic criteria established by the APA, one must engage in this behavior at least two times a week for a period of 3 months. Patients with bulimia nervosa, similar to those suffering from anorexia nervosa, have an impaired body image and a fear of losing control over their body weight. Both anorexia nervosa and bulimia nervosa should be considered life-threatening disorders.

Binge eating disorder is characterized by consuming large amounts of food in short periods of time (4). Unlike bulimia nervosa, binge eating is not associated with purging. Binge episodes are often initiated by emotional/psychological cues (e.g., loneliness, anxiety) rather than by physical hunger. These binges typically occur when the person is alone and may be followed by feelings of shame, guilt, and depression. To achieve a clinical diagnosis of binge eating disorder, a person must engage in at least two periods of bingeing per week for 6 months (4). The prevalence of binge eating disorder in the general population has been estimated at 2%. In contrast, 25 to 70% of obese individuals seeking treatment for weight loss may suffer from this disorder (27).

Recognition of the signs of disordered eating is necessary for successful intervention. The box on page 201 lists some of the common signs of disordered eating. If the HFI notices these signs, the issue should be discussed in a nonconfrontational manner. However, many people when approached about this issue will deny the existence of a problem. Asking gentle questions about the client's health (e.g., "How are you feeling?" or "You look a little tired") is one way to attempt to break the ice on this very delicate subject. Successful intervention for eating disorders requires a multidisciplinary approach combining medical, nutritional, and psychological professionals. A knowledge of local support groups or professionals who work with patients who have eating disorders will allow the HFI to recommend places for clients to receive help.

6 In Review

Eating disorders can significantly impair health and may even result in death. Anorexia nervosa, bulimia nervosa, and binge eating disorder are three eating disorders recognized by the APA. Intervention for eating disorders should be multidisciplinary and should include psychological counseling.

Strategies for Gaining Weight

Before concluding this chapter it is important to mention that some individuals struggle to increase their body weight. The HFI should encourage these individuals to attempt to accumulate fat-free mass rather than all-fat weight. This will necessitate adding resistance training to one's exercise routine. Various nutritional supplements are touted as "guaranteed" ways to increase muscle mass. However, as mentioned in chapter 7, even those who are training intensely need only about 1.5 g of protein per kilogram of body weight. Supplements such as creatine phosphate may contribute somewhat to weight gain, but much of the change will be attributable to greater water retention in the muscle.

Signs of Disordered Eating

A preoccupation with food, calories, and weight
Repeatedly expressed concerns about being or feeling fat, even when weight is average or below average
Increasing self-criticism of one's body
Secretly eating or stealing food
Eating large meals, then disappearing or making trips to the bathroom
Consumption of large amounts of food not consistent with the individual's weight
Bloodshot eyes, especially after trips to the bathroom
Swollen parotid glands at the angle of the jaw, giving a chipmunk-like appearance
Vomitus, or odor of vomitus in the bathroom
Wide fluctuations in weight over short periods of time
Periods of severe caloric restriction
Excessive laxative use
Compulsive, excessive exercise that is not part of the individual's training regimen
Unwillingness to eat in front of others
Expression of self-deprecating thoughts after eating
Wearing baggy or layered clothing
Mood swings
Appearing preoccupied with the eating behavior of others
Continuous drinking of diet soda or water

Adapted from Johnson (14).

The following box provides some tips for increasing weight over time. When individuals continually lose weight or struggle to gain weight, a physician should be consulted about the possibility of underlying conditions.

7 In Review

The additional calories needed to increase weight should come from increasing the number of healthy snacks and/or the size of meals. The addition of resistance training to one's exercise routine may help increasing muscle mass.

Tips for Gaining Weight

Increase caloric intake by 200 to 1000 kcal per day. This can be done by increasing meal size, number of meals, or number of between-meal snacks.
Increase the number of healthy snacks consumed. Choose bread, fruit, granola, and other nutritious foods.
The majority of additional calories consumed should be complex carbohydrates (e.g., pasta, bread, rice, potatoes).
Add resistance training to the daily routine. Weight training is an effective means for increasing the body's fat-free mass.
When training intensely, ensure that 1.5 g of protein for each kilogram of body weight is consumed daily.
Increase consumption of milk and fruit juices. These excellent choices not only provide additional calories but also provide essential nutrients.

Case Study

You can check your answers by referring to appendix A.

11.1

A 52-year old female comes to your facility for an initial evaluation. She complains that she has gained 15 pounds in the last 3 years, and she wants to lose that extra weight. She is 5′5″ and weighs 160 pounds. She is currently a non-exerciser and has a sedentary job. Calculate her estimated Resting Metabolic Rate and Daily Caloric Need.

Source List

1. American College of Sports Medicine. (2000). *ACSM's guidelines for exercise testing and prescription* (6th ed.). Philadelphia: Lippincott Williams & Wilkins.
2. American College of Sports Medicine. (2001). Appropriate intervention strategies for weight loss and prevention of weight regain for adults. *Medicine and Science in Sports and Exercise, 33*(12), 2145-2156.
3. American Dietetic Association. Daily Nutrition Tips. [Online] Available: www.eatright.org/ermprev.html [July 10, 2002].
4. American Psychiatric Association. (1994). *Diagnostic and statistical manual of mental disorders*. Washington, DC: American Psychiatric Press.
5. Bouchard, C., Perusse, L., Leblanc, C., Tremblay, A., & Theriault, G. (1988). Inheritance of the amount and distribution of human body fat. *International Journal of Obesity, 12*, 205-215.
6. Cottrell, R.R. (1992). *Weight control*. Guilford, CT: Dushkin.
7. Cunningham, J.J. (1991). Body composition as a determinant of energy expenditure: A synthetic review and a proposed general prediction equation. *American Journal of Clinical Nutrition, 54*, 963-969.
8. DiPietro, L. (1999). Physical activity in the prevention of obesity: Current evidence and research issues. *Medicine and Science in Sports and Exercise, 31*(11, Suppl.), S542-S546.
9. Flegal, K.M. (1999). The obesity epidemic in children and adults: Current evidence and research issues. *Medicine and Science in Sports and Exercise, 31*(11, Suppl.), S509-S514.
10. Grundy, S.M., Blackburn, G., Higgins, M., Lauer, R., Perri, M.G., & Ryan, D. (1999). Physical activity in the prevention and treatment of obesity and its comorbidities: Roundtable consensus statement. *Medicine and Science in Sports and Exercise, 31*(11, Suppl.), S502-S508.
11. Hill, J.O., & Melanson, E.L. (1999). Overview of the determinants of overweight and obesity: Current evidence and research issues. *Medicine and Science in Sports and Exercise, 31*(11, Suppl.), S515-S521.
12. Holden, J.H., Darga, L.L., Olson, S.M., Stettner, D.C., Ardito, E.A., & Lucas, C.P. (1992). Long-term follow-up of patients attending a combination very-low calorie diet and behaviour therapy weight loss programme. *International Journal of Obesity, 16*, 605-613.
13. Israel, D. (2001). Nutrition. In J.L. Roitman (Ed.), *ACSM's resource manual for guidelines for exercise testing and prescription* (4th ed., pp. 401-407). Philadelphia: Lippincott Williams & Wilkins.
14. Jebb, S.A., & Moore, M.S. (1999). Contribution of a sedentary lifestyle and inactivity to the etiology of overweight and obesity: Current evidence and research issues. *Medicine and Science in Sports and Exercise, 31*(11, Suppl.), S534-S541.
15. Johnson, M.D. (1994). Disordered eating. In R. Agostini (Ed.), *Medical and orthopedic issues of active and athletic women* (pp. 141-151). Philadelphia: Hanley & Belfus.
16. Lavery, M.A., & Loewy, J.W. (1993). Identifying predictive variables for long-term weight change after participation in a weight loss program. *Journal of the American Dietetic Association, 93*, 1017-1024.
17. Lichtman, S.W., Pisarska, K., Berman, E.R., Pestone, M., Dowling, H., Offenbacher, E., Weisel, H., Heshka, S., Matthews, D.E., & Heymsfield, S.B. (1992). Discrepancy between self-reported and actual caloric intake and exercise in obese subjects. *New England Journal of Medicine, 327*, 1893-1898.
18. Mokdad, A.H., Serdula, M.K., Dietz, W.H., Bowman, B.A., Marks, J.S., & Koplan, J.P. (1999). The spread of the obesity epidemic in the United States, 1991-1998. *Journal of the American Medical Association, 282*(16), 1519-1522.
19. Molé, P.A. (1990). Impact of energy intake and exercise on resting metabolic rate. *Sports Medicine, 10*, 72-87.
20. Montoye, H.J., Kemper, H.C.G., Saris, W.H.M., & Washburn, R.A. (1996). *Measuring physical activity and energy expenditure*. Champaign: Human Kinetics.
21. Must, A., Spandano, J., Coakley, E.H., Field, A.E., Colditz, G., & Dietz, W.H. (1999). The disease burden associated with overweight and obesity. *Journal of the American Medical Association, 282*(16), 1523-1529.
22. National Heart, Lung, and Blood Institute. (1998). *Clinical guidelines on the identification, evaluation, and treatment of overweight and obesity in adults* (NIH Publication No. 98-4083). Bethesda, MD: National Institutes of Health—National Heart, Lung, and Blood Institute.
23. National Institute of Diabetes and Digestive and Kidney Diseases. Weight loss and control. [Online]. Available: www.niddk.nih.gov/health/nutrit/nutrit.htm [July 10, 2002]
24. Prentice, A.M., & Jebb, S.A. (2000). Physical activity level and weight control in adults. In C. Bouchard (Ed.), *Physical activity and obesity* (pp. 247-261). Champaign, IL: Human Kinetics.
25. Salbe, A.D., & Ravussin, E. (2000). The determinants of obesity. In C. Bouchard (Ed.), *Physical activity and obesity* (pp. 69-102). Champaign, IL: Human Kinetics.
26. Stunkard, A.J., Sørensen, T.I.A., Hanis, C., Teasdale, T.W., Chakraborty, R., Schull, W.J., & Schulsinger, F. (1986). An adoption study of human obesity. *New England Journal of Medicine, 314*, 193-198.
27. Wadden, T.A., & Stunkard, A.J. (1993). Psychosocial consequences of obesity and dieting: Research and clinical findings. In A.J. Stunkard & T.A. Wadden (Eds.), *Obesity: Theory and therapy* (pp. 163-177). New York: Raven Press.
28. Welle, S., Forbes, G.B., Statt, M., Barnard, R.R., & Amatruda, J.M. (1992). Energy expenditure under free-living conditions in normal-weight and overweight women. *American Journal of Clinical Nutrition, 55*, 14-21.
29. Westerterp, K.R. (2000). The assessment of energy and nutrient intake in humans. In C. Bouchard (Ed.), *Physical activity and obesity* (pp. 133-149). Champaign, IL: Human Kinetics.
30. Williamson, D.F., Madans, J., Anda, R.F., Kleinman, J.C., Kahn, H.S., & Byers, T. (1993). Recreational physical activity and ten-year weight change in a US national cohort. *International Journal of Obesity, 17*, 279-286.
31. Wing, R.R., & Hill, J.O. (2001). Successful weight loss maintenance. *Annual Review of Nutrition, 21*, 323-341.

twelve

Exercise Prescription for Muscular Strength and Endurance Training

Avery D. Faigenbaum and Kyle J. McInnis

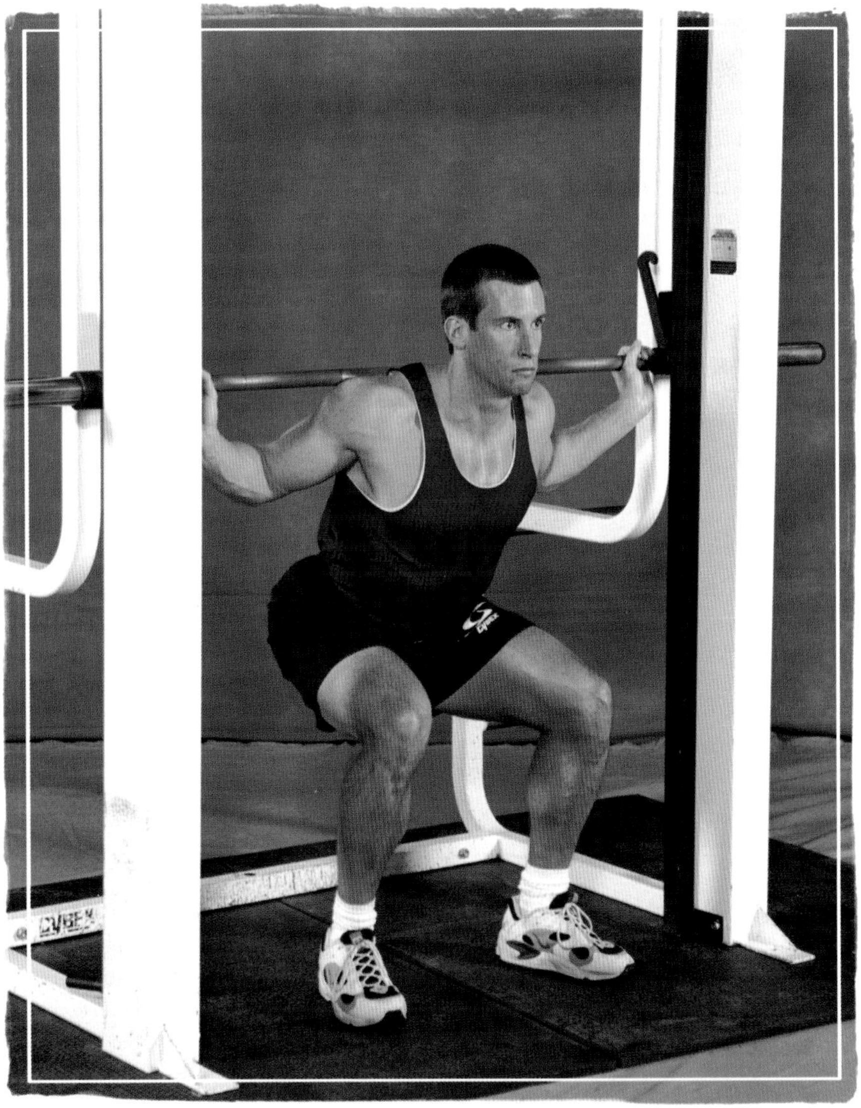

Objectives

The reader will be able to do the following:

1. Explain the physiological principles of overload, specificity, and progressive resistance and understand how they relate to exercise programming.
2. Describe the following methods of strength training: isometrics, dynamic constant external resistance training, variable resistance training, isokinetics, and plyometrics.
3. Describe the different modes of strength training.
4. Discuss the health and fitness benefits of strength training and understand precautions to enhance participant safety.
5. Describe the acute program variables that are used to design strength training programs and discuss the relationship between the number of repetitions, training intensity, number of sets, and rest period between sets.
6. Understand the concept of periodization and its application to the design of exercise programs, and differentiate between overreaching and overtraining.
7. Describe the following systems of strength training: single set, multiple set, circuit training, pre-exhaustion, and assisted training systems.
8. Discuss the safety, benefits, and recommendations of strength training for youth, seniors, pregnant women, and adults with CHD.
9. Identify safe and effective exercises designed to enhance the muscular fitness of specific muscle groups.

For many years, **strength training** was used primarily by adult athletes to enhance sports performance and increase muscle size. However, over the past decade, strength training has become recognized as an important method of enhancing the health and fitness of males and females of all ages and abilities. Like aerobic training, moderate-intensity strength training provides a wide variety of health and fitness benefits (see table 12.1). Today, strength training is performed by children, older adults, women in advanced stages of pregnancy, and patients with chronic disease conditions. For the HFI, the ability to design safe and effective strength training programs for individuals with a range of ages, fitness levels, and health conditions is a valuable professional asset. This chapter focuses on strength training guidelines and principles that can be used to develop general exercise programs for enhancing muscular fitness. Recommendations for developing speed, strength, and power for elite athletes are available elsewhere (9, 15, 54).

In this chapter, the term *strength training* (also known as resistance training) refers to a method of conditioning designed to increase one's ability to exert or resist force. This term encompasses a wide range of resistive loads (from light manual resistance to plyometric jumps) and a variety of training modalities including free weights (barbells and dumbbells), weight machines, elastic tubing, medicine balls, stability balls, and body weight. Strength training should be distinguished from the competitive sports of **weightlifting**, **powerlifting**, and **bodybuilding**. The term *local muscular endurance* refers to the ability of a muscle or muscle group to perform repeated contractions against a submaximal resistance. *Power* refers to the rate of performing work and is the product of strength and speed of movement. For ease of discussion, the terms *children* and *youth* are broadly defined in this chapter to include the preadolescent and adolescent years, and the terms *older* and *senior* have been arbitrarily defined to include individuals over 65 years of age.

Table 12.1 Comparison of Effects of Aerobic Endurance Training With Strength Training on Health and Fitness Variables

Variable	Aerobic Exercise	Resistance Exercise
Bone mineral density	↑↑	↑↑
Body composition		
% Fat	↓↓	↓
LBM	↔	↑↑
Strength	↔	↑↑↑
Glucose metabolism		
Insulin response to glucose challenge	↓↓	↓↓
Basal insulin levels	↓	↓
Insulin sensitivity	↑↑	↑↑
Serum lipids		
HDL	↑↔	↑↑↔
LDL	↓↔	↓↔
Resting HR	↓↓	↔
Stroke volume, resting and maximal	↑↑	↔
BP at rest		
Systolic	↓↔	↔
Diastolic	↓↔	↓↔
$\dot{V}O_2$max	↑↑↑	↑↑↔
Submaximal and maximal endurance time	↑↑↑	↑↑
Basal metabolism	↑	↑↑

Note. ↑ = values increase; ↓ = values decrease; ↔ = values remain unchanged; single arrow = small effect; double arrows = medium effect; triple arrows = large effect; LBM = lean body mass; HDL = high-density lipoprotein cholesterol; LDL = low-density lipoprotein cholesterol; HR = heart rate; BP = blood pressure.

From Pollock et al. (2000).

Fundamental Principles

Muscular performance will improve only if the conditioning program is based on sound training principles. Although factors such as initial level of fitness, heredity, nutritional status (e.g., diet composition and hydration), health habits (e.g., sleep), and motivation will influence the rate and magnitude of adaptation that occurs, three fundamental principles that determine the effectiveness of all strength training programs are the principles of overload, progressive resistance, and specificity.

Overload Principle

For more than a century, the overload principle has been a basic tenet of strength training. The overload principle states that to enhance muscular performance, the body must exercise at a level beyond that at which it is normally stressed. For example, an adult male who can easily complete 10 **repetitions** with 20 lb while performing a barbell curl exercise must increase the weight, the repetitions, or the number of **sets** if he wants to increase his arm strength. Otherwise, if the training stimulus is not increased beyond the level to which the muscles are accustomed, training adaptations will not occur. Overload is typically manipulated by changing the exercise intensity, duration, or frequency.

Principle of Progressive Resistance

The principle of progressive resistance refers to continually and progressively placing demands on the body that are greater than that to which it is normally accustomed. As a muscle becomes stronger, it will adapt to the stress that is placed on it. To make long-term gains in muscular fitness, the training stimulus must be increased consistently at a rate that is compatible with the training-induced adaptations that are occurring. A reasonable guideline is to increase the training weight about 5% and decrease the repetitions by 2 to 4 when a given load can be performed for the desired number of repetitions with proper exercise technique. For example, if an adult female can easily perform 12 repetitions of the chest press exercise using 100 lb, she should increase the weight to 105 lb, decreasing the repetitions to 8, if she wants to continually make gains in muscle strength. Alternatively, she could increase the number of sets, increase the number of repetitions, or add another chest exercise to her exercise routine. Although every training session does not have to be more intense than the last session, the principle of progressive resistance states that the training stimulus needs to be increased continually if additional gains are desired. Once the desired level is achieved, gains in muscular fitness can be maintained with a modified training program provided that the individual continues to lift the same amount of weight.

Principle of Specificity

The principle of specificity refers to the distinct adaptations that take place as a result of the training program. This principle is often referred to as the SAID principle (which stands for specific adaptations to imposed demands). In essence, every muscle or muscle group must be trained to make gains in strength and/or local muscular endurance. Exercises such as the squat and leg press can be used to enhance lower body strength, but these exercises will not affect upper body strength. Furthermore, the adaptations that take place in a muscle or muscle group will be as simple or as complex as the stress placed on them. For example, because basketball requires multiple-joint and multiplanar movements (e.g., frontal, sagittal, and transverse planes), it seems prudent for basketball players to perform complex exercises that closely mimic the movements of their sport. The specificity principle also can be applied to the design of strength training programs for individuals who want to enhance their abilities to perform activities of daily life such as stair climbing and house cleaning that also require multiple-joint and multiplanar movements.

1 In Review

Gains in muscular strength and local muscular endurance will occur only if the overload placed on a muscle or muscle group is greater than that to which it is normally accustomed. To make continual gains, the athlete must increase the overload by varying the intensity, duration, and/or frequency of training. The design of the strength training program will influence the specific training-induced adaptations that occur. A sport-specific or activity-specific strength training program should include exercises that meet specific training objectives.

Program Design Consideration

Similar to exercise programs that enhance cardiorespiratory fitness, strength training programs should be based on the participant's interests, current fitness level, health needs, clinical status, and individual goals as well as the fundamental principles of strength training. By assessing the needs of each participant and applying basic training principles to the program design, safe and effective strength training programs can be developed for each individual. However, because the magnitude of adaptation to a given exercise stimulus will vary among individuals, it is prudent to be aware of interindividual differences and be prepared to alter the program to reduce the risk of injury and optimize gains.

Health Status

The health status of each participant should be assessed before participating in a strength training program. As discussed in chapter 3, a health and medical questionnaire such as the PAR-Q should be completed by each participant and reviewed to make decisions about further medical evaluation. Additional questions on the preparticipation health screening questionnaire regarding past strength training experiences, previous musculoskeletal injuries, and personal interests can also aid in the design of the strength training program.

Fitness Level

An important factor to consider when designing strength training programs is the participant's current fitness status or previous experience strength training. This is sometimes referred to as one's training age. Those who are the least experienced in strength training tend to have a greater capacity for improvement compared with experienced lifters. Although any reasonable strength training program can be used to increase the strength of untrained individuals, more intense and higher volume programs are often needed to produce desirable adaptations in strength-trained athletes. For example, a 22-year-old football player with 5 years of strength training experience (i.e., a training age of 5 years) may not achieve the same strength gains in a given period of time as a 35-year-old client who has no experience strength training (i.e., a training age of zero). This is based on the observation that the potential for adaptation gradually decreases as training age increases.

Training Goals

After the pre-exercise screening, it is important to establish realistic short- and long-term goals. The results of a muscular fitness evaluation (see chapter 8) along with the participant's interests can be used to help set realistic and measurable goals. To improve compliance, these goals ideally are set by the individual with guidance from a knowledgeable fitness professional. Typical goals are to increase muscle strength and decrease body fat. An effort to establish realistic goals and increase confidence to achieve those goals is important because it may help to avoid unrealistic expectations that ultimately can lead to discouragement and poor adherence. Periodic fitness testing and reviewing individualized workout logs can help the HFI assess training progress and modify the training program. Last, understanding that training programs designed to improve health and fitness are quite different from training programs designed to enhance sports performance will further promote the development of and adherence to programs ideally suited to the individual's needs.

Types of Strength Training

Different types of strength training can be used to enhance muscular strength and local muscular endurance. Although each method has advantages and disadvantages, there are several important factors to consider when selecting one type of training over another or including multiple types within a given training program. The most common types of strength training include isometrics, dynamic constant external resistance training, variable resistance training, isokinetics, and plyometrics.

Isometrics

Isometric training or static strength training refers to a type of muscle action in which muscle length does not change. This type of training is usually performed against an immovable object such as a wall or a weight machine loaded with a heavy weight. The concept of isometric training was popularized in the 1950s when Hettinger and Muller reported remarkable gains in muscle strength resulting from one daily 6-s isometric contraction at two-thirds of maximal force (38). Although subsequent studies also reported gains in strength resulting from isometric training, the reported gains were substantially less than those reported earlier (30).

An advantage of isometric training is that specialized equipment is not required and the cost is minimal. Increases in strength and muscle **hypertrophy** can occur from this type of training. However, a major limitation of isometric training is that the strength gains that occur are specific to the joint angle at which the training occurred. For example, if isometric training of the elbow flexors is performed at a joint angle of 90°, muscle strength will be increased at this joint angle but not necessarily at other angles. Even though there seems to be about 20° of carryover on either side of the joint angle, to increase strength throughout the full ROM the same isometric exercise must be performed at varying joint angles. Isometric training may help to maintain muscle strength and prevent muscle **atrophy** when a limb is immobilized in a cast, but gains in functional strength (e.g., stair climbing) and motor performance ability (e.g., sprinting and jumping) as a result of isometric training are unlikely to occur if isometric training takes place only at one joint angle.

Factors such as the number of repetitions performed, duration of the contractions, intensity of the contraction, and frequency of training can influence the strength gains resulting from isometric training. In general, isometric training characterized by maximal voluntary muscle actions performed for 3 to 5 s for 15 to 20 repetitions at least 3 times per week tends to optimize strength gains (29). Because of the nature of isometric training, it is particularly important for individuals who train isometrically to avoid the "breath-holding" Valsalva maneuver, which reduces venous return to the heart and increases SBP and DBP. During all types of strength training, regular breathing patterns (i.e., exhale while lifting and inhale while lowering) should be encouraged.

Dynamic Constant External Resistance (DCER) Training

Strength training that involves a lifting and lowering phase is called dynamic. Exercises using free weights (e.g., barbells and dumbbells) and weight machines are dynamic because the weight is lifted and lowered through a predetermined ROM. Although the term *isotonic* traditionally was used to describe this type of training, this term literally means constant (*iso*) tension (*tonic*). Because tension exerted by a muscle as it shortens varies with the mechanical advantage of the joint and the length of the muscle fibers at a particular joint angle, the term isotonic does not accurately describe this method of training. As shown in figure 12.1, when a barbell curl is performed, the elbow flexors are strongest at

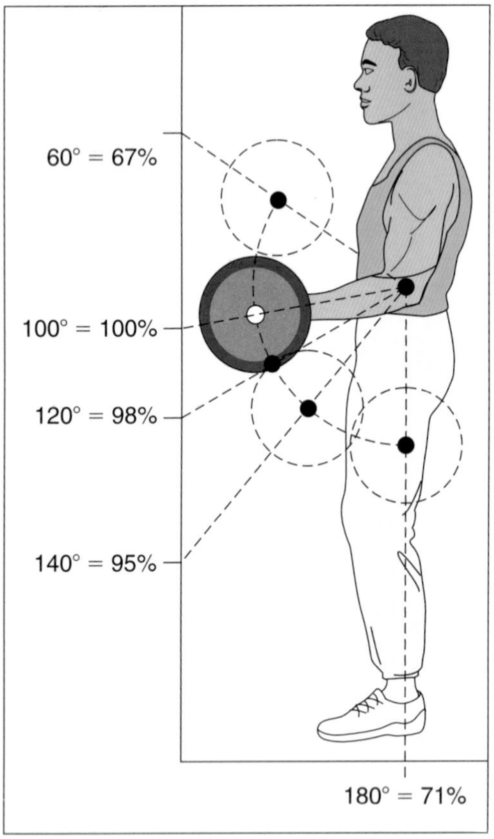

Figure 12.1 Variation in strength relative to the angle of the elbow flexors during the biceps curl.
Reprinted from Wilmore and Costill 1994.

approximately 100° and weakest at 60° (elbows fully flexed) and at 180° (elbows fully extended). The same principle applies to other muscle groups. DCER better describes a type of strength training in which the weight lifted does not change during the lifting (**concentric**) and lowering (**eccentric**) phase of an exercise.

DCER training is the most common method of strength training for enhancing health and fitness. Endless combinations of sets and repetitions and different types of training equipment can be used for DCER training. Although there is not enough scientific evidence to make any specific recommendations regarding the most effective speed for DCER training (e.g., 4 s or 14 s per repetition), proper form and technique should be used on all exercises. Weight machines generally limit the user to fixed planes of motion. However, they are easy to use and are ideal for isolating muscle groups. Free weights are less expensive and can be used for a wide variety of different exercises that require greater proprioception, balance, and coordination. Several free weight exercises (e.g., barbell squat and bench press) require the use of a spotter who can assist the lifter in case of a failed repetition. In addition to improving health and fitness, DCER training is also used to enhance motor performance skills and sports performance.

Research Insight

Individuals beginning a strength training program often focus on the concentric phase of the exercise and underestimate the value of the eccentric phase. Hawkins et al. (37) studied the effects of concentric and eccentric strength training on the bone mineral density of adult females (ages 20-23) and concluded that eccentric muscle action increases the site-specific osteogenic response. Subjects trained one leg concentrically and one leg eccentrically three times a week for 18 weeks. The strength training protocol for each leg consisted of three sets of three or four maximal repetitions on an isokinetic training machine. Although both legs increased muscle strength, only the eccentrically trained leg significantly increased lean body mass and bone mineral density. These findings are particularly important for adults who want to prevent or offset age-related declines in musculoskeletal health.

During DCER training, the weight lifted does not change throughout the ROM. Because muscle tension can vary significantly when a DCER exercise is performed, the heaviest weight that can be lifted throughout a full ROM is limited by the strength of a muscle at the weakest joint angle. As a result, DCER exercise provides enough resistance in some parts of the movement range but not enough resistance in others. For example, during the barbell bench press exercise, more weight can be lifted during the last part of the exercise than in the first part of the movement when the barbell is being pressed off the chest. This is a limitation of DCER training that should be recognized when choosing starting weights for beginners.

In an attempt to overcome this limitation, mechanical devices that operate through a lever arm or cam have been designed to vary the resistance throughout the exercise's ROM (see figure 12.2). These devices, called variable resistance machines, theoretically force the muscle to contract maximally throughout the ROM by varying the resistance to match the exercise strength curve. These machines can be used to train all the major muscle groups, and

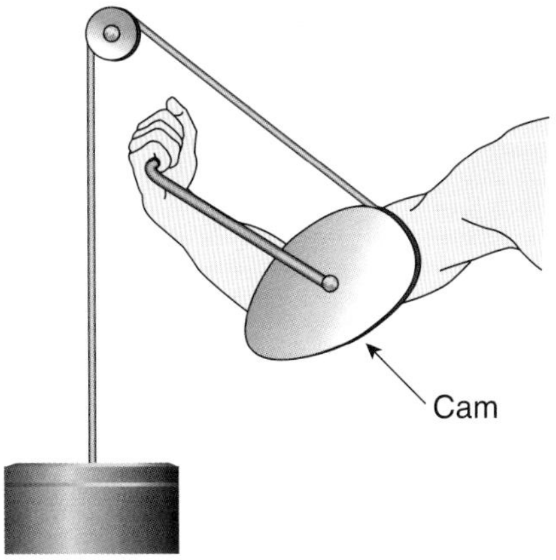

Figure 12.2 A variable resistance device for the biceps muscle in which a cam alters the resistance throughout the ROM.

Modified from Wathen and Roll 1994.

by automatically changing the resistive force throughout the movement range, they provide proportionally less resistance in weaker segments of the movement and more resistance in stronger segments of the movement. Like all weight machines, variable resistance machines provide a specific movement path, which makes the exercise easier to perform compared with free weight exercises, which require balance, coordination, and the involvement of stabilizing muscle groups. These features make variable resistance machines a popular mode of strength training for people who desire safe and simple exercise sessions.

Isokinetics

The term *isokinetics* refers to a muscular action performed at a constant angular limb velocity. Isokinetic training involves specialized and expensive equipment, and most isokinetic devices are designed to train only single-joint movements. Isokinetic machines generally are not used in fitness centers, but this type of training is used by physical therapists and athletic trainers for injury rehabilitation. Unlike other types of strength training, in isokinetics the speed of movement—rather than the resistance—is controlled. During isokinetic training, any force applied to the isokinetic machine is met with an equal reaction force. Although it is theoretically possible for a muscle to contract maximally through an exercise's full ROM, this seems unlikely during isokinetic training because of the acceleration at the beginning and deceleration at the end of the ROM.

Isokinetic training studies have generally found that strength increases are specific to the training velocity (12). Isokinetic training at a slow movement velocity (e.g., 60-180°/s) will increase strength at that velocity, but strength gains at faster velocities are unlikely to occur. If the purpose of the training program is to increase strength at higher velocities (e.g., for enhanced sports performance), performing high-speed isokinetic training appears prudent. Although further research is warranted, the best approach may be to perform isokinetic training at slow, intermediate, and fast velocities to develop increased strength and power at different movement speeds.

Plyometrics

Plyometric training was first known simply as "jump training" and refers to a specialized method of conditioning designed to enable a muscle to reach maximal force in the shortest possible time. This type of exercise is characterized by quick, powerful movements involving a prestretch and the stretch-shortening cycle (15). Exercises that involve jumping, skipping, hopping, and throwing movements performed explosively can be considered plyometrics. Although plyometric exercises often are associated with high-intensity drills such as depth jumps (i.e., jumping from a box to the ground and then immediately jumping upward), common activities such as jumping jacks and hopscotch also can be considered a type of plyometric exercise, because every time the feet hit the ground, the quadriceps go through a stretch-shortening cycle. Both mechanical factors (i.e., increased stored elastic energy) and neurophysiological factors (i.e., change in the muscle's force velocity characteristics) contribute to the increased force production resulting from plyometric training (56).

Since the 1970s, plyometric exercises have been performed by elite athletes in many sports such as volleyball and track and field. More recently, this type of training has become popular in group exercise classes and fitness programs. Plyometric training typically involves different types of jumps and hops for the lower extremities and medicine ball exercises for the upper extremities. Plyometric exercises can be grouped as low intensity (e.g., squat jump), moderate intensity (pike jump), or high intensity (single-leg hop). To date, few controlled studies have investigated the effects of different plyometric training programs on the development of strength and speed.

Plyometric exercises place a great amount of stress on the involved muscles, connective tissues, and joints and thereby increase the risk of musculoskeletal injury. As such, the risk of performing plyometric training may outweigh any benefits for untrained individuals enrolled in fitness programs. Because plyometric exercises are not required to enhance health and fitness, the appropriateness of plyometric training for each individual should be assessed before initiating this type of conditioning. It seems prudent to restrict plyometric training to individuals who have developed a solid foundation of muscle strength by first participating in a basic strength training program or simply to begin plyometric training with lower intensity drills and gradually progress to higher intensity drills over time.

Other considerations for plyometric training include proper footwear, adequate space, and a shock-absorbing landing surface (e.g., wrestling mat, suspended floor, or grass playing field). Research has yet to determine the minimal training threshold for plyometric exercise that is necessary to achieve the desired outcomes of improved strength and power. However, it seems reasonable for strength-trained adults to begin low-intensity plyometric training with 1 to 3 sets of 6 to 10 repetitions on one upper body and one lower body exercise performed twice per week on nonconsecutive days. Because of the apparent higher risk of injury in untrained individuals, it is recommended that all exercise sessions be supervised by qualified fitness professionals with experience in plyometric training. Additional training guidelines and examples of plyometric drills are available elsewhere (15).

2 In Review

Different types of strength training can be used to increase muscle strength, local muscular endurance, and power. The effects of isometric training are generally limited to the joint angle at which the training occurs. Dynamic constant external resistance training refers to exercises performed throughout a ROM with free weights and weight machines. Isokinetic training occurs at a constant limb velocity with maximal force exerted throughout the joint's ROM. Plyometric training enables a muscle to reach maximal strength as quickly as possible.

Modes of Strength Training

Different modes of strength training can be used to accommodate the needs of youth, adults, and seniors. Provided that the fundamental principles of training are adhered to, almost any mode of strength training can be used to enhance muscular fitness. Some types of equipment are relatively easy to use and others require balance, coordination, and high levels of skill. A decision to use a certain type of mode of strength training should be based on each client's needs, goals, and abilities. The major modes of strength training are weight machines, free weights (barbells and dumbbells), body weight exercises, and a broadly defined category of balls, bands, and elastic tubing. Table 12.2 summarizes the advantages and disadvantages of different modes of strength training.

Weight machines are designed to train all the major muscle groups and can be found in most fitness centers. Both single-joint (e.g., leg extension) and multiple-joint (e.g., leg press) exercises can be performed on weight machines, which are relatively easy to use because the exercise motion is controlled by the machine and typically occurs in only one anatomical plane. This may be particularly important to consider when designing strength training programs for sedentary or inexperienced individuals. Also, several weight machines exercises such as the lat pull-down and leg curl are difficult to mimic with free weights. Weight machine are designed to fit the average male or female, although smaller individuals may not be able to properly position themselves on the equipment. A seat pad or back pad can be used to adjust body position to allow for a better fit. Some companies now manufacture weight training machines specifically designed for children. These machines are smaller versions of adult-sized machines and have weight increments that are appropriate for younger populations.

Free weights are also popular in fitness centers and come in a variety of shapes and sizes. Although it may take longer to master proper exercise technique when using free weights compared with weight machines, there are several advantages of free weight training. For example, proper fit is not an issue with adjustable barbells and dumbbells because "one size fits all." Free weights also offer a greater variety of exercises than weight machines because they can be moved in many different directions. Another important benefit of using free weights is that they require the use of additional stabilizing and assisting muscles to hold the correct body position during an exercise. As such, free weight training can occur in different planes. This is particularly true with dumbbells, because they train each side of the body independently.

Table 12.2 Comparison of Different Modes of Strength Training

	Weight machines	Free weights	Body weight	Ball and cords[a]
Cost	High	Low	None	Very low
Portability	Limited	Variable	Excellent	Excellent
Ease of use	Excellent	Variable	Variable	Variable
Muscle isolation	Excellent	Variable	Variable	Variable
Functionality	Limited	Excellent	Excellent	Excellent
Exercise variety	Limited	Excellent	Excellent	Excellent
Space requirements	High	Variable	Low	Low

[a]Medicine balls, stability balls, and elastic cords.

In general, free weights allow the participant to train "functionally" by encouraging different muscle groups to work together. However, unlike weight machines, several free weight exercises require the aid of a spotter who can assist the lifter in case of a failed repetition. The use of a spotter is particularly important on the bench press exercise. Tragically, there have been at least six documented deaths associated with weight training equipment, and at least half involved the home bench press or other supine free weight exercises (46). Accidents such as these underscore the importance of close supervision and an appropriate progression of training loads when training with free weights.

Body weight exercises such as push-ups, pull-ups, and curl-ups are some of the oldest modes of strength training. Obviously, a major advantage of body weight training is that equipment is not needed and a variety of exercises can be performed. Conversely, a limitation of body weight training is the difficulty in adjusting the body weight to the individual's strength level. Sedentary or overweight participants may not be strong enough to perform even one repetition of a push-up or pull-up. In such cases, prescribing body weight exercises not only may be ineffective but may have a negative effect on program compliance. Exercise machines that allow individuals to perform body weight exercises such as pull-ups and dips by using a predetermined percentage of their body weight are available. These machines provide an opportunity for participants of all abilities to incorporate body weight exercises into their strength training program and feel good about their accomplishments.

Stability balls, medicine balls, and elastic tubing are safe and effective alternatives to weight machines and free weights. Medicine balls were popular in the 1950s, and stability balls and elastic tubing have been used by therapists for many years. Now fitness professionals are using balls and bands for strength training and conditioning. Not only are stability balls, medicine balls, and elastic tubing relatively inexpensive, but they can be used to enhance strength, local muscular endurance, and power. In addition, exercises performed with balls and tubing can be proprioceptively challenging, which carries added benefit.

Stability balls are lightweight, inflatable balls (about 45 to 75 cm in diameter) that add the elements of balance and coordination to any exercise while targeting selected muscle groups. Although many exercises can be performed with a stability ball, these balls are used most often to develop core (i.e., abdominal and lower back) strength and improve posture. In terms of positioning, when sitting on a stability ball, the participant's feet should be at a 90º angle; the firmer the ball, the more difficult the exercise will be. Figure 12.3 illustrates the performance of an abdominal curl exercise on a stability ball.

Medicine balls come in different shapes and sizes (about 1 kg to more than 10 kg) and are a safe and effective alternative to free weights and weight machines. In addition to squatting or chest pressing with a medicine ball, participants can use these balls in throwing drills—such as throwing from participant to instructor or against the wall—to enhance upper body explosive power. Fast-speed medicine ball training can add a new dimension to a strength training workout that can be particularly beneficial for athletes.

Strength training with an elastic rubber cord involves performing an exercise against the force required to stretch the cord and then returning it to its unstretched state. A variety of exercises can be performed by holding the ends of the cord with both hands or attaching one end of the cord to a fixed object. Incorporating exercises with stability balls, medicine balls, and elastic tubing into a workout session can be challenging, motivating, and beneficial.

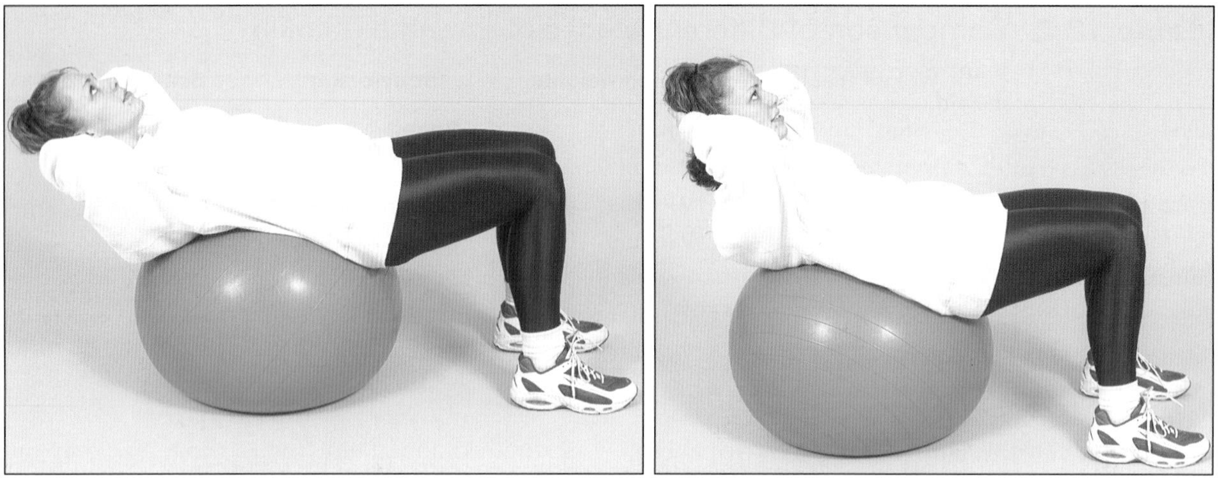

Figure 12.3 An individual performing an abdominal curl on a stability ball.

3 **In Review**

Weight machines, free weights, body weight exercises, medicine balls, stability balls, and elastic cords can be used to enhance muscular fitness. When designing strength training programs, HFIs should evaluate the advantages and disadvantages of each training mode to meet individual needs, goals, and abilities.

Safety Issues

Strength training programs should be designed by health and fitness professionals who are knowledgeable of safe and effective training methods. Although all strength training activities have some degree of medical risk, the chance of injury can be reduced by following established training guidelines and safety procedures. Most acute injuries are the result of improper exercise technique, excessive loading, or inadequate supervision. The following box presents general safety recommendations for designing and instructing strength training programs.

Safety Recommendations for Strength Training

- Review participants' health/history questionnaires before they begin strength training.
- Provide adequate supervision and instruction when necessary.
- Regularly practice emergency procedures.
- Encourage participation in warm-up and cool-down activities.
- Move carefully around the strength training area, and don't back up without looking first.
- Fix broken or malfunctioning equipment immediately or put an "out of order" sign on it.
- Use collars on all plate-loaded barbells and dumbbells
- Be aware of proper spotting procedures and offer assistance when needed.
- Model appropriate behavior and do not allow "horseplay" in the fitness center.
- Demonstrate correct exercise technique and do not allow participants to train improperly.
- Periodically check all strength training equipment.
- Ensure the training environment is free of clutter and appropriately maintained.
- Stay up to date with current strength training guidelines and safety procedures for special populations.

Supervision and Instruction

Individuals who want to participate in strength training activities should first receive guidance and instruction from qualified fitness professionals who understand strength training principles and genuinely appreciate individual differences. Fitness professionals should be able to correctly perform the exercises they prescribe and should be able to modify exercise form and technique if necessary. The HFI should know the exercises that require spotters and should be prepared to offer assistance in case of a failed repetition. When working in a health/fitness facility, the staff should be attentive and should try to position themselves with a clear view of the training center so that they can have quick access to individuals who need assistance. In addition, the fitness staff is responsible for enforcing safety rules (e.g., proper footwear, safe storage of weights, and no foolish play in the fitness center) and safe training procedures (e.g., emphasizing proper exercise technique rather than the amount of weight lifted).

Research Insight

Although personal training has become popular in the fitness industry, the effects of one-on-one supervision on strength training adaptations have not been scientifically examined. Mazzetti et al. (48) compared changes in muscle performance after 12 weeks of periodized strength training in adult men who exercised in a closely supervised program or an unsupervised program. Although both groups followed the same training protocol, subjects who worked with a personal trainer made significantly greater gains in maximal strength than subjects who trained without supervision. These findings suggest that personal trainers can help clients maximize gains in strength performance provided that the training program is appropriately designed.

Training Environment

If exercise is to take place in a public, community, worksite, or school-based fitness center, the strength training area should be well-lit and large enough to handle the number of individuals exercising in the facility at any given time. The facility should be clean and the equipment should be well maintained. Equipment pads that come in contact with the skin should be cleaned daily, and cables, guide rods, and chains on machines should be checked weekly. Equipment should be spaced to allow easy access to each strength training exercise, and equipment such as free weights and collars should be returned to the proper storage area after each use. Recommended temperature (68-72° F), humidity (60% or less), and air circulations (at least 8-12 air exchanges per hour) should be maintained in the strength training area (5). Additional recommendations for fitness facility maintenance and risk management are available elsewhere (5).

Warm-Up and Cool-Down

Strength training should be preceded by warm-up activities. A proper warm-up increases body and muscle temperature, increases blood flow, and may decrease the likelihood of injury (17, 35). A general warm-up typically includes 5 to 10 min of low- to moderate-intensity aerobic exercise such as slow jogging or stationary cycling. A general warm-up before stretching is recommended to enhance the benefits of stretching. The increase in muscle temperature resulting from the general warm-up will allow for a greater amount of flexibility. A specific warm-up involves movements that are the same as (or similar to) the strength training exercises that are about to be performed. For example, after a general warm-up, a lifter could perform a light set of 10 repetitions on the chest press exercise before attempting a heavy set. It makes sense to physically and mentally prepare for the demands of strength training by spending a few minutes warming up. After a strength training workout, it's a good idea to cool down with general calisthenics and static stretching exercises. A cool-down can help to relax the body and possibly reduce muscle stiffness and soreness.

4 In Review

Qualified supervision and instruction, a safe training environment, and adherence to established training guidelines will help to minimize the risk of injury during strength training. The HFI should educate participants about safe strength training procedures that are consistent with each individual's needs and abilities and should encourage participation in warm-up and cool-down activities.

Strength Training Guidelines

Guidelines for strength training are not as universally accepted as recommendations for enhancing aerobic fitness. Although sports medicine organizations recognize the importance of strength training for health and fitness, there has been considerable debate regarding the training volume (i.e., sets × repetitions × weight lifted). In particular, the efficacy of performing either single or multiple sets has captured the interest of some exercise scientists (14, 29). Yet, despite various claims about the best training approach to take, there does not appear to be one "optimal" combination of sets, repetitions, and exercises that will promote long-term adaptations in muscular fitness for all individuals. Rather, many program variables may be altered to achieve desirable outcomes provided that fundamental training principles are followed.

There are many factors to consider when designing a strength training program. In the 1980s, Kraemer identified five acute program variables that affect the design of a strength training workout (42). The choice of exercise, order of exercise, training weight (which will determine the number of repetitions), number of sets, and rest periods between sets and exercises are the five program variables that describe all possible single exercise sessions. Because individuals will respond differently to the same strength training program, sound decisions must be made based on an understanding of exercise science, individual needs, and personal goals. The following box summarizes ACSM's strength training guidelines for apparently healthy adults.

Choice of Exercise

A limitless number of exercises can be used to enhance muscle strength, power, and local muscular endurance. It is important to select exercises that are appropriate for an individual's exercise technique experience and training goals. Also, the choice of exercises should promote muscle balance across joints and between opposing muscle groups (e.g., quadriceps and hamstrings). Selected weight machine and free weight exercises and the primary muscle groups strengthened are listed in table 12.3.

Exercises generally can be classified as single-joint (i.e., body-part specific) or multiple-joint (i.e., structural). The dumbbell biceps curls and leg extension are examples of single-joint exercises that isolate a specific body part (biceps and quadriceps, respectively), whereas squats and deadlifts are multiple-joint exercises that involve two or more primary joints. Exercises also can be classified as closed kinetic chain or open kinetic chain. Closed kinetic chain exercises are those in which the distal joint segment is stationary (e.g., squat), whereas open chain exercises are those in which the terminal joint is free to move (e.g., leg extension). Closed kinetic chain exercises more closely mimic everyday activities and include more functional movement patterns (18).

Single-joint exercises and many machine exercises are often used by individuals who have limited experience strength training or by those who simply enjoy this mode of training. This type of training is also beneficial in activating specific muscles (e.g., during injury rehabilitation). With most machines, the path of movement is fixed and therefore the movement is stabilized. Conversely, exercises with free weights require additional muscles to stabilize the movement and are therefore more challenging. Also, dual-limb exercises with free weights (e.g., dumbbell lateral raise) may be particularly beneficial for individuals who need to strengthen a weaker limb. It is important to eventually incorporate multiple-joint exercises into a strength training program to promote the coordinated use of

Summary of ACSM's Strength Training Guidelines for Apparently Healthy Adults

- Perform a minimum of 8 to 10 exercises for each of the major muscle groups.
- Perform a minimum of 1 set of 8 to 12 repetitions.
- Strength train 2 to 3 days per week.
- Perform each exercise in a controlled manner through the full range of motion.
- Maintain a normal breathing pattern.
- Exercise with a partner for assistance and motivation.

Adapted from ACSM (2000).

Table 12.3 Selected Weight Machine and Free Weight Exercises and the Primary Muscle Group(s) Strengthened

Weight machine exercise	Free weight exercise	Primary muscle group(s) strengthened
Leg press	Barbell squat	Quadriceps, gluteus maximus
Leg extension	Dumbbell lunge	Quadriceps
Leg curl	Barbell standing hip extension	Hamstrings
Chest press	Barbell bench press	Pectoralis major
Pec dec	Dumbbell fly	Pectoralis major
Front pull-down	Dumbbell pullover	Latissimus dorsi
Seated row	Dumbbell one-arm row	Latissimus dorsi
Overhead press	Dumbbell press	Deltoids
Biceps curl	Barbell curl	Biceps
Triceps extension	Lying triceps extension	Triceps

Note. A description of the proper exercise technique for each exercise is available elsewhere (1, 10).

multiple-joint movements. When a participant is learning a new multiple-joint exercise, such as the squat, it is important to start with a light weight (e.g., unloaded barbell or wooden dowel) so that the individual can master the technique of the exercise before weight is added to the bar. Regardless of the type of exercise performed, the concentric and eccentric phases of each lift should be performed in a controlled manner with proper exercise technique.

Another issue concerning the choice of exercise is the inclusion of exercises for abdominal and low back musculature. It is not uncommon for beginners to focus on strengthening their chest and biceps and not spend adequate time strengthening their abdominals and low back. Strengthening the midsection not only may improve force output and enhance body control during free weight exercises such as the squat but also may decrease the risk of injury. Thus, "prehabilitation" exercises for the low back and abdominals should be included in all strength training programs. That is, exercises that may be prescribed for the rehabilitation of an injury should be performed before injury occurs as a preventive health measure. Exercises such as abdominal curl-ups and back extensions are useful, but they only train muscles that control trunk flexion and extension. Multidirectional exercises that involve rotational movements and diagonal patterns performed with one's own body weight or a medicine ball can be effective in strengthening the abdominals and low back. Depending on the needs and goals of the individual, other prehabilitation exercises (e.g., internal and external rotation for the rotator cuff musculature) can be incorporated into the exercise session.

Order of Exercise

There are many ways to arrange the sequence of exercises in a training session. Traditionally, large muscle group exercises are performed before smaller muscle group exercises, and multiple-joint exercises are performed before single-joint exercises. Following this exercise order will allow heavier weights to be used on the multiple-joint exercises because fatigue will be less of a factor. It is also helpful to perform more challenging exercises earlier in the workout when the neuromuscular system is less fatigued. However, in some cases (injury prevention or rehabilitation), it may be appropriate to follow a reverse order of training in which the smaller muscle groups are trained first. In general, it seems reasonable to follow the priority system of training in which exercises that will most likely enhance health and fitness are performed early in the training session. Also, power exercises such as plyometrics should be performed before strength exercises so that the individual can train for maximal power without undue fatigue. A sample strength training program is illustrated in Form 12.1.

Number of Repetitions

One of the most important variables in the design of a strength training program is the amount of weight used for an exercise (51). Gains in strength, power, and local muscular endurance are influenced by the amount of weight lifted, which is inversely related to the number of repetitions that can be performed. As the weight increases, the number of repetitions that can be performed decreases. By definition, the

form 12.1

Weekly 3 to 5 Day Weight Training Log

Name John Doe
Week of training 4th

	Day 1			Day 2			Day 3			Day 4			Day 5			Training goal
	Wt	Rep	Set	Wt	Rep	Set	Wt	Rep	Set	Wt	Rep	Set	Wt	Rep	Set	Comments
Leg extension	50	6	3				59	6	3				50	6	3	Slight soreness in midportion of triceps
Leg curl	55	6	3				55	6	3				55	6	3	
Chest press	No wt	35	3				No wt	35	3				No wt	35	3	
Lat pulldown	180	6	3				180	6	3				180	6	3	
Biceps curl	100															
Triceps extension	60	6	3				60	6	3				60	6	3	
Back extension	90	6	3				90	6	3				45	6	3	
Abdominal curl	45	6	3				45	6	3				45	6	3	

Wt = weight
Rep = repetitions

amount of weight that can be lifted with proper technique for only one repetition is called the one repetition maximum (or 1RM). Similarly, the amount of weight that can be lifted with proper technique for 10 but not 11 repetitions is called the 10 repetition maximum (or 10RM). To maximize gains in muscle strength, it is recommended that training sets be performed to volitional fatigue (defined as the inability to complete a repetition because of temporary fatigue) using the appropriate resistance.

The use of RM loads is a relatively simple method to prescribe strength training intensity. Research studies suggest that RM loads of 6 or less have the greatest effect on developing muscle strength, whereas RM loads of 20 or more have the greatest impact on developing local muscular endurance (29). RM loads in the middle of this continuum (e.g., 8-12RM) seem to be best for developing strength and local muscular endurance (see figure 12.4). Using weights that exceed an individual's 6RM capacity will have a minimal impact on local muscular endurance, whereas training with very light weights (e.g., above 20RM loads) will result in only small gains in strength. The ACSM recommends a range of 8 to 12 repetitions for apparently healthy adults (7).

A percentage of an individual's 1RM also can be used to determine the strength training intensity. If the 1RM on the chest press exercise is 100 lb, a training intensity of 75% would be 75 lb. In general, most individuals can perform about 10 repetitions using 75% of their 1RM. Obviously, this method requires the evaluation of the 1RM on all exercises used in the training program. In many cases this is not realistic because of the time required to perform 1RM testing correctly on 8 to 10 different exercises. Furthermore, maximal strength testing for small muscle group assistance exercises (e.g., biceps curl and lying triceps extension) typically is not performed.

The relationship between the percentage of the 1RM and the number of repetitions that can be performed varies with the amount of muscle mass required to perform the exercise. For example, studies have shown that at a given percentage of the 1RM (e.g., 60%), adults can perform more repetitions on a large muscle group exercise such as the leg press compared with a smaller muscle group exercise such as the leg curl (39). Therefore, prescribing a strength training intensity of 70% of 1RM on all exercises warrants additional consideration because at 70% of the 1RM, an individual may be able to perform 20 or more repetitions on a large muscle group exercise and this may not be ideal for enhancing muscle strength. If a percentage of the 1RM is used for prescribing strength training activities, the prescribed percentage of the 1RM for each exercise may need to be changed to maintain a desired training range (e.g., 8-12RM).

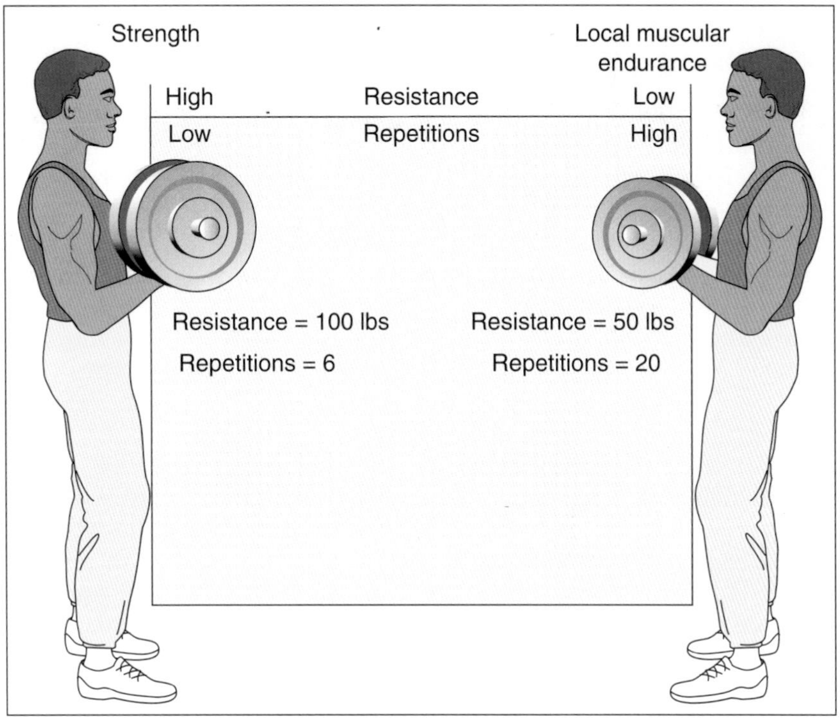

Figure 12.4 The strength/endurance continuum. The use of heavy weights/low repetitions has the greatest effect on strength and power, whereas the use of light weights/high repetitions has the greatest effect on local muscular endurance.

Adapted, by permission, from Powers and Dodd 1996.

Number of Sets

A set refers to a group of repetitions performed continuously and is an important training variable. The number of sets performed in a workout is directly related to the training volume, which can be determined by multiplying the number of sets times the number of repetitions by the weight lifted. For example, if an individual performs 2 sets of 10 repetitions with 100 lb, the training volume would be 2000 lb ($2 \times 10 \times 100 = 2000$). Although there has been much debate regarding the number of sets performed per exercise, not every exercise needs to be performed for the same number of sets. The ACSM recommends that apparently healthy adults perform a minimum of one set on each exercise to achieve muscular fitness goals (7).

In general, one-, two-, and three-set protocols have proven to be equally effective for untrained individuals during the first 2 to 3 months of training if the programs are not periodized (34, 40, 50). However, the results of some—but not all (36)—long-term studies (≥24 weeks) suggest that multiple-set periodized programs may result in superior gains in strength, power, hypertrophy, and local muscular endurance compared with low-volume single-set programs (44, 45, 47). Additional long-term training studies are needed to explore the effects of single- and multiple-set training protocols on muscular fitness in trained and untrained subjects.

When you are prescribing a strength training program for beginners, it is sensible to begin with a single-set program and gradually increase the number of sets depending on personal goals and time available for training. Clearly, a single-set protocol reduces training time and may therefore provide a practical approach for individuals who do not strength train regularly. However, it is also possible that a multiple-set protocol can be a time-efficient method of training. For example, instead of performing 1 set on 12 different exercises during every workout, individuals can perform 2 sets on 6 exercises or 3 sets on 4 exercises. With a careful selection of multiple-joint exercises, all muscle groups can be trained each exercise session regardless of the number of sets or exercises performed. Different combinations of sets and exercises are not only effective and time efficient, but they also allow the participant to vary the training stimulus, which may be vital for long-term gains.

Rest Periods Between Sets and Exercises

The length of the rest period between sets and exercises is an important but often overlooked training variable. In general, the length of the rest period will influence energy recovery and the training adaptations that take place. For example, if the primary goal of the program is muscular strength, heavier weights and longer rest periods (e.g., 3-4 min) are needed, whereas if the goal is muscular endurance, lighter weights and shorter rest periods (e.g., 30-60 s) are required. Obviously, the heavier the weight lifted, the longer the rest period should be. In general, a rest period of 1 to 2 min between sets and exercises is appropriate for most individuals. Short rest periods (<30 s between sets and exercises) are not recommended for beginners because of the discomfort and high blood lactate concentrations (10-14 mmol/L) associated with this type of training (43). However, over time, the rest periods can be reduced gradually to provide ample opportunity for the body to tolerate increased muscle and blood acid levels.

Strength Training Frequency

Adequate recovery between exercise sessions is vital for maximizing training-induced adaptations. A strength training frequency of 2 to 3 times per week on nonconsecutive days typically is recommended for beginners. This frequency will allow for adequate recovery between sessions and minimize muscle soreness. There should be at least 48 hr of rest between sessions that stress the same muscle groups. Depending on individual goals, exercise tolerance, and time available for training, the frequency can be increased. If individuals strength train on two consecutive days, different muscle groups should be trained each day to avoid overtraining. The type of training in which different muscles are trained on different days is called a split routine.

Periodization

Periodization is used to achieve specific goals, avoid overtraining, and keep the program effective and challenging. In essence, periodization is a systematic process of planned variations in the training program over a period of time. Over the past 10 years the concept of periodization has increased in popularity, and more recently our understanding of the benefits of periodized training programs compared with nonperiodized programs has increased (27).

Periodically varying the strength training program by changing the choice of exercise or the combination of sets and repetitions can optimize gains in muscle performance as well as prevent boredom and thus enhance compliance. In addition, a periodized strength training program may help to decrease the risk of injury (28). For example, if an individual's lower body routine typically consists of the squat, leg extension, and leg curl exercises, performing the dumbbell lunge, hip abduction, and hip adduction exercises on alternate workout days will likely add to the effectiveness and enjoyment of the strength training program. Furthermore, varying the volume and intensity of training can help to prevent training plateaus, which are not uncommon in health and fitness centers. Many times a strength plateau can be avoided by decreasing the training intensity to allow ample opportunity for the individual to recover from high-intensity training. In the long term, this recovery will allow the body to make even greater gains during the next high-intensity training period. The underlying concept of periodization is based on Selye's general adaptation syndrome, which proposes that after a period of time, adaptations to a new stimulus will no longer take place and "staleness" may result. Periodization can be used to avoid staleness and to make continual gains.

Although there are many models of periodization, the general concept is to prioritize training goals and then develop a long-term plan that varies throughout the year. In general, the year is divided into specific training cycles (e.g., a **macrocycle**, a **mesocycle,** and a **microcycle**) with each cycle having a specific goal (e.g., hypertrophy, strength, or power). The classic periodization model is referred to as a linear model because the volume and intensity of training gradually change over time. For example, at the start of a macrocycle, the training volume may be high and the training intensity may be low. As the year progresses, the volume is decreased as the intensity of training increases.

Research Insight

Which is preferable, low-volume circuit or high-volume periodized resistance training? Previous studies have reported similar strength gains in subjects who participated in single-set and multiple-set training programs during the initial 7 to 12 weeks of training. Marx et al. (47) compared training adaptations to single-set circuit weight training versus multiple-set periodized strength training in untrained adult women who strength trained 3 times a week for 24 weeks. After the first 12 weeks of training, both exercise groups made significant improvements in muscular performance. However, only the subjects who followed a multiple-set periodized strength training program made significant gains in muscle strength, power, and local muscular endurance during the next 12 weeks of the training program. These findings suggest that single- and multiple-set training protocols may be effective during the initial adaptation period, but periodized, multiple-set training programs appear to keep the training stimulus effective for longer periods of time.

Although this type of training originally was designed for weightlifters and track-and-field athletes who attempted to peak for a specific competition, this model can be modified for fitness enthusiasts. For example, individuals who routinely perform the same combination of sets and repetitions on all exercises may benefit from gradually increasing the weight and decreasing the number of repetitions as strength improves. The classic periodized model, which consists of four distinct phases, is outlined in table 12.4. After the four-phase program is complete, individuals should be encouraged to participate in recreational activities or low-intensity strength training to reduce the likelihood of overtraining. This period of restoration is called active rest and typically lasts for 1 to 3 weeks. After active rest, individuals can then return to Phase 1 of their training program with more energy and vigor.

Another model of periodization is referred to as a nonlinear or undulating model because of the daily fluctuations in training volume and intensity. For example, an individual may perform 2 sets of 10 repetitions with a moderate load on Monday, 3 sets of 6 repetitions with a heavy load on Wednesday, and 1 set of 15 repetitions with a light load on Friday. Whereas the heavy training days will maximally activate the trained musculature, selected muscle fibers will not be maximally taxed on light and moderate training days. By alternating training intensities, the participant can minimize the risk of overtraining and maximize the potential for maintaining training-induced strength gains (33). A sample nonlinear periodized workout plan for a trained adult is presented in table 12.5. In addition, fitness professionals should consider an individual's vacation schedule or travel plans when incorporating periods of active rest into the year-long training schedule. Periods of restoration lasting from 1 to 3 weeks will allow for physical and psychological recovery from the strength training sessions. A detailed review of periodization and specific examples of periodized programs are available elsewhere (28).

5 In Review

Designing a safe and effective strength training program involves an understanding of exercise science along with an appreciation of the "art" of prescribing exercise. The choice of exercise, order of exercise, weights used, number of sets and rest periods between sets, and exercises are the acute program variables that contribute to the design of a training session. Periodization refers to varying the acute program variables over time to achieve specific goals, prevent overtraining, and decrease boredom.

Table 12.4 Sample Linear Periodized Workout for Maximizing Strength Gains in Healthy Adults

	Phase 1 General preparation	Phase 2 Hypertrophy	Phase 3 Strength	Phase 4 Peaking
Intensity	12–15RM	8–12RM	6–8RM	4–6RM
Sets	1–2	2	2–3	3
Rest period between sets	60–120 s	60 s	60–120 s	120–180 s

Note. The workout is for major muscle group exercises performed each phase; each phase lasts about 6–8 weeks. RM = repetition maximum.

Table 12.5 Sample Nonlinear Periodized Workout for a Trained Adult

	Monday	Wednesday	Friday
Intensity (RM)	8–10RM	4–6RM	13–15RM
Sets	2	3	1
Rest period between sets and exercises	2 min	3 min	1 min

[a]This plan is for the major muscle group exercises performed each day.

Overreaching and Overtraining

Overtraining syndrome is caused by an excessive frequency, volume, and / or intensity of training combined with inadequate rest and recovery. In essence, overtraining syndrome may occur when the exercise training stimulus exceeds the rate of adaptation. Overtraining syndrome typically includes a plateau or decrease in performance. Other observable manifestations of overtraining include decreased body weight, loss of appetite, sleep disturbances, decreased desire to train, muscle tenderness, and an increased risk of infection (58).

Overtraining on a short-term basis has become known as overreaching (33). Unlike overtraining syndrome, which can last for months, recovery from overreaching can occur within a few days. In fact, overreaching is sometimes a planned part of conditioning programs as individuals train at higher volumes and intensities. Nevertheless, overreaching should be considered the first stage of overtraining and therefore warrants attention because not all individuals recover quickly from overreaching. Individuals may need to decrease the intensity and volume of their training program to recover from overreaching.

A downfall of many fitness programs is not allowing for adequate recovery between workouts. For example, if an individual strength trains on Monday, Wednesday, and Friday and jogs on Tuesday and Thursday, the chronic forces placed on the lower body can injure muscles and connective tissue and decrease performance in the weight room and on the track. Overtraining can result from poor programming characterized by frequent training sessions without adequate rest and recovery between workouts. From a practical perspective, it is important to consider an individual's training age as well as all the fitness activities regularly performed. Periodization can help to avoid overtraining and promote long-term gains in muscular fitness.

6 In Review

Strength training programs should be characterized by an appropriate overload combined with planned periods of rest and recovery. Overreaching is often the first stage of the overtraining syndrome, which typically is characterized by a decrease in performance and other physical and psychological effects. Adequate rest and recovery between workouts can help to avoid overtraining syndrome.

Strength Training Systems

Many different strength training systems can be used to enhance muscular fitness. Some systems have been scientifically proven to be effective, whereas others are based on anecdotal evidence. The wide variety of strength training systems clearly illustrates the type of programs that can be developed by manipulating the acute program variables. Five of the most common strength training systems are the single-set system, multiple-set system, circuit training system, pre-exhaustion system, and assisted training system.

Single-Set System

This system of strength training is one of the oldest systems and consists of performing a single set of a predetermined number of repetitions (e.g., 8-12) until volitional fatigue. More recently, the single-set approach has become known as the high-intensity training (HIT) system. This effective and time-efficient method of strength training is popular among some fitness professionals.

Multiple-Set System

The multiple-set system is an effective training method for enhancing strength and power. This system of training became popular in the 1940s and originally consisted of 3 sets of 10 repetitions with increasing weights. For example, the classic multiple-set protocol used by Delorme in his pioneering rehabilitation work involved performing the first set of 10 repetitions at 50% of the 10RM, the second set of 10 repetitions at 75% of the 10RM, and the third set of 10 repetitions at 100% of the 10RM (19). Over the years, many different multiple-set programs using different combinations of sets and repetitions have been shown to be effective. For example, the pyramid system is a multiple-set system in which the weight is increased progressively over several sets so that fewer and fewer repetitions can be performed (see table 12.6).

Table 12.6 Example of a Light to Heavy Pyramid Training System

Set number	Repetitions	Intensity (% 1RM)
1	10	75
2	8	80
3	6	85

Circuit Training System

This system of training involves a series of strength exercises performed in a circuit with minimal rest (e.g., about 30 s) between exercises (see figure 12.5). Generally, moderate weights are used (about 60% of the 1RM), and 10 to 15 repetitions are performed at each exercise station. In addition to increasing muscular strength and local muscular endurance, circuit training also can improve cardiovascular fitness. However, gains in maximal oxygen consumption resulting from aerobic training are far greater than those resulting from circuit training. Starting with a 1-min rest period between exercises and gradually reducing the rest period to the desired range as the body adapts is recommended when an individual is beginning a circuit training program. A sample circuit strength training program is illustrated in figure 12.5

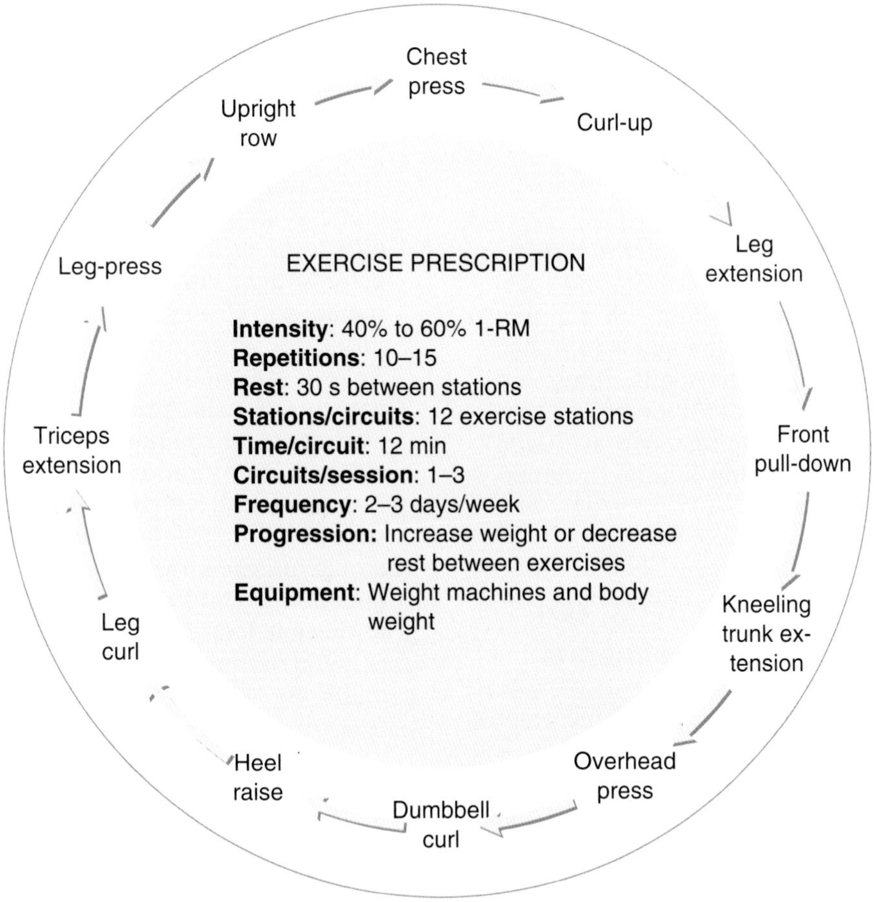

Figure 12.5 Sample circuit weight training program.

Adapted from Heyward 1991.

Pre-Exhaustion System

This training method generally consists of performing successive sets of two different exercises for the same target muscle or muscle group. For example, after performing one set to volitional fatigue on the bench press exercise, the individual immediately performs another set of dumbbell flys to facilitate chest development. This type of training forces the target muscle group (e.g., pectoralis major) to work longer and harder and is often used to increase muscle hypertrophy.

Assisted Training System

As the name implies, this method of training requires the assistance of another individual who, after several repetitions of an exercise are performed to volitional fatigue, can provide just enough assistance to allow the lifter to complete 3 to 5 additional repetitions. Because muscles are stronger eccentrically than concentrically, assistance may not be needed during the eccentric phase of the forced repetitions. Although this advanced training system will enhance muscular fitness, it is not recommended for beginners because it typically results in muscle soreness attributable to the reliance on heavy eccentric muscle actions.

7 **In Review**

Different strength training systems can be used to enhance strength, power, and local muscular endurance. Although all training systems can be effective, the key is to match the training system with the needs, goals, and abilities of each individual for long-term success. The strength training system that is used will influence the training-induced adaptations that take place.

Strength Training for Special Populations

Strength training can be a safe, effective, and beneficial method of conditioning for males and females of all ages and abilities. Although most of the research on strength training has been done on trained adults, a growing body of evidence indicates that children, seniors, pregnant women, and individuals with heart disease can participate safely in a strength training program provided that appropriate training guidelines are followed.

Children

Despite previous concerns that children would not benefit from strength training because of inadequate levels of circulating androgens, research studies conducted over the past decade clearly demonstrate that boys and girls can benefit from strength training. The ACSM (7), the American Academy of Pediatrics (2), and the National Strength and Conditioning Association (23) support children's participation in strength training activities provided that the program is appropriately designed and competently supervised. In addition to increasing strength and local muscular endurance, regular participation in a youth strength training program may favorably influence several measurable indexes of health, including body composition, cardiovascular fitness, and bone mineral density (22). Furthermore, because many children who enter sports programs may be ill-prepared for the demands of sport training and competition, participation in a preseason strength training program may decrease the risk of sport-related injuries (57).

Research Insight

A traditional concern associated with children participating in sports and activities characterized by high-impact loading is that this type of stress may harm the developing musculoskeletal system. Morris et al. (52) studied the effects of 10 months of supervised physical activity (i.e., high-impact aerobic workouts, dance, and strength training performed three times per week) on 38 girls (age 9-10 years). An age-matched group of 33 girls served as control subjects. After the training period, the exercise group gained significantly more lean mass, muscle strength, and bone mineral content compared with the controls. These results suggest that strength-building exercises enhance muscle strength and bone mineral acquisition in children. This may be particularly important for girls who appear to be at increased risk for developing osteoporosis later in life.

Although there is no minimum age requirement for participation in a youth strength training program, all children should have the emotional maturity to accept and follow directions and understand the benefits and risks associated with this type of training. In general, if children are ready for organized sports, then they are ready for some type of strength training. As a point of reference, many 7- and 8-year-old boys and girls have participated in closely supervised youth strength training programs (24). Although some observers may be concerned about the stress that strength training exercises place on the developing musculoskeletal system, the sport-specific forces placed on the joints of children may be greater in both duration and magnitude than those resulting from moderate intensity strength training. Furthermore, injury to the epiphyseal plate or growth cartilage has not been reported in any prospective youth strength training study. Nevertheless, HFIs should follow age-specific training guidelines to decrease the likelihood of an accident or injury while youth perform strength exercises.

Children should begin strength training at a level that is commensurate with their physical abilities. No matter how big or strong a child is, adult training programs and training philosophies (e.g., "No pain, no gain") should not be imposed on children. The focus of youth strength training programs should be on learning proper form and technique on a variety of exercises. During each session, fitness professionals should listen to each child's concerns and closely monitor each child's ability to handle the prescribed training weight. Different combinations of sets and repetitions and a variety of training modes from child-size weight machines to body weight exercises have proven to be effective. According to the ACSM, children should perform 1 to 2 sets of 8 to 12 repetitions on 8 to 10 different exercises (7).

When working with children, remember that the goal of the program should not be limited to increasing muscle strength. Teaching children about their bodies and promoting a lifelong interest in physical activity are equally important. The following program design considerations should be followed when developing strength training programs for children:

- Parents or legal guardians should complete a health history questionnaire for each child.
- Qualified instructors should supervise youth fitness activities.
- The exercise area should be free of clutter and adequately ventilated.
- Children should use a light weight or wooden stick when learning a new exercise.
- Participants should increase the weight gradually (5-10%) as strength improves.
- Two or three nonconsecutive training sessions per week are recommended.
- When necessary, adult spotters should be nearby in case of a failed repetition.
- Children should stay hydrated before, during, and after each exercise session.
- Fitness programs for children should include activities that enhance strength, endurance, flexibility, agility, and balance.

Seniors

The number of men and women over the age of 65 is increasing, and research studies and clinical observations indicate that seniors can benefit from strength training programs (6, 59). Even individuals over the age of 90 can enhance their muscular fitness by strength training (25). Regular participation in a strength training program can help to offset the age-related declines in bone, muscle mass, and strength that often make activities of daily life—such as climbing stairs—more difficult. Bones become more fragile with age because of a decrease in bone mineral content that results in an increase in bone porosity. Advancing age also is associated with a loss of muscle mass, which has been termed *sarcopenia* (21). This includes a proportional loss of both the type 1 (slow twitch) and type 2 (fast twitch) fibers, with the type 2 fibers having the greatest loss in cross-sectional area. Evidence indicates that seniors who strength train can improve muscle strength, muscle power, gait speed, and balance, which in turn can enhance overall function and reduce the potential for injury caused by falls (26, 32).

Seniors can adapt readily to strength training exercises. If the training intensity is adequate, seniors can make relative gains in strength that are equal to or greater than those of younger individuals. Research studies using computerized tomography and muscle biopsy analysis have reported evidence of muscle hypertrophy in seniors who strength train (32), and others have reported that strength training can increase the resting metabolic rate (13) and bone mineral density (53) of older adults who strength train. Although both aerobic and strength exercise is important for seniors, only strength training can increase muscle strength and muscle mass. These potential benefits may be particularly important for seniors who are at increased risk for osteoporotic fractures. However, seniors will retain the beneficial effects of strength training only as long as they continue their exercise program. During prolonged periods of inactivity, adaptive changes in skeletal muscle strength and bone will return to pre-exercise levels (20). This is sometimes referred to as the principle of reversibility.

The ACSM recommends that older (approximately 50-60 years of age) or more frail individuals strength train with a moderate load that can be performed for 10 to 15 repetitions (7). Additional program design considerations for seniors include the following:

- Participants should undergo careful preparticipation health screening, particularly because many seniors have a variety of known, coexisting medical conditions.
- All strength training activities should be preceded by a 5- to 10-min warm-up period of low-intensity aerobic exercise and stretching.
- Seniors should learn proper breathing patterns and should be cautioned about performing the Valsalva maneuver.
- Participants should begin with 1 set of 10 to 15 repetitions on 8 to 10 exercises.
- Initially, seniors should use a light weight to allow for connective tissue adaptations.
- Given a choice, seniors should begin training on weight machines and gradually progress to free weight exercises, which require more balance, skill, and coordination.
- Participants should strength train at least twice per week and allow at least 48 to 72 hr of recovery between sessions.
- Exercises should be performed within a pain-free ROM.
- At least during the initial phase of training, qualified fitness professionals should provide guidance and offer assistance as needed.

Pregnant Women

An increasing body of evidence suggests that regular exercise during pregnancy poses little risk to either the mother or the fetus (4, 16). In fact, strength training during pregnancy may be particularly beneficial because it enhances muscle strength, which allows activities of daily life to be performed with greater ease, and it may minimize low back pain, which is common during pregnancy. Along with aerobic exercise, strength training at an appropriate intensity, duration, and frequency may contribute to enhanced overall fitness and feelings of well-being during pregnancy.

However, exercise is not advised for all women who are pregnant, especially those who have medical complications. Thus, pregnant women should consult with their personal physician or qualified medical care provider about activities that may or may not be appropriate during pregnancy. The American College of Obstetricians and Gynecologists established the following absolute contraindications for exercise during pregnancy: hemodynamically significant heart disease, restrictive lung disease, incompetent cervix / cerclage, multiple gestation at risk for premature labor, persistent second to third trimester bleeding placenta previa after 26 weeks of gestation, premature labor during the current pregnancy, ruptured membranes, and preeclampsia / pregnancy-induced hypertension.

Limited data are available regarding strength training for pregnant women. Although most women who strength train and become pregnant can continue to lift weights during pregnancy (with modifications for comfort level and specific symptoms), women who have never participated in a strength training program before may not be ideally suited to begin such a program. General guidelines for exercising while pregnant are discussed elsewhere in this textbook (chapter 21) and generally include maintaining adequate hydration, wearing appropriate clothing, and exercising at a comfortable intensity. Also, pregnant women who exercise should be particularly careful to maintain adequate calories and a well-balanced diet (4, 16).

The following program design considerations are appropriate for pregnant women:

- Avoid ballistic exercises, which may increase susceptibility to injury.
- Practice proper breathing patterns and avoid the Valsalva maneuver while lifting weights.
- Use a weight that can be performed for 12 to 15 repetitions without undue fatigue.
- Avoid exercise in the supine position after the first trimester.
- Gradually increase the weight as strength improves.
- Stop exercise in the event of any feelings of discomfort or complications such as vaginal bleeding, abdominal pain or cramping, ruptured membranes, or abnormal or excessive increase in blood pressure or heart rate.

Adults With CHD

Cardiac rehabilitation programs traditionally have emphasized aerobic exercise to maintain and improve cardiorespiratory fitness. However, muscular strength and local muscular endurance are also important to prepare the patient for return to work and leisure-time activities (49, 55). Many activities of daily living, as well as most occupational tasks, place demands on the cardiovascular system that closely resemble strength exercise. Because many cardiac patients are deconditioned and lack the strength and confidence to perform common activities involving muscular effort, the addition of strength training to an overall physical activity program provides patients with an opportunity to restore or gain optimal physiologic function. The ACSM (7), the American Heart Association (55), and the American Association of Cardiovascular and Pulmonary Rehabilitation (3) recommend strength training as part of a comprehensive cardiac rehabilitation program.

For many years, many medical and health practitioners believed that strength training activities were potentially harmful to cardiac patients and would "strain" the cardiovascular system (8, 31). However, research accumulated over the past decade or so indicates that the majority of cardiac patients can safely engage in strength training activities provided that the program is appropriately designed and carried out within the prescribed guidelines (11, 41). Regular participation in a strength training program may favorably affect muscle strength, local muscular endurance, cardiorespiratory endurance, cardiac risk factors, and psychosocial well-being. Furthermore, strength-trained patients also may experience reduced myocardial oxygen demands for a given load after training, because these patients could perform any submaximal load at a lower percentage of the maximal voluntary contraction, and thus HR and BP response would be attenuated after training (49).

Each patient's personal physician should review his or her health and medical history before initiating a strength training program. Although many low- to moderate-risk patients can safely participate in a strength training program, the safety and appropriateness of strength training for patients with low fitness levels or severe left ventricular dysfunction should be decided on an individual basis. In some cases, strength training is not advised or should be carried out only in a medically supervised environment. The ACSM has identified the following contraindications to strength training for cardiac patients: unstable angina, uncontrolled arrhythmias, left ventricular outflow obstruction, a recent history of congestive heart failure that has not been evaluated and treated effectively, severe valvular disease, and uncontrolled hypertension (SBP ≥160 mm Hg and DBP ≥105 mm Hg) (7).

It was previously was suggested that cardiac patients should avoid strength training for several months after the initial event (e.g., MI, cardiac surgery). Although recent findings indicate that most cardiac patients can begin strength training activities even 3 weeks after MI, after being appropriately screened, the decision to begin strength training activities should be based on a patient's health and medical status as determined by a qualified medical care provider as well as individual needs, interests, and goals. The guidelines for designing a strength training program for individuals with known or occult heart disease who have been medically cleared for participation are the same as those for older adults. Namely, experts recommend one set of light to moderate loads for 10 to 15 repetitions for each of the major muscle groups performed 2 to 3 nonconsecutive days per week. Patients recovering from coronary artery bypass graft surgery may need to avoid exercises that cause pulling on the sternum for the first 3 months after surgery (55).

Program Design Considerations for Cardiac Patients

- A physician should review each patient's health and medical history.
- Strength training should begin with a light weight and focus on slow, controlled movements.
- The patient should begin with 1 set of 10 to 15 repetitions on 8 to 10 different exercises.
- The patient should strength train 2 to 3 times per week on nonconsecutive days.
- Weight should be increased gradually as strength improves (2-5 lb for an upper body exercise and 5-10 lb for a lower body exercise).
- The patient should avoid breath holding and the Valsalva maneuver by exhaling during the concentric (i.e., lifting) phase.
- The patient should not grip the weight handles or bars tightly, because this will cause an excessive BP response.
- Exercise should be stopped in the event of any warning signs or symptoms such as dizziness, abnormal shortness of breath, or chest pain.

8 In Review

Strength training can be a safe and beneficial component of a comprehensive fitness program for individuals of all ages and those with medical conditions provided that appropriate guidelines are followed and qualified instruction is available. Despite previous concerns, children, seniors, pregnant women, and CHD patients can benefit from participation in a well-designed strength training program. Individuals should first be appropriately screened to identify those who may be contraindicated for strength training as determined by a qualified medical care provider.

Exercise Prescription Summary for Strength Training

Strength training is an important part of a well-designed fitness program. Strength training performed at a moderate intensity can enhance musculoskeletal strength, power, and local muscular endurance. Strength training refers to the use of any one or a combination of training modalities and training systems that overload the musculoskeletal system. If the fundamental principles of overload, progression, and specificity are followed, strength training can be a safe and effective method of physical conditioning for men and women of all ages and health status including children, pregnant women, seniors, adults with CHD, and many others.

Factors to consider when designing a strength training program include the choice of exercise, order of exercise, weight loads, number of sets, and rest periods between sets or between exercises. In addition, individual preferences, goals, presence of coexisting medical conditions, and time available for training should be considered when designing a strength training program. Because individuals respond differently to any exercise training program, HFIs should take a personalized approach to designing and modifying the program as strength training improves. Although any reasonable program can increase the strength of untrained individuals, it becomes more challenging to enhance the muscular fitness of strength-trained individuals. After the initial period of rapid strength gains, additional improvements occur at a slower rate and require a modification of the initial training stimulus. Periodization refers to varying the volume and intensity of training and is important for maximizing gains in muscular fitness and promoting long-term exercise compliance.

Case Studies

You can check your answers by referring to appendix A.

12.1

An adult member at your fitness center has been strength training for 6 months and claims to have made significant gains in strength. He performs 1 set of 8 to 12 repetitions on 10 weight machines 2 to 3 times per week. However, over the past 8 weeks he notices that he isn't making the gains that he used to. What advice would you give this member regarding his strength training program?

12.2

Your fitness director wants to increase usage of the strength training center between the hours of 3 and 5 P.M., when attendance at the club is usually low. She asks you to develop a proposal for two different afternoon workout classes at your facility. One class would be a physical activity program for children, and the other class would focus on strength-building activities for seniors living at the local nursing home. Comment on the safety and appropriateness of strength training for children and seniors. What are important program design considerations to include in your proposal to the fitness director?

Appendix

Selected Strength Training Exercises for the Major Muscle Groups

Leg Press

Prime muscle movers: Quadriceps, gluteus maximus
Exercise technique: The exerciser starts in a sitting position with the knees bent at 90º and the feet placed about shoulder-width apart on the footpad. The torso should be erect and the back should be pressed against the back of the seat. The participant extends his or her legs almost completely (without "locking" the knees) and then slowly returns to the starting position and repeats.

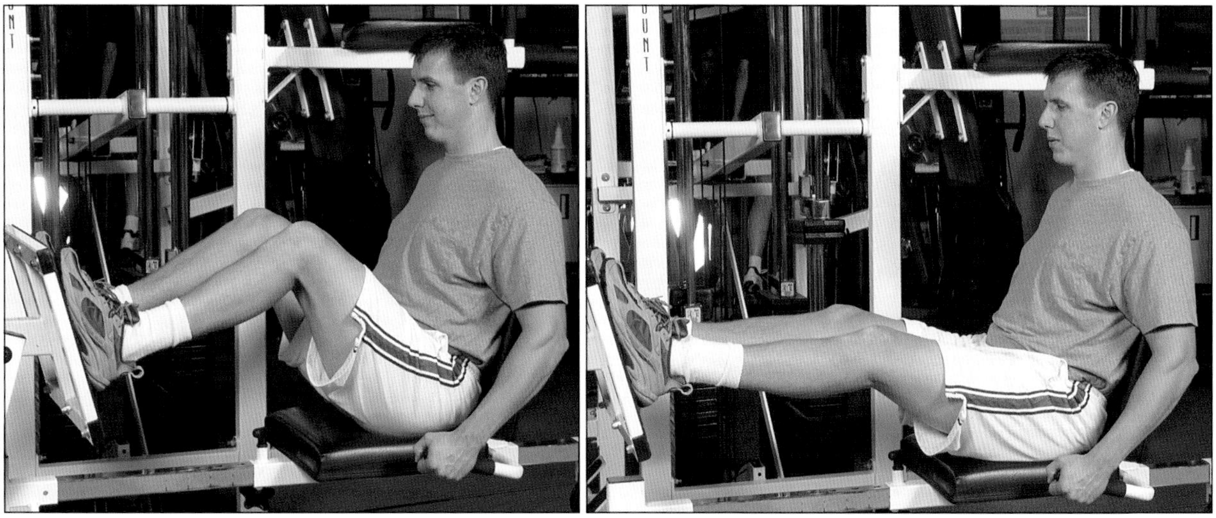

Leg Curl

Prime muscle movers: Hamstrings
Exercise technique: The participant lies face down on the bench with the kneecaps just over the edge of the board and the ankles under the padded exercise bar. He or she should grasp the handles and rest the head on the bench. The participant bends both knees and pulls the lower legs toward the buttocks and then slowly returns to the starting position and repeats.

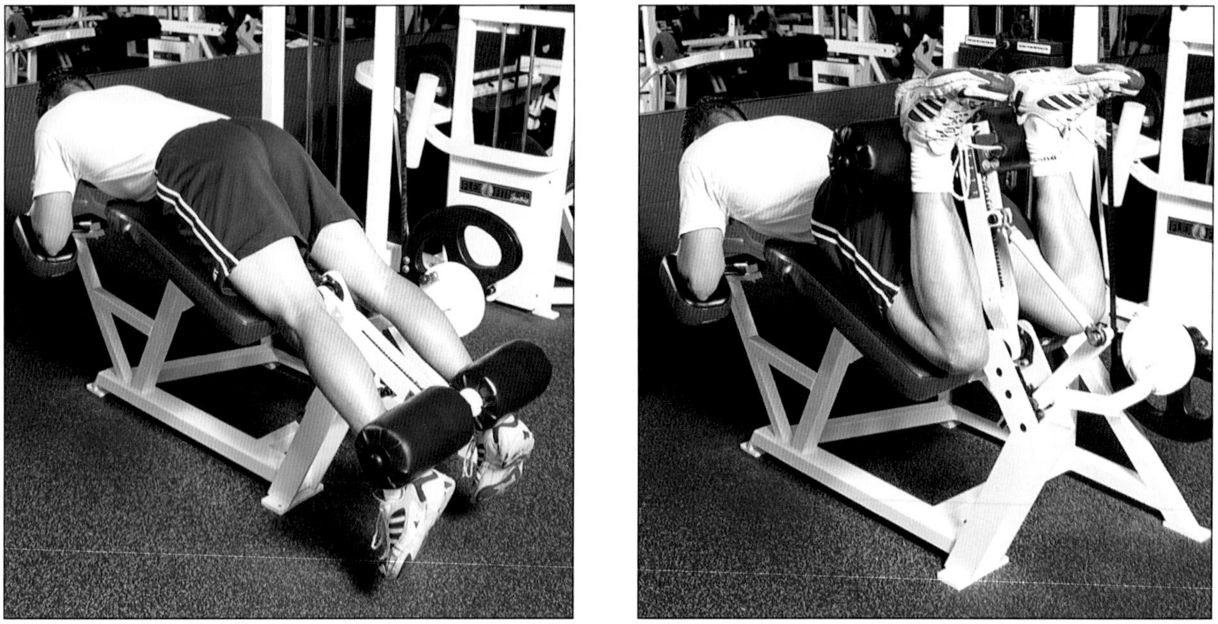

Dumbbell Heel Raise

Prime muscle movers: Gastrocnemius, soleus
Exercise technique: The participant stands with a dumbbell in the right hand hanging at arm's length and places the left hand on a wall for support. The left foot is lifted off the floor. The participant raises the heel of the right foot as high as possible and then slowly lowers to the starting position and repeats. This exercise should be performed on both sides of the body. The participant should concentrate on keeping the torso and knees straight to avoid upper leg involvement. To increase the ROM, a 1- to 2-in. board can be placed under the ball of the exercising foot. If this is too difficult, this exercise can be performed with both feet on the floor or board.

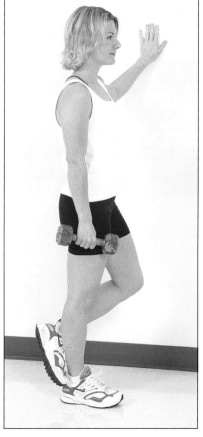

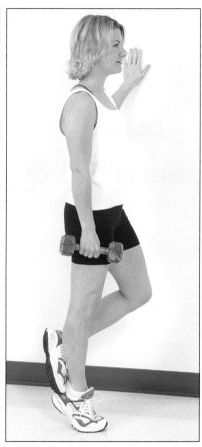

Bench Press

Prime muscle movers: Pectoralis major, anterior deltoid, and triceps
Exercise technique: The participant lies flat on the bench and holds the barbell with a wider than shoulder-width grip directly above the chest, with arms straight and feet flat on the floor. The participant should slowly lower the barbell to the chest and then press the barbell back up to the starting position. The exercise is repeated for the desired number of repetitions. The barbell should not be bounced on the chest, and a spotter should stand by in case of a failed repetition.

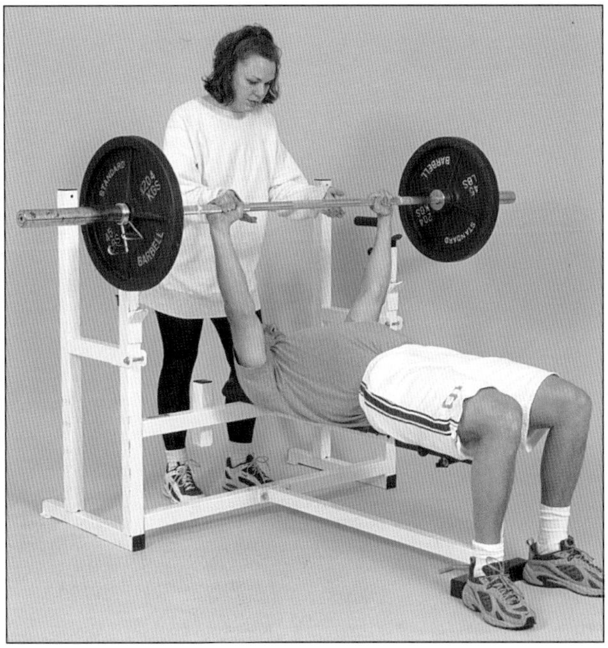

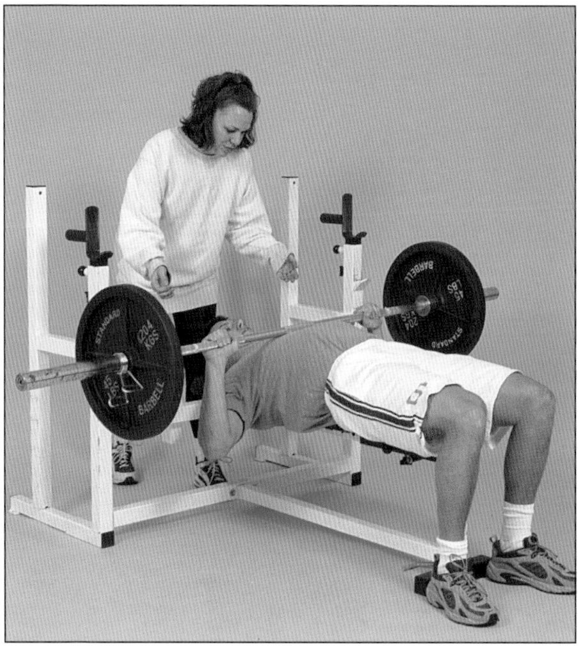

Front Pull-down

Prime muscle movers: Latissimus dorsi, biceps
Exercise technique: The participant should sit on the seat with the arms fully extended and place both knees under the exercise pad. The participant grips the bar underhand (palms toward the face) using a shoulder-width grip. Keeping the upper body erect, the participant slowly pulls the bar downward just under the chin and then allows the bar to return slowly until the arms are fully extended. The exercise is repeated for the desired number of repetitions.

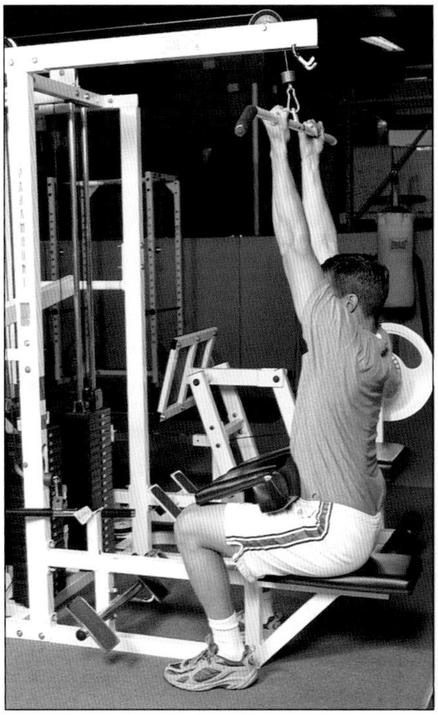

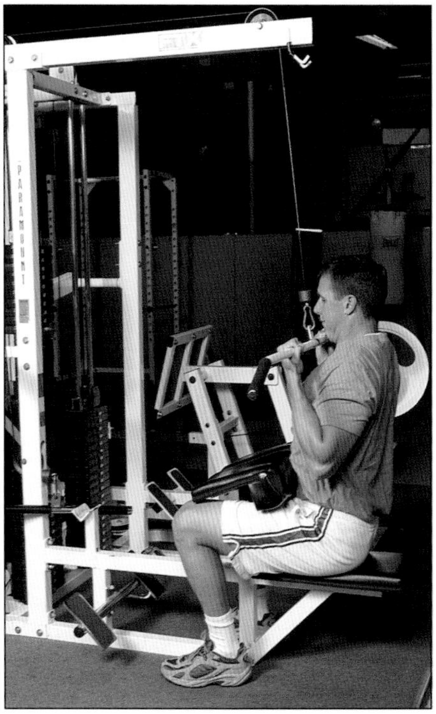

Dumbbell Overhead Press

Prime muscle movers: Deltoids, triceps

Exercise technique: In the standing position, the participant holds a dumbbell in each hand at shoulder level with palms facing forward. The participant should press the weights overhead to a straight arm position and then slowly return to the starting position and repeat. The participant should not bend or sway the back to complete a repetition.

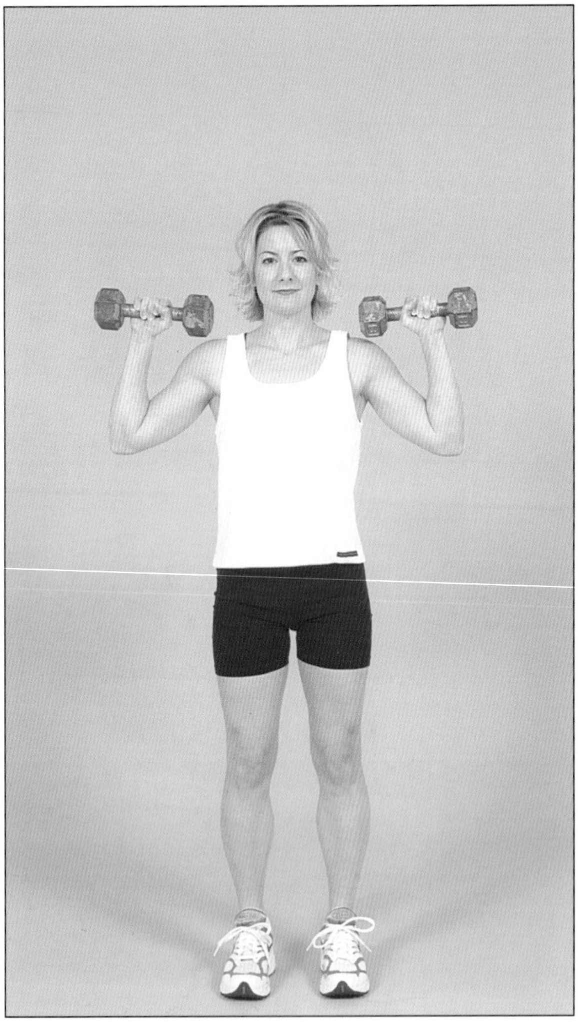

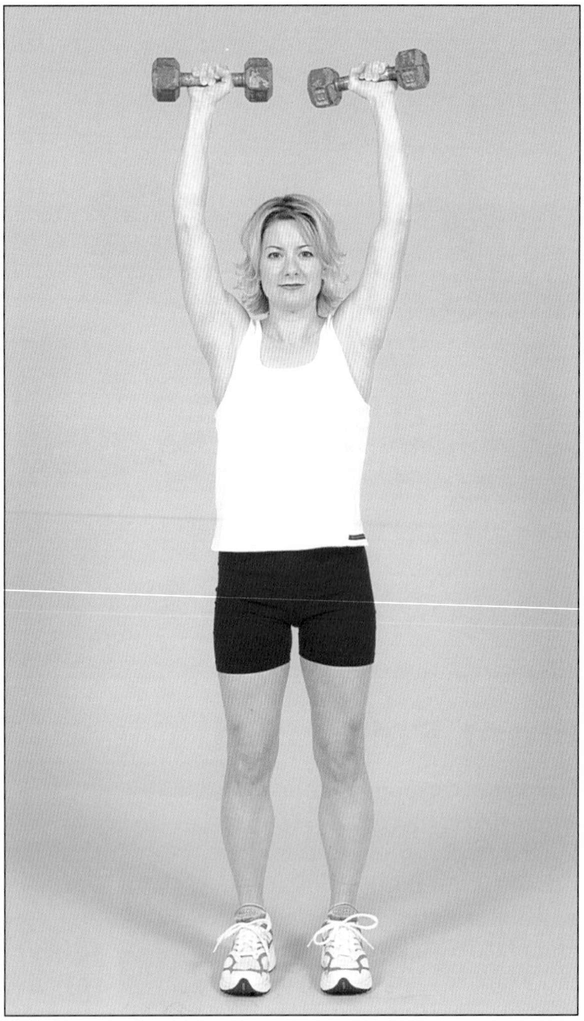

Dumbbell Curl

Prime muscle movers: Biceps
Exercise technique: The participant stands with a dumbbell in each hand (palms facing forward) and the arms at his or her sides. The participant bends the elbows to bring the weights toward the shoulders and then slowly returns to the starting position and repeats. The back should not be bent or swayed to complete a repetition.

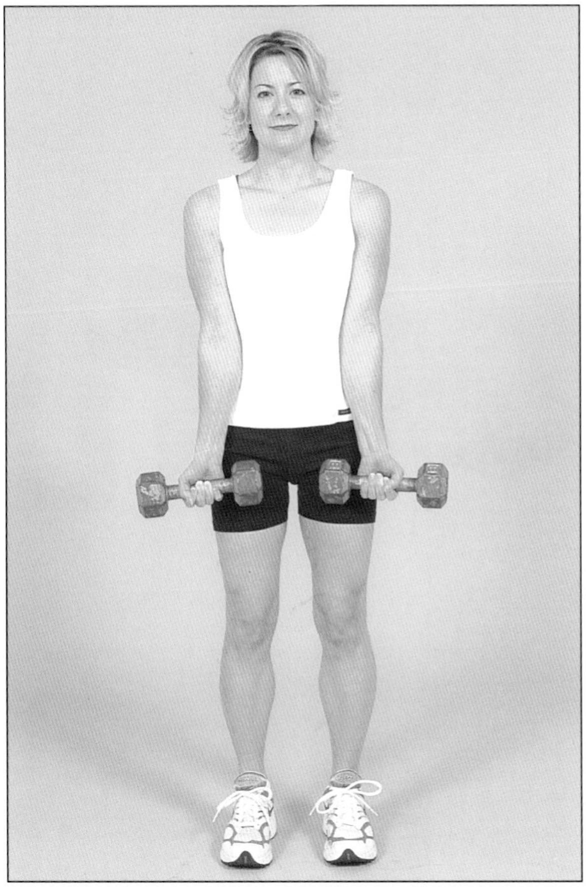

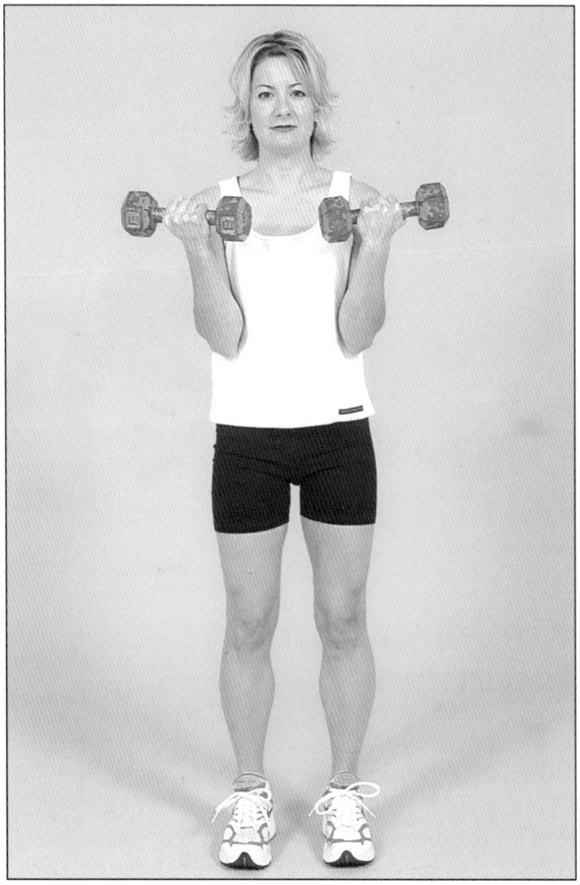

Lying Triceps Extension

Prime muscle movers: Triceps
Exercise technique: The participant lies on his or her back on a flat exercise bench and holds a dumbbell in each hand with arms straight over shoulders and palms facing each other. The participant lowers both dumbbells to the side of the head by bending only at the elbows, then slowly returns to the starting position and repeats. The upper arm should not be swayed to complete a repetition.

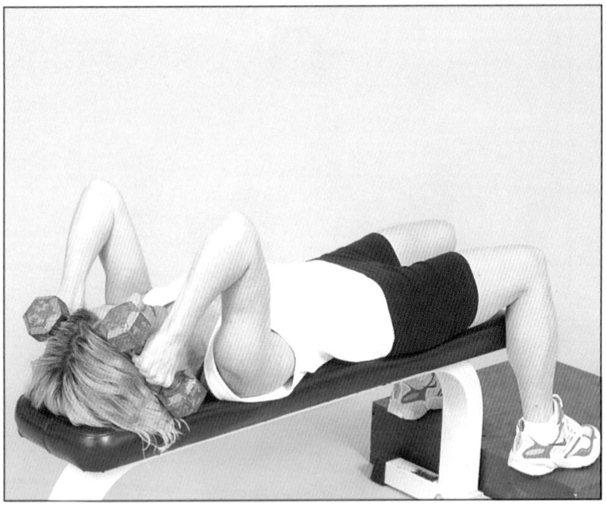

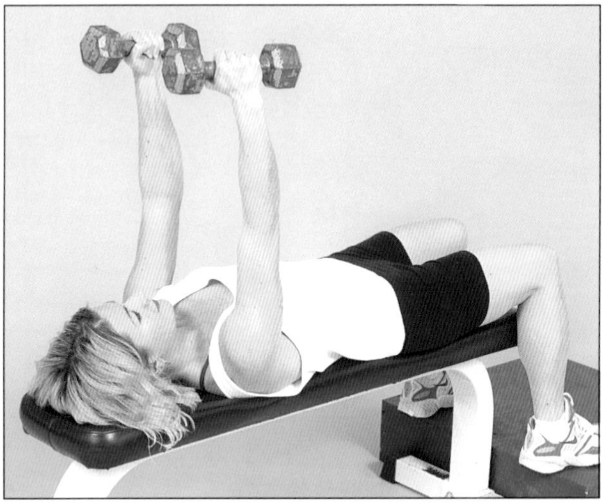

Kneeling Trunk Extension

Prime muscle mover: Erector spinae
Exercise technique: The participant kneels on the floor and supports the body on both hands and both knees. The participant extends the right leg backward until it is parallel to the floor, pauses briefly, returns to the starting position, and then extends the left leg backward. To make this exercise more challenging, the participant can raise the left arm parallel to the floor while extending the right leg (and vice versa).

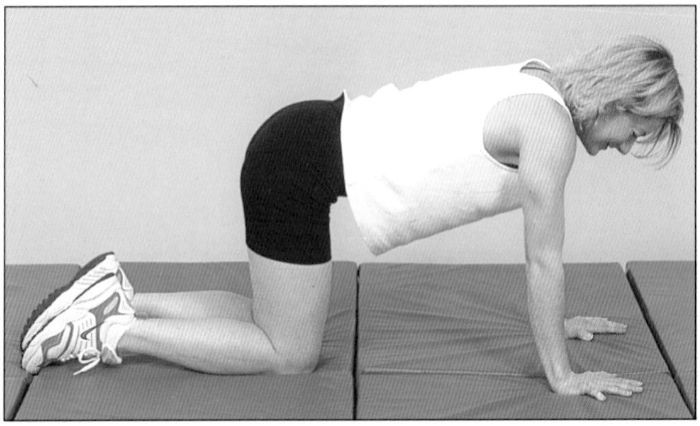

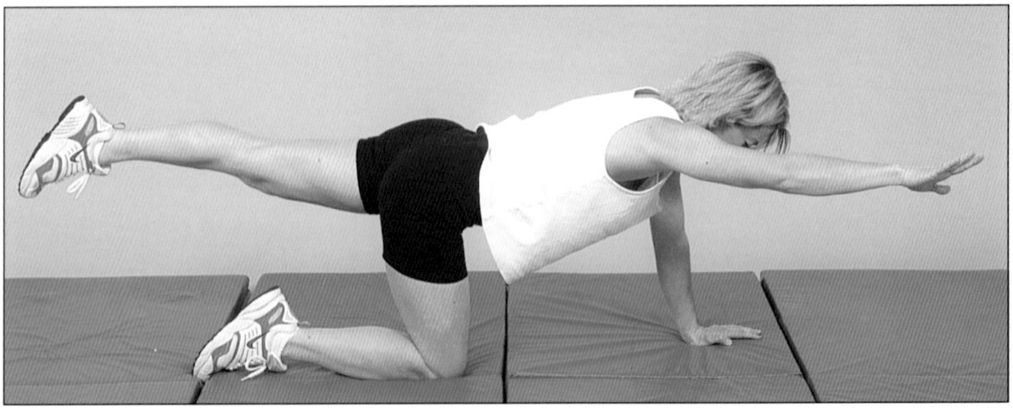

Abdominal Curl

Prime muscle mover: Rectus abdominis
Exercise technique: The participant lies on his or her back with the knees bent, feet about 12 to 15 in. from the buttocks, and hands placed on the thighs (or behind the head). Leading with the chin, the participant lifts the shoulders and upper back off the mat (about 30-45º) moving the hands toward the knees, pauses briefly, and then returns to starting position and repeats. If the hands are placed behind the head, the participant must not pull the head forward with the hands during this exercise.

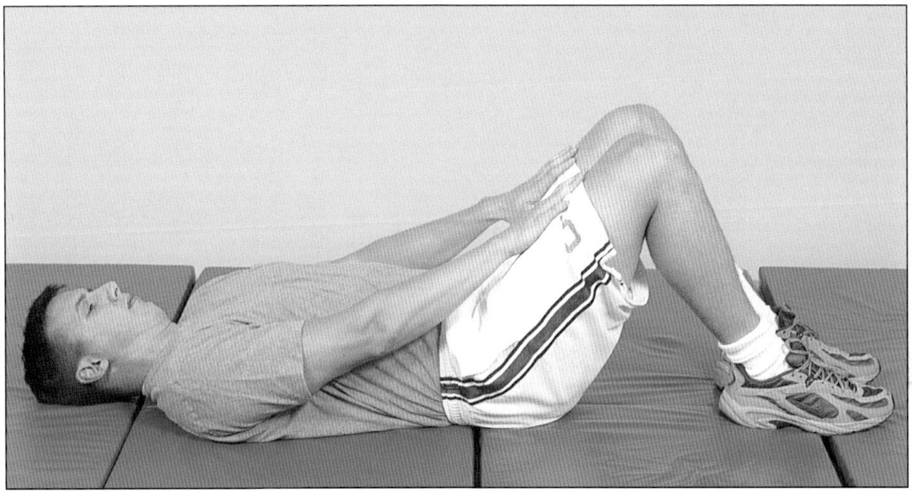

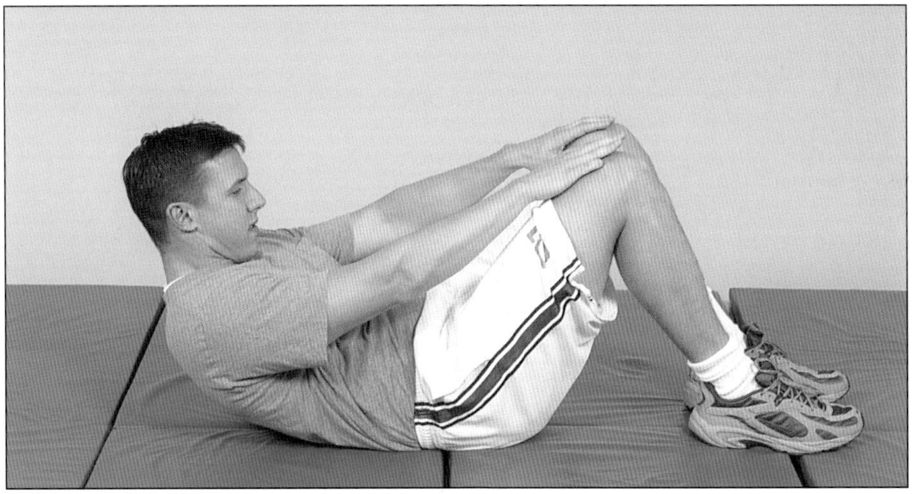

Source List

1. Aaberg, E. (1988). *Muscle mechanics*. Champaign, IL: Human Kinetics.
2. American Academy of Pediatrics. (2001). Strength training for children and adolescents. *Pediatrics, 107,* 1470-1472.
3. American Association of Cardiovascular and Pulmonary Rehabilitation. (1999). *Guidelines for cardiac rehabilitation and secondary prevention programs* (3rd ed.). Champaign, IL: Human Kinetics.
4. American College of Obstetricians and Gynecologists. (2002). *Exercise during pregnancy and the postpartum period* International Journal of Gynecology and Obstetrics, 77, 79-81.
5. American College of Sports Medicine. (1997). *ACSM's health/fitness facility standards and guidelines* (2nd ed.). Champaign, IL: Human Kinetics.
6. American College of Sports Medicine. (1998). Exercise and physical activity for older adults. *Medicine and Science in Sports and Exercise, 30,* 992-1008.
7. American College of Sports Medicine. (2000). *ACSM's guidelines for exercise testing and prescription* (6th ed.). Philadelphia: Lippincott Williams & Wilkins.
8. Atkins, J., Matthews, O., Blomqvist, C., & Mullins, C. (1976). Incidence of arrhythmias induced by isometric and dynamic exercise. *British Heart Journal, 38,* 465-471.
9. Baechle, T., & Earle, R. (2000). *Essentials of strength training and conditioning* (2nd ed.). Champaign, IL: Human Kinetics.
10. Baechle, T., & Graves, B. (1994). *Weight training instruction: Steps to success*. Champaign, IL: Human Kinetics.
11. Beniamini, Y., Rubenstein, J., Faigenbaum, A., Lichtenstein, A., & Crim, M. (1999). High intensity strength training of patients enrolled in an outpatient cardiac rehabilitation program. *Journal of Cardiopulmonary Rehabilitation, 19,* 8-17.
12. Brown, L. (2000). *Isokinetics in human performance*. Champaign, IL: Human Kinetics.
13. Campbell, W., Crim, M., Young, V., & Evans, W. (19940. Increased energy requirements and changes in body composition with resistance training in older adults. *American Journal of Clinical Nutrition, 60,* 167-175.
14. Carpinelli, R., & Otto, R. (1998). Strength training: Single versus multiple sets. *Sports Medicine, 26,* 73-84.
15. Chu, D. (1996). *Explosive power and strength*. Champaign, IL: Human Kinetics.
16. Clapp, J. (1996). The effects of continuing regular endurance exercise on the physiologic adaptations to pregnancy outcomes. *American Journal of Sports Medicine, 24,* S28-S29.
17. Cross, K., & Worrell, T. (1999). Effects of a static stretching program on the incidence of lower extremity musculotendinous strains. *Journal of Athletic Training, 34,* 11-14.
18. Davies, G. (1995). The need for critical thinking in rehabilitation. *Journal of Sport Rehabilitation, 4,* 1-22.
19. DeLorme, T., & Watkins, A. (1948). Techniques of progressive resistance exercise. *Archives of Physical Medicine and Rehabilitation, 29,* 263-273.
20. Drinkwater, B. (1995). Weight-bearing exercise and bone mass. *Physical Medicine and Rehabilitation Clinics of North America, 6,* 567-578.
21. Evans, W. (1995). What is sarcopenia? *Journal of Gerontology, 50A,* 5-8.
22. Faigenbaum, A. (2001). Strength training and children's health. *Journal of Physical Education, Recreation and Dance, 72,* 24-30.
23. Faigenbaum, A., Kraemer, W., Cahill, B., Chandler, J., Dziados, J., Elfrink, L., Forman, E., Gaudiose, M., Micheli, L., Nitka, M., & Roberts, S. (1996). Youth resistance training: Position statement paper and literature review. *Strength and Conditioning, 18,* 62-75.
24. Faigenbaum, A., & Westcott, W. (2000). *Strength and power for young athletes*. Champaign, IL: Human Kinetics.
25. Fiatarone, M.A., Marks, E.C., Ryan, N.D., Meredith, C.N., Lipsitz, L.A., & Evans, W. (1990). High-intensity strength training in nonagenarians: Effects on skeletal muscle. *Journal of the American Medical Association, 263,* 3029-3034.
26. Fiatarone, M., O'Neill, E., Ryan, N., Clements, K., Solares, G., Nelson, M., Roberts, S., Kehayias, J., Lipsitz, L., & Evans, W. (1990). Exercise training and nutritional supplementation for physical frailty in very elderly people. *New England Journal of Medicine, 330,* 1769-1775.
27. Fleck, S. (1999). Periodized strength training: A critical review. *Journal of Strength and Conditioning Research, 13,* 82-89.
28. Fleck, S., & Kraemer, W. (1996). *Periodization breakthrough*. New York: Advanced Research Press.
29. Fleck, S., & Kraemer, W. (1997). *Designing resistance training programs* (2nd ed.). Champaign, IL: Human Kinetics.
30. Fleck, S., & Schutt, R. (1985). Types of strength training. *Clinics in Sports Medicine, 4,* 150-169.
31. Flessas, A.P., Connelly, G.P., Handa, S., Tilney, C.R., Kloster, C.K., Rimmer, R.H., Keefe, J.F., Klein, M.D., Ryan, T.J. (1976). Effects of isometric exercise on the end diastolic pressures, volumes and function of the left ventricle in man. *Circulation, 59,* 839-847.
32. Frontera, W., Meredith, C., O'Reilly, K., Knuttgen, H., & Evans, W. (1988). Strength conditioning of older men: Skeletal muscle hypertrophy and improved function. *Journal of Applied Physiology, 42,* 1038-1044.
33. Fry, A., & Kraemer, W. (1997). Resistance exercise overtraining and overreaching. *Sports Medicine, 23*(2), 106-129.
34. Graves, J., Pollock, M., Leggett, S., Braith, R., Carpenter, D., & Bishop, L. (1988). Effect of reduced frequency on muscular strength. *International Journal of Sports Medicine, 9,* 316-319.
35. Hartig, D., & Henderson, J. (1999). Increasing hamstring flexibility decreases lower extremity overuse injuries in military basic trainees. *American Journal of Sports Medicine, 27,* 173-176.
36. Hass, C., Garzarella, L., De Hoyos, D., & Pollock, M. (2000). Single versus multiple sets in long-term recreational weightlifters. *Medicine and Science in Sports and Exercise, 32,* 235-242.
37. Hawkins, S., Schroeder, E., Wiswell, R., Jaque, S., Marcell, T., & Costa, T. (1999). Eccentric muscle action increases site-specific osteogenic response. *Medicine and Science in Sports and Exercise, 31,* 1287-1292.
38. Hettinger, R., & Muller, E. (1953). Muskelleistung und muskeltraining (Muscle achievement and muscle training). *Arbeits Physiologie, 15,* 111-126.
39. Hoeger, W., Barette, S., Hale, D., & Hopkins, D. (1987). Relationship between repetitions and selected percentages on the one repletion maximum. *Journal of Applied Sport Science Research, 1,* 11-13.
40. Jacobson, B. (1986). A comparison of two progressive weight training techniques on knee extensor strength. *Athletic Training, 21,* 315-319.
41. Kelemen, M.H., Stewart, K., Gillilan, R.E., Ewart, C.K., Valenti, S.A., Manley, J.D., Kelemen, M.D. (1986). Circuit weight training in cardiac patients. *Journal of the American College of Cardiology, 7,* 38-42.
42. Kraemer, W. (1983). Exercise prescription in weight training: Manipulating program variables. *National Strength and Conditioning Association Journal, 5,* 58-59.
43. Kraemer, W., Noble, B., Culver, B., Clark, M. (1987). Physiologic responses to heavy resistance exercise with very short rest periods. *International Journal of Sports Medicine, 8,* 247-252.
44. Kraemer, W., Ratamess, N., Fry, A., Triplett-McBride, T., Koziris, P., Bauer, J., Lynch, J., & Fleck, S. (2000). Influence of resistance training volume and periodization on physiological and performance adaptations in collegiate women tennis players. *American Journal of Sports Medicine, 28*(5), 626-632.
45. Kramer, J., Stone, M., O'Bryant, H., Conley, M., Johnson, R., Nieman, D., Honeycutt, D., & Hoke, T. (1997). Effects of single vs. multiple sets of weight training: Impact of volume, intensity and variation. *Journal of Strength and Conditioning Research, 11*(3), 143-147.
46. Lombardi, V. (2000). 1998 U.S. weight training injuries and deaths. *Medicine and Science in Sports and Exercise, 32,* S346.
47. Marx, J., Ratamess, N., Nindl, B., Gotshalk, L., Volek, J., Dohi, K., Bush, J., Gomez, A., Mazzetti, S., Fleck, S., Hakkinen, K., Newton, R., & Kraemer, W. (2001). Low volume circuit versus high volume periodized resistance training in women. *Medicine and Science in Sports and Exercise, 33,* 635-643.
48. Mazzette, S., Kraemer, W., Volek, J., Duncan, N., Ratamess, N., Gomez, A., Newton, R., Hakkinen, K., & Fleck, S. (2000). The influence of direct supervision of resistance training on strength performance. *Medicine and Science in Sports and Exercise, 32,* 1175-1184.
49. McCartney, N. (1998). Role of resistance training in heart disease. *Medicine and Science in Sports and Exercise, 30*(10, Suppl.), S396-S402.
50. McGee, D., Jessee, T., Stone, H., & Blessing, D. (1992). Leg and hip endurance adaptations to three weight training programs. *Journal of Applied Sport Science Research, 6,* 92-95.
51. Mikesky, A., Gidding, C., Mathews, W., & Gonyea, W. (1991). Changes in muscle fiber size and composition in response to heavy-resistance exercise. *Medicine and Science in Sports and Exercise, 23,* 1042-1049.
52. Morris, F., Naughton, G., Gibbs, J., Carlson, J., & Wark, J. (1997). Prospective ten-month exercise intervention in premenarcheal girls: Positive effects on bone and lean mass. *Journal of Bone and Mineral Research, 12,* 1453-1462.
53. Nelson, M., Fiatarone, M., Morganti, C., Trice, I., Greenberg, R., & Evans, W. (1994). Effects of high intensity strength training on multiple risk factors for osteoporotic fractures. *Journal of the American Medical Association, 272,* 1909-1914.
54. Pearson, D., Faigenbaum, A., Conley, M., & Kraemer, W. (2000). The National Strength and Conditioning Association's basic guidelines for the resistance training of athletes. *Strength and Conditioning Journal, 22*(4), 14-27.
55. Pollock, M., Franklin, B., Balady, G., Chaitman, B., Fleg, J., Fletcher, B., Limacher, M., Pina, I., Stein, R., Williams, M. Bazzarre, T. (2000). Resistance exercise in individuals with and without cardiovascular disease: Benefits, rationale, safety and prescription. *Circulation, 101*(7), 828-833.
56. Potach, D., & Chu, D. (2000). Plyometric training. In T. Baechle & R. Earle (Eds.), *Essentials of strength training and conditioning* (2nd ed., pp. 427-440). Champaign, IL: Human Kinetics.
57. Smith, A., Andrish, J., & Micheli, L. (1993). The prevention of sports injuries of children and adolescents. *Medicine and Science in Sports and Exercise, 25*(Suppl. 8), 1-7.
58. Stone, M., Keith, R., Kearney, J., Fleck, S., Wilson, G., & Triplett, N. (1991). Overtraining: A review of signs and symptoms. *Journal of Applied Strength and Conditioning Research, 5,* 35-50.
59. Westcott, W., & Baechle, T. (1999). *Strength training for seniors*. Champaign, IL: Human Kinetics.

thirteen

Exercise Prescription for Flexibility and Low Back Function

Wendell Liemohn

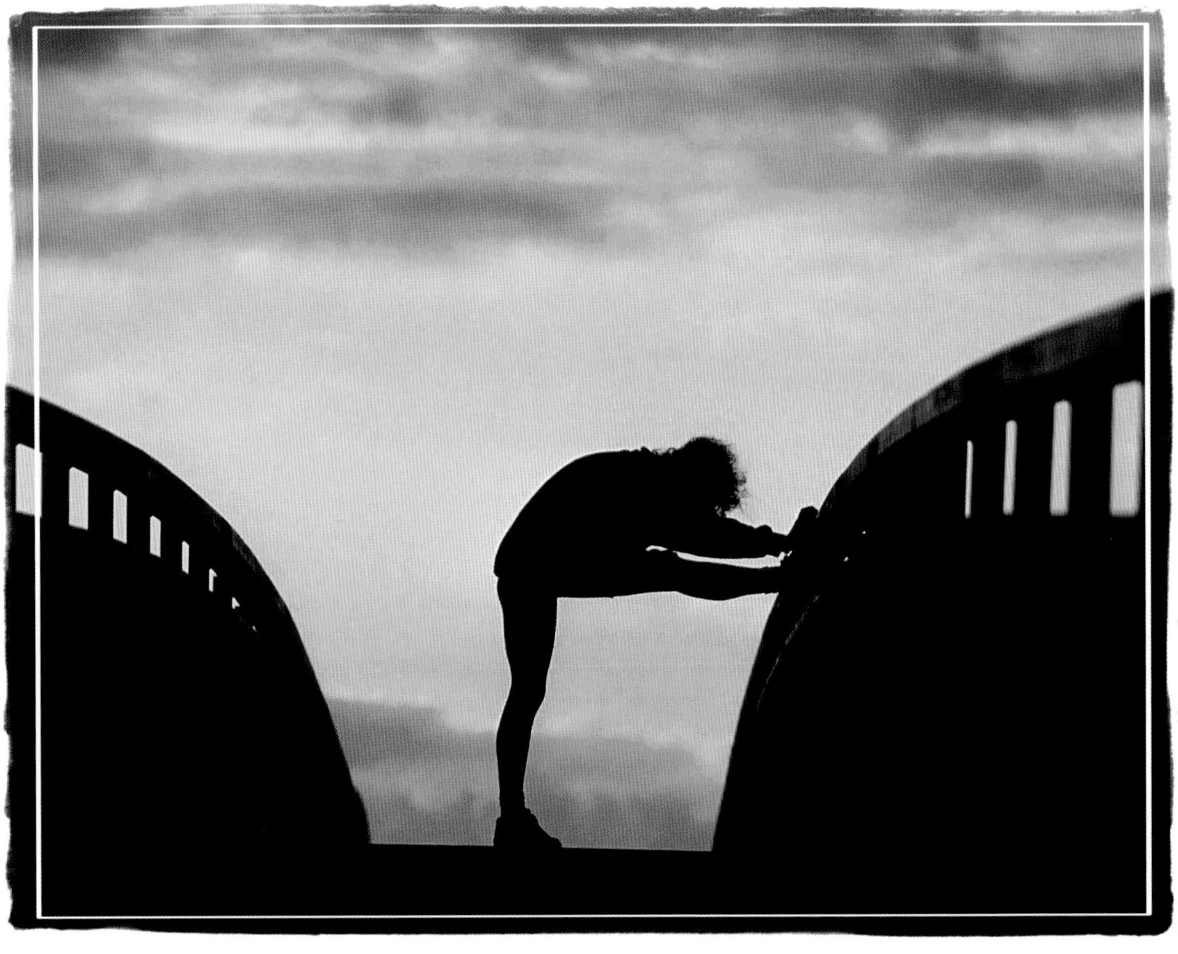

Objectives

The reader will be able to do the following:

1. Describe a motion segment, the shock absorbers of the spine, and the role of the facet joints.
2. Differentiate between functional and structural spinal curves and describe limitations that either may impose on exercise programs for the afflicted individual.
3. Explain why it is important that the muscles of the trunk be able to control pelvic positioning.
4. Differentiate between the low back problems typically seen in adults and those seen in youth.
5. Describe how the anatomical limitations of ROM should be a factor as you prescribe ROM exercises for your clients.
6. Explain what is meant by core strength and describe how the muscles of the trunk can work together as a dynamic corset and how they can be strengthened.
7. Describe exercises that will increase the strength and endurance of those muscles that are fundamental to the development of core strength.

Low back pain (LBP) is one of the most common complaints among adults in the United States; it accounts for more lost person-hours than any other type of occupational injury and is the most frequent cause of activity limitation in individuals under age 45. The discussion of LBP in this chapter begins with a review of select anatomical and biomechanical concepts of the trunk and spine. The types of LBP seen in adults versus those seen more often in youth are then explored. A discussion follows on potential stresses to the spine and how they can produce symptoms related to LBP. This is followed by a discussion on core strength. The last section describes exercises that can be used to improve flexibility and low back function.

Anatomy of the Spine

The spine is depicted in figures 27.2 and 27.9. In our discussion of LBP, the emphasis is on the five lumbar vertebrae stacked on the sacrum; the latter is also the posterior wall of the pelvis. When LBP is discussed, the fundamental unit of the lumbar spine is the **motion segment**; it consists of two vertebrae and their intervening **disc** (figure 13.1). The bodies of the vertebrae and their intervening disc are sometimes referred to as the anterior aspect of the motion segment. The posterior aspect of the motion segment is attached to the anterior aspect by the pedicles; the latter provide the lateral boundary of the foramen (vertical passageway) for the spinal cord. In addition to the transverse and spinous processes, the posterior elements of the vertebrae include the superior and inferior articular processes; each of their junctions is referred to as a zygapophyseal or **facet joint**. In addition to assisting in supporting loads on the spine, the facet joints control the amount and the direction of vertebral movement.

A series of ligaments provide additional reinforcement for the vertebrae of the spine. The anterior and posterior longitudinal ligaments provide stability for the anterior portion of the motion segments; they run the length of the spine on the anterior and posterior surfaces of the bodies of the vertebrae as well as the intervertebral discs. The ligaments that support the posterior aspect of the motion segment include the ligamentum flavum; it is located immediately behind the spinal cord and serves as its posterior boundary. Also reinforcing the posterior aspect of the motion segments are the facet joint capsular ligaments; they span the synovial joints formed by the superior and inferior articular processes between each vertebral pair. The posterior aspects of each motion segment are reinforced further by the interspinous and supraspinous ligaments; they of course are attached to the spinous

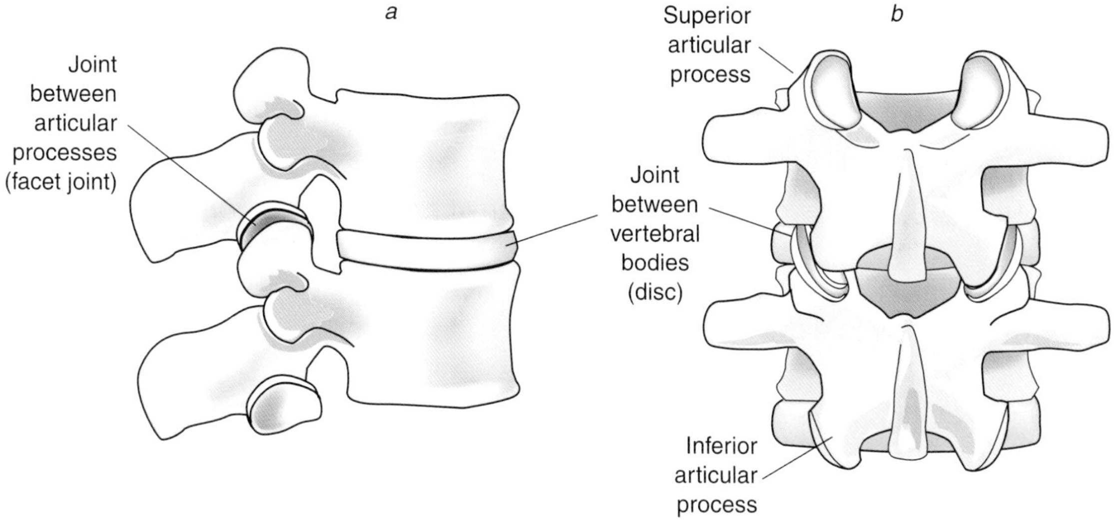

Figure 13.1 Lumbar vertebral motion segment. Note how the facet joints (i.e., the junction of the superior and inferior articular processes) are positioned to provide stability and control the amount and direction of movement.

processes. All of these ligaments have pain receptors; therefore, a sprain to any of them can signal a potential back problem.

The discs enable each vertebra to be more mobile (figure 13.2). Each intervertebral disc consists of a centrally placed nucleus (nucleus pulposus) surrounded by a sheath of connective tissue fibers (anulus fibrosis); a disc is somewhat analogous to a jelly donut (i.e., the disc has a nucleus and periphery). Intervertebral discs act as spacers and shock absorbers; when compressive forces are placed on the spine (e.g., carrying a load), the nucleus of the disc exerts pressure in all directions to help absorb the force. The disc most vulnerable to injury in the low back is the one between the fifth lumbar vertebra and the sacrum (i.e., L5–S1 disc); this is logical because its load is greater than that of any of the other discs. The next most often injured disc in the low back is the one between L4 and L5.[1] Except for their periphery, the discs do not have pain receptors; however, if the nucleus of a disc breaks through its normal boundaries, the disc's peripheral pain receptors will be activated. (The pain receptors in the ligaments of the spine can also quickly tell the body when something is wrong in a ligament or in an adjacent damaged disc that exceeds its normal confines.) If a disc is diseased or injured, its ability to withstand stress is adversely affected and the motion segment to which it belongs may become unstable.

The disc is avascular (i.e., without a blood supply); its nutrition is enhanced by motion occurring in the spine (e.g., motion enables the disc to absorb nutrients through the vertebral end plates). Long-term bed rest and smoking similarly decrease nutrition to the disc (2). However, when we sleep, discs imbibe fluid and actually become "tighter" than they were at the end of the day; for this reason back injuries often occur in the mornings when these fuller discs permit less movement. Slow warm-ups before strenuous exercise or work are desirable.

The curvatures of the spine as viewed from the side are described as lordotic when they are concave and **kyphotic** when they are convex; cervical and lumbar curves are normally lordotic and the thoracic curve is kyphotic. Exaggerations of these curves are not desirable. For example, an increased anterior (or forward) pelvic tilt would increase the lordotic curve in the lumbar area; this posture increases stresses on ligaments, discs, vertebrae, and the musculature of the spine. A small lumbar lordotic curve is natural and, along with the cervical lordosis and thoracic kyphosis curves, assists the discs in cushioning compressive forces occurring to the spine in activities of daily living. Although some believe that an excessive lordosis is a risk factor for low back pain, not all research supports this contention. Factors such as being overweight, wearing high heels often, or lack of appropriate muscle length or strength can affect the degree of lordosis. With respect to the latter, tightness in the hip flexors (e.g., the iliopsoas) can increase the lordotic curve by causing an anterior pelvic tilt; conversely, tightness in the hamstrings can reduce the lordosis (see figures 9.5 and 27.10).

[1] Disc pathology also occurs in the cervical spine. Poor sitting postures can contribute to this condition too; however, in cervical dysfunction a motion segment of the neck corresponding to the brachial plexus is the site of the problem.

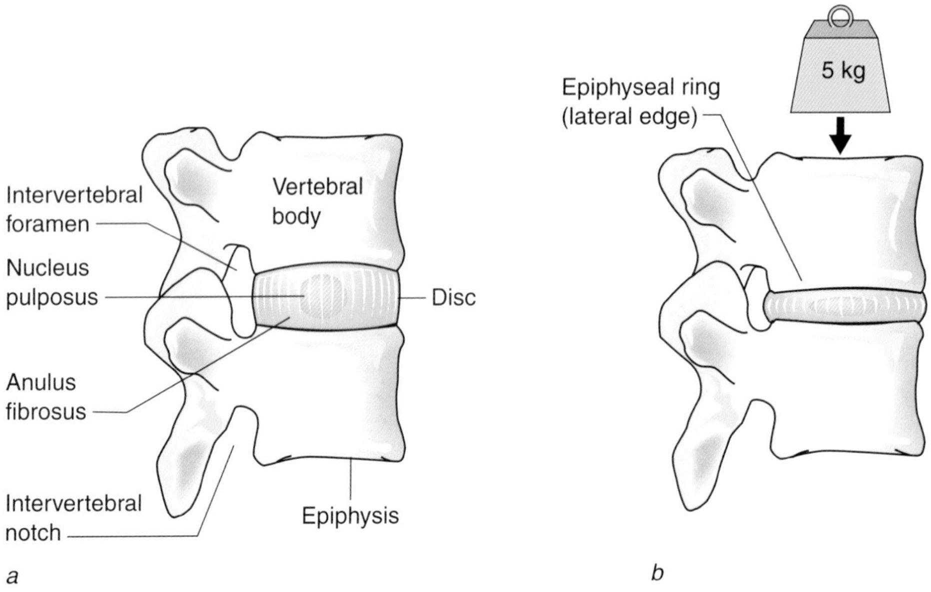

Figure 13.2 Discs allow flexibility and act as shock absorbers. In adults, most low back problems start in the disc. When weight is added (in this case perpendicular to the disc), the force is absorbed in all directions; however, if the external force were applied obliquely, the pressure within the disc would be away from the direction of the applied force.

1 In Review

The fundamental unit of the spine is the motion segment; it consists of two vertebrae and their intervening disc.The spinal discs absorb shock to the vertebral column by exerting pressure in all directions to help absorb the force. Most back problems begin in the disc; the disc most often injured is the one between L5 and S1. Natural curvatures of the spine assist the discs in cushioning compressive forces. Although the facet joints aid in supporting loads, one of their primary responsibilities is controlling the amount and direction of spinal movement such as that seen in rotation.

Spinal Movement

Chapter 9 provides a general review of spinal movement constraints. This section discusses flexion, spinal curvature, extension, and lateral movement.

Flexion

The flexion movements seen in curl-up and crunch-type exercises are discussed in chapter 27. In these exercises, each lumbar vertebra rotates from its backward tilted position to a neutral or **end-ROM** (straightened lumbar) position. After the lumbar spine is straightened in the up movement of the curl-up or crunch, for example, no further spinal flexion can take place (see figure 9.3). If the crunch movement is continued until a full sit-up position is reached, the movement must occur at the hip joint. Then the muscles crossing this joint (e.g., psoas and iliacus) would be the prime movers as the abdominals contract statically; the drawbacks to this type of movement are discussed later in this chapter.

Functional/Structural Spinal Curves

Spinal curves are called **functional** if the curve can be removed by assuming a posture that takes away the force responsible for the curve. Figure 13.3 provides an example of how leg posture affects the pull of the psoas musculature on the lumbar spine (figure 13.3*a*); when the paired psoas are relaxed (figure 13.3*b*), the lordotic curve is reduced. Habitually tight hip flexors, however, will cause an anterior tilt of the pelvis and thus reduce ROM at the hip joint; if this happens, a functional curve may become **structural**. A structural curve would not be amenable to easy reduction; such curves result from an unhealthy posture assumed over a period of years. For example, if the individual in figure 13.3 had a

a

b

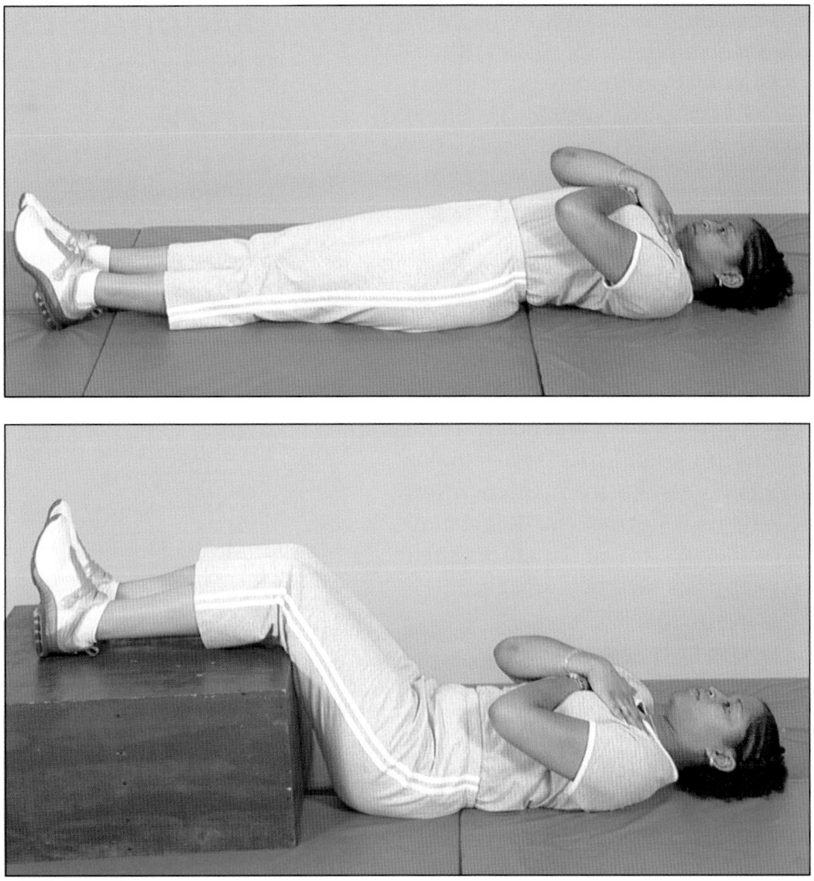

Figure 13.3 *(a)* When the supine posture is assumed, the pull of the psoas muscle can produce an exaggerated lordotic curve. *(b)* When the legs are supported, the psoas relaxes and the lordotic curve flattens if it is a functional curve. However, if the lordosis were a structural curve, a curve similar to that seen in (*a*) would be seen in (*b*) despite the absence of muscle tension.

structural lumbar lordosis, the lordotic curve would be retained regardless of whether the legs were supported.

A person with a structural lumbar lordosis would have extreme difficulty in doing crunches because of lack of mobility in the **lumbosacral** area. Although this person might be able to do sit-ups by using the hip flexors if the feet were held, this could exacerbate the problem. It would be far better for the exercise leader to provide a substitute abdominal exercise such as isometric holds for an individual with this mobility problem.

Extension

As discussed in chapter 9, spinal extension movements / postures are used less often than spinal flexion ones in most activities of daily living; therefore, it should not be any surprise that with aging there is often a greater loss in extension ROM than flexion ROM. For example, an individual sitting for many hours each day at a computer terminal often assumes a "slumping" posture for much of this time; an increase in thoracic kyphosis, round shoulders, and a decrease in lumbar lordosis might be the result of continued use of such a poor posture (see figure 9.1). If this individual does not extend the spine or retract the shoulders periodically, the capability of doing these movements may be lessened and the poor posture may become structural. Sitting postures are usually more stressful on the spine than standing postures because the lordotic curve is usually diminished; when this happens the individual may "hang" on his or her ligaments (i.e., posterior ligaments of the lumbar spine) or use the back musculature to hold this posture. Another factor is that most individuals spend much more time sitting, whether at a desk, work station, or in a vehicle, than they do standing. The end result is that greater compressive forces are placed on intervertebral discs. The slump posture shown in figure 9.1 is an example of a person hanging in end-ROM. Hanging in end-ROM can lengthen the ligaments and increase the compressive forces placed on intervertebral discs. Keeping the spine in a neutral position (e.g., midway between maximum flexion and extension) is much more desirable.

Lateral Flexion and Rotation

Because some of the most forceful stresses are placed on the discs in movements that combine bending and rotation, exercises involving these movements should always be done under muscle control. In other words, exercises involving intervertebral movement should not be done ballistically (e.g., movements in which momentum plays a major role). If the movement results from momentum rather than muscle control, normal end-ROM may be exceeded and connective tissue structures such as spinal ligaments or discs may be damaged.

Lateral Curvatures

When the spine is viewed from the back, ideally a straight vertical line is seen; however, minor lateral deviations are prevalent and may be related to something so nominal as hand dominance. Therapeutic exercise alone is not very effective in correcting major lateral curves (e.g., a scoliosis). Moreover, inappropriate exercise prescription can make a scoliotic condition worse. Therefore, it is imperative that exercise leaders obtain advice from a physical therapist, an orthopedic surgeon, or other appropriate medical personnel before giving or prescribing exercises in an attempt to straighten or correct a scoliotic curve. In young individuals with a scoliosis, bracing is the mainstay of nonoperative therapy. However, because bracing is not always effective and rarely is effective for adults, internal fixation devices often are implanted surgically (5). The exercise program for the scoliotic patient with either external bracing or internal fixation would have to incorporate the limitations that either device presents on ROM and general mobility.

2 In Review

Functional curves can be removed by assuming a posture that reduces the force that caused the curve. Structural curves usually develop over a period of years and are not easily removed.

Mechanics of the Spine and Hip Joint

For this discussion, the reader is encouraged to refer to figures 9.3, 9.5, and 27.9. The muscles crossing the hip joint can be viewed as guy wires bracing the pelvis; if any of these guy wires are too tight, the abdominal musculature will have difficulty in controlling pelvic positioning. Because the sacral portion of the pelvis is the foundation for the "kinetic chain" of 24 vertebrae stacked on it, pelvic positioning is important to the integrity of the spine. For example, tightness in the hamstrings can severely affect the ability of the pelvis to be tilted anteriorly, and thus pelvic ROM is diminished. If the body subsequently were subjected to an unplanned stress (e.g., stepping in a hole or slipping on ice), body parts are obligated to give with the resulting force. If the hamstrings cannot give, connective tissue structures of the spine may have to absorb the stress. If there is tearing or other damage to spinal ligaments, discs, or both, a step toward an acute low back problem has been made. A shortened I-T band or a tightened piriformis also might create a problem; however, it has been contended that the "piriformis syndrome" is usually caused by other pathology (19), More in-depth discussions of biomechanical stresses to the spine appear elsewhere (4, 10, 15, 17, 19).

3 In Review

The pelvis serves as the foundation for the spine, so the ability of the trunk muscles to control pelvic positioning is essential to having a healthy back. It is essential that neither the hip flexors nor hip extensors are too tight. Because the body is a kinetic chain, tightness in other lower extremity muscles can affect static and dynamic postures.

Low Back Pain: A Repetitive Microtrauma Injury

Even though some individuals might remember a specific movement that they believe caused their low back problem, this is not generally the case. Rather, the analogy of the straw that breaks the camel's back usually better describes the occurrence of a low back problem.

Low Back Problems Seen in Adults

It has been contended that most cases of acute LBP in adults are caused by damage to the intervertebral discs (6). However, one incorrect movement seldom causes injury to a disc. LBP such as a disc injury typically is caused by a succession of the same type of inappropriate movements occurring over time; because of this, LBP often is called either a repetitive microtrauma condition or repetitive motion injury.

If one takes a paper clip and bends it once, it is still quite strong; however, its molecular makeup has been changed and it will never be the same again. The paper clip can be further bent and remain strong, but with each successive bend it becomes weaker; with continual bending it eventually breaks. Similarly, one could use poor biomechanics in lifting an object; however, the one maneuver is not apt to cause a back problem. If poor biomechanics in lifting objects are repeated hundreds of times, however, connective tissue structures of the spine can weaken like the paper clip and eventually yield to even a nominal stress (e.g., bending to the floor to pick up a paper clip). It might not be until this time that acute symptoms are noted.

Cumulative repetitive microtrauma affects the disc's homeostasis, and eventually it adversely alters the disc's pivotal responsibility as a shock absorber of the spinal unit. For example, minor tears in the periphery of the disc can be painful and can forewarn of more serious problems. Eventually, the jelly-like nucleus may leak out of its normal confines and cause an unstable motion segment; this would be analogous to a radial tire losing air pressure and its effect on cornering ability. When a disc is affected, specific movements may be exceedingly painful and the condition will get worse unless appropriate interventions are made. Thus, what started as a minor problem can evolve into a major one. The key is to never let the problem get started; maintaining good physical fitness and strengthening the trunk musculature with appropriate exercises are keys to decreasing the chances of having LBP.

Low Back Problems Seen in Youth

In youth, low back problems are not typically seen in the disc, as in adults, but rather in the part of the vertebrae posterior to the spinal cord, including the superior and inferior articular processes (refer to figure 13.1). The part of a vertebra between the superior and inferior articular processes is called the **pars interarticularis**. Stress to this area can lead to complications such as **spondylolysis** and **spondylolisthesis**. The former condition is essentially a stress fracture in the pars interarticularis on one side; sometimes it evolves into a frank (complete) fracture on both sides of a spinous process, either because the bone does not unite properly or because it fails to withstand the stress to which it is subjected. Then the condition is called spondylolisthesis, and the body of the vertebra is apt to slip over the vertebra below. This injury usually occurs at the lumbosacral junction (i.e., L5 slipping over S1).

Although the causes of spondylolisthesis might include genetic ties, stresses resulting from participation in activities such as weightlifting or gymnastics could also be the cause. Appropriate coaching and guidance in athletic activities for youth are important for avoiding unhealthy stresses on growing bones. Not all cases of spondylolysis and spondylolisthesis necessarily begin before skeletal maturity; although the exact age of onset might be unknown, many professional football players have this condition (16). Spondylolisthesis has been cited as the most likely cause of LBP in patients under 26 years of age, but it is rarely the sole cause of LBP in individuals over 40 (5).

Repetitive hyperextension can also damage the facet joints. They are synovial joints and their articular cartilage can be subject to injury in this type of movement. Although this may happen in youth, damage to articular cartilage could eventually lead to arthritic problems.

4 In Review

LBP is often referred to as a repetitive microtrauma or repetitive motion injury because its development occurs over a period of time as opposed to being the result of one traumatic incident. Low back problems in adults usually originate in the disc; in youth, low back problems usually originate in the posterior elements of the vertebrae.

Exercise Considerations: Preventive and Therapeutic

"Stepped-up" versions of the exercises viewed as being therapeutic often can be used as prophylactic (preventive) exercises. Ideally ROM, strength, or both should be improved before their deficiencies cause a problem.

ROM and Low Back Function

As discussed in chapter 9, ROM deficiencies in the spine and its supporting structures have been viewed as prognostic indicators of LBP. Good ROM can decrease the probability of a low back problem; once LBP occurs, good ROM can reduce the severity of the problem.

As displayed in figure 27.9, a limited degree of spinal mobility in the sagittal plane (e.g., flexion, extension) and the coronal plane (e.g., lateral flexion) is present in the cervical and lumbar segments. Although rotation is restricted in the lumbar and thoracic regions, a considerable amount is present in the cervical region, particularly between C1 and C2.

Extension of the spine is an issue often ignored or misinterpreted in exercise programs. Although it is acknowledged that ballistic-extension movements of the spine (and ballistic-rotation movements) are totally inappropriate, as discussed in chapter 9, slow and controlled extension movements are appropriate and should be included in exercise programs.

Trunk Strength and Low Back Function

The trunk is sometimes referred to as the core of the body; thus, the musculature of the spine and the abdominal wall is positioned to contribute to core strength and thus to core stability. Core strength and stability have been the focus of much attention in recent years. Individuals with good core strength and endurance are less apt to have LBP; moreover, having good core stability can enhance performance in athletic as well as in work-related activities. The large muscles of the spine that contribute to core stability include the erector spinae, multifidus, and quadratus lumborum (see figure 13.4). The abdominal muscles that contribute to core stability include the rectus abdominis, internal and external obliques, and transversus abdominis. The role of the transversus abdominis in core stability particularly has been emphasized in the past few years.

Although the popular literature often indicts weakened abdominal musculature as a prime cause of LBP, the musculature of the spine is proportionately weaker than the abdominal musculature in low back patients (3). Moreover, in our review of exercise intervention research in which good randomized, controlled trial designs were followed in treating chronic LBP, three studies were found and each emphasized development of extensor muscles of the spine (10). However, before accepting this at face value, one should realize that dependent on the specific diagnosis of the spine malady, extension-biased exercises might be appropriate for one diagnosis and contraindicated for another. This notwithstanding, the strength of the abdominal muscles is also vital to the maintenance of a healthy spine; therefore, exercises that will be discussed include strengthening exercises for the major trunk muscles believed to be important for core stability.

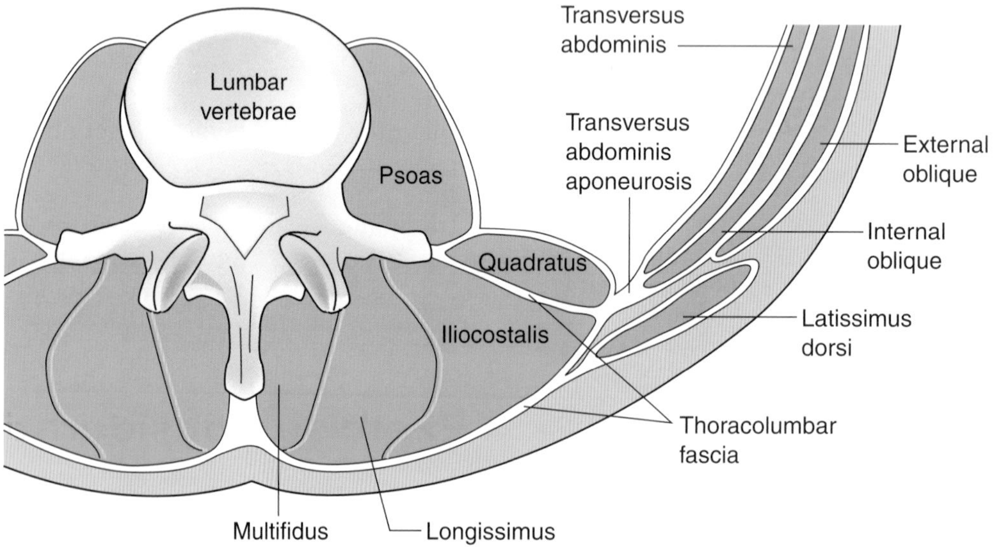

Figure 13.4 Cross-section of the major muscles of the trunk that contribute to core stability. Note in particular how the transversus abdominis attaches to the connective tissue sheath that houses the erector spinae (ilio costalis and longissimus) and multifidus; with the obliques, this muscle envelopes the rectus abdominis anteriorly as their respective sides meet at the linea alba. Although the internal oblique also attaches to this sheath, its attachment is quite narrow and hence it cannot exert as much of a lateral stabilizing force (hoop tension) as the transversus abdominis.

An Examination of Exercises That Involve Muscles of the Spine

One of the exercises that has gained in popularity in recent years both as a therapeutic exercise in the clinic as well as an exercise that can be used in conditioning programs is the quadruped (see appendix). Although it is not considered a challenging strength-development exercise for the back musculature, it can improve the endurance of these important muscles; moreover, the compression force that it places on the discs is nominal. (Disc compression forces are discussed in more detail later in this chapter.) If the contralateral limbs are raised, the bird dog exercise becomes more difficult and requires additional bracing of the abdominal muscles; thus, it is an exercise not only for the erector spinae and multifidus but also for the lateral abdominals. Another often recommended exercise for the development of spinal musculature is back extension on the Roman chair. A modification of this piece of equipment called the variable angle Roman chair is appropriate for those who are too weak to use a regular Roman chair, have an acute LBP condition, or are recovering from surgery. A comparable back extension exercise can be done from a table or therapy ball with assistance (see appendix). When undertaking trunk extension exercises to develop back extensor muscle strength, the exerciser should never exceed his or her normal lordosis when doing the trunk raise (i.e., the exerciser should not hyperextend the spine). Another key point is that back muscle endurance appears to be more important than back muscle strength relative to risk factors for LBP.

A muscle of the spine that in the past received little emphasis but is now deemed important to spine function and core stability is the quadratus lumborum (figure 13.5). Because its origin is on the posterior part of the iliac crest and the iliolumbar ligament and its insertion is on the last rib and the transverse processes of the upper four lumbar ver-

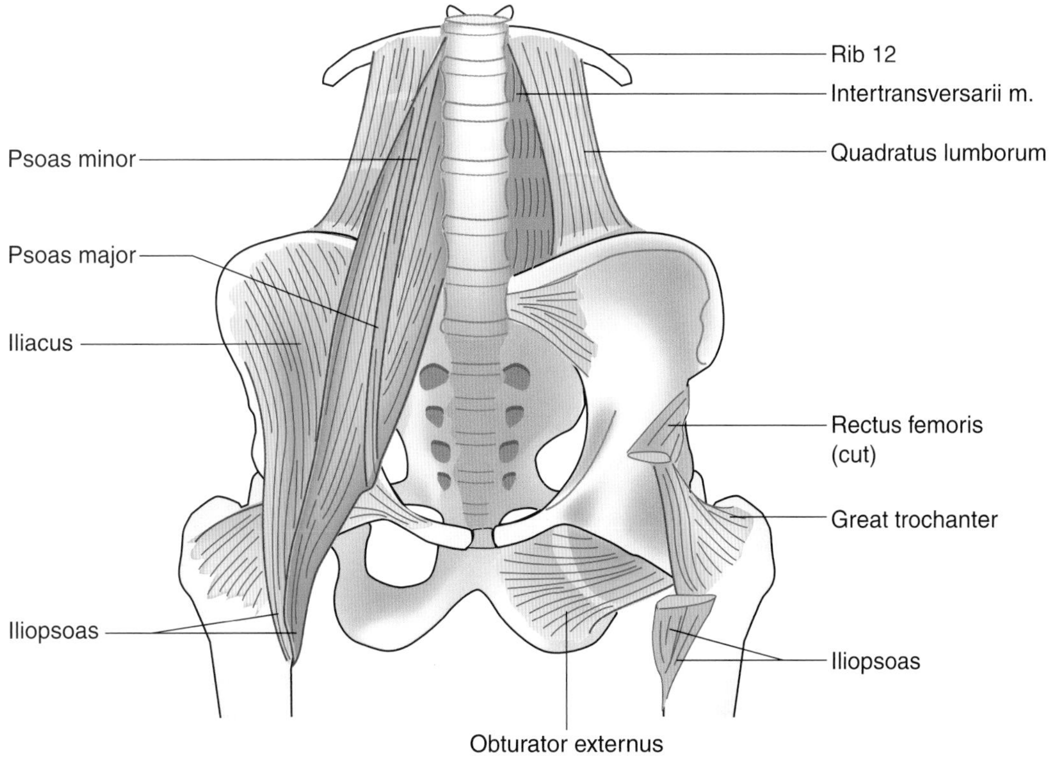

Figure 13.5 The fibers of the quadratus lumborum run vertically from the crest of the ilia to the 12th rib; this muscle is aligned to act in the frontal plane to laterally flex or to control lateral flexion. In the latter role it is a strong contributor to core stability. (Note also the direction of the fibers of the psoas; although the psoas is a strong flexor at the hip joint, its fibers are aligned to exert strong compression forces on the lumbar intervertebral discs. For this reason it is most important to consider these compressive forces when prescribing abdominal strengthening exercises.)

tebrae, it is well positioned to provide core stability in the frontal plane. An exercise that develops not only the quadratus lumborum but also the lateral abdominals is the horizontal isometric bridge (see appendix). Because this exercise involves only nominal contraction of the psoas, it does not place much compressive pressure on the intervertebral discs of the lumbar vertebrae (1, 9).

5 In Review

Lack of strength and particularly insufficient endurance in the back musculature often are seen in individuals with LBP. Moreover, in those individuals, the back musculature often is proportionately weaker than the abdominal musculature; in part this might be attributable to neglect of extensor muscle strength in exercise programs. In performing dynamic extension exercises, the participant should not exceed the normal lumbar lordosis. Some of the exercises designed to improve the strength and endurance of the muscles of the spine are also good exercises for the lateral abdominal muscles.

An Examination of Exercises That Involve the Muscles of the Abdominal Wall

Even though the back musculature may be disproportionately weaker in LBP patients, it is still imperative that the abdominal muscles not be neglected. For example, the rectus abdominis is in a position to control the tilt of the pelvis directly (figure 9.5); this is an important consideration in maintaining a healthy spine. Development of the rectus abdominis is emphasized in crunch-type activities. To repeat the discussion appearing earlier in this chapter, it is only necessary to lift the shoulders off the exercise surface; it is most important, particularly for the less fit, to minimize the role of the hip flexors (e.g., the paired psoas) in any trunk flexion exercise. Unfortunately, many individuals have thought that bending the knees reduces the role of the psoas muscles; this is not so, particularly if the feet are supported. Moreover, the psoas muscles place extreme compressive forces on the discs of the lumbar motion segments of the vertebral column in activities such as sit-ups or bilateral leg lifts.

Posterior rotation of the pelvis is often incorporated into abdominal strengthening exercises; for someone with disc disease, this is not always appropriate. Posterior rotation of the pelvis typically removes the lumbar lordosis; such a movement can prompt the nucleus of the intervertebral disc to migrate posteriorly. If the disc is damaged, pressure can be placed on the damaged tissue and its pain receptors or even on spinal nerves. McGill (12) suggested that to rectify this potential problem in a person with disc disease, the exerciser should (a) keep one leg extended while bending the contralateral knee and (b) place the palm of one hand on the exercise surface under the lumbar lordotic curve (i.e., the small of the back).

In standard crunch-type activities, the rectus abdominis does most of the work and the lateral abdominal muscles seldom are called into play. The lateral abdominal muscles (i.e., transversus abdominis, internal and external obliques) also should be developed because by their attachments both anteriorly (i.e., where they ensheathe the rectus abdominis) and posteriorly (i.e., where they attach to extensive connective tissue structures of the spine that ensheathe the erector spinae and the multifidus), the lateral abdominal muscles can enhance both anterior and posterior muscle groups. Strong lateral abdominal muscles are in a position to brace and splint the trunk; this can help prevent undesirable rotary motion in addition to protecting the back as heavy objects are lifted. From a biomechanical perspective, the lateral abdominal muscles are extremely important to attain and maintain a healthy low back.

A good way to involve the lateral abdominals in crunch-type exercises is to hollow the abdominal area: in other words, bring the navel toward the spine before performing the crunch. The latter technique reduces the role of the rectus abdominis and puts more emphasis on the lateral abdominals. Exercises that will enhance the development of the lateral musculature also include diagonal crunches and isometrics. Besides doing the diagonal curl dynamically, the participant can perform the diagonal curl isometrically by using challenging lengths of isometric holds (e.g., 5-30 s). Although isometric exercises may be considered passé for limb movements because of lack of specificity of training, in reality isometrics are most specific to the stabilization of the spine (13). The previously mentioned horizontal isometric side bridge is also an excellent exercise. With strong lateral abdominals it is much easier to stabilize and brace the spine; if one has a strong core, she or he will be much less susceptible to the repetitive microtrauma that can lead to serious cases of LBP.

Two recently published and excellent studies discussed trunk flexion exercises from a cost-benefit perspective (1, 9). In essence, these studies determined the percentage of maximal voluntary contraction (MVC) of select muscles used in common abdominal strengthening activities. Concurrently they determined either indirectly or directly the amount of compressive force each exercise placed on intervertebral discs (i.e., which would indicate psoas activity). Ideally, there should be a high percentage of MVC of the abdominal muscles; this would be a benefit. However, a high level of psoas activity would be a cost because the paired psoas can put an extreme amount of compression force on the discs of the spine, which can damage them. The trunk-flexion strengthening exercises presented in the appendix (for both sagittal and frontal planes) were selected because the MVC of the psoas was found to be relatively low and the MVC of one or more of the abdominal muscles was high (9). However, another consideration should be factored into exercise selection: the client's physical fitness level. Obviously, some exercises may be beneficial to athletes in excellent condition but could be inappropriate for other people; thus, sometimes the quality of the movement should be considered along with the physical condition of the exerciser (11).

6 In Review

In individuals with low back problems, the back musculature often is proportionately weaker and/or has less endurance than the abdominal musculature; in part, this might be attributable to neglect of extensor muscle strength in exercise programs. The trunk musculature can work together as a dynamic corset; the lateral abdominal muscles "tie" the flexors and extensors of the spine together and facilitate a strong core. Although the erector spinae, multifidus, and the rectus abdominis are important trunk muscles, the lateral abdominals and the quadratus lumborum warrant special attention to develop a strong core.

Prophylactic Exercises for Enhancing Low Back Function

Even though many injuries and diseases of the low back can be treated conservatively with therapeutic exercise, the diversity and complexity of low back problems are such that they preclude making a simple diagnosis and presenting an exercise regimen for that diagnosis. Moreover, arming a person with a set of therapeutic exercises who does not concurrently understand the nuances of different low back conditions could be dangerous. Because it is beyond the scope of this chapter to discuss these countless nuances, the emphasis in this discussion is on the presentation of sound exercises that enhance low back function. Nevertheless, the exercises presented in the appendix are often used by physical therapists in treating low back patients. For more in-depth information in this area, other sources are available (7, 8, 14).

Exercises to Enhance Flexibility

This chapter's appendix describes exercises recommended for low back flexibility. The guy-wire concept discussed in chapter 9 (see figure 9.5) is helpful to consider when exploring exercises for low back flexibility. Although the trunk musculature (e.g., the abdominals and the erector spinae) is crucial to controlling pelvic positioning, the ability to control the pelvis is reduced or negated if either the hip flexors or the hip extensors are too tight. The bottom line is that having good hip-joint mobility is fundamental to having a healthy spine. Several exercises that can be used to improve ROM in joints and structures relevant to the low back are presented in this chapter's appendix.

Exercises to Develop the Trunk Musculature

This chapter's appendix also describes additional exercises recommended for developing the musculature of the trunk. Key points to remember in doing spinal extension movements is that exercisers should not exceed their normal lumbar lordosis when moving into extension.

Posterior pelvic tilts and crunches are basic to the exercise programs of many individuals for the development of the abdominal musculature. As previously mentioned, when individuals do these exercises, the rectus abdominis often does most of the work and the lateral abdominal muscles are involved minimally.

7 In Review

Maintenance of good hip-joint ROM is essential for a healthy spine. An exerciser should not exceed the normal lordotic curve when doing active back extension exercises. The ROM capabilities of the trunk are quite nominal; keep this in mind when setting up exercise programs for clients. Isometric holds can nicely supplement regular crunches as well as diagonal crunches.

Case Studies

You can check your answers by referring to appendix A.

13.1

An exercise leader is using a double-leg lowering task with a group of relatively fit adults, ostensibly to improve the strength of the abdominals. When questioned about the use of this exercise, he advises you that physical therapists have often used a similar activity to test the abdominal strength of their patients, even those who are symptomatic for LBP. Discuss the appropriateness or inappropriateness of the use of such an exercise.

13.2

An exercise leader is using the sit-and-reach (or standing toe-touch) exercise presumably to improve hip-joint flexibility. Because she is aware that ballistic stretches are usually contraindicated, the exercise leader strongly admonishes her group to perform the exercise with slow and easy stretches. Discuss the appropriateness or inappropriateness of these directions.

13.3

An exercise leader prescribes oblique (diagonal) curls that require the exerciser to maintain a 15-s isometric contraction after at least one shoulder blade is raised from the exercise surface. Discuss the appropriateness or inappropriateness of this activity.

Appendix

Flexibility, Strength, and Endurance Exercises to Improve Low Back Function

Flexibility Exercises to Improve ROM

In performing limb flexibility exercises, the participant should first stretch to symmetry; after symmetry is achieved, the participant should work on improving flexibility in both limbs. Static stretches held for 30 to 60 s are recommended; these can be repeated twice during the exercise period. However, for those areas in which extreme tightness is noted, ideally there should be several exercise bouts each day.

Hip Flexor Stretch (Standing)

The participant grasps the contralateral ankle and raises the leg while keeping the trunk straight (a). Note incorrect technique of individual on the right (b); tilting the pelvis precludes stretching the hip flexors.

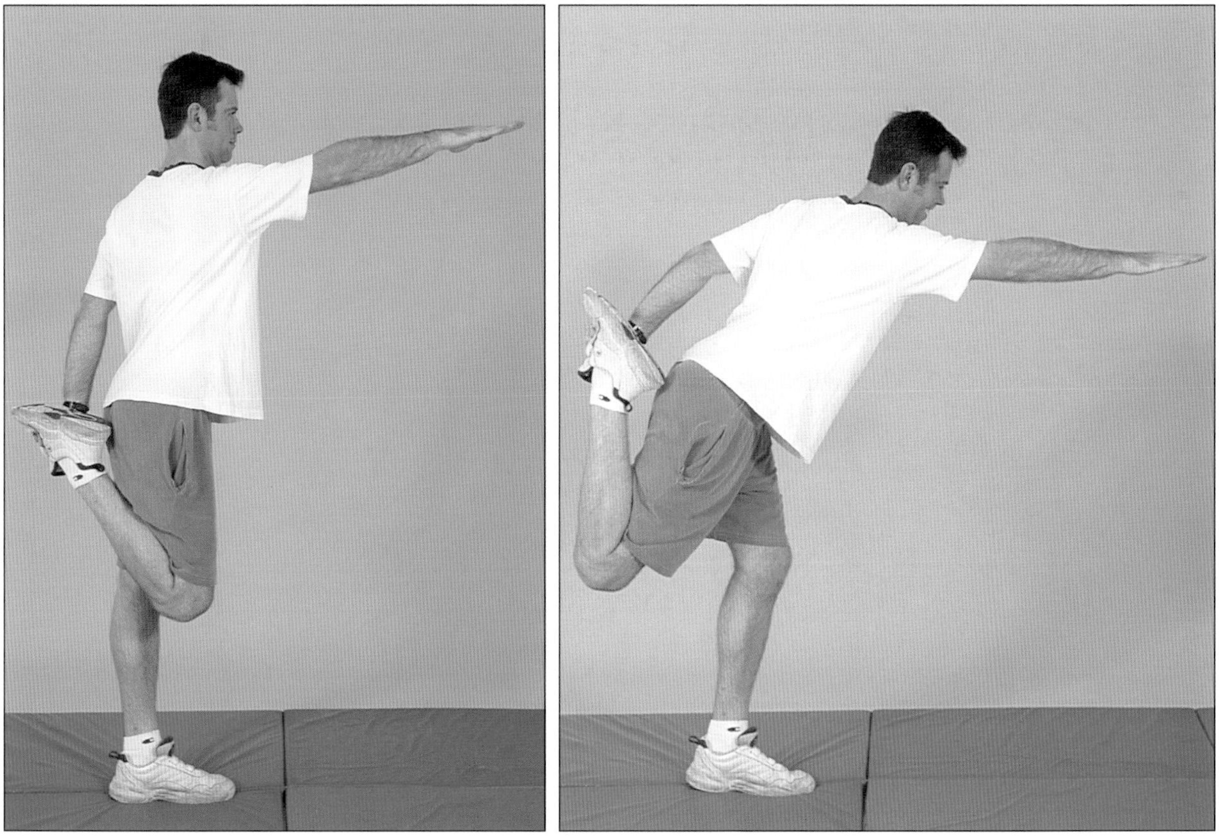

a *b*

Hip Flexor Stretch (Supine)

The participant assumes the Thomas test position and pulls the contralateral leg back as far as possible; this posterior rotation of the pelvis can place added tension on the contralateral hip flexors.

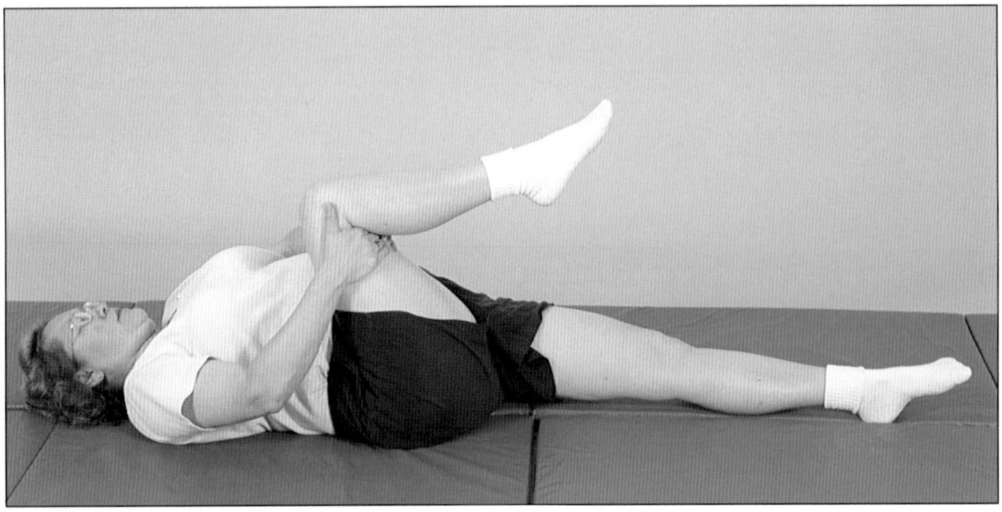

I-T Band Stretch

With hips stacked, the exerciser places the ankle of the lower leg on the lateral distal thigh; by outwardly rotating the thigh of lower leg, the I-T band of upper leg is stretched. (In some cases, gravity alone may be an effective stretch of the I-T band from this position.)

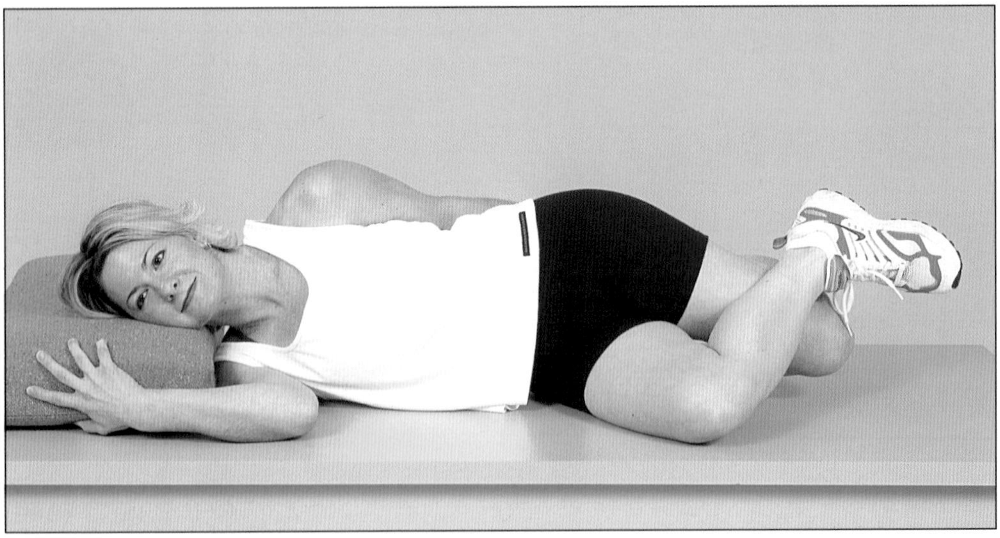

Piriformis Stretch

The piriformis of the right leg is being stretched in this maneuver. This posturing is markedly similar to that achieved while sitting at a chair and placing the lateral malleolus (ankle) of one leg on distal femur of contralateral leg.

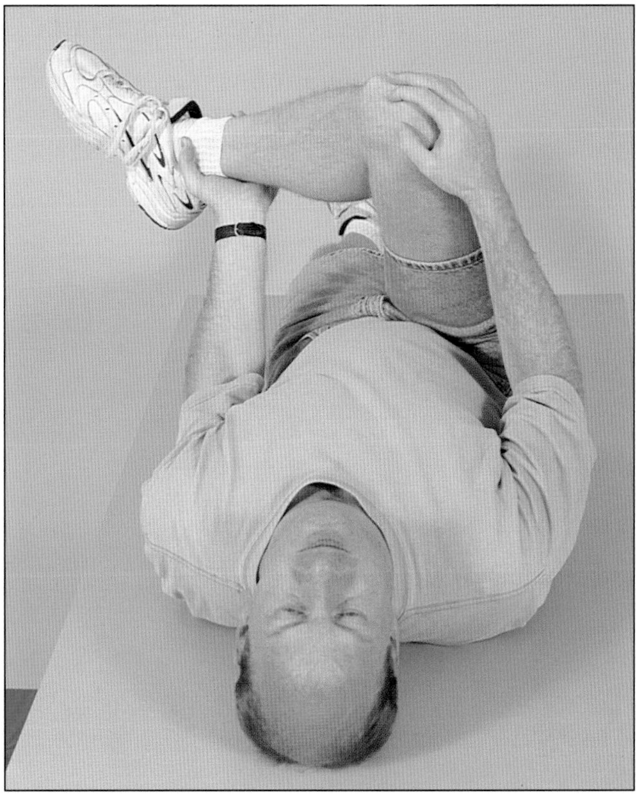

Cailliet Stretch

The exerciser should lean forward until tension is felt in the hamstrings and then hold this position. The sequence is repeated for each leg 3 to 4 times. If the hamstrings are tight (e.g., sacral angle less than 80°), stress could be placed on structures of the spine; this is not desirable. To avoid this, the back should be kept straight and the movement emphasis should be at the hip joint.

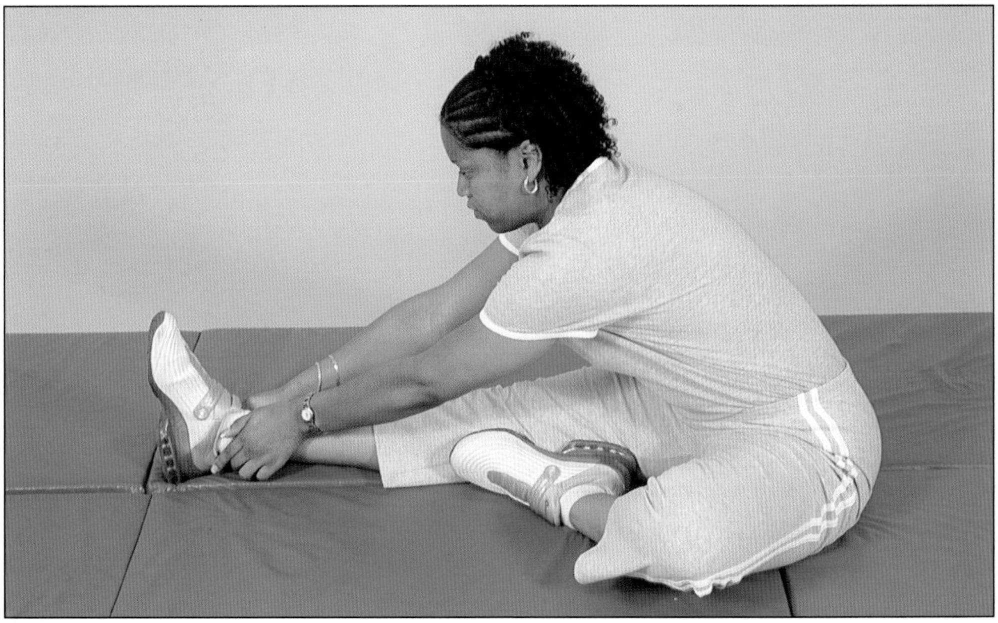

Step/Chair Stretch

This stretch can be more effective if the trunk is "splinted" and the participant emphasizes movement at the hip joint rather than using the more slouched posture also depicted (*b*). In (*a*) the hamstrings can be isolated in the stretch if the movement is made only at the hip joint. Although the hamstrings can also be stretched in (*b*), the soft tissue structures of the lower back are also stretched. A more appropriate stretch for the lower back is presented in the next figure.

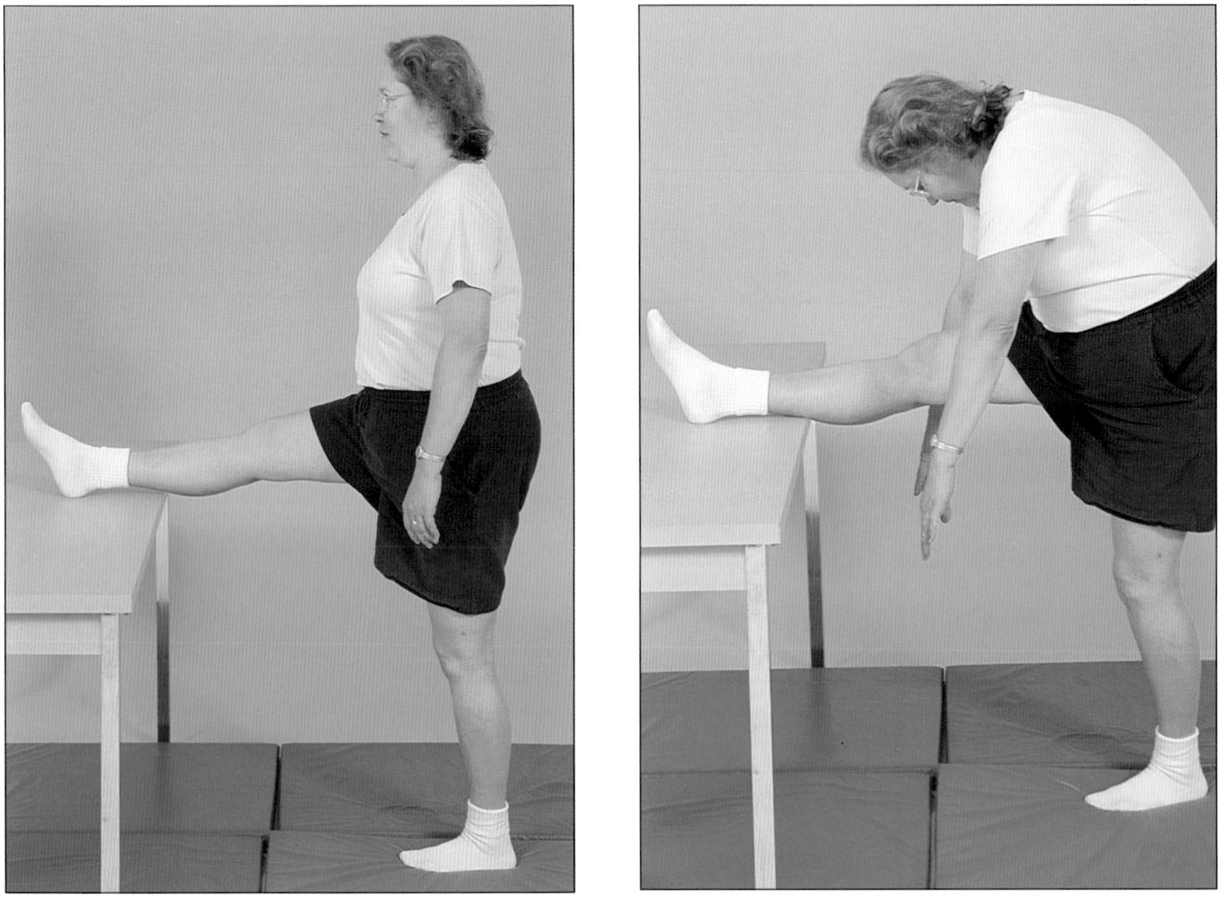

a *b*

Mad Cat Stretch

The exercise involves slowly cycling through full spine flexion to full extension. This exercise is not used for increasing ROM but rather for spine mobility; it would be a particularly appropriate morning exercise when the discs tend to be distended and tight, because the spinal loading is minimal.

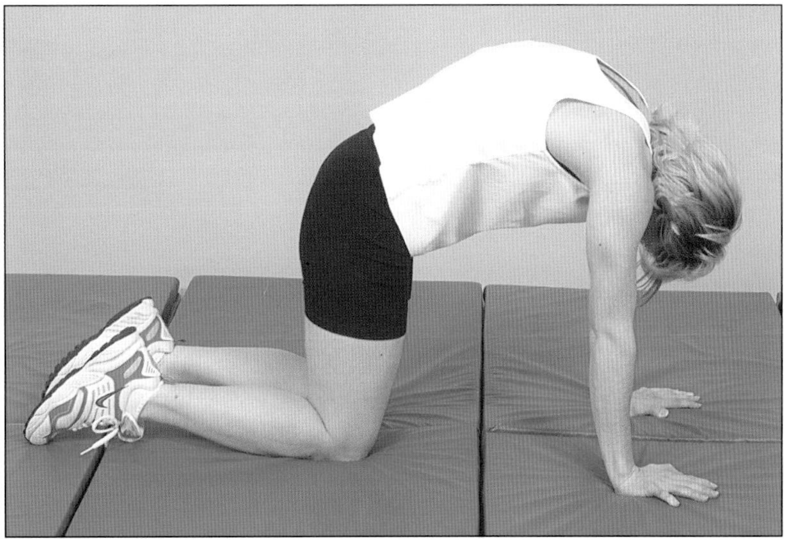

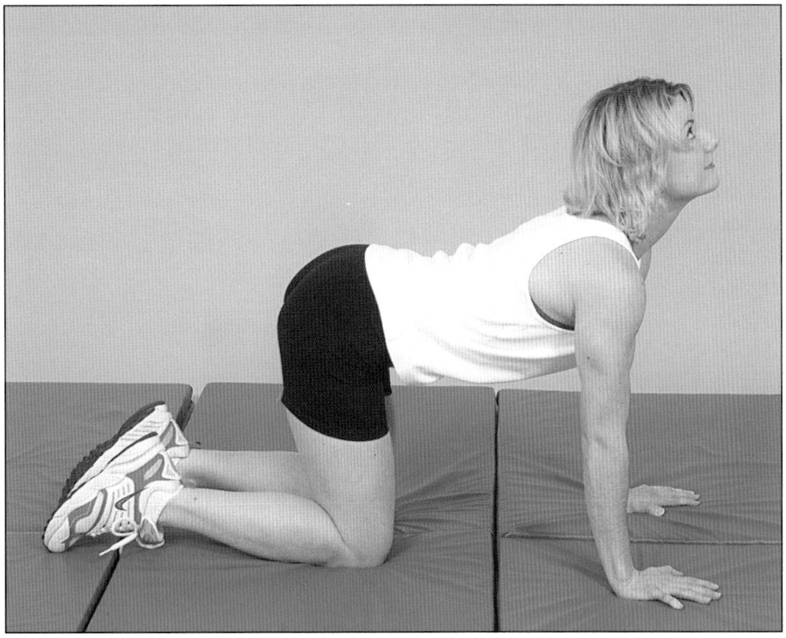

Trunk Flexion

The participant pulls one (*a*) and eventually both (*b*) knees toward the shoulders. Some disc patients might experience problems with (*b*) because in some flexion-type movements, the nucleus of the disc is pushed posteriorly.

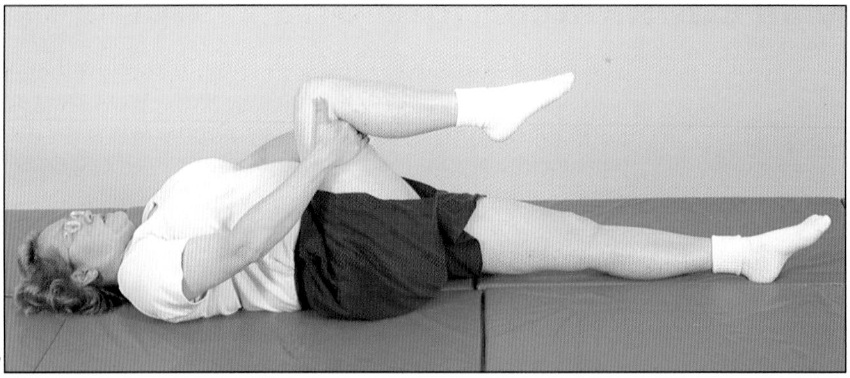

a

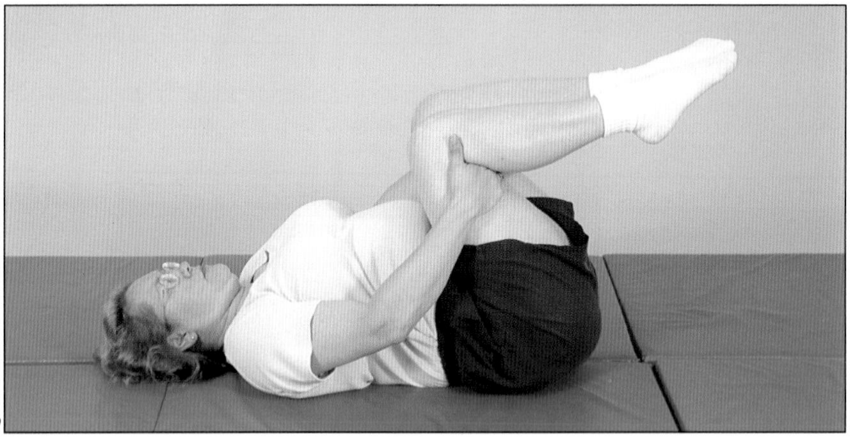

b

Trunk Extension

The exerciser places the hands under shoulders and slowly extends the arms while keeping the pelvis in contact with the floor (back muscles are kept relaxed).

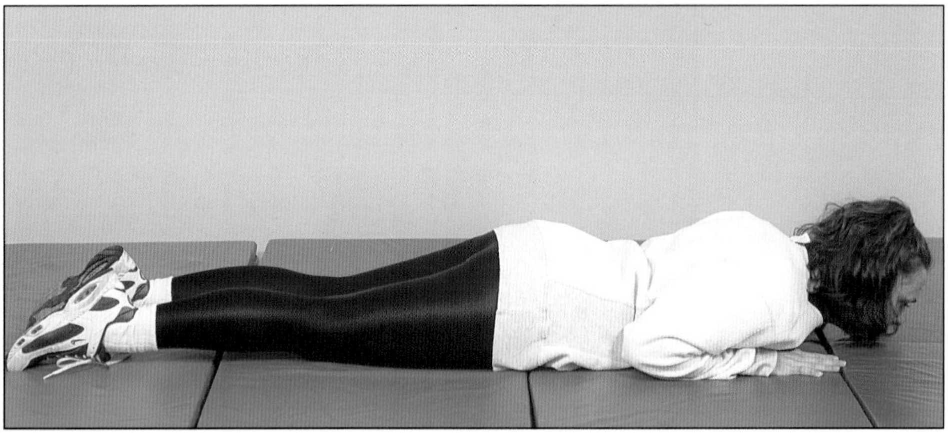

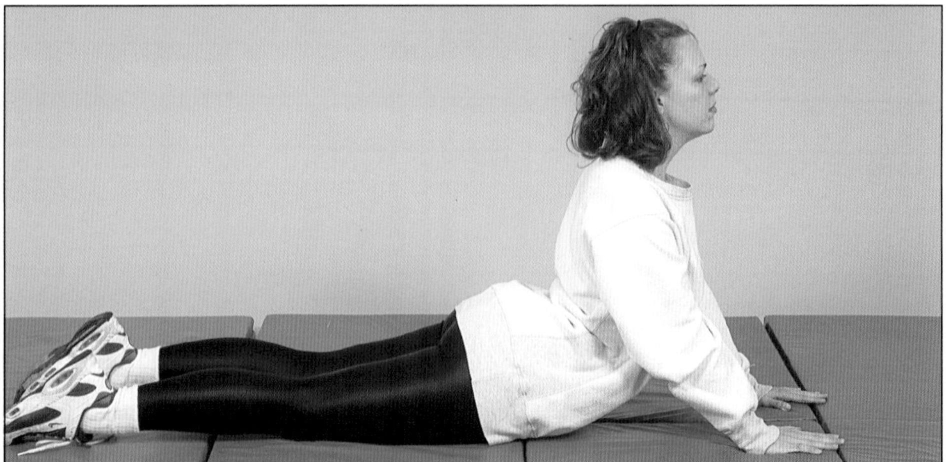

Trunk Strength and Endurance Exercises

In these, as in any other strength-training exercises, overload must be achieved. Strength can be developed by doing, for example, 10 to 15 repetitions of each exercise (or until overload is reached); however, workouts can also be varied by doing most of the exercises with 30- to 60-s isometric holds and fewer repetitions. The latter can be advantageous for the development of trunk muscle endurance, which is critical for attaining good core stability.

Quadruped

Initially this exercise is done one limb at a time and then it is advanced if the exerciser raises contralateral limbs; it can be done dynamically or isometrically. Abdominal bracing and core stability requirements are increased when two limbs are raised. When back patients perform this exercise, it is important that it be done in pain-free ROM and with the shoulders and hips level. There should not be any bobbing or other trunk movement during this exercise; this is important!

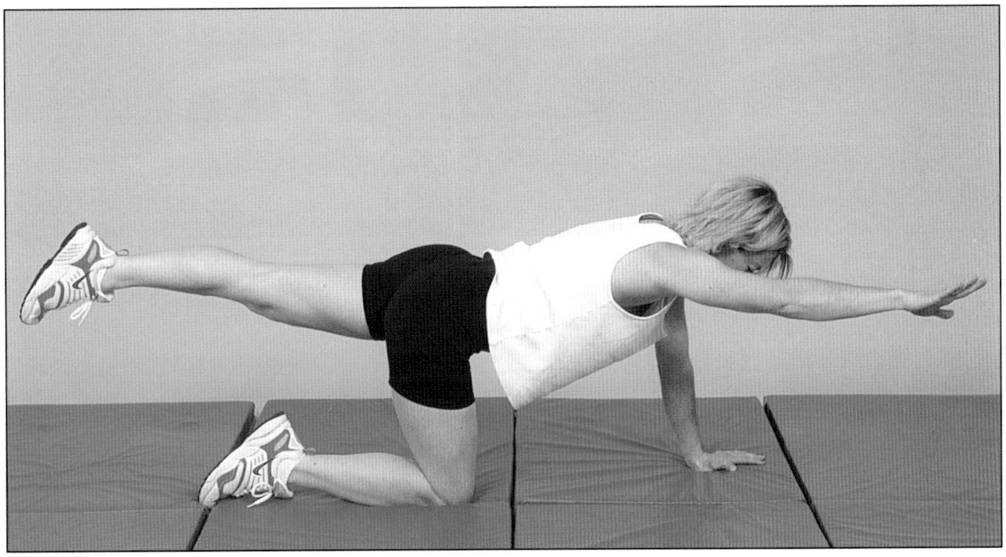

Roman Chair

This is a very effective exercise for the lumbar erector spinae and the multifidus. For individuals with less strength, the activity depicted in the bottom figure is appropriate.

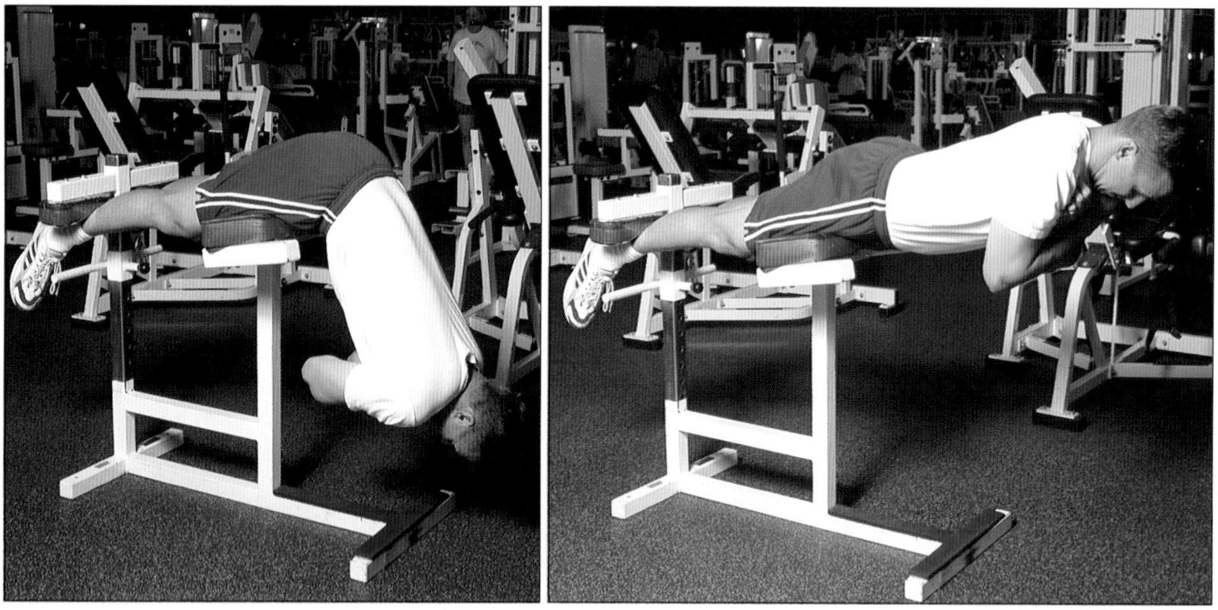

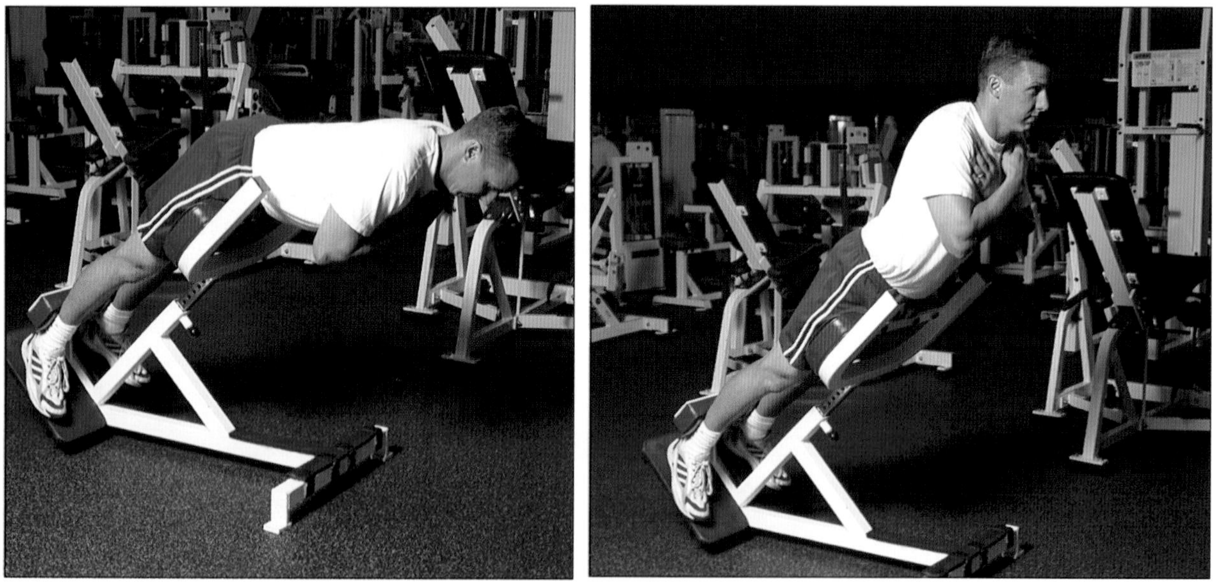

Posterior Pelvic Tilt

This exercise can be done by itself or as the first phase of a crunch. The participant posteriorly rotates the pelvis from starting position (*a*) until the low back is snug against the floor (*b*). (This exercise may not be appropriate for individuals with disc pathology.)

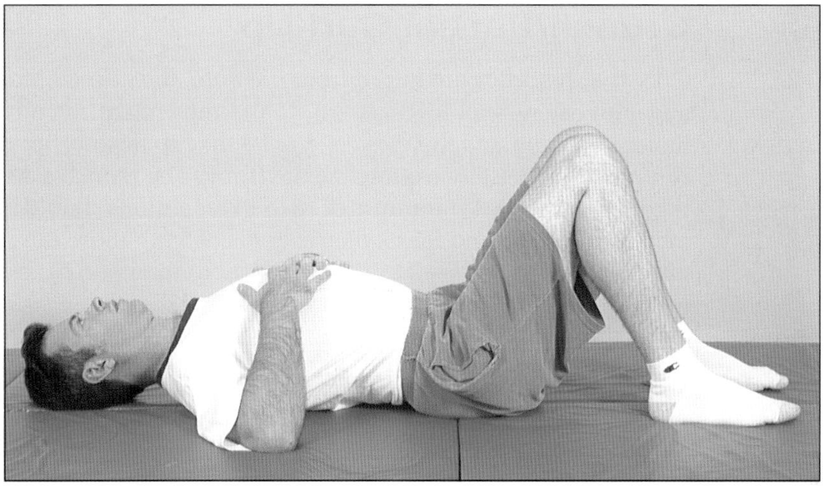

a

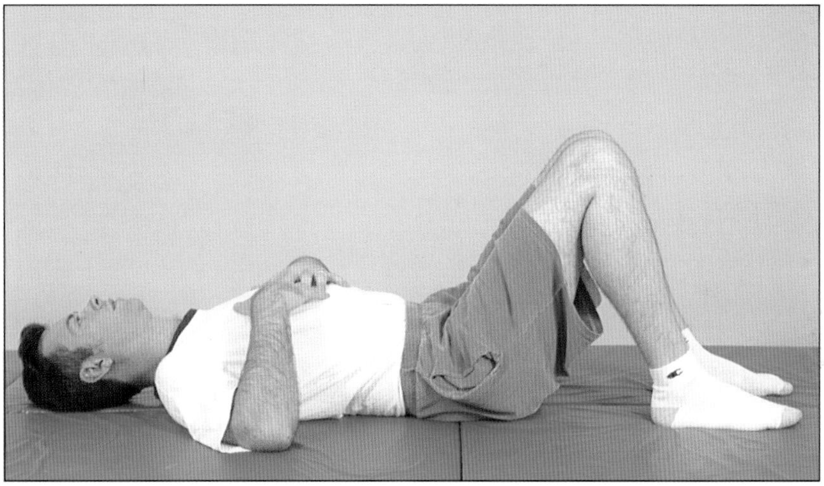

b

For the following abdominal wall exercises, research is cited that indicates the degree of MVC seen for the musculature involved. As discussed previously, it is desirable as much as possible to minimize psoas activity while concurrently maximizing abdominal wall activity. The only exercises included here are those that the author thought best met these criteria in the exercises examined in the cited source. Other exercises may be appropriate for a specific population.

Crunch/Partial Curl Up

Once the shoulders are raised from the floor, the normal lordosis has been straightened and movement should cease (*a*). If the movement is continued, it will occur at the iliofemoral joint and the movers will be the hip flexors, because the abdominal muscles contract isometrically to stabilize the trunk. The crunch also can be performed with the thighs vertical (*b*). A minimum of 10 to 15 repetitions should be the goal. Two or three sets may be repeated, and / or isometric holds of 5 s or more can be incorporated with the up position. MVC: psoas—7 to 10%, rectus abdominis—62%, external oblique—68%, internal oblique—36%, transversus abdominis—12% (9).

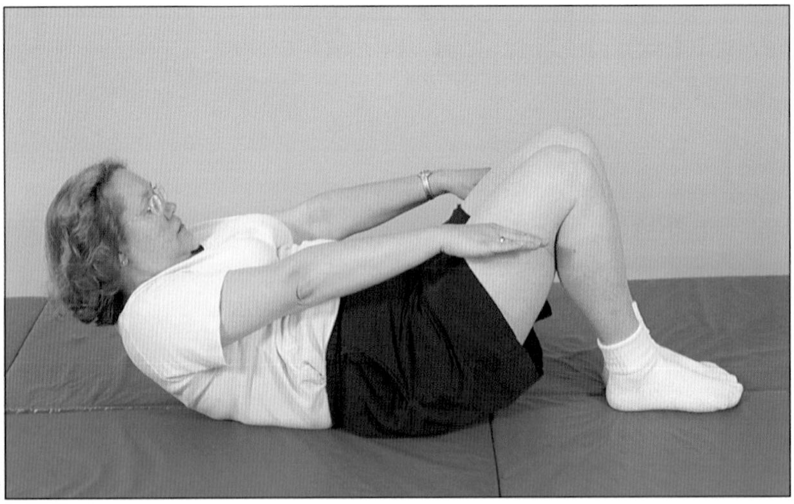

a

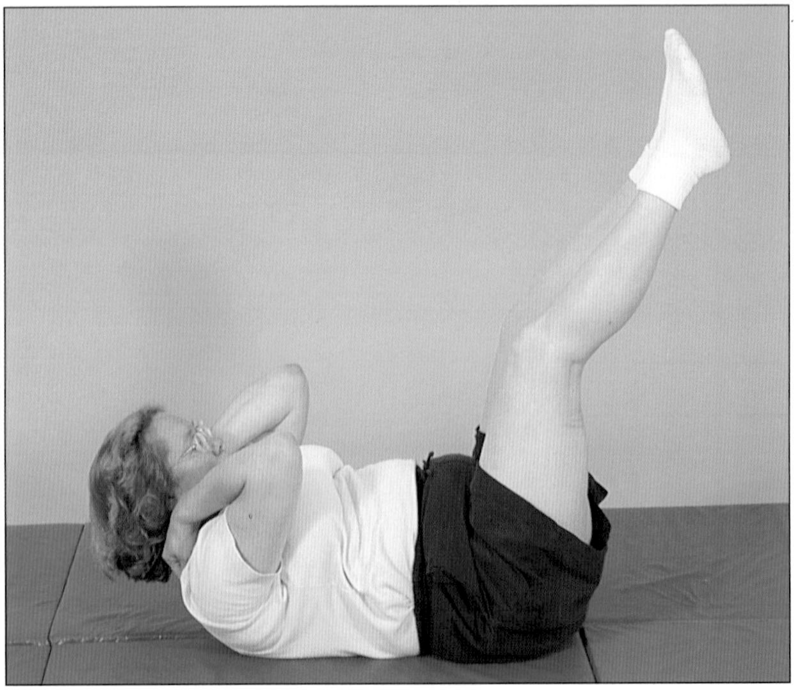

b

Cross Curl-Up

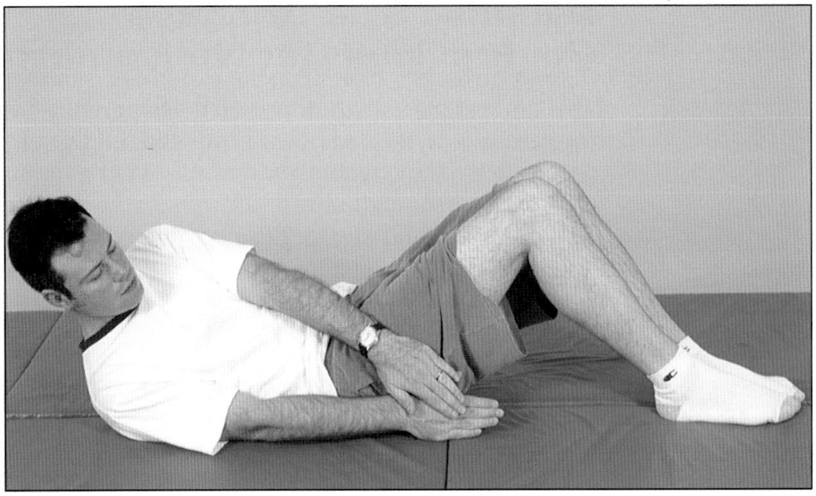

This exercise ensures greater involvement of the internal and external oblique musculature. A minimum of 10 to 15 repetitions should be the goal. Two or three sets may be repeated, and/or isometric holds of 5 s or more can be incorporated with the up position. MVC: psoas—4 to 5%, rectus abdominis—62%, external oblique—68%, internal oblique—36%, transversus abdominis—12% (9).

Horizontal Isometric Side Bridge

This can be done with either the knees or the feet on the floor. The latter is more difficult and would increase the spine load over figures cited. MVC: psoas—12 to 21%[2], rectus abdominis—21%, external oblique—43%, internal oblique—36%, transversus abdominis—39% (9).

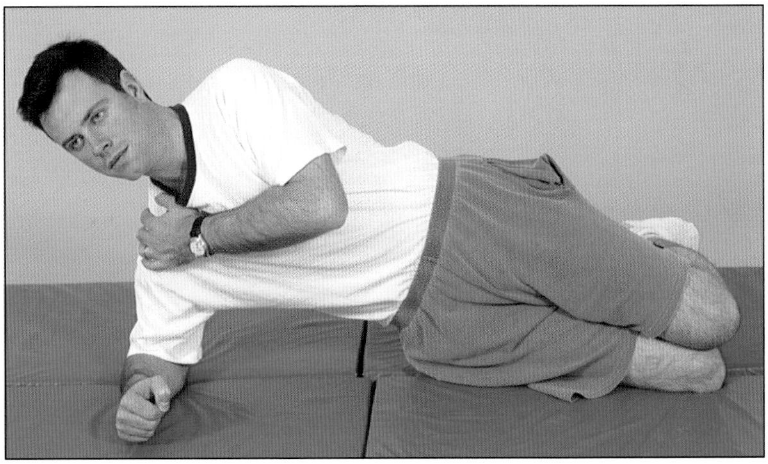

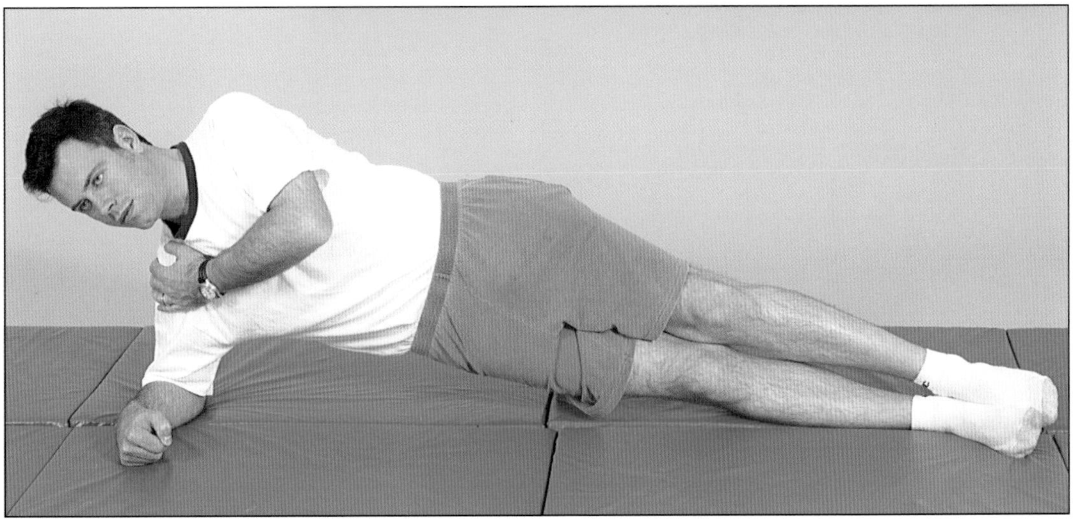

[2] Indwelling electrodes were inserted in two psoas cites.

Dynamic Side Bridge (As Previous But No Isometric Hold)

This can be done with the knees on the floor or the feet. The latter is more difficult and also increases the spine load over figures cited. If this exercise were done dynamically, MVC: psoas—13 to 26%, rectus abdominis—41%, external oblique—44%, internal oblique—42%, transversus abdominis—44% (9). In the dynamic version of this bridge exercise, the hips are raised and lowered respectively.

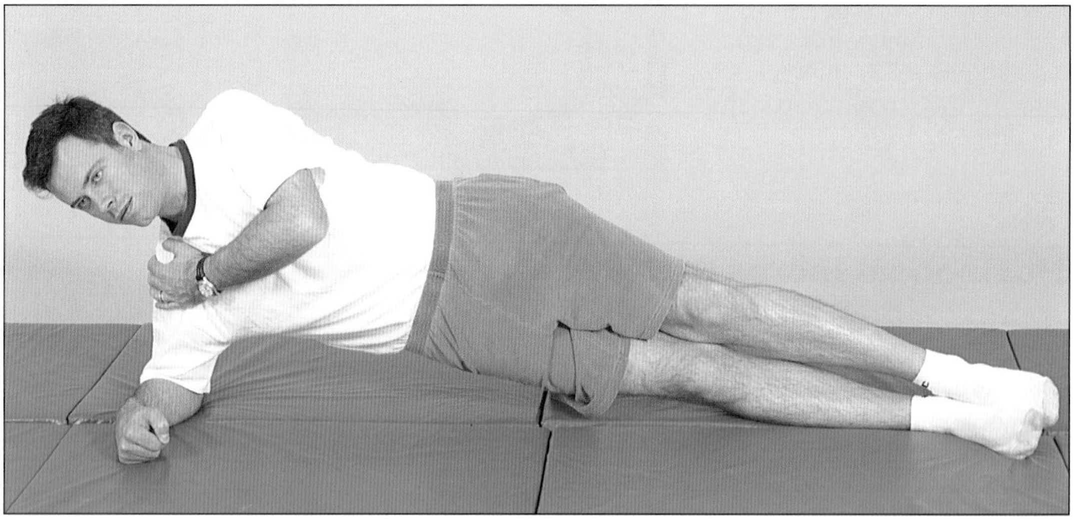

Source List

1. Axler, C.T., & McGill, S.M. (1997). Low back loads over a variety of abdominal exercises: Searching for the safest abdominal challenge. *Medicine and Science in Sports and Exercise, 29*(6), 804-811.
2. Battie, M.C., Videman, T., Gill, K., Moneta, G.B., Nyman, R., Kaprio, J., Koskenvut, M. (1991). Smoking and lumbar intervertebral disc degeneration: An MRI study of identical twins. *Spine, 16*(9), 1015-1021.
3. Biering-Sorensen, F. (1984). Physical measurements as risk indicators for low-back trouble over a one-year period. *Spine, 9*(2), 106-119.
4. Bogduk, N. (1998). *Clinical anatomy of the lumbar spine and sacrum*. London: Churchill Livingstone.
5. Borenstein, D.G., & Wiesel, S.W. (1989). *Low back pain—Medical diagnosis and comprehensive management*. Philadelphia: Saunders.
6. Cailliet, R. (1988). *Low back pain syndrome*. Philadelphia: Davis.
7. Donelson, R. (1991). The McKenzie method. In A.H. White & R. Anderson (Eds.), *Conservative care of low back pain* (pp. 97-104). Baltimore: Williams & Wilkins.
8. Fritz, J.M., & Hicks, G.E. (2001). Exercise protocols for low back pain. In W. Liemohn (Ed.), *Exercise prescription and the back* (pp. 167-181). New York: McGraw-Hill Medical.
9. Juker, D., McGill, S., Kropf, P., Steffen, T. (1998). Quantitative intramuscular myoelectric activity of lumbar portions of psoas and the abdominal wall during a wide variety of tasks. *Medicine and Science in Sports and Exercise, 30*(2), 301-310.
10. Liemohn, W., & Gagnon, L.H. (2001). Efficacy of therapeutic exercise in low back rehabilitation. In W. Liemohn (Ed.), *Exercise prescription and the back* (pp. 229-240). New York: McGraw-Hill Medical.
11. Liemohn, W., Haydu, T., Phillips, D. (1999). Questionable exercises. *PCPFS Physical Activity and Fitness Research Digest, 3*(8), 1-8.
12. McGill, S.M. (2001). Low back stability: From formal description to issues for performance and rehabilitation. *Exercise and Sport Sciences Reviews, 29*(1), 26-31.
13. Nachemson, A.L., Andersson, B.J., Schultz, A.B. (1986). Valsalva maneuver biomechanics: Effects on lumbar trunk loads of elevated intraabdominal pressures. *Spine, 11*, 476-479.
14. O'Sullivan, P.B., Twomey, L., Allison, G.T. (1997). Dynamic stabilization of the lumbar spine. *Critical Reviews in Physical and Rehabilitation Medicine, 9*(3 & 4), 315-330.
15. Porterfield, J.A., & DeRosa, C. (1998). *Mechanical low back pain—Perspective in functional anatomy*. Philadelphia: Saunders.
16. Sinaki, M., Lutness, M.P., Ilstrup, D.M., Chu, C.P., Gramse, R.R. (1989). Lumbar spondylolisthesis: Retrospective comparison and three-year follow-up of two conservative treatment programs. *Archives in Physical Medicine and Rehabilitation, 70*(8), 594-598.
17. Waddell, G. (1998). *The back pain revolution*. Edinburgh, UK: Churchill Livingstone.
18. White, A.A., & Panjabbi, M.M. (1990). *Clinical biomechanics of the spine*. Philadelphia: Lippincott Williams & Wilkins.
19. Zuhosky, J.P., & Young, J.L. (2001). Functional physical assessment for low back injuries in the athlete. In W. Liemohn (Ed.), *Exercise prescription and the back* (pp. 67-88). New York: McGraw-Hill Medical.

fourteen

Exercise Leadership for Health and Fitness

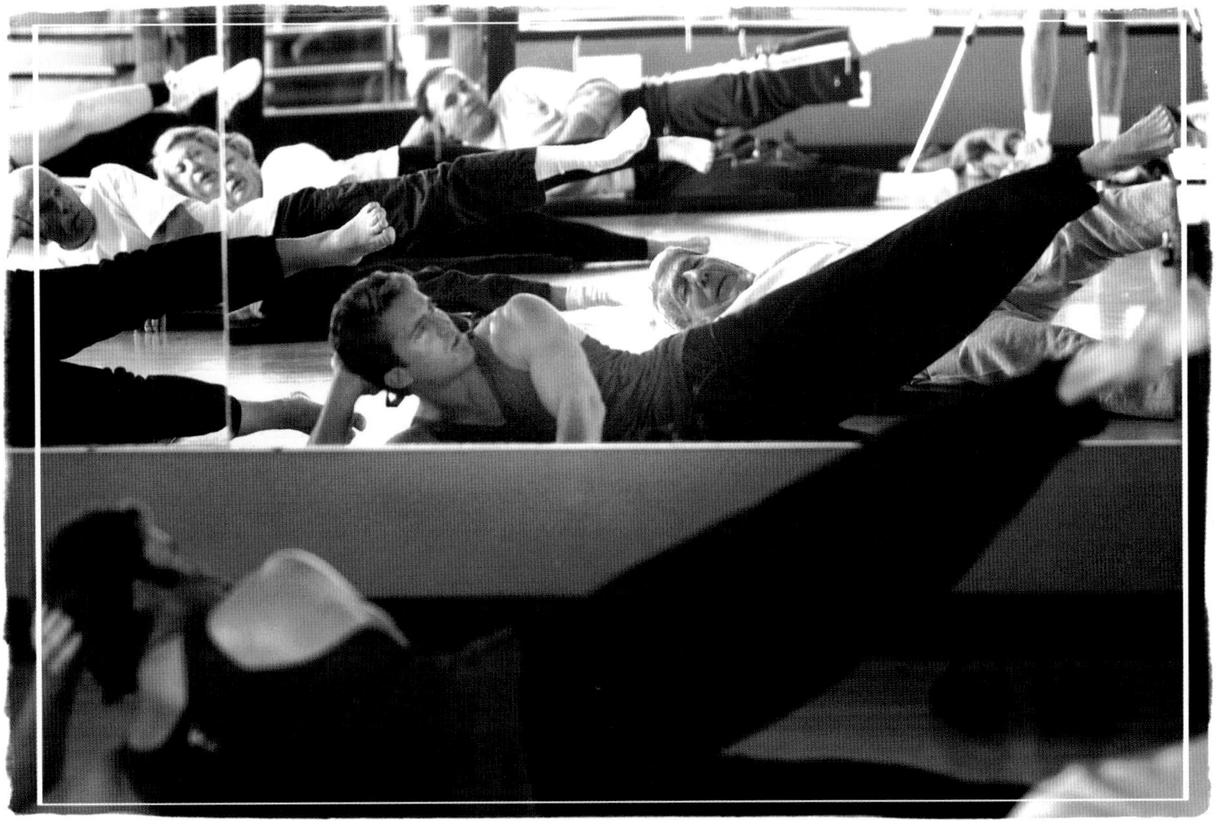

Objectives

The reader will be able to do the following:

1. Distinguish between guidelines for moderate-intensity exercise programs recommended for everyone and systematically structured exercise programs for people interested in improving functional capacity.
2. Describe the factors related to a high and low probability of participation.
3. Describe the characteristics of a good exercise leader.
4. Describe safety and clothing considerations relative to walking and jogging programs.
5. Explain the balance between duration and intensity in a typical walking program, and indicate activities used in walking programs to improve enjoyment and adherence.
6. Outline appropriate walk/jog/walk intervals used at the beginning of a jogging program.
7. Describe exercise recommendations for cycling that improve cardiorespiratory fitness.
8. List the elements of games that provide effective fitness benefits.
9. Describe the activities done in a swimming pool, other than lap swimming, that can be an effective part of an aerobic exercise program.
10. Provide recommendations for beginners starting low- and high-impact dance exercise programs, and indicate the typical kinds of exercises included in such programs.
11. Recommend appropriate beginning goals for people using exercise equipment.
12. Describe a circuit training program that uses aerobic and strength training equipment.

The purpose of a fitness program must be kept uppermost in the HFI's mind. The HFI is trying to help people include appropriate physical activity as a vital part of their lifestyles. This assumes that the participants understand what type of physical activity is appropriate, have sufficient skills to achieve satisfaction from the activities, and have the intrinsic motivation to continue to be active for the rest of their lives. Thus, HFIs try to help people increase their physical fitness levels in ways that are psychologically, mentally, and socially relevant and appealing.

Effective Leadership

Individuals need to do 30 min of moderate-intensity physical activity daily to achieve health goals. To obtain and maintain cardiorespiratory fitness, a person must participate in vigorous, dynamic aerobic exercise at least 3 days per week. Yet, about 4 in 10 Americans are completely sedentary, less than 25% do periodic vigorous exercise, and only 15% do 30 min of daily moderate activity. Less than one in five is involved in muscular strength and endurance activities, and less than one third do flexibility exercises (19). At the same time, more than half of the people who start a formal exercise program drop out within a few months (2).

1 In Review

Moderate-intensity exercise (30 min daily) is recommended for all people. Vigorous aerobic exercise should be done at least 3 days a week to improve and maintain cardiorespiratory fitness.

Figure 14.1 summarizes the factors related to a high probability and a low probability of participation. The HFI and the exercise leader must understand that a wide variety of factors affect people's involvement in personal or supervised exercise programs. In general, better-educated, self-motivated individuals who enjoy physical activity and believe in the health outcomes associated with physical activity are more likely to exercise regularly. In contrast, individuals with a high risk of CHD who also hold blue-collar jobs are less likely to be involved in formal exercise. It appears that the people with the greatest need to exercise are the least likely to become involved. More than personal characteristics, however, are involved in the decision.

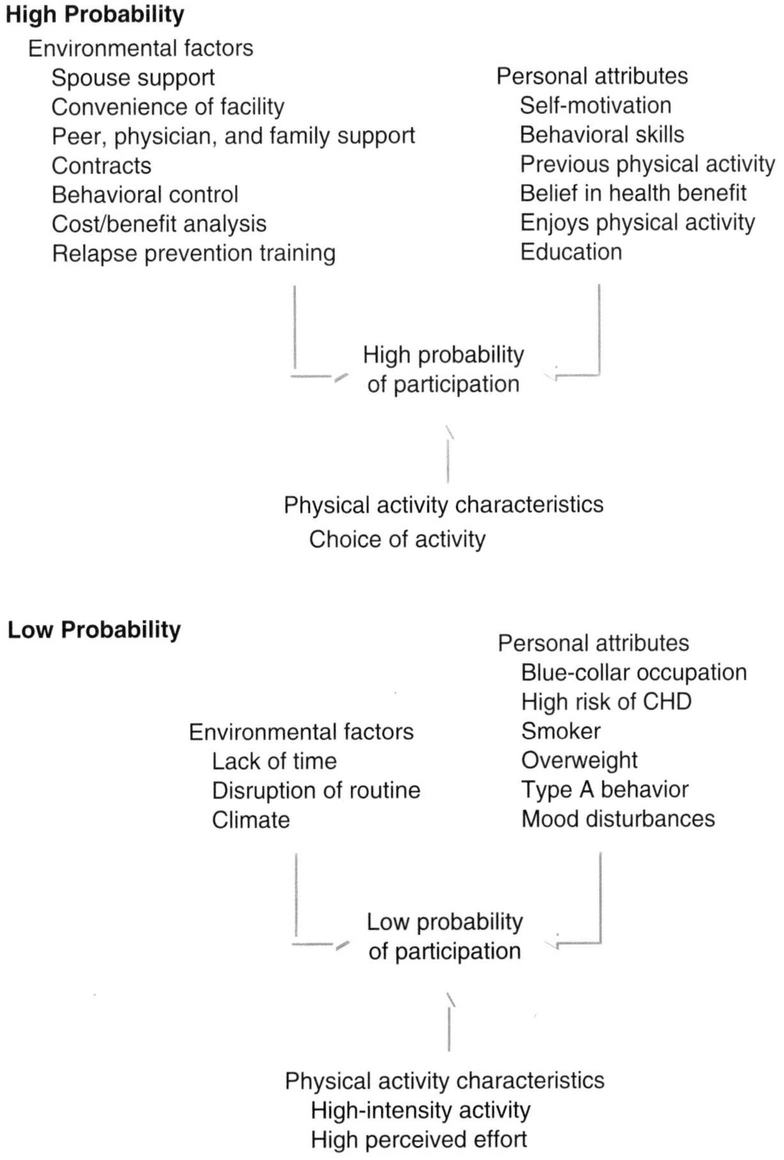

Figure 14.1 High and low probability of participation.

2 In Review

Different environmental factors, personal attributes, and physical activity characteristics can predict the probability of an individual's participating in an exercise program. See figure 14.1.

Support from one's spouse or partner, family, physician, and peers seems to drive involvement, but this must be viewed against the variable of perceived convenience of facilities. People with poor time-management and goal-setting skills are less likely to be successful. What does this say about the HFI's role in providing exercise leadership? It is clear that exercise leadership involves much more than exercise!

Henry Kissinger is cited as saying that a leader is one who can take people from where they are to where they have not been (15). This is true for the exercise leader, who must counter the negative influences bearing on the portion of the population most in need of physical activity. We normally think that an HFI does the following:

- Screens individuals relative to health status.
- Evaluates various fitness components.
- Prescribes activities at the appropriate intensity, duration, and frequency consistent with test results and personal goals.
- Leads individuals or groups in appropriate activities.
- Monitors participants' responses within an exercise session.
- Modifies activities depending on environmental and other factors.
- Records progress and problems.
- Responds to emergencies.
- Refers problems to appropriate health professionals.

Leadership, however, means more than simply taking a class through its paces. HFIs also must make the participant feel welcome, motivate the person or group, and be a friend. To do all these things, the exercise leader must develop interpersonal skills. These leadership abilities are summarized in the box below.

Since 1980, a variety of organizations have developed certification and education programs to promote exercise programming in preventive and rehabilitative settings. One of the earliest to do so was the ACSM. Qualification in these certification areas requires the applicant to have a specific knowledge base and demonstrate specific behaviors. The current certification programs include the following:

Exercise Specialist®

Health/Fitness Instructor$_{\text{SM}}$

Registered Clinical Exercise Physiologist®

These certifications are considered the standard by many in the fields of fitness and cardiac rehabilitation. However, there are a variety of other respected certification programs.

Relationship-Oriented Abilities Associated With Effective Leadership

Listening skills

Attention to individual needs

Concern regarding integration of new participants

Acceptance to group interaction

Educational skills

Motivational skills with participants and staff

Rapport and empathy leading to sensitivity

Consistency/honesty/tactfulness

Skilled at opening avenues of communication between participants and staff

Reprinted from Oldridge, 1988, Qualities of an exercise leader. In *Resource manual for guidelines for exercise testing and prescription*. By permission of Lea & Febiger.

- American Council on Exercise (ACE)—Aerobics Instructor, Personal Trainer, and Lifestyle & Weight Management Consultant (ACE; 4851 Paramount Drive, San Diego, CA 92123)
- Aerobics and Fitness Association of America (AFAA)—AFAA Fitness Practitioner™ (AFAA; 15250 Ventura Boulevard, Suite 200, Sherman Oaks, CA 91403)
- National Strength and Conditioning Association (NSCA)—Certified Strength and Conditioning Specialist, and Personal Trainer (1955 N. Union Boulevard, Colorado Springs, CO 80909)
- YMCA—YMCA Exercise Instructor, YMCA Exercise Instructor Trainer, and their advanced counterparts (YMCA of the USA; 101 North Wacker Drive, Chicago, IL 60606-7386)

In addition to these certification programs, certifications for unique aspects of exercise leadership are presented later in this chapter. Next, the responsibilities of the HFI are examined in greater detail.

Role Model

The authors of this book clearly support the notion that the HFI should be an inspiring role model for his or her clients. The idea of an overweight, out-of-shape exercise leader is one whose time has passed. A leader must plan appropriate activities, evaluate the progress of the participants, and provide incentives, but the leadership associated with many exercise programs is in the form of quiet, subtle value statements that do not require words. The HFI's presence and behaviors, consistent with a healthy lifestyle, add much meaning and value to her or his words and programs.

Program Planning

All activity programs must have daily, weekly, and monthly plans to provide appropriate activities, meet the needs of the participants, and reduce the possibility of boredom. This planning allows the HFI to judge the usefulness of the activity and encourage systematic modification from one month to the next. If the HFI is working with individuals who exercise on their own, the need for specific exercise recommendations becomes obvious. The value of the feedback received from these individuals depends on the information they were given at the start of their program. The following considerations can be applied to both group and individual exercise programs.

Vary the Program

Variety should be a cornerstone of every exercise program. Some elements are a part of each exercise session: warm-up and stretching, a stimulus phase, and a cool-down. The variety comes in the form of different exercises used in each part of a session, short educational messages presented to the class while they are stretching or cooling down, or the use of games to add spice to routine exercises. The most important thing is to plan the activity sessions far enough in advance to minimize repetition and maximize variety.

Accommodate Individual Differences

A participant should be able to choose from a variety of activities. A program must address the needs, interests, and limitations of the group being served. The choice of equipment, the activities, and the pace of the class must be considered when planning for young / old, less fit / very fit, and more skilled / less skilled participants (12). Offer different options from which people may choose (e.g., 1-lb vs. 5-lb weights, low-impact vs. high-impact moves, 1-mile fast walks vs. 3-mile jogs).

Maintain Control

The exercise leader must have control over the exercise session. This is especially true in the use of games (e.g., indoor soccer), where the intensity is not as easily controlled as in jogging. Control implies an ability to modify the session as needed to meet the THR and total work goals of each individual. Some people will have to slow down; others may need encouragement to increase their intensity. The element of control (at a distance) for people who exercise without direct supervision can be provided by using written guidelines about what to do and when to move from one stage to the next. In addition, specific information should be provided about symptoms that indicate inappropriate responses to exercise.

Monitor Progress and Keep Records

Keeping track of a participant's response to the exercise session will give clues about that individual's adaptation to that particular session and about overall, day-to-day changes. This information is important for updating exercise prescriptions and answering specific questions the participant may raise. Each exercise class should have regular pauses to check HR and determine whether individuals are close to their THRs. Rather than keeping track of a large number of 10-s THRs, ask each participant to indicate the number of beats over or under the 10-s goal. This increases the participant's awareness of the THR and indicates how the intensity of the exercise should be adjusted to stay on target.

Each person's HR response is probably the best and most objective indicator of his or her adjustment to an exercise session, but do not stop with that. Elicit information about how the participant feels in general; ask about any new pains, aches, or strange sensations. Record keeping should include a daily attendance check, a weekly weighing, a regular BP check (if appropriate), and a column asking for comments (e.g., THR, any aches or pains). An example of such a form is the Daily Activity Form (see form 14.1). This information allows the HFI to make better recommendations about the participants' exercise programs and refer them to appropriate professionals if needed.

The point we have emphasized throughout this section on exercise leadership is the need for the leader to help the participant. The behavioral strategies list on page 268 suggests ways for HFIs to become better leaders.

3 In Review

The effective fitness professional must develop relationship-oriented abilities, serve as a role model for others, understand the importance of variety, accommodate differences, control the environment for safety, and monitor and record clients' progress. Asking for participants' HR, RPE, and any unusual responses to the exercise are ways to monitor exercise intensity during an exercise session.

Progression of Activities

Sedentary people who want to begin a fitness program should follow a logical sequence of fitness activities. Moderate-intensity activities are encouraged for everyone, but a systematic program of activities should be provided to help participants increase functional capacity. The following paragraphs summarize our recommendations on how this can be accomplished.

Phase 1: Regular Walking

The first phase, for sedentary individuals, is to include exercise as a part of their weekly patterns. The major fitness goal is to increase the exercise that can be done comfortably, so no emphasis on intensity is necessary at this point. The person starts with the distance that can be walked easily without pain or fatigue and then gradually increases the distance and pace until about 4 miles can be walked briskly every other day. People with an orthopedic limitation can substitute a weight-supported activity such as cycling, rowing, or swimming.

Phase 2: Recommended Work Levels for a Change in Fitness

Once Phase 1 is accomplished, the person is taught about recommended levels of work for fitness changes (see chapter 10). A work-relief, interval training program is introduced—jogging is the work, and walking is the relief. So the person walks, jogs a few steps, then walks, and so forth. Gradually, jogging covers more distance than walking, until the person can jog continuously for 2 to 3 miles at THR. People interested in cycling and swimming (see later in this chapter) also can use interval training. People interested in aerobic dance should transition from the walking program to a low-intensity, low-impact class.

Phase 3: Variety of Fitness Activities

The first two phases are generally recommended for everyone (with alternative activities for people who cannot or choose not to jog—such as cycling, dancing, or running in water). Phase 3, on the other hand, is quite individualized, based on the person's interests. The purpose is to promote the continued activity habit by participation in an activity that the person naturally enjoys. Some people prefer to continue to stretch, walk, and jog; some prefer to exercise alone; and others (the majority) enjoy working out with others. Some people like cooperative and relatively low-level competitive activities, and others like the thrill of competition. Some enjoy a variety of different movement forms; others enjoy repeating the same type of activity. The HFI must provide an atmosphere where people feel free to try new things without embarrassment and allow individuals to choose from among a variety of options for their fitness activities.

form
14.1

Daily Activity Form

Name: ____

Target weight: _________________ Target heart rate zone: _________________

Week	Day	Weight	Resting BP	Resting HR	Exercise HR	RPE	Signs, symptoms, comments
1	Mon	______	______	______	______	____	_______________
	Wed	______	______	______	______	____	_______________
	Fri	______	______	______	______	____	_______________
2	Mon	______	______	______	______	____	_______________
	Wed	______	______	______	______	____	_______________
	Fri	______	______	______	______	____	_______________
3	Mon	______	______	______	______	____	_______________
	Wed	______	______	______	______	____	_______________
	Fri	______	______	______	______	____	_______________
4	Mon	______	______	______	______	____	_______________
	Wed	______	______	______	______	____	_______________
	Fri	______	______	______	______	____	_______________

Behavioral Strategies of the Effective Exercise Leader

1. Show a sincere interest in the participants. Learn why they have chosen your program and what they would really like to achieve.
2. Be enthusiastic in your instruction and guidance.
3. Develop a personal relationship with each participant.
4. Consider the various reasons why adults exercise (e.g., health, recreation, weight loss, social, personal appearance) and allow for individual differences.
5. Initiate participant follow-up (i.e., postcards or telephone calls) when several unexplained absences occur in succession. Novice exercisers should be advised that an inevitable slip in attendance does not imply failure.
6. Practice what you preach. Participate in the exercise sessions yourself. Good posture and grooming are essential to projecting the desired self-image. Cigarette smoking should be prohibited, and drinking soda or eating candy on the gymnasium floor also is unacceptable.
7. Honor special days (e.g., birthdays) or exercise accomplishments with extrinsic rewards such as T-shirts, ribbons, or certificates.
8. Attend personally to orthopedic and musculoskeletal problems. Provide alternatives to floor exercise.
9. Counsel participants on proper foot apparel and exercise clothing.
10. Avoid constant references to complicated medical or physiological terminology, but don't ignore it altogether. Concentrate on a few selected terms to provide a little education at a time.
11. Arrange for occasional visits by personal physicians.
12. Provide a constant flow of newspaper or magazine articles to the participants on topics related to physical activity and other pertinent information.
13. Encourage an occasional visitor or participant to lead activity.
14. Have a designated area for participant counseling. Avoid trying to converse with clients while performing another task simultaneously.
15. Display your continuing education certifications and educational degrees. You are more likely to be successful at modifying behavior if you are perceived to be an expert.
16. Introduce first-time exercisers on the gymnasium floor or in the locker room. This orientation will encourage a sense of belonging to the group.
17. Reinforce participants by complimenting them on their appearance as they are exercising. Your conversation during exercise also can serve as a distracter from any unpleasant sensations that they may be experiencing.
18. Consider entering city- or business-sponsored road races to pace your participants. Exercise leaders also can show their interest and enthusiasm by cheering clients at community fitness events.

Reprinted from Franklin et al. 1990. Courtesy of Barry A. Franklin, PhD.

Walk/Jog/Run Programs

While walking, the participant keeps at least one foot on the ground at all times. In jogging and running, more muscular force is exerted to propel the body completely off the ground, causing a nonsupport phase. The distinction between jogging and running is not as clearly defined. Some people view the speed as being the difference, but no single criterion for speed is commonly accepted. Others distinguish between the two by the intent of the participant—a jogger is simply interested in exercise, whereas a runner trains to achieve performance goals in road races.

General Safety Considerations

A variety of safety factors common to both walking and jogging should be mentioned before we discuss how to institute walking and jogging programs.

Footwear

Any comfortable pair of good, well-supported shoes can be worn for a beginning walking program. The serious walker and all joggers should invest in appropriate shoes having well-padded heels that are higher than the soles and a fitted heel cup. The shoes should be flexible enough to bend easily. The same kind of socks that will be worn while exercising should be worn during the fitting to ensure a comfortable and proper fit. Only the serious competitive runner needs racing shoes, which are a lighter weight and offer less cushioning.

Clothing

The weather conditions and vigorousness of the activity determine the amount and type of clothing to be worn. Warm weather dictates light, preferably cotton, loose-fitting clothing. Nothing should be worn that prevents perspiration from reaching the outside air. A brimmed hat should cover the head on hot, sunny days. For the jogger, long pants are probably not needed until the temperature (wind-chill factor considered) drops below 40° F.

In cold weather, the walker or jogger should dress in layers for the flexibility of removing or adding clothing when necessary. Wool and polypropylene fabrics are good choices for extreme cold, but most joggers tend to overdress. A hat, preferably a wool stocking cap that can be pulled down over the forehead and ears, and gloves or mittens also should be worn. Cotton socks worn as mittens are useful not only to keep hands warm but also to act as "wipers" for the sniffling nose that often accompanies cold-weather walking and jogging.

Surface

The surface for walkers is not as crucial as it is for joggers, although some walkers (especially those with orthopedic problems) should exercise on a soft surface such as grass or a running track with a shock-absorbent surface. Many people prefer exercising off of the track for visual stimulation and interest, but regular jogging on hard surfaces such as concrete or blacktop can lead to stress problems in the ankle, knee, and hip joints and in the lower back. Joggers need to observe special precautions when running on the road: Jog facing traffic, assume cars at crossroads do not see joggers, and beware of cracks and curbs. Running cross-country usually means running on a softer surface, but joggers must be aware of the uneven terrain and the increased potential for ankle injuries.

Safety Tips

Educate participants that for safety when walking or jogging they should practice the following:

- Move toward the oncoming traffic.
- Yield the right of way to cars.
- Listen to music only while exercising on a very quiet street, and always listen for and be aware of traffic.
- Choose well-lighted streets or running tracks on school grounds.
- Walk or jog with a partner if you must exercise at night.

4 In Review

Walkers and joggers should have supportive and flexible shoes and should wear clothing that accommodates weather conditions and exercise intensity. They should follow rules of the road and walk or jog in safe areas at safe times.

Walking

The advantages of walking include its convenience, practicality, and naturalness. Walking is an excellent activity, especially for people who are overfat and poorly conditioned and whose joints cannot handle the stresses of jogging.

As with all exercise programs, the participants begin with warm-up activities and perhaps some static stretching before the actual walk. The walk should begin at a slow speed and gradually increase to a pace that feels comfortable to the participant. The arms should swing freely, and the trunk should be kept erect with a slight backward pelvic tilt. The feet should point forward at all times. Many walkers have taken to malls, which provide air-conditioned comfort, safety, and a smooth surface and are usually within a short, convenient drive.

Walking programs can progress by increasing the distance and/or the speed. Participants should gradually increase their distances until they can easily walk 4 miles at a brisk pace. It is not appropriate to begin jogging or attempt to achieve THR in an aerobic dance class until the 4-mile walking goal can be reached. The walking program below is graduated and leads to an activity level suitable for beginning a jogging program.

How do you make walking interesting for a class of 30 to 40 participants? An exercise leader must emphasize variety to keep interest high in such situations. There are several ways you might do this:

- Have participants follow the leader over hill and dale, up and down steps or slopes, with the walking speed changing from time to time.
- Have the group do "line-walking" on a track, in which the person at the end of the line must walk faster to catch up to the front of the line, which, as a whole, moves at a steady pace—giving each person an interval-type workout.
- Add a ball to the front of the line-walking line, and have participants pass it to the side or

Walking Program

Rules

1. Start at a level that is comfortable to you.
2. Be aware of new aches or pains.
3. Don't progress to the next level if you are not comfortable.
4. Monitor and record your HR.
5. It is healthful to walk at least every other day.

Stage	Duration	HR	Comments
1	15 min		
2	20 min		
3	25 min		
4	30 min		
5	30 min		
6	30 min		
7	35 min		
8	40 min		
9	45 min		
10	45 min		
11	45 min		
12	50 min		
13	55 min		
14	60 min		
15	60 min		
16	60 min		
17	60 min		
18	60 min		
19	60 min		
20	60 min		

Reprinted from Franks and Howley 1998.

overhead until it reaches the end of the line, at which time the last person dribbles to the front and restarts the process.

- Vary the activity used to reach the front of the line-walking line, with people skipping, jogging, and so on.
- Vary the length of the line-walking line so that "teams" can be formed, and control the overall pace by balancing the teams and checking the THR.
- Plan a game of "tag" in a gym or field where all participants must walk, with the leader exerting control by defining the boundaries.
- Establish a distance goal for a 15-week walking class—such as "we will walk from here to Nashville" (a total of 180 miles walked over the 15 weeks)—and use a large map to monitor each participant's progress from week to week, using stick pins. Award T-shirts or hold a country-western party when everyone finishes. Longer distances can be used along with the class total of miles walked to focus on group accomplishments.

5 In Review

Walking programs should begin at a slow speed and gradually increase the speed to a comfortable pace. Distance should be increased gradually until 4 miles can be walked at a brisk pace. The previous list details activities that improve enjoyment and, consequently, adherence to the program.

Jogging

No single factor determines when an individual can begin jogging. A person who can walk about 4 miles briskly but is unable to reach the THR range by walking should consider a jogging program to make additional improvements in CRF. A slow to moderate walker whose HR is within the THR zone should increase the distance and / or speed of walking rather than begin jogging. Also, the ability of the individual's joints to withstand the additional stresses of jogging should be considered. Remember, walking may be the first and only activity for a large number of people, and it is more important that they stay active than move up the scale to more intense activities.

The techniques of jogging are basically the same as walking. Jogging requires a greater flexion of the knee of the recovery leg, and the arms are bent more at the elbows. The arm swing is exaggerated slightly but should still be in the forward / backward direction. The heel makes the first contact with the ground; then the foot immediately rolls forward to the ball of the foot and then to the toes. As speed increases, the landing foot may contact the ground closer to a flat-footed position. Breathing is done through both the nose and mouth. Common faults of the beginning jogger include breathing with the mouth closed, insufficiently bending the knee during the recovery phase, and swinging the arms across the body.

Many people begin jogging at too high a speed, which results in an inability to continue for a sufficient length of time to accomplish the desired amount of total work; often this causes people to dislike jogging. This problem can be prevented by jogging at a speed slow enough to allow conversation and using work-relief intervals, which for beginners is slow jogging for a few seconds, then walking, then slow jogging, and so forth. Participants should be reassured that they will be walking less and jogging more as they become more fit. An example of such a progression is shown in the jogging program on page 272.

6 In Review

Stages 1 through 5 of the jogging program are appropriate walk/jog intervals to use at the beginning of a jogging program.

After a person can jog 2 or 3 miles continuously within the THR zone, several approaches to a jogging program are available. A person can simply jog 3 or 4 times a week, with the only plan being to exercise at an intensity that will elevate the HR to the training zone for a predetermined minimum length of time (or distance), with the option to go longer (or farther) on days when so desired. Other people do better with a specific program that includes progressive speed and distance goals, even if they do not plan to compete.

As with the walking class mentioned earlier, the HFI should include variety in a jogging program, and the same types of modifications cited earlier for the walking program would be appropriate. In addition, in some communities where there are established exercise or fitness trails, one can combine

Jogging Program

Rules

1. Complete the walking program before starting this program.
2. Begin each session with walking and stretching.
3. Be aware of new aches and pains.
4. Don't progress to the next level if you are not comfortable.
5. Stay at the low end of your THR zone; record your HR for each session.
6. Do the program on a work-a-day, rest-a-day basis.

Stage 1	Jog 10 steps; walk 10 steps. Repeat five times and take your HR. Stay within THR zone by increasing or decreasing walking phase. Do 20 to 30 min of activity.
Stage 2	Jog 20 steps; walk 10 steps. Repeat five times and take your HR. Stay within THR zone by increasing or decreasing walking phase. Do 20 to 30 min of activity.
Stage 3	Jog 30 steps; walk 10 steps. Repeat five times and take your HR. Stay within THR zone by increasing or decreasing walking phase. Do 20 to 30 min of activity.
Stage 4	Jog 1 min; walk 10 steps. Repeat three times and take your HR. Stay within THR zone by increasing or decreasing walking phase. Do 20 to 30 min of activity.
Stage 5	Jog 2 min; walk 10 steps. Repeat two times and take your HR. Stay within THR zone by increasing or decreasing walking phase. Do 30 min of activity.
Stage 6	Jog 1 lap (400 m, or 440 yd) and check your HR. Adjust pace during run to stay within the THR zone. If HR is still too high, go back to the Stage 5 schedule. Do 6 laps with a brief walk between each.
Stage 7	Jog 2 laps and check HR. Adjust pace during run to stay within the THR zone. If HR is still too high, go back to Stage 6 activity. Do 6 laps with a brief walk between each.
Stage 8	Jog 1 mile and check HR. Adjust pace during the run to stay within THR zone. Do 2 miles.
Stage 9	Jog 2 to 3 miles continuously. Check HR at the end to ensure that you were within THR zone.

Reprinted from Franks and Howley 1998.

walking/jogging with specific exercises for all parts of the body. "Fun runs" are held in many communities; the goal is to finish the distance, and a small prize is usually awarded.

Joggers who are not fast enough to compete successfully in road races may enjoy other types of competition, such as prediction runs, in which speed does not determine the winner. The purpose of a prediction run is to see which jogger comes closest to her or his predicted time of finishing, which is declared before the race. A "handicapped" run requires joggers to know and declare their previous fastest times for the distance. A percentage (80-100%) of the time difference between the fastest runner's declared time and each other runner's time is subtracted from each runner's actual finish time. For example, suppose runner A's fastest previous time is 18 min for 3 miles; runner B's is 19 min; and runner C's is 20 min. Forty-eight seconds (0.8 [80%] $\times$ 60-s difference between A and B) is subtracted from B's finish time, and 96 s (0.8 $\times$ 120-s difference) is subtracted from runner C's. Suppose runner A completes the race in 17:50, runner B in 18:30, and C in 20:10. The adjusted finish times would be runner A = 17:50 (actual time), runner B = 17:42 (18:30 – 48), and runner C = 18:34 (20:10 – 96). Runner B is the winner. Another method of handicapping a race is to stagger the start according to each jogger's previous best time, with the slowest runner starting first and the fastest last. The first one over the finish line is the winner. Teams can be formed in which each four-member team, for example, could have one runner from each of four groups classified by running speed.

Competitive Running

Almost all communities have road races sponsored by track clubs and service organizations as a means of raising funds, many for worthy purposes. Each entrant pays a registration fee, and most of the races have sex and age divisions, with prizes awarded to the top finishers, both overall and in each division. Usually every finisher receives an award such as a certificate or T-shirt. The race distances range between 1 mile (often considered a "fun run") and 100 miles, but the most common are the 5K (3.1 miles) and 10K (6.2 miles). Remember that fitness participants should not be pressured to enter road races by those who enjoy them. The HFI should consider entering races with interested participants to help them select a starting spot and establish a pace and to provide encouragement. This may help them make a good transition from a jogging group to an individualized jogging program.

Those who train for performance goals will be working at the top part of the THR range, 6 to 7 days per week, and for more than 30 to 40 min per exercise session. Such programs are bound to result in more injuries, and the HFI should encourage participants pursuing such goals to have an alternative activity that they can enjoy when they are recovering from injuries.

Cycling

Riding a bicycle or stationary exercise cycle is another good fitness activity. Some people who have problems walking, jogging, or playing sports may be able to cycle without difficulty. The cycling program below follows the guidelines for making CRF improvements (see chapter 10). Although bicycles and terrain vary widely, checking THR allows the cyclist to adjust the speed so that she or he is working at the appropriate intensity. Generally, a person covers 3 to 4 times the distance cycling compared with jogging (e.g., a person works up to 3 miles jogging or 9-12 miles cycling per workout). The seat should be comfortable, and its height should be adjusted so that the knee is slightly bent at the bottom of the pedaling stroke.

Cycling Program

Rules

1. Adjust the seat so that it is comfortable for you.
2. Use either a regular bicycle or a stationary exercise cycle.
3. If you are starting at Stage 1, simply get used to riding 1 or 2 miles. Don't be concerned about time or reaching the lower end of your THR zone.

Stage	Distance (miles)	THR (%HRmax)	Time (min)	Frequency (days/week)
1	1-2	—	—	3
2	1-2	60	8-12	3
3	3-5	60	15-25	3
4	6-8	70	25-35	3
5	6-9	70	25-35	4
6	10-15	70	40-60	4
7	10-15	80	35-50	4-5

Reprinted from Franks and Howley 1998.

7 In Review

In general, one should cycle 3 to 4 times the distance compared with jogging for an equivalent caloric expenditure and cardiorespiratory workout.

Games

One of the wonderful characteristics of children that is often lost in adulthood is a sense of playfulness. A child does not feel a need to justify spending time playing a game just for the fun of it. One of the attributes that seem to be present in coronary-prone behavior is the inability to appreciate play for its own sake. Perhaps one of the things a good fitness program can do for people is provide them with activities that increase both fitness and playfulness.

For games to be an effective part of a fitness program, certain elements must be present:

- Competition—Competition is not to be avoided, but little emphasis should be put on winning; the game should not be used to exclude people from participating.
- Cooperation—Having small groups solve problems together to accomplish fitness tasks can be enjoyable and healthy.
- Enjoyment—Enjoyment requires a balance of cooperation and competition, continued participation by everyone, and the chance for everyone to be a winner.
- Inclusion—A key ingredient for a fitness game is that everyone is included. This may mean modifying the rules.
- Skill—Some fitness games may require certain minimum levels of skill that can be taught as part of the fitness program.
- Vigor—The main body of the workout should include games in which all participants are continuously active in the THR range.

Special Considerations

Participants at any fitness level can do the warm-up and cool-down activities of most games. The more vigorous games, however, usually involve high-intensity bursts, stopping, starting, and quickly changing directions. They are not recommended for the early stages of a fitness program. Some additional stretching and easy movements in different directions should be included as part of the warm-up for games. Obviously, the space, number of people, and equipment have to be considered in the selection of activities. The leader must emphasize safety and should change the rules immediately when something is not working. A variety of games should be offered, so that people with different skill levels can participate. When large groups are involved in activities, the activities should be changed frequently to maintain interest. In addition to warm-up and cool-down activities, higher and lower intensity activities should be alternated to prevent undue fatigue. People should be encouraged to go at their own pace. THR should be checked periodically to ensure that people are within their ranges.

Fitness Games

Fitness games and activities are summarized on the next page. In general, the level of control varies from that associated with circle and line activities to those with few rules, such as "keep-away." Games can involve diverse muscle groups and use the body weight as a resistance. Simultaneously, games encourage the continued development of balance and coordination, which are not necessarily outcomes of walking, jogging, or exercising with fixed equipment. *The Sport Ball Exercise Handbook* (4), a book written specifically to encourage games in a fitness setting, should be a part of every exercise leader's library. *The New Games Book* (13), a classic in this area, and *Inclusive Games: Movement Fun for Everyone* (8) provide a playful, fun, and inclusive approach to games for various numbers of people. In games, as with all activities, the HFI needs to include individuals with disabilities by modifying or adapting the activities (17).

8 In Review

Effective games for a fitness program should be enjoyable, inclusive, vigorous, cooperative, competitive, and skill-related.

Aquatic Activities

Aquatic activities can be a major part of a person's exercise program or can be the needed relief from other forms of exercise, especially when a person is injured. The intensity of the activity can be graded to suit the needs of the least and the most fit, from the recent post-MI patient to the endurance athlete. HR can be checked at regular intervals to see whether THR has been reached, and a caloric expenditure

Fitness Games and Activities

1. Skills and games with balls of various sizes. The size and type of ball can lead to innovative use—for instance, the cage ball can be used as a substitute for a basketball. Examples of other balls include tennis balls, volleyballs, playground balls, basketballs, medicine balls, handballs, softballs, mush balls, and Nerf balls.
2. Activities with apparatus. Examples include hula hoops, Frisbees, paddle rackets, skip ropes, skittles, "quoits," surgical tubing, culverts, and play buoys.
3. Chasing games. Examples include tag, chain tag, fox and geese, and dodge ball.
4. Relays with and without apparatus. Examples include running, hopping, rolling, crawling, and dribbling with hands and feet.
5. Stunts and contests. Examples are dual activities such as balancing stunts, forward rolls, backward rolls, strength moves, push-ups, sit-ups, and limited combatives such as rooster fights and partner sparring.
6. Lead-up games for major sport games. Examples are soccer, tennis, basketball, volleyball, handball, and football, often with rules adjusted to fit the level of skill and capacity of the participants.
7. Children's games. Activities include skittle ball, four square, and bounce ball.

Adapted from Giese, 1988, Organization of an exercise testing session. In *Resource manual for guidelines for exercise testing and prescription*. By permission of Lea & Febiger.

goal can be achieved, given the high-energy requirement associated with aquatic activities. Individuals with orthopedic problems who cannot run, dance, or play games can exercise in water. The water supports the person's body weight, and problems associated with weight-bearing joints are minimized.

Target Heart Rate

One consistent finding is that the maximal HR response to a swimming test is about 18 beats · min^{-1} lower than that found in a maximal treadmill test. This suggests that for swimming, THR should be shifted downward (2 beats less for a 10-s count) to achieve the 60 to 80% $\dot{V}O_2$max goal associated with an endurance training effect (10).

Progression

Swimming activities can be graded not only by varying the speed of the swim but also by varying the activity. A post-MI patient with an extremely low functional capacity benefits from simply walking through the water. People with recent bypass surgery benefit from moving the arms as they walk across the pool. Following are examples of activities that can be used in aquatic exercise programs. The reader is referred to *Water Fitness After 40* (18) and *YMCA Water Fitness for Health* (16) for detailed information on aquatic exercise.

Side-of-Pool Activities

A wide variety of activities can be done while holding on to the side of the pool with one or both hands. These range from simply moving the legs to the side, front, or back to practicing a variety of kicks that ultimately can be used while swimming. ROM-type movements in the pool are a good way to warm up before undertaking the more vigorous activities of walking or jogging across the pool.

Walking and Jogging Across the Pool

A person with a low functional capacity can begin an aquatic program by simply walking across the shallow end of the pool. The water offers resistance to the movement while supporting the body weight, resulting in a reduced downward load on the ankles, knees, and hips. The arms can be involved in the activity to simulate a swimming motion; this increases the ROM of the arms and shoulder girdle. The speed and form of the walk can be changed as the person becomes accustomed to the activity. The person can walk with long strides with the head just above the water or do a side-step across the pool. Last, the person can practice jogging across the pool with the water at chest height. Remember to check whether THR has been achieved.

Flotation Devices

People with limited skill can use flotation devices (e.g., a life jacket or kickboard). The extra resistance offered by the jacket compensates for the extra buoyancy it provides. The participant should stop periodically to determine whether THR has been reached.

Lap Swimming

The participant must be skilled to use swimming as a substitute activity for running or cycling. An unskilled swimmer operates at a very high energy cost, even when moving slowly, and may become too fatigued to last through the whole workout. But this doesn't mean that swimming should be eliminated as an option in personal fitness programs. A person can learn to swim over a period of several months, gradually adjusting during that time to the exercise. After learning to swim, the person becomes able to use swimming as the primary activity, even if elementary strokes are used. Increasing the number of activities a person can do increases the chance that the person will remain active when something interferes with a primary activity.

Lap swimming should be approached the same way as lap running: warming up with stretching activities, starting slowly, taking frequent breaks to check the pulse rate, and gradually increasing the distance. Remember, the caloric cost of swimming compared with the cost of running is about a 1:4 ratio. If jogging a total distance of 1 mile is a reasonable goal in someone's physical activity program, then swimming 400 m (1/4 mile) is equivalent in terms of energy expenditure. The swimming program below describes a series of stages that could be included in an endurance swimming program, beginning with walking across the pool. All steps assume that a warm-up has preceded the activity and that a cool-down follows.

Swimming Program

Rules

1. Start at a level that is comfortable for you.
2. Don't progress to the next stage if you are not comfortable with the current one.
3. Monitor and record your HR.

Stage 1	In chest-deep water, walk across the width of the pool four times and see if you are close to THR. Gradually increase the duration of the walk until you can do two 10-min walks at THR.
Stage 2	In chest-deep water, walk across and jog back. Repeat twice and see if you are close to THR. Gradually increase the duration of the jogging until you can complete four 5-min jogs at THR.
Stage 3	In chest-deep water, walk across and swim back (any stroke). Use a kickboard or flotation device if needed. Repeat this cycle twice and see if you are at THR. Keep up this pattern of walk-swim to do about 20 to 30 min of activity.
Stage 4	In chest-deep water, jog across and swim back (any stroke); repeat and check THR. Gradually decrease the duration of the jog and increase the duration of the swim until four widths can be completed within the THR zone. Accomplish 20 to 30 min of activity per session.
Stage 5	Slowly swim 25 yd; rest 20 s. Slowly swim another 25 yd and check THR. On the basis of the HR response, change the speed of the swim and/or the length of the rest period to stay within the THR zone. Gradually increase the number of lengths you can swim (e.g., three, then four) before checking THR.
Stage 6	Increase the duration of continuous swimming until you can accomplish 20 to 30 min without a rest.

Reprinted from Franks and Howley 1998.

The HFI should not view the stages in the swimming program as discrete steps that must be followed in a particular order. Two stages can be combined, or games can be introduced, to make the walk-and-jog and width swims more enjoyable. The major goal is to gradually increase the intensity and duration of the aquatic activities.

9 In Review

Various aquatic activities include doing upright activities (e.g., walking and jogging across the pool, using flotation devices) as well as swimming. Exercises also can be done holding on to the side of the pool, such as moving the legs from front to back or practicing a paddle kick.

Exercising to Music

Moving to the rhythm of music is an enjoyable way to exercise. One can join a group at a fitness club, do individual workouts with a personal fitness trainer, or exercise at home with videotapes.

Advantages

Exercise to music provides an enjoyable fitness activity for many participants—young and old, male and female. Since the mid-1970s, aerobics has evolved from the traditional high-intensity and low-impact classes to a variety of specialized classes to fit everyone's tastes and fitness levels. The use of water, steps, slides, tubing, resistance balls, martial arts, and boxing provides numerous opportunities to cross-train or learn new techniques. Fortunately, certification and continuing education programs to support this expansion have developed in conjunction with these trends (see later in this chapter).

Getting Motivated

Working out to music is a great way to motivate people to continue exercising. The variety of tempos and rhythms of the different songs keeps the workout exciting and challenging for participants. Familiar lyrics often distract from the feeling of fatigue. Music makes routine exercises fun, and the class setting helps to promote camaraderie and regular participation.

Achieving THR

Aerobic dance programs can develop all the fitness components. The recommended frequency, intensity, and total work (see chapter 10) can be achieved in exercise-to-music programs and can increase $\dot{V}O_2max$ (20). THR can be monitored easily after a music segment, but beginners need to be cautioned about doing too much too soon. A recent review indicated that THR can be achieved with either low- or high-impact routines. Although the energy cost of high-intensity, high-impact aerobic dance is higher than that of low-impact programs for the same routines and music, the activities are not very different in terms of caloric expenditure when multidirectional movements are included in the low-impact routines (20).

Low Skill Requirement

Movement to music can be adapted to any skill level because no competition is involved. The only rule is to keep moving at a pace needed to achieve THR. The routines can also be adapted for all ages. Most aerobics classes provide participants with an appropriate workout routine within a safe environment (assuming instructors are certified and emphasize safe exercises). Warm-ups are structured to provide low-impact movements and dynamic stretching before the 30 to 40 min of the cardiovascular portion of the workout. Gradual progression within each session, as well as from one workout to the next, is provided to enhance enjoyment.

The HFI should be familiar with the types of aerobic dance programs offered in his or her community, because some (e.g., Jazzercize®) may require more knowledge and skill of "dance" movements than other forms. HFIs should also be aware of the programs that would be appropriate for different age, skill-level, and interest groups.

Disadvantages

Injury is always a potential risk in fitness programs, and aerobic dance is no different. One review found that about 44% of students and 76% of instructors reported injuries resulting from aerobic dance, with the injury rate being 1 injury per 100 hr of activity for students and 0.22 to 1.16 injuries per 100 hr for the instructors. The severity of the injuries, however, was such that only once in 1092 to 4275 hr of participation did an individual have to seek medical attention (6). It is our recommendation that people should participate in aerobic dance programs only after they can walk about 4 miles without discomfort. They should move from low-intensity, low-impact sessions to more strenuous sessions using THR as a guide. Furthermore, introductory classes to step or other specialized forms of aerobics should be taken to develop the skills needed for participation in the regular classes.

It is not uncommon for individuals to experience muscle soreness, as well as a variety of acute soft-tissue injuries, because of regular participation in aerobic activities. In addition, evidence shows that chronic conditions may develop because of improper form or simply from doing large numbers of repetitions of a specific exercise. These can include the following:

- Chronic shoulder soreness from too many overhead pulls
- Elbow or wrist pain from the use of hand-held weights in aerobics classes
- Achilles tendinitis and plantar fasciitis from high-impact forces and improper step techniques
- Groin pulls and shin splints from improper slide technique
- Low back problems from exercising with weak abdominals (anterior pelvic tilt) and doing improper stretching
- Knee problems from using a step that is too high

It is also common for instructors and participants to experience some hearing losses from music played too loudly. See chapter 25 for advice on how to prevent and deal with acute and chronic problems associated with participation in exercise.

Here are some suggestions to minimize the risk of injury in exercise-to-music classes:

1. Participants should warm up with low-impact activity and dynamic stretching, and cool down with static stretches of the following muscles: calf, anterior tibialis, quadriceps, hamstrings, hip flexors, low back area, and shoulders.
2. Participants should avoid hypertension of the neck.
3. Instruct participants to avoid forward flexion of the spine unless supported by a bent knee balanced directly over the heel.
4. Participants should practice correct standing posture (i.e., pelvis in neutral position, buttocks tight, head and chin up, shoulders back).
5. Deep-knee bends should be avoided; participants should not squat to where the thighs are below parallel and the knees are over the toes rather than placed properly over the middle of the foot.
6. Participants should wear good shoes with good cushioning and support.
7. Participants should work all muscle groups evenly to achieve a balanced workout.
8. Instruct participants that they should not stop in the middle of a routine, because this can cause venous pooling in the lower legs.
9. The leader should practice routines to ensure that movement transitions are smooth, safe, and easy to follow. Teach basic movements before using them in combination.
10. The leader should monitor the class at all times. Use eye contact, emphasize safe movements by making corrections while leading, and check THR or RPE regularly.

Music Selection

Selection of music for different phases of the exercise session sets the tone for the appropriate intensity of warm-up, aerobic phase, and cool-down (9, 11). The music can vary, depending on choice, from top-40 hits to instrumental Muzak. The warm-up starts slowly, with the music tempo about 100 beats $\cdot$ min^{-1}. The cardiorespiratory endurance phase includes increasingly intense aerobic exercises at a faster pace (no more than 160 beats $\cdot$ min^{-1}), whereas the muscle conditioning phase (typically including abdominal work) is set to a slower tempo (usually 118-130 beats $\cdot$ min^{-1}). Step classes are limited to 118 to 125 beats $\cdot$ min^{-1}, and slide classes are restricted to <140 beats $\cdot$ min^{-1}. In the final cool-down, the music tempo and volume are decreased for a relaxing conclusion.

The leader should consider purchasing music selections from one of the many aerobic music companies in the fitness market. They sell professionally mixed music selections with appropriate tempos for each class. Not only are the tapes made for specific classes (e.g., step, slide, low-impact), but most companies pay the licensing fees that protect the instructor from suits related to fraud. The music should be changed periodically to provide variety.

Components

There are no set routines; the instructor can individualize the program. Suggested components of an exercise session include a full-body warm-up (including low-impact and dynamic flexibility exercises); exercises for cardiorespiratory endurance using a variety of muscle groups; an active standing recovery cool-down; exercises for muscular endurance and strength for the arms, legs, and abdominals; and a final cool-down.

An easy progression for beginners would include 25 to 30 min of mostly flexibility activities, with light muscular and cardiorespiratory endurance activities. A more advanced program would last 45 to 60 min, with longer duration for all of the fitness components. The phases of an exercise-to-music class are discussed next.

Warm-Up

For a gradual progression, the program should begin with low-impact movements and dynamic stretching for the whole body. Dynamic flexibility includes exercises such as arm circles, side bends, back rolls, half-knee bends, stationary lunges, toe taps, and Achilles curls. The warm-up should continue for 5 to 10 min, gradually increasing the HR and preparing the body for the cardiorespiratory workout to come.

Cardiorespiratory Endurance

In this segment, movements concentrate on the large muscles of the legs, with arm movements adding flair and extra cardiorespiratory intensity (arm movements are optional). This segment is specific to the type of class. For the high-intensity/low-impact classes, marches, step-touches, hops, strides, skips, knee lifts, hamstring curls, jumping jacks, step-hops, cross-over steps, toe-heel kicks, and so forth are used to elevate the HR within the target zone. The instructor can individualize the style from a calisthenics workout to a funky dance routine.

If the class uses a step or slide, the leader should be knowledgeable and trained in that form of movement to provide safe instruction. It is most important for an aerobics instructor to hold a national certification and be able to lead a class with smooth transitions before instructing a class on her or his own.

The duration of the cardiorespiratory section is 15 to 40 min, with THR taken about every 15 min. The intensity of this segment can be increased by using more vigorous arm movements or higher hops (power jumps), and it can be decreased by lowering the arms, slowing the pace, and walking rather than jogging through the movement. It is recommended that one stay within the safety guidelines for speed of music, height of step, and width of slide. This element of control will enhance the participant's safety.

Recovery Cool-Down

A 2- to 5-min active-standing cool-down should follow the cardiorespiratory segment. It should begin by lowering the intensity of the previous activities (e.g., walking) to decrease the HR. Dynamic stretches should be repeated, followed by static stretches.

Muscular Endurance

Once the recovery cool-down is completed, the muscular endurance exercises can be performed for 10 to 20 min. It is recommended that these activities begin with exercises done in the standing position, with a gradual movement to the floor. Many classes end with abdominal work in the supine position.

Final Cool-Down

The final cool-down consists mainly of static stretches done lying on the floor. The stretches are held for at least 10 s. Incorporate every muscle group, especially those specifically worked on in the class, with special focus on the hamstrings and low back.

Aerobic Dance Organizations

Here are some of the many aerobic dance organizations that provide opportunities to be certified as well as educational and professional support materials:

- Aerobics and Fitness Association of America (AFAA), 15250 Ventura Boulevard, Suite 200, Sherman Oaks, CA 91403
- American Council on Exercise (ACE), 4851 Paramount Drive, San Diego, CA 92123
- Jazzercize, 2808 Roosevelt Boulevard, Carlsbad, CA 92008

10 In Review

Beginning dance exercisers should be able to walk 4 miles without discomfort before participating in aerobic dance programs. Components of an exercise session include a full-body warm-up; exercises for cardiorespiratory endurance using a variety of muscle groups; an active-standing recovery cool-down; exercises for muscular endurance and strength for the arms, legs, and abdominals; and a final cool-down.

Exercise Equipment

The traditional walk, jog, run, and dance programs offered by an exercise leader have been supplemented in many fitness clubs by exercise equipment. The equipment includes treadmills, cycle ergometers, ski machines, rowers, climbing ergometers, and stepping devices. The variety of equipment can help a participant stay with an exercise program as well as provide feedback about the number of calories used. Participants with orthopedic limitations can choose weight-supported activities (e.g., cycle ergometers). People training for specific performance goals can do so in air-conditioned comfort, although air conditioning may be a problem for participants who plan to engage in races scheduled for hot days. The issue of acclimatization to a hot environment must be addressed for reasons of performance and safety (see chapters 10 and 25).

If a participant plans to buy exercise equipment for home use, the HFI can help with the decision by encouraging experimentation with all types of equipment and, within each type (e.g., rowing machines), as many brands as possible. The cost of the equipment may appear high in the short term, but it may be a wise investment in the long run in terms of healthcare costs, if the person uses it.

Generally, fitness clubs provide a variety of strength training equipment that can be used as part of an overall workout or as a separate strength training workout on another day. Recommendations for gains in muscular strength and endurance were presented in chapter 12. The emphasis at the start of a program must be on endurance, low resistance, and high repetitions. As strength and interest increase, some participants may shift the emphasis to high-resistance, low-repetition workouts. It is more important to work all the major muscle groups evenly, rather than concentrate on gaining strength in only a few muscle groups.

11 In Review

Appropriate beginning goals for people using exercise equipment are to emphasize endurance, low resistance, and high repetitions. Encourage beginners to use a variety of equipment and to be sure to work all major muscle groups.

Circuit Training

Circuit training can be an effective way to conduct an exercise program. The point is to maximize the variety of exercise, distribute the work over a larger muscle mass than could be accomplished with a single form of exercise, and include exercises for all aspects of a fitness session. Circuits can include the following:

- Moving from one piece of exercise equipment to another with a brief rest period between each. A person might exercise for 5 to 10 min (or 50-100 kcal) on a cycle ergometer, then on a treadmill, then on a rower, then on a bench step, and so on.
- A typical workout for muscular strength and endurance, in which one "set" is done on a specific machine before moving to the next, and the rotation is repeated 2 to 3 times (see chapter 12).
- A circuit set up around the perimeter of a large room with signs posted describing specific exercises that the participant should do during one trip around the circuit. The circuit could include warm-up activities, flexibility activities, strengthening exercises using body weight as a resistance, and, of course, aerobic activities. Beginning, intermediate, and advanced goals specifying the number of repetitions (or duration) can be posted at each station. Include a station to check the THR after the aerobic exercise stations.

Good examples of walk/jog/run circuits have been in place for the past decade. Many communities have set up jogging trails that have signposts along the way indicating specific exercises to do at each stop. They can be found in many cities, and they provide a break in the regular routine of steady jogging or running while focusing attention on flexibility and strengthening exercises.

12 In Review

Circuit training programs offer variety and can include exercises in all aspects of fitness (e.g., cardiorespiratory, muscle strength/endurance, flexibility). The preceding list suggests a few circuit training possibilities.

Case Studies

You can check your answers by referring to appendix A.

14.1

You are making a presentation to a group of adults who have their own neighborhood walking program. What topics should you address to emphasize safety and comfort?

14.2

A participant who has been involved in your walking program for the past 10 weeks asks your advice regarding an aerobic dance class. What would you recommend?

Source List

1. American College of Sports Medicine. (2000). *ACSM's guidelines for exercise testing and prescription* (6th ed.). Philadelphia: Lippincott Williams & Wilkins.
2. Dishman, R.K. (1990). Determinants of participation in physical activity. In C. Bouchard, R.J. Shephard, T. Stephens, J.R. Sutton, & B.D. McPherson (Eds.), *Exercise, fitness, and health* (pp. 75-101). Champaign, IL: Human Kinetics.
3. Franklin, B.A., Oldridge, N.B., Stoedefalke, K.G., & Loechel, W.E. (1990). *On the ball*. Carmel, IN: Benchmark Press.
4. Franklin, B.A., Oldridge, N.B., Stoedefalke, K.G., & Loechel, W.E. (2001). *The sport ball exercise handbook*. Monterey, CA: Exercise Science.
5. Franks, B.D., & Howley, E.T. (1998). *Fitness leaders' handbook* (2nd ed.). Champaign, IL: Human Kinetics.
6. Garrick, J.G., & Requa, R.K. (1988). Aerobic dance—A review. *Sports Medicine, 6*, 169-179.
7. Giese, M.D. (1988). Organization of an exercise session. In S.N. Blair, P. Painter, R. Pate, L.K. Smith, & C.B. Taylor (Eds.), *Resource manual guidelines for exercise testing and prescription* (pp. 244-247). Philadelphia: Lea & Febiger.
8. Kasser, S.L. (1995). *Inclusive games: Movement fun for everyone*. Champaign, IL: Human Kinetics.
9. Kisselle, J., & Mazzeo, K. (1983). *Aerobic dance*. Englewood, CO: Morton.
10. Londeree, B.R., & Moeschberger, M.L. (1982). Effect of age and other factors on maximal heart rate. *Research Quarterly for Exercise and Sport, 53*, 297-304.
11. Mazzeo, J.W. (1984). *Shape-up*. Englewood, CO: Morton.
12. McSwegin, P.J., & Pemberton, C.L. (1993). Exercise leadership: Key skills and characteristics. In J.L. Durstine, A.C. King, P.L. Painter, J.L. Roitman, L.D. Zwiren, & W.L. Kenney (Eds.), *ACSM's resource manual for guidelines for exercise testing and prescription* (2nd ed., pp. 319-326). Philadelphia: Lea & Febiger.
13. New Games Foundation. (1976). *The new games book*. Garden City, NY: Dolphin Books.
14. Oldridge, N.B. (1988). Qualities of an exercise leader. In S.N. Blair, P. Painter, R.R. Pate, L.K. Smith, & C.B. Taylor (Eds.), *Resource manual for guidelines for exercise testing and prescription* (pp. 239-243). Philadelphia: Lea & Febiger.
15. Peters, T.J., & Waterman, R.H. (1982). *In search of excellence*. New York: Warner Books.
16. Sanders, M.E. (Ed.). (1999). *YMCA water fitness for health*. Champaign, IL: Human Kinetics.
17. Seaman, J. (1999). Physical activity and fitness for persons with disabilities. *PCPFS Physical Activity and Fitness Research Digest, 3*(5).
18. Sova, R. (1995). *Water fitness after 40*. Champaign, IL: Human Kinetics.
19. U.S. Department of Health and Human Services (2000). *Healthy people 2010*. Washington, DC: Author.
20. Williford, H.N., Scharff-Olson, M., & Blessing, D.L. (1989). The physiological effects of aerobic dance—A review. *Sports Medicine, 8*, 335-345.

part four

Special Populations

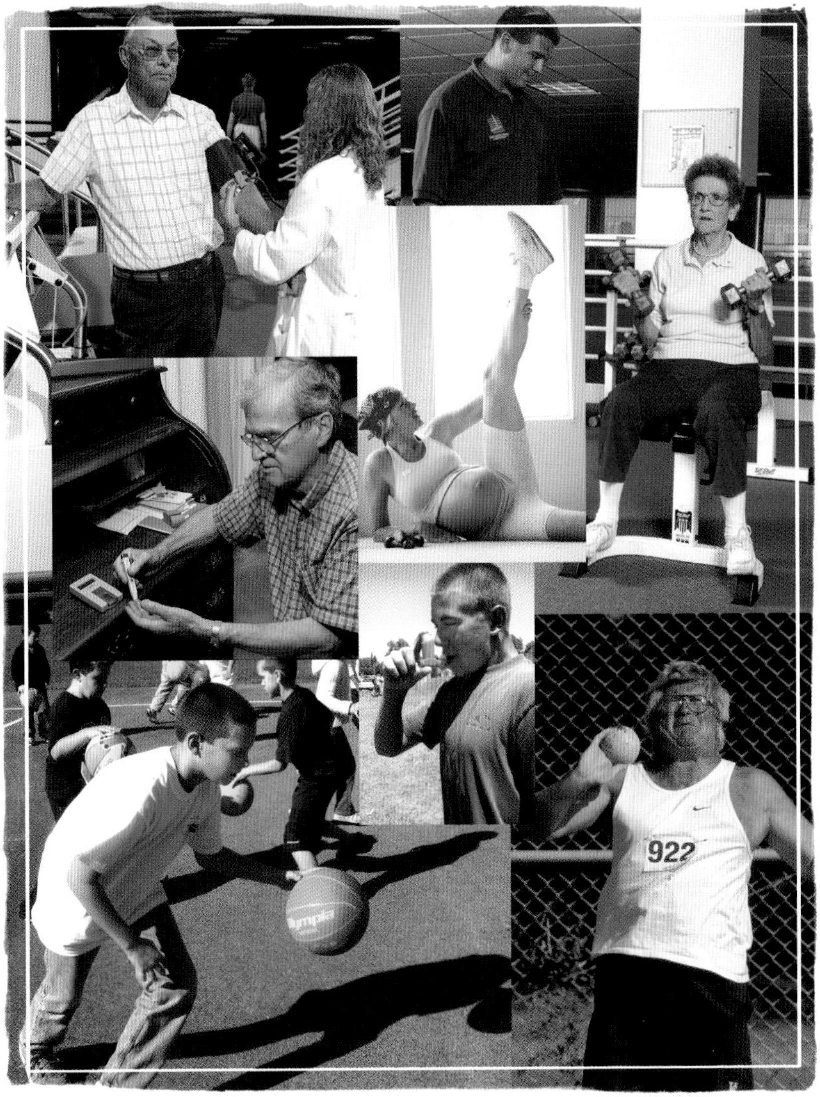

This new section for the fourth edition the *Health Fitness Instructor's Handbook* is based on several interrelated factors:

- Physical activity is beneficial for individuals of both sexes, all ages, and with a variety of medical conditions.
- Recommendations for physical activity need to be modified for individuals based on several factors.
- Behavior modification strategies need to be appropriate for different groups.
- HFIs and PFTs are increasingly expected to work with individuals with a variety of clinical conditions.

In chapters 15, 16, and 21 we explain special characteristics and health challenges for children, older individuals, and women, respectively. In chapters 17, 18, 19, and 20, we'll give you recommendations for safe and effective physical activity for some of the major health problems we face today, including

- heart disease and hypertension **(chapter 17)**,
- obesity, the new public health epidemic **(chapter 18)**,
- diabetes **(chapter 19)**, and
- asthma and other pulmonary problems **(chapter 20)**.

Any one of these topics could take a complete book in and of itself. Our purpose is to help fitness professionals gain an appreciation for the importance of these populations, understand the role of physical activity in the quality of life for all people, and provide practical guidelines for special screening, testing, supervision, and activity modifications that are recommended for each population.

fifteen

Exercise and Children and Youth

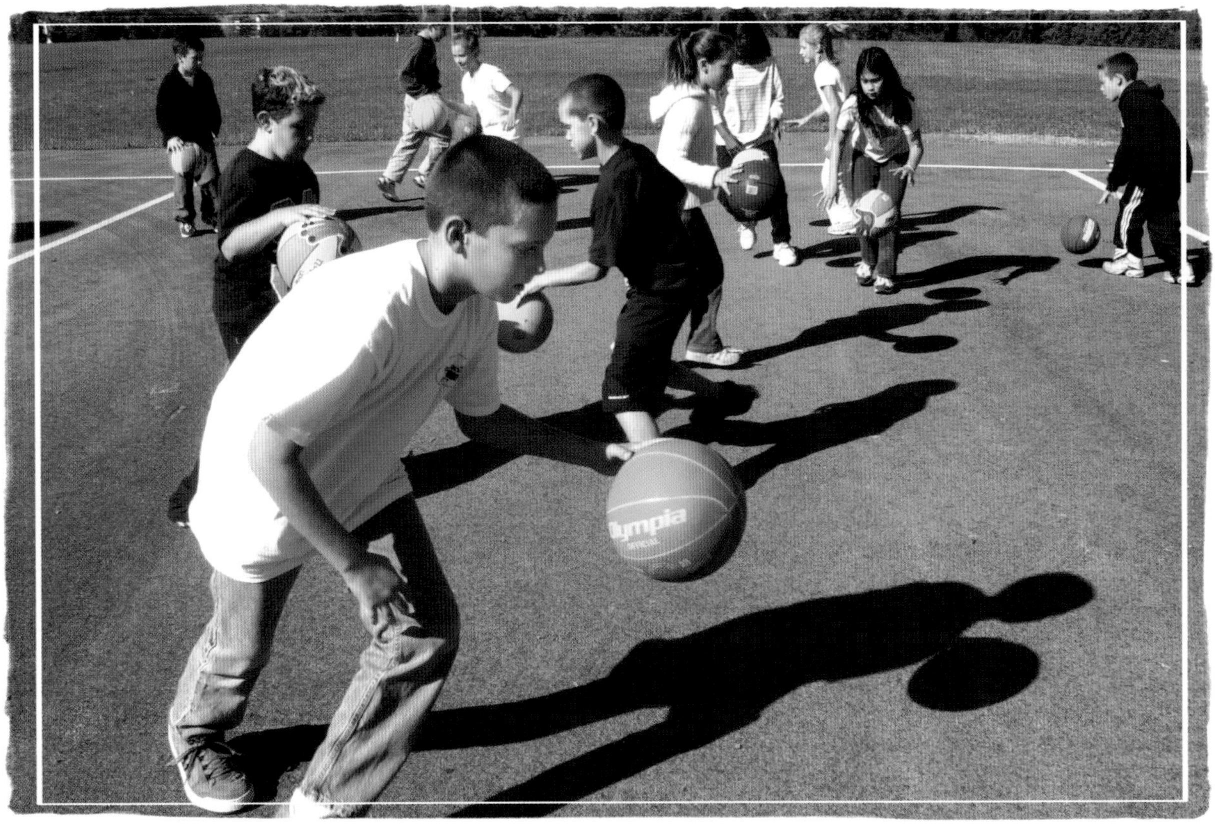

© HUMAN KINETICS

Objectives

The reader will be able to do the following:

1. Understand the importance of physical activity for children and youth.
2. Compare the responses of children, youth, and adults to acute and chronic exercise.
3. Prescribe physical activity for children and youth.
4. Describe health-related physical fitness testing for children and youth.
5. Describe special precautions for exercise and testing for children and youth.

It is increasingly evident that physical activity is essential for the highest quality of life throughout the lifespan; however, most of the experimental research related to the effects of exercise on fitness has been conducted on young adults. Most of the epidemiological research on the role of physical activity for improved health outcomes has emphasized older adults. One of the common conclusions drawn from all types of research is that regular physical activity needs to be an integral part of one's lifestyle. It is recommended that this active lifestyle begin early in life. Although the correlations for tracking physical activity across various ages are not very high, Malina (11) concluded, "Allowing for the different methods for estimating habitual physical activity, change associated with normal growth and maturation, and lack of control for important covariates in studies of tracking, physical activity tracks reasonably well from childhood into young adulthood" (p. 7). There is increasing evidence that physical activity also enhances the health and fitness of children and youth.

There is increasing emphasis on motivating people of all ages to begin and continue regular physical activity (30). In addition, physical fitness testing for children and youth is a part of many physical education programs.

This chapter deals with how to implement regular physical activity programs for children and youth and the role of fitness testing in the young. We focus on school-aged children and youth. Although not covered in this chapter, physical development is vitally important in preschool infants and children (15, 32). The emphases during the first years of life are primarily on motor development and healthy growth and are very individualized.

1 In Review

Regular physical activity is essential for the highest quality of life throughout the lifespan. It is important that children and youth include physical activity as an integral part of their lifestyle.

Response to Exercise

This section reviews the immediate (acute) and long-term (chronic) effects of physical activity for children and youth, contrasting their reactions to those of adults (see chapter 28).

Acute

Zwiren (33) comprehensively described the differences between children and adults in terms of acute response to exercise. Following are some of the most relevant differences:

Relative to adults, children are similar in terms of

- $\dot{V}O_2max$ in ml · kg^{-1} · min^{-1} (endurance tasks can be performed well), and
- creatine phosphate + ATP (children can deal well with very brief, intense exercise).

Children are lower in terms of

- capacity to generate ATP via glycolysis (children have a lower capacity to do intense activity lasting 10-90 s),
- ability to dissipate heat via evaporation and acclimatize to heat (children have an increased potential for heat-related illness), and

- economy of walking and running (children require more oxygen to walk or run at the same speed; standard equations listed in chapter 4 for estimating energy expenditure of walking and running cannot be used).

Children are better in terms of

- achieving a steady state in oxygen uptake (children experience a smaller oxygen deficit and faster recovery; they are well suited to intermittent activities).

2 In Review

Children have similar acute responses to exercise compared with adults. They are well suited for intermittent activities and should use caution in extreme environmental conditions.

Chronic

The box below illustrates that children and youth experience many of the same health and fitness benefits from regular physical activity as do adults. An active lifestyle seems to be natural for children. It is thought to be a normal and essential part of the growth and development that take place during these years (32). This chapter emphasizes the fitness and health aspects of activity for children and youth, but the achievement of fundamental motor skills (e.g., moving, throwing, catching) is an important aspect of the active lifestyle (33).

3 In Review

Chronically active youth not only prepare for active lifestyles as adults but also derive health and fitness benefits during their childhood and adolescence.

Special Considerations

Children and youth with various medical problems obviously need special attention (3). Young children need to be protected from an overemphasis on one specific sport or activity and the intense training that often accompanies it, which can lead to physical or emotional problems. Children and youth should be encouraged to choose many different activities in an enjoyable and fun atmosphere. Young children do not adapt to extreme environmental conditions; thus, more precautions need to be taken for very hot or cold conditions (1, 33).

Although exercise-related deaths are rare in children, they are most often linked to congenital heart defects (i.e., abnormalities of the heart resulting in imperfect oxygenation of the blood manifested by cyanosis and breathlessness) or acquired myocarditis (i.e., inflammation of the myocardium). Children with these conditions should avoid intense activities. Children (as well as youth and adults) with other medical conditions (see chapters 17-20) need to modify their activities, but in almost all cases activity can still be healthful. Children and their parents should work with healthcare professionals to make reasonable modifications in activities (e.g., longer warm-up and cool-down, lower intensity).

Benefits of Chronic Physical Activity: Children and Youth

Health
- Fun and enjoyment
- Improved self-esteem and self-efficacy
- Reduced risk factors for heart disease
- Reduced anxiety and stress
- Enhanced bone formation
- Weight management
- More social interaction

Fitness
- Greater strength and endurance
- Improved aerobic endurance
- Increased skill development

Adapted from ACSM, 2000, p. 220.

4 In Review

Children and youth should be screened for cardiovascular problems that might cause exercise-related deaths. Other medical problems can be addressed with commonsense modifications in activity. The exercise leader should emphasize a variety of enjoyable activities with less emphasis on intense training for and competition in one specific sport.

Testing

Concern for the fitness of our children and youth goes back over 100 years. Park's (16) historical review of the topic of fitness and fitness testing indicates that physical education leaders in the latter part of the 19th century were convinced of the connections among exercise, fitness, and health. Not surprisingly, fitness testing was a part of the process. Initially, testing was concerned more with anthropometry, strength, and sometimes a medical exam. Tests of motor ability also were developed, but it was a long time before a national test battery of fitness tests became a reality.

The driving force in fitness promotion in the first half of the 20th century was war or the threat of war, attributable to the concern raised when a large number of young men could not pass an induction exam into the armed forces. In the early 1950s, a new alarm was sounded when a study showed that a large percentage of American children could not pass basic flexibility and power tests. In response to this concern, President Eisenhower established the President's Council on Youth Fitness. Soon after that, the American Association of Health, Physical Education, and Recreation published its Youth Fitness Test, with fitness test items such as the pull-up, sit-up, shuttle run, standing broad jump, 50-yd dash, softball throw for distance, and 600-yd run-walk. This test battery emphasized "skill-related" fitness with an emphasis on muscular power (16).

In the early 1980s, the publication of *Healthy People* and *Promoting Health/Preventing Disease: Objectives for the Nation* shifted the focus to health-related fitness. In support of this health-related focus, the American Alliance of Health, Physical Education, Recreation and Dance published the *Health-Related Physical Fitness Test Manual* with the emphasis on testing fitness components related to health, including the 1-mile run for cardiorespiratory fitness, skinfold measurements to evaluate body composition, and the sit-and-reach and the sit-up to evaluate low back function. Following this publication, the introduction of criterion-referenced standards was advocated to focus on health-related goals rather than maximal performance (16). The criterion-reference standard for cardiorespiratory fitness is 42 $ml \cdot kg^{-1} \cdot min^{-1}$ for males ages 5 to 17 years. For females, the standards are 40 $ml \cdot kg^{-1} \cdot min^{-1}$ for ages 5 to 9, with a decrease of 1 $ml \cdot kg^{-1} \cdot min^{-1}$ per year until age 14, at which the standard becomes 35 $ml \cdot kg^{-1} \cdot min^{-1}$ (9). In short, these standards are not very different from those recommended for adults.

Physical Fitness

There are two major physical fitness tests for children and youth (see table 15.1), namely, the FITNESSGRAM (7) and the President's Challenge Physical Activity and Fitness Awards Program (18). Both test for cardiorespiratory fitness, muscular strength/endurance, and flexibility. The FITNESSGRAM and the health-related part of the PCPFS test also test for body composition. The President's Challenge Physical Fitness test includes a test of agility.

Table 15.1 Physical Fitness Test Items

Fitness component	FITNESSGRAM[a]	PCPFS[b] fitness	PCPFS health-related
Cardiovascular	1-mile run[c]	1-mile run[d]	1-mile run[d]
Strength/endurance	Curl-up; Push-up	Curl-up; Push-up[e]	Curl-up; Push-up
Flexibility	Sit and reach[f]; trunk lift	Sit and reach[f]	Sit and reach
Body composition	Skinfolds or BMI	—	BMI
Agility	—	Agility run	—

Note. PCPFS = President's Council on Physical Fitness and Sports; BMI = body mass index. [a]Cooper Institute for Aerobic Research (7). [b]President's Council on Physical Fitness and Sports President's Challenge (18). [c]Or the PACER (7). [d]Shorter distances for younger children (18). [e]Uses one leg at a time (7). [f]Or V-sit (18).

The FITNESSGRAM and the health-related portion of the President's challenge use health criteria as standards for the tests, whereas the physical fitness portion of the President's challenge uses percentiles (by age and sex) for its standards.

Clinical Testing

In addition to the contraindications to exercise testing for adults (see chapter 5), Zwiren (33) listed the following reasons not to test children:

- Dyspnea at rest (or forced expiratory volume less than 60% of predicted value)
- Acute renal disease or hepatitis
- Insulin-dependent diabetes (in subjects who do not take insulin as prescribed) or ketoacidosis
- Acute rheumatic fever with carditis
- Severe pulmonary vascular disease
- Poorly compensated heart failure
- Severe aortic or mitral stenosis
- Hypotrophic cardiomyopathy with syncope

Cardiorespiratory Fitness

Measuring $\dot{V}O_2$max in children using both the cycle ergometer and the treadmill has a sound historical foundation (2, 19). The GXT format is used for children, and one must match the characteristics of the test (initial grade / speed on the treadmill, increments per stage) to the child in the same way as for the adult (see chapter 5). Treadmill testing may be easier because of the role that children's shorter attention span can play in completing a cycle protocol. In addition, local muscle fatigue may shorten a cycle ergometer test before the child reaches maximum aerobic power. If a cycle is used for young children, adjustments must be made to the handlebars, seat height, crank length, and resistance scale (33). Table 15.2 lists the ACSM's recommendations for suitable treadmill and cycle ergometer protocols to follow when testing children (1).

5 In Review

Fitness testing of children and youth is a part of many school and youth agency programs. The emphasis has usually been on field tests of health-related components of physical fitness. Children and youth can be tested on GXTs with minor modifications.

Table 15.2 Protocols Suitable for Graded Exercise Testing of Children

Modified Balke treadmill protocol

Subject	Speed (mile · hr^{-1})	Initial grade (%)	Increment (%)	Stage duration (min)
Poorly fit	3.00	6	2	2
Sedentary	3.25	6	2	2
Active	5.00	0	2.5	2
Athlete	5.25	0	2.5	2

McMaster cycle test

Height (cm)	Initial load (W)	Increments (W)	Step duration (min)
<120	12.5	12.5	2
120-139.9	12.5	25	2
140-159.9	25	25	2
≥160	25	50 (boys) 25 (girls)	2

Reprinted from American College of Sports Medicine 2000.

Recommendations for Physical Activity

As seen on page 287, children and youth enhance their health and well-being through regular physical activity. At a time when many "adult" diseases are increasingly diagnosed in children and youth, we must be concerned with one's health throughout the lifespan. Risk factors for heart disease are increasingly appearing in children and youth, including obesity, hypertension, and type 2 diabetes (30). The recent increase in childhood obesity is considered a public health epidemic (26, 28). Both healthy and unhealthy behaviors often begin early in life and are more difficult to acquire or change as one ages. Thus, encouraging children and youth to include physical activity as a part of their daily life may provide the basis for a lifetime of this healthy habit (11). It is now well established (29, 30) that regular physical activity can reduce the risk of developing a wide variety of health problems at all ages.

Currently, the trend is to emphasize the physical activity behavior more than the fitness test scores. The major question is, what kinds of physical activities should children do?

Childhood is a period in which most motor skills (e.g., throwing, jumping, running, riding, swimming) develop. Children are inherently active, and one of the most important elements adults must provide is an opportunity to play (32). This need for children to develop motor skills must be kept in mind when attending to fitness goals (33).

Both national physical fitness testing programs (7, 18) now recognize the behavior of physical activity (ACTIVITYGRAM and Presidential Active Lifestyle Award). This allows teachers and youth leaders to reward both the behavior of regular physical activity and the physical fitness outcomes. The ACTIVITYGRAM (7) provides a profile of the type, amount, and intensity of activity. It recommends at least 45 min (in three segments) for children and 30 min for adolescents (in two segments). The Presidential Active Lifestyle Award (18) provides an award for participating in at least 60 min of activity, 5 days a week for 6 weeks. Both are based on the child's self-report of activity. The ACTIVITYGRAM provides more information about the type of activity, although the Presidential Active Lifestyle Award is easier to use.

There are three major reasons for emphasizing an active lifestyle for children and youth:

- Enhancing health and fitness for children and youth
- Beginning an active lifestyle that can be continued
- Reducing risks for health problems throughout life

Exercise Prescription for Children (Preadolescents)

The recommendations for adult physical activity can be applied to older, postpubescent adolescents. Children and younger youth (prepubescent and pubescent) need to be considered separately—as is often said, they are not miniature adults.

The following box summarizes the physical activity recommendations for children (6, 8, 14, 17, 33).

Cardiorespiratory Fitness

In general, the same exercise prescription for CRF for adults (see chapter 10) can be used for children. Corbin and Pangrazi (8) recommended more physical activity for children, recognizing that there will be some decline in activity with age. There is some disagreement about whether the standard prescription will increase $\dot{V}O_2max$. The prescription may be effective in increasing $\dot{V}O_2max$ in pubescent and postpubescent children but less so in younger

Physical Activity Recommendations for Children

1. Extended periods of inactivity are inappropriate!
2. An accumulation of 60 min to several hours of age and developmentally appropriate activity is encouraged per day.
3. Some of the activity should include moderate to vigorous activities lasting 10 min or more, usually on an intermittent basis with periods of lighter activity or rest in between.
4. A variety of activities is recommended.
5. The emphasis should be on fun and enjoyment.

Adapted from 8, 14, 17, 33.

children (32, 33). This suggests that attention should be directed toward health-related benefits of aerobic exercise rather than simply on $\dot{V}O_2$max. When the focus is on health-related benefits, the use of a wide variety of continuous physical activities (e.g., cycling, running, in-line skating), team sports (e.g., basketball, soccer), individual and dual sports (e.g., tennis, racquetball), and recreational activities (e.g., hiking) can contribute to energy expenditure and its associated benefits. Parents, schools, and communities must (a) provide opportunities for children to have safe places to walk, run, and cycle; (b) provide organized programs for children to learn and play sports; and (c) focus on personal achievement rather than on winning at all costs.

6 In Review

Children should emphasize health-related physical activity, with a variety of endurance activities appropriate for their age level. Long periods of inactivity should be avoided.

Strength

Muscular strength and endurance of children can be improved by participating in formal weight training programs. Safety precautions must be taken, however, because children are anatomically, physiologically, and psychologically immature (4, 21, 33). The following guidelines are offered (adapted from 1, 33):

- Ensure that trained personnel supervise each session.
- Adapt equipment to children.
- Include adequate warm-up.
- Teach proper lifting techniques, with no breath holding.
- Stress controlled lifting techniques; avoid ballistic movements.
- Have children perform 1 or 2 sets of 8 to 10 different exercises (with 8-12 reps per set), and include major muscle groups.
- Use multiple-joint exercises.
- Limit training sessions to 2 times per week (with 2-3 days rest in between).
- Encourage other activities.
- Do not use a resistance that cannot be lifted at least 8 times; overload by first increasing the number of repetitions and then the absolute resistance.
- Do not allow children to perform exercises to the point of momentary muscle fatigue, because this can harm developing bone and joint structures.
- Include flexibility exercises.

7 In Review

Children can benefit from resistance training. The emphasis should be on safety, supervision for proper form, and muscular endurance (i.e., less resistance and more repetitions).

Exercise Prescription for Youth (Pubescent and Postpubescent)

Rowland (20) pointed out that the motivation for activity shifts from a biological one in children to a more psychosocial one in adolescence. Many of these influences have a negative influence on physical activity, resulting in the well-known decline in physical activity, especially among females. Although the recommendations for physical activity are essentially the same as for adults (25), the strategy for enhancing motivation must be directed at these adolescent psychosocial factors (22). Youth sports can fill that need for some. An increasing number of females are participating in sports (27), from less than 300,000 in 1971 to more than 2 million in 1995; however, that is still only 63% of the number of male participants. Both Bunker (5) and Weiss (31) emphasized a wide variety of accessible activities that promote self-esteem and can be done in an enjoyable atmosphere.

As Morrow and Jackson (13) indicated, physical education plays an important part in promoting physical activity for children and adolescents. A number of programs, such as Coordinated School Health (12), SPARK (23), and PATH (10), have shown that physical education programs can have a very positive effect on both children (23) and youth (10). In addition, the increased time spent on physical education does not diminish achievement in other subject matter areas (24).

8 In Review

Young people can benefit from adult exercise prescription; however, motivation for physical activity shifts toward peers.

Case Studies

You can check your answers by referring to appendix A.

15.1

A parent has read that for major strength gains, one should use a resistance that can only be lifted for 3 to 6 repetitions. He knows that strength is important for some of the sports his 9-year-old son wants to play, so he asks for your advice.

15.2

A parent's group is recommending that additional reading and math be included in the schools with a reduction of physical education and recess. The school board has asked you to respond to this recommendation.

Source List

1. American College of Sports Medicine. (2000). *ACSM's guidelines for exercise testing and prescription* (6th ed.). Philadelphia: Lippincott Williams & Wilkins.
2. Åstrand, P-O. (1952). *Experimental studies of physical working capacity in relation to sex and age*. Copenhagen: Ejnar Munksgaard.
3. Bar-Or, O. (1995). Health benefits of physical activity during childhood and adolescence. *PCPFS Research Digest, 2*(4).
4. Bar-Or, O., & Malina, R.M. (1995). Activity, fitness, and health of children and adolescents. In L.W.Y. Cheung & J.B. Richmond (Eds.), *Child health, nutrition, and physical activity* (pp. 79-123). Champaign, IL: Human Kinetics.
5. Bunker, L.K. (1998). Psycho-physiological contributions of physical activity and sports for girls. *PCPFS Research Digest, 3*(1).
6. Centers for Disease Control and Prevention. (1997). Guidelines for school and community programs to promote lifelong physical activity among young people. *Morbidity and Mortality Weekly Report, 44*(RR-6), 1-36.
7. Cooper Institute for Aerobic Research. (1999). *FITNESSGRAM: Test administration manual* (2nd ed.). Champaign, IL: Human Kinetics.
8. Corbin, C.B., & Pangrazi, R.P. (1994). Toward an understanding of appropriate physical activity levels for youth. *PCPFS Research Digest, 1*(8).
9. Cureton, K.J., & Warren, G.L. (1990). Criterion-referenced standards for youth health-related fitness tests: A tutorial. *Research Quarterly for Exercise and Sports, 61*, 7-19.
10. Fardy, P., & Azzollini, A. (1998). The PATH program. *Active youth: Ideas for implementing CDC physical activity promotion guidelines* (pp. 81-85). Champaign, IL: Human Kinetics.
11. Malina, R.M. (2001). Tracking of physical activity across the lifespan. *PCPFS Research Digest, 3*(14).
12. McKenzie, F.D., & Richmond, J.B. (1998). Linking health and learning: An overview of coordinated school health programs. In E. Marx, S. Frelick Wooley, with D. Northrop (Eds.), *Health is academic: A guide to coordinated school health programs* (pp. 1-14). New York: Teachers College Press.
13. Morrow, J.R., Jr., & Jackson, A.W. (1999). Physical activity promotion and school physical education. *PCPFS Research Digest, 3*(7).
14. National Association for Sport and Physical Education. (1998). *Physical activity for children: A statement of guidelines*. Reston, VA: Author.
15. National Center for Education in Maternal and Child Health. (2001). *Bright futures in practice: Physical activity*. Arlington, VA: Author.
16. Park, R.S. (1989). *Measurement of physical fitness: A historical perspective*. Washington, DC: ODPHP National Health Information Center.
17. Pate, R. (1998). Physical activity for young people. *PCPFS Research Digest, 3*(3).
18. President's Council on Physical Fitness and Sports. (2002). *President's Challenge Physical Activity and Fitness Award Program*. Washington, DC: Author.
19. Robinson, S. (1938). Experimental studies of physical fitness in relation to age. *Arbeitsphysiologie, 10*, 251-323.
20. Rowland, T.W. (1999). Adolescence: A "risk factor" for physical inactivity. *PCPFS Research Digest, 2*(4).
21. Rowland, T.W. (1990). *Exercise and children's health*. Champaign, IL: Human Kinetics.
22. Sallis, J.F. (1994). Influences on physical activity of children, adolescents, and adults or determinants of active living. *PCPFS Research Digest, 1*(7).
23. Sallis, J.F., McKenzie, T.L., Alcaraz, J.E., Kolody, B., Faucette, N., & Hovell, M. (1997). The effects of a 2-year physical education program (SPARK) on physical activity and fitness on elementary school students. *American Journal of Public Health, 87*, 45-50.
24. Sallis, J.F., McKenzie, T.L., Kolody, B., Lewis, M., Marshall, S., & Rosegard, P. (1999). Effects of health-related physical education on academic achievement: Project SPARK. *Research Quarterly for Exercise and Sport, 70*, 127-134.
25. Sallis, J.F., Patrick, K., & Long, B.L. (1994). An overview of international consensus conference on physical activity guidelines for adolescents. *Pediatric Exercise Science, 6*, 299-301.
26. Satcher, D. (1998). Opening remarks. *Childhood obesity: Causes and prevention* (CNPP-6). Washington, DC: U.S. Department of Agriculture Center for Nutrition Policy and Promotion.
27. Seefeldt, V.D., & Ewing, M.E. (1997). Youth sports in America: An overview. *PCPFS Research Digest, 2*(11).
28. U.S. Department of Agriculture. (1999). *Childhood obesity: Causes and prevention. Symposium proceedings* (CNPP-6). Washington, DC: U.S. Department of Agriculture Center for Nutrition Policy and Promotion.
29. U.S. Department of Health and Human Services. (1996). *Physical activity and health: Report of the Surgeon General*. Atlanta: U.S. Department of Health and Human Services, Centers for Disease Control and Prevention, National Center for Chronic Disease Prevention and Health Promotion.
30. U.S. Department of Health and Human Services. (2000). *Healthy people 2010*. Washington, DC: Author.
31. Weiss, M.R. (2000). Motivating kids in physical activity. *PCPFS Research Digest, 3*(11).
32. Williams, M.A. (2001). Human development and aging. In J.L. Roitman (Ed.), *ACSM's resource manual for guidelines for exercise testing and prescription* (4th ed., pp. 513-519). Philadelphia: Lippincott Williams & Wilkins.
33. Zwiren, L.D. (2001). Exercise testing and prescription considerations throughout childhood. In J.L. Roitman (Ed.), *ACSM's resource manual for guidelines for exercise testing and prescription* (4th ed., pp. 520-528). Philadelphia: Lippincott Williams & Wilkins.

sixteen

Exercise and Older Adults

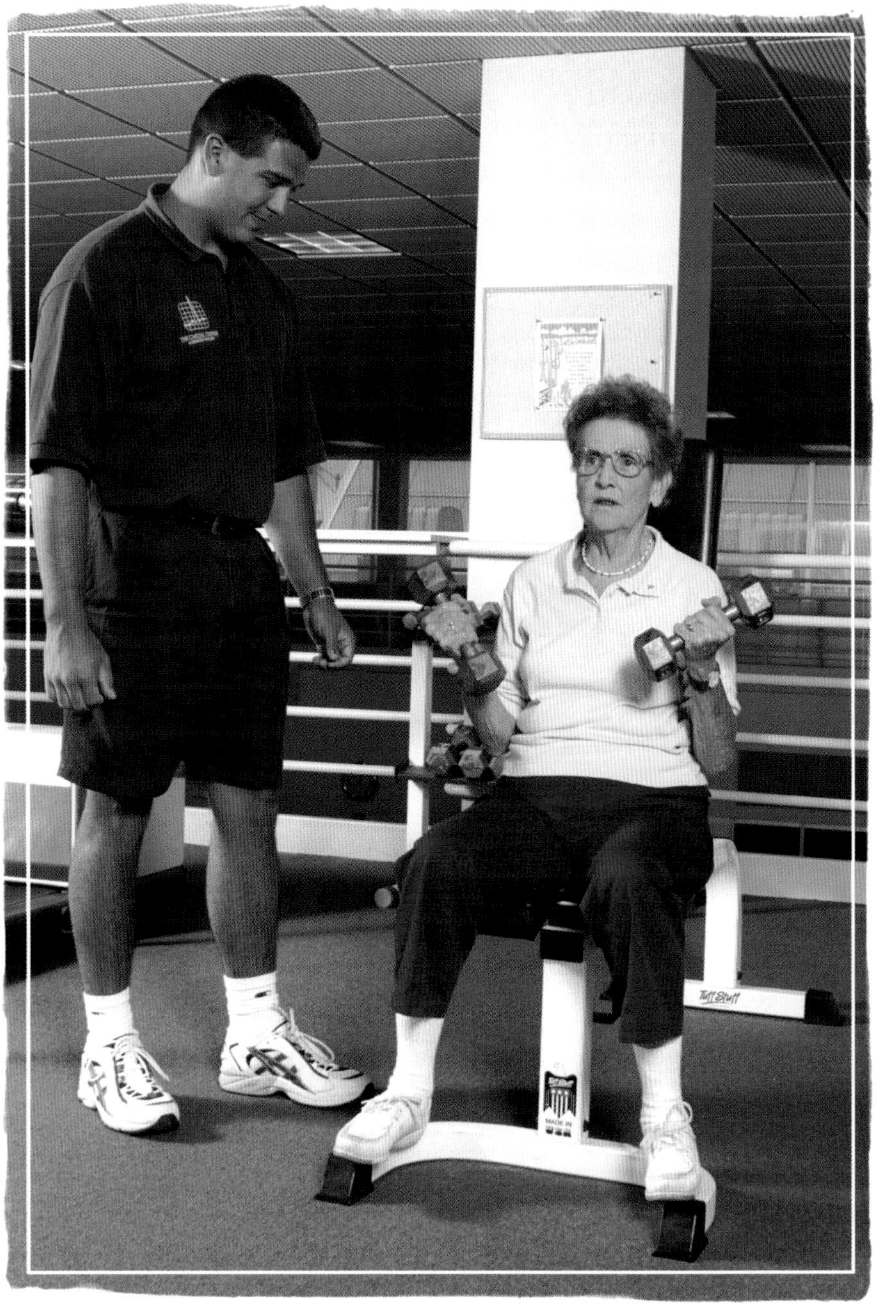

© Human Kinetics

Objectives

The reader will be able to do the following:

1. Describe the changes taking place in the number of individuals >65 years old during the first three decades of the 21st century, and provide a brief profile of the older population, indicating factors that would affect the delivery of fitness-related programs.
2. Describe the typical changes in $\dot{V}O_2$max, strength, body composition, and flexibility with age and the effect of exercise training on each.
3. Describe modifications to exercise tests to accommodate typical limitations seen in the older population.
4. Describe "functional tests" used to evaluate the different component of fitness.
5. Explain why one must address "individual differences" in the older population relative to exercise prescription.
6. Provide general guidelines for exercise prescription for cardiorespiratory fitness, muscular fitness, and flexibility for the older population.

A constant theme throughout this text is the importance of physical activity and exercise in leading a healthy and fit life. This message is especially important for the elderly, the fastest growing segment of the population. The "baby boom" generation (those born between 1946 and 1960) represented a spike in the birth rate in the United States after World War II; these individuals are now coming to full maturity. Figure 16.1 shows the changes in the number of persons over 65 years of age, projected to the year 2030 (26). The number actually doubles between 2000 and 2030 because of the baby boom generation. In addition, because of advances in hygiene and medicine over the past century, life expectancy has increased in general and with it the numbers of individuals living to advanced ages. Shephard (21) described age classifications and characteristics of those 40 to 85+ years of age:

Middle age—40 to 65 years of age; 10 to 30% loss of biological functions.

Old age—also called young old age; 65 to 75 years of age; further loss of function.

Very old age—typically, 75 to 85 years of age; substantial impairment in function but can still lead independent life.

Oldest old age—over 85 years of age; institutional or nursing care typically is needed.

Currently, there are 16 and 34 times more persons in the 75 to 84 and 85+ age groups than in 1900, respectively (26). These latter age groups already have had a major impact on health delivery systems, the financing of health care, family issues in caring for parents and grandparents, and, in general, concerns about quality-of-life issues for those contemplating retirement. These changes also affect the role of the HFI and personal fitness trainer in providing appropriate physical activity and exercise programs to increase and maintain health and fitness in these older individuals. Are fitness clubs ready to welcome older individuals, when the focus has been on a younger, healthier age group? Are the personnel trained to service the special needs of this older age group? This chapter summarizes important information related to this age group; however, we recommend the following references to provide a more complete understanding: *Physical Dimensions of Aging* (23), *Aging, Physical Activity, and Health* (21), ACSM's "Exercise and Physical Activity for the Older Adult" (1), and Holloszy and Kohrt's review on aging and exercise in the *Handbook of Physiology* (13).

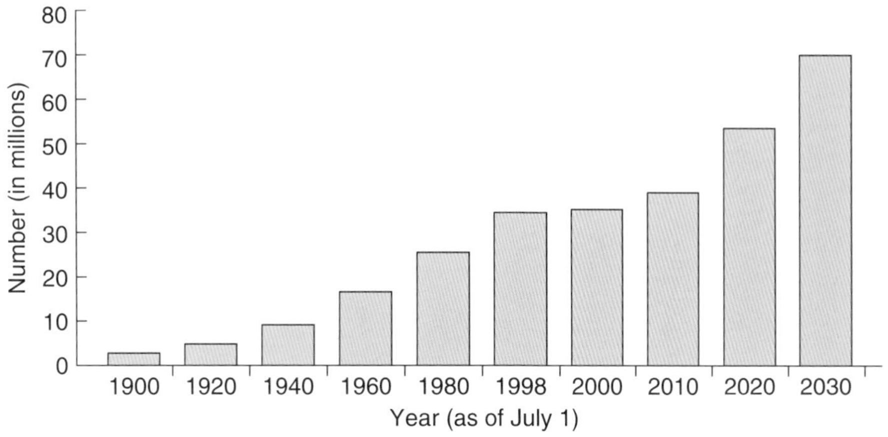

Figure 16.1 Number of persons 65 years and older, from 1900 to 2030.

Note: Increments in years are uneven.

From: U.S. Department of Health and Human Services. (2000). A profile of older Americans: 2000. Washington, D.C.

Overview

A variety of demographic and physiological characteristics of this older (>65 years of age) population affect planning fitness facilities, developing programming options, and anticipating emergencies. The following, from *A Profile of Older American: 2000* (26), provides some insights into the population as a whole:

- There are four times as many widows as widowers in this age group.
- The majority live in a family setting; however, as the population ages, the number living alone or in an institution increases.
- In 1996, 26% of older white Americans rated their health as fair or poor, versus 41.6% for African Americans and 35.1% for Hispanic Americans.
- Physical activity limitations increase with age. Thirty percent of those 65 to 74 years old report limitations, in contrast to 50% of those >75 years. More than half of those over 65 years report one disability, and a third report a severe disability. The disabilities interfered with their capacity to carry out activities of daily living (ADLs) and instrumental activities of daily living (IADLs), that is, preparing meals, shopping, and doing housework.
- Most older persons have at least one chronic condition and many have several. These include arthritis (49%), hypertension (36%), hearing impairments (30%), heart disease (27%), cataracts (17%), orthopedic impairments (18%), and diabetes (10%).

This brief demographic profile indicates that fitness programs must address issues related to screening and the need for socialization, provide more joint-protective activities, emphasize prevention or treatment of chronic diseases, and focus on pragmatic goals to maintain independent living (21). However, it is important to remember that these characteristics (i.e., type and severity of disease, physical limitations, fitness) are not uniformly distributed across the older population and that we must attend to individual differences. We address this issue in the sections dealing with exercise prescription.

1 In Review

The number of older individuals in the United States is increasing as the baby boom generation comes to full maturity. Older individuals present special challenges to fitness professionals because of the presence of chronic diseases and physical activity limitations. Programs must address prevention and reduction of the progression of chronic diseases as one ages as well as increasing or maintaining fitness to allow one to live independently.

Effects of Aging on Fitness

There is no question that physiological function decreases with age; however, some systems and functions age faster than others. Further compounding the issue, each individual displays a unique rate of aging that is influenced by genetic and environmental (e.g., education, health care, economic status, nutrition, exercise) factors (23). Consequently, it is not uncommon to find someone who is intellectually "young" but physically "old," or a 70-year-old who has the physiological capacity of a 50-year-old.

In general, the common chronic diseases that contribute to morbidity in older individuals respond to exercise interventions in a manner similar to that of younger adults. Endurance training (1)

- improves blood lipids (linked more to a reduction in body fatness rather than exercise),
- lowers blood pressure to the same degree as shown for younger individuals with hypertension, and
- improves glucose tolerance and insulin sensitivity.

As described earlier in the text, the primary fitness components (cardiorespiratory fitness, muscular fitness, body composition, and flexibility) affect our ability to perform work and engage in recreational pursuits at any age. Although "natural" changes in these fitness components occur with age, the evidence is overwhelming that regular exercise maintains them at considerably better levels than does a sedentary lifestyle. The following sections address each of these fitness components.

Cardiorespiratory Fitness

Figure 16.2 shows that maximal aerobic power ($\dot{V}O_2$max) decreases at the rate of about 1% per year in healthy men and women after the age of 20 (12). This decrease is due to both inactivity and weight gain as well as to an "aging" effect. Some studies show that this rate of decline is reduced by half in men who maintain a vigorous exercise program, but not without exception (2, 13). Women show a 10% decline per decade independent of activity status (8); however, trained women, as expected, have a higher $\dot{V}O_2$max at any age compared with their sedentary counterparts. It should be no surprise that the decrease in $\dot{V}O_2$max with age affects endurance performance. Average running speed in distance races decreases about 1% per year, suggesting a link between the decrease in $\dot{V}O_2$max and distance running performance. However, a variety of other factors (e.g., running economy, lactate threshold, joint trauma) also might affect running performance (13).

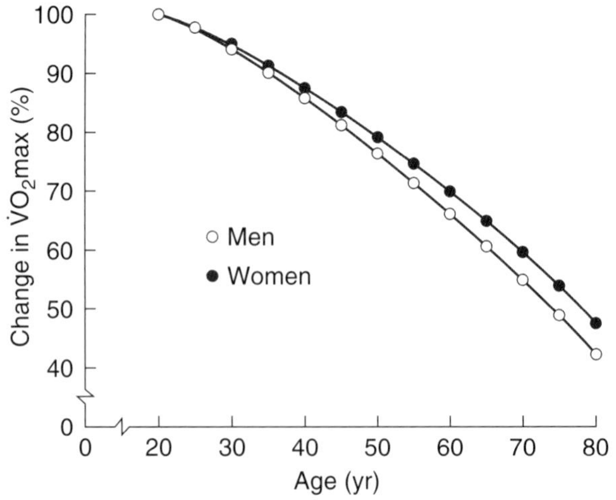

Figure 16.2 Percent change in $\dot{V}O_2$max in men and women with age.

From: Holloszy, J.O., & Kohrt, W.M. (1995). Exercise. In *Handbook of Physiology*, E.J. Masoro, ed. pp. 633-666. New York: Oxford Press.

Effect of Training

The fact that all people experience a decline in $\dot{V}O_2$max with age means that by the time of retirement, one's ability to engage in routine physical activities has been compromised. This reduced capacity for work can further reduce physical activity, setting up a vicious cycle leading to lower and lower levels of cardiorespiratory fitness. This may result in an individual not being able to perform ADLs, which would affect one's quality of life and independence (23).

Maximal oxygen uptake (see chapter 28) is equal to the product of maximal cardiac output (maximal HR times maximal stroke volume) and maximal oxygen extraction (systemic arteriovenous oxygen difference). There is no question that maximal HR decreases with age (e.g., 220 – age) and is the major contributor to the age-related decrease in maximal cardiac output. The Frank-Starling mechanism appears to compensate for the lower maximal HR in middle age to reduce the magnitude of change in maximal cardiac output, but it is less effective in old age (1, 13). Maximal oxygen extraction is also lower in the elderly compared with younger sedentary adults, but it is probably attributable more to their level of inactivity than a true "aging" effect. Endurance training increases $\dot{V}O_2$max about 10 to 30% in older individuals, similar to that of young adults (1, 13). The increase in $\dot{V}O_2$max is due to an increase in both maximal cardiac output and oxygen extraction in older men but is due almost entirely to an increase in oxygen extraction in older women. This may be related to the observation that older women show little or no increase in left ventricle mass, end diastolic volume, or maximal stroke volume after endurance training. The increase in oxygen extraction is due to increases in capillary number and mitochondrial enzymes, just as in younger adults (13, 20).

2 In Review

$\dot{V}O_2$max decreases about 1% per year in sedentary men and women because of a decrease in both maximal cardiac output and maximal oxygen extraction. Endurance training increases $\dot{V}O_2$max in older adults similar to what is observed in younger adults. The increase in $\dot{V}O_2$max is due to increases in both maximal cardiac output and oxygen extraction in men but is due solely to an increase in oxygen extraction in women.

Muscular Strength and Endurance

Muscular strength begins to decline at about age 30, but the majority of the decrease occurs after age 50 when it falls at the rate of 15% per decade, with a more rapid decrease of 30% per decade after age 70 (15, 20). The loss of strength is related directly to a loss of muscle mass (sarcopenia), with the latter attributable primarily to a loss of muscle fibers (motor units) and secondarily to an atrophy of those muscle fibers (primarily type 2) that remain (see figure 16.3). However, fiber type distribution is maintained across age, as is strength per cross-sectional area of muscle (1, 13, 15, 20).

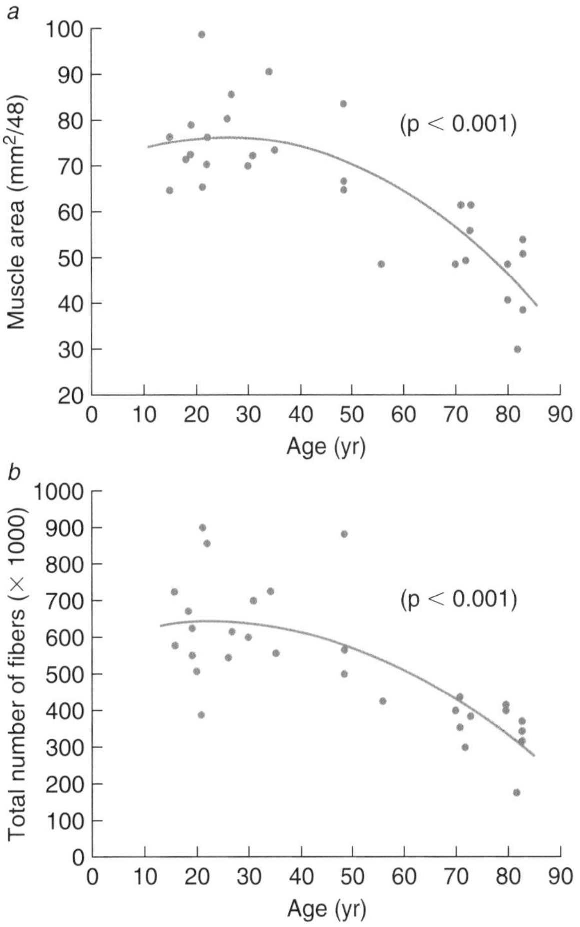

Figure 16.3 *(a)* Relationship between age and muscle area of whole vastus lateralis muscle cross sections. *(b)* Relationship between total number of fibers and age in whole vastus lateralis muscle.

Copied from: Rogers, M.A., and Evans, W.J. (1993). Changes in skeletal muscle with aging: Effects of exercise training. *Exercise and Sport Sciences Reviews*, 21, 65-102.

Effect of Training

Maintenance of muscle mass is important, not only for our ability to carry out daily activities but because it is linked to our resting metabolic rate (see chapter 11) and the risks of type 2 diabetes and hypertension (2, 20). A considerable body of evidence shows that an intense (~80% 1RM) resistance training program increases both muscle mass and strength in 60- to 96-year-old individuals (7, 11). These training programs resulted in modest increases in muscle fiber area (10-30%) but very large increases (>100%) in 1RM strength. The disproportionate increase in strength is similar to what is observed when young adults participate in intense resistance training programs (see chapter 12) and is ascribed to neural adaptations. There is also evidence that strength training programs can increase $\dot{V}O_2$max in this population (10). Interestingly, for the frail elderly, it is recommended that strength training should precede aerobic conditioning because one must be able to rise from a chair and maintain balance and posture to walk (1).

3 In Review

Muscular strength decreases with age because of a loss of motor units (muscle mass) as well as a reduction in the size of the muscle fibers that remain. Intense resistance training programs (~80% 1RM) cause large (>100%) increases in strength, attributable primarily to neural factors, because muscle fiber size increases only 10 to 30%.

Body Composition

Chapters 6 and 11 provided detail associated with health risks, measurement issues, and approaches to dealing with body composition. In general, body fatness increases from about 16% and 25% in 25-year-old males and females to 28% and 41% in 75-year-olds, respectively. This amounts to a gain of about 10 kg of fat for both groups over that time frame. Fat-free mass is stable until about 40 years of age but decreases 3% and 4% per decade between 40 and 60 years of age and 6% and 10% per decade from 60 to 80 years of age, for men and women, respectively (13).

Effect of Training

Evidence indicates that the increase in body weight (and fat) is related to a sedentary lifestyle rather than to an increase in food intake or an "aging" effect. Cross-sectional and longitudinal studies on older male and female athletes suggest that regular vigorous exercise is associated with a stable weight as one ages (13). However, observations of highly trained athletes indicate that body fatness still increases about 2% per decade. Consequently, vigorous exercise attenuates, but does not prevent, the increase in body fatness with age. An important aspect of the change in body composition in the elderly attributable to exercise intervention programs is that most of the body fat is lost from central stores, which reduces the risk of metabolic and cardiovascular diseases (13). Exercise is also important in dealing with the loss of bone mineral density with age, but there is more to the story (see the box below).

4 In Review

An increase in body fat with age is attributed more to a decrease in physical activity than an increase in caloric intake. Vigorous exercise is associated with a stable body weight as one ages, and exercise intervention programs result in the loss of body fat from central stores, which is associated with reduced risk of cardiovascular and metabolic diseases.

Bone

Bone mineral density (BMD), a measure of bone mass, decreases with age at about the same rate as the fat-free mass; however, in women bone loss is accelerated after menopause (13). The latter is a major concern because the risk of fractures increases as the BMD decreases. Bloomfield (5) provided concise recommendations for dealing with this problem: maximize BMD through adequate calcium intake and physical activity before age 30, and then reduce the rate of loss from that point in time. Hormone levels (estrogen and testosterone), calcium intake, and physical activity affect the rate of loss of BMD. The higher rate of loss of BMD after menopause can be prevented by hormone replacement therapy. Vigorous exercise and calcium intake are important in maintaining BMD but cannot substitute for hormone replacement therapy. Older individuals need additional calcium (see chapter 7) to help maintain BMD and possibly to realize the full benefits of increased physical activity. The most effective exercise programs for bone health in older women include activities that

- involve a wide variety of muscle groups and movement directions,
- use fast rather than slow movements and provide some impact (e.g., walking, jogging), and
- generally exceed 70% of maximal capacity for both strength or endurance.

However, in older individuals with severe osteoporosis, impact-producing and forward spinal flexion exercises should be avoided (5).

Flexibility

The ability to move a joint through its normal ROM is an important factor related to one's ability to carry out daily activities and to the risk of low back pain (see chapter 9). Joint motion is influenced by the condition of the muscle, connective, and cartilage tissues associated with the joint. In general, the increase in collagen cross-linkages in tendons and ligaments and a degradation of articular cartilage contribute to the reduction in joint ROM with age (1). However, in evaluating the health of a joint it is difficult to separate "aging" effects from those associated with chronic inactivity.

Effect of Training

Because of the variability in the number of subjects, the types of research design, and the methods of assessment in studies investigating the effect of training on flexibility, it is difficult to provide a general profile of the training effect as was done for $\dot{V}O_2$max and strength (1, 18, 23). However, both general programs of physical activity and special ROM exercise programs have been shown to improve flexibility in the very old (21). Clearly, additional research is needed in this area.

5 In Review

Adequate flexibility throughout old age contributes to one's ability to perform ADLs and maintain independence. Flexibility can be improved through general programs of physical activity and special ROM exercises.

Special Considerations Regarding Exercise Testing

Age is a risk factor because the likelihood of a serious condition increases with age. The passage of time allows the consequences of poor health behaviors (e.g., smoking, high-fat diet, inactivity) to add up and manifest themselves as some major medical problem (e.g., lung cancer, atherosclerosis, glucose intolerance). Consequently, one must follow the ACSM risk stratification guidelines (3) closely when working with the elderly (1).

Risk stratification provides clear guidance for test selection and personnel requirements. Clearly, with the higher incidence of cardiovascular disease in the older age groups, diagnostic exercise testing may be used as part of a medical exam. However, standard submaximal CRF tests (see chapter 5) may be used as part of a fitness assessment. Independent of the reason for testing, modifications may have to be made to address certain limitations (3, 7, 22):

Instrumentation

- A cycle ergometer may be a better choice for those with arthritis of the knee or hip or those with balance problems.
- Tracking cadence may be a problem unless an electronic cycle ergometer is available.
- If a treadmill is used, additional practice may be needed, with emphasis on slow walking speeds.

Intensity/Progression

As mentioned in chapter 5, for deconditioned persons with low $\dot{V}O_2$max values, the initial intensity of a GXT should be low, increments per stage should be small, and perhaps a longer time (3 versus 2 min) per stage should be allowed so a steady state can be achieved.

Exercise Prescription

The Surgeon General's report on physical activity and health (25) documented that many adults do not participate in any leisure-time physical activity and that the problem gets worse with age. Clearly, the general recommendation that adults should participate in moderate physical activity on most, preferably all, days of the week is an essential message for all ages, but especially for older individuals, who are positioned to gain substantially from an increase in physical activity (17). However, an activity that might constitute "moderate" work for a younger, more fit adult may be classified as "very heavy" for an older individual (see figure 10.8) (14).

What's Old?

The only thing two 65-year-old men in your fitness class may have in common is their age! They may differ substantially in their health risk (chronic diseases), cardiorespiratory fitness ($\dot{V}O_2$max), and experience with exercise. Scientists and clinicians (9, 19, 23) have developed a variety of classification schemes to deal with this reality; Rimmer's (19) classification scheme is representative:

Level I	*Healthy*: No major medical problems; in relatively good condition for age; has exercised the past 5 years.
Level II	*Ambulatory/nonactive*: No major medical problems; has never participated in a structured exercise program.
Level III	*Ambulatory/disease failure:* Diagnosed as having severe coronary artery disease, arthritis, diabetes, or chronic obstructive pulmonary disease.
Level IV	*Frail elderly*: Relies on partial assistance from professional staff for ADLs; can stand or walk short distances (usually less than 100 ft) with an assistive device; spends most of the day sitting.
Level V	*Wheelchair-dependent*: Relies on total assistance from professional staff for ADLs; cannot stand or walk.

These classifications should be viewed as a continuum of abilities and problems, rather than discrete categories. As one moves across the continuum:

Risk of disease increases.

- Need for supervision by medical personnel is greater.
- Use of medication increases.
- Testing moves from fitness to diagnostic to "functional" (see box below).

Fitness level decreases.

- Range of suitable fitness activities decreases.
- The HFI must be creative and adapt conventional activities to the limitations of the individual.
- The HFI must incorporate socialization as part of the activity.

Personnel needs change.

- Personnel need more education in gerontology, pathophysiology, and pharmacology.
- Staff mix may include fitness, nursing, physical therapy, and therapeutic recreation personnel.

Functional Testing

A common method to evaluate the capabilities of older individuals involves a series of performance tests that are linked to underlying fitness components. The Senior Fitness Test, developed by Rikli and Jones (18), evaluates the different fitness components with the following tests:

Chair stand	Number of times a person can stand from a seated position in 30 s, with arms folded across the chest (assesses lower body strength).
Arm curl	Number of curls that can be completed in 30 s with a 5-lb (women) or 8-lb (men) dumbbell (assess upper body strength), while participant is in a seated position.
6-min walk	Number of yards one can walk in 6 min around a 50-yd course (assesses aerobic endurance).
2-min step	Number of full steps the participant can complete in 2 min while raising knee to midway between knee and hip, while standing in place. This is an alternate for the 6-min walk.
Chair sit-and-reach	Number of inches between extended fingertips and tip of toes when the participant is sitting in a chair with legs extended and hands reaching toward toes (assesses lower body flexibility).
Back scratch	Number of inches between the extended middle fingers when the participant reaches with one hand over the shoulder and the other hand up the back (assesses upper body flexibility).
8-foot up-and-go	Number of seconds required to get up from seated position, walk 8 ft, turn, and return to seated position (assesses agility and dynamic balance).
Height and weight	Used to calculate BMI.

These tests have been shown to be valid and reliable, and normative data are provided for ages 60 to 94 years for men and women (18). These practical and easy tests can be used to track progress over the course of a training program or document loss of function that might necessitate additional medical attention.

Cardiorespiratory Fitness

A formal program of activities aimed at improving CRF should be built on a base of moderate-intensity activities that are tied to an individual's lifestyle (1). Like any workout, it should begin with a formal warm-up and end with a cool-down, during which flexibility exercises can be done. It is crucial to adapt the activities to the levels of ability of the individuals in the group. Those at the high end of the fitness continuum can participate in a wide variety of activities similar to those used for younger individuals. Those who have the $\dot{V}O_2max$ of cardiac patients (5-7 METs) can follow a routine of exercises that would not be too different from those used in a cardiac rehabilitation program (see chapter 17). However, prescribing activities for those at the low end of the functional continuum, in whom $\dot{V}O_2max$ may be only 2 to 4 METs, demands special creativity and attention to safety. Exercises can be done standing with support, seated on a chair, or in the water (4, 18). Because of the prevalence of joint-related problems, modes of exercise should be chosen that do not aggravate the problem. The needs for additional assistance with balance and attention to safety relative to the risk of a fall should be incorporated into the routine (see box below).

The general exercise prescription is similar to what was described in chapter 10 for the typically sedentary individual (2, 3):

- Intensity: THR can be used to set the exercise intensity, but measured maximal HR is preferred to predicted maximal HR. Intensity guidelines are similar to those of younger adults, but the low end of the THR zone should be emphasized at the beginning of the program, and RPE also should be used to determine whether the intensity is suitable.
- Duration: If the client is extremely deconditioned, the exercise sessions should be divided into segments (5-10 min) that can be done throughout the day (or within the context of a single class period). Some may not be able exercise for 30 min continuously.
- Frequency: Moderate activity daily. Formal exercise training sessions should be done 3 times per week, with a rest day between the exercise days.

Muscular Strength and Endurance

The exercise prescription for increasing strength is described in chapter 12. It is highlighted here (3):

- Instruct participants on safety, proper lifting technique, and breathing.
- Participants should perform 8 to 10 exercises that use the major muscle groups.
- Participants should stay within the pain-free ROM.
- Participants should not exercise if an arthritic joint is painful or inflamed (see box on page 302).
- Each set should involve 10 to 15 repetitions that elicit an RPE of about 12 to 13.
- Participants should perform the workout at least twice a week with 48 hr between sessions.

Flexibility

Tai chi and yoga programs can be used to achieve and maintain flexibility goals. However, for most individuals, flexibility goals can be achieved within the context of a regular exercise class. Elements of the program include the following (3):

- Slow movements through pain-free ROM, with static stretches held for 10 to 30 s
- At least four repetitions per muscle group
- Performed 2 to 3 days per week as part of the warm-up and cool-down

Balance and Falls

Loss of balance can lead to a fall, with dire consequences. The lower bone density in elderly people predisposes them to fractures, and ~50% are not able to return to regular walking after a fracture (23). The ability to maintain balance is influenced by a wide variety of factors, such as strength, vision, proprioception, medications, illnesses, flexibility, and environmental hazards (23). A considerable body of information shows that exercise programs improve balance and reduce falls, but not without exception (1, 21). The general recommendation is to include activities for balance training, resistance exercise, walking, and weight transfer (1). However, medications, environmental hazards, and vision also must be addressed to reduce the risk of falls (23).

Osteoarthritis

Osteoarthritis, a common problem in many older adults, is a degenerative joint disease associated with damage to the articular cartilage that lines joint structures. The swelling and pain associated with osteoarthritis affect joint ROM and may prevent an individual from participating in physical activity. A variety of over-the-counter and prescription medications can reduce pain and inflammation and allow one to participate in physical activity. Activity programs should not provide an excessive load to the involved joint (e.g., the participant with a knee or hip problem should perform stationary cycling or pool work instead of jogging or stair climbing). Gradual warm-up and flexibility exercises should be included, and the intensity and duration of the program should be at the low end of the spectrum. A work/relief interval-training program also can be appropriate for individuals with osteoarthritis (16).

6 In Review

The exercise prescription for older individuals is similar to that of younger adults, with additional attention to risk stratification, level of CFR, and limitations related to chronic or degenerative (e.g., osteoarthritis) diseases. Exercises should be selected to minimize joint trauma, provide an additional measure of safety, and accomplish fitness goals in a socially supportive environment.

Epilogue

This chapter has focused on the fact that regular participation in physical activity is associated with better health (lower risk of chronic diseases) and fitness (cardiovascular function, strength, body composition, and flexibility) as one ages. However, regular participation in physical activity also has been shown to improve both psychological and social functioning to achieve a sense of well-being (1, 6, 24, 27). This is a good example of how regular physical activity affects the whole person, leading to a more active and fulfilling life. The World Health Organization (27) has summarized the immediate and long-term benefits of physical activity on psychological and social functioning:

Immediate benefits
(associated with the current exercise session)

- Enhanced relaxation
- Reduced stress and anxiety
- Enhanced mood state
- Empowered to be more independent and self-sufficient
- Enhanced social and cultural integration, especially from small-group programs

Long-term benefits
(attributable to regular participation over time)

- Improved general well-being
- Improved mental health
- Improved cognitive function: better central nervous system processing speed and reaction time
- Improved motor control and performance for both fine and gross motor skills
- Increased skill acquisition: new skills can be learned
- Enhanced integration: the person is less likely to withdraw from society
- Formation of new friendships, particularly in small groups and other social environments
- Widened social and cultural networks
- Role maintenance and new role acquisition: the person remains active in society
- Enhanced intergenerational activity: diminishes stereotypic perceptions about aging and the elderly

Case Study

You can check your answers by referring to appendix A.

16.1

A 67-year-old male who has been actively involved in jogging and tennis most of his life has developed arthritis in his left knee. The problem has caused him to reduce his jogging, and his lack of "fitness," as he calls it, is affecting his tennis game, which he is determined to continue. He comes to your health club for testing and advice about what he can do to increase and maintain his fitness.

Source List

1. American College of Sports Medicine. (1998). Exercise and physical activity for older adults. *Medicine and Science in Sports and Exercise, 30,* 992-1008.
2. American College of Sports Medicine. (1998). The recommended quantity and quality of exercise for developing and maintaining cardiorespiratory and muscular fitness, and flexibility in healthy adults. *Medicine and Science in Sports and Exercise, 30,* 975-991.
3. American College of Sports Medicine. (2000). *ACSM's guidelines for exercise testing and prescription* (6th ed.). Baltimore: Lippincott Williams & Wilkins.
4. American Council on Exercise. (1998). *Exercise for the older adult*. Champaign, IL: Human Kinetics.
5. Bloomfield, S.A. (2001). Optimizing bone health: Impact of nutrition, exercise, and hormones. *Gatorade Sports Science Institute: Sports Science Exchange, 14*(3), 82.
6. Chodzko-Zajko, W.J. (1998). Physical activity and aging: Implications for health and quality of life in older persons. *PCPFS Physical Activity and Fitness Research Digest, 3*(4).
7. Criswell, D.S. (2001). Human development and aging. In *ACSM's Health & Fitness Certification Review*. pp. 31-47. Baltimore: Lippincott Williams & Wilkins.
8. Fiatarone, M.A., Marks, E.C., Ryan, N.D., Meredith, C.N., Lipsitz, L.A., & Evans, W.J. (1990). High-intensity strength training in nonagenarians. *Journal of the American Medical Association, 263,* 3029-3034.
9. Fitzgerald, M.D., Tanaka, H., Tran, Z.V., & Seals, D.R. (1997). Age-related declines in maximal aerobic capacity in regularly exercising vs. sedentary women: A meta-analysis. *Journal of Applied Physiology, 83,* 160-165.
10. Fitzgerald, P.L. (1985). Exercise for the elderly. *Medical Clinics of North America, 69,* 189-196.
11. Frontera, W.R., Meredith, C.N., O'Reilly, K.P., & Evans, W.J. (1990). Strength training and determinants of VO_2max in older men. *Journal of Applied Physiology, 68,* 329-333.
12. Frontera, W.R., Meredith, C.N., O'Reilly, K.P., Knuttgen, H.G., & Evans, W.J. (1988). Strength conditioning in older men: Skeletal muscle hypertrophy and improved function. *Journal of Applied Physiology, 64,* 1038-1044.
13. Holloszy, J.O., & Kohrt, W.M. (1995). Exercise. In E.J. Masoro (Ed.), *Handbook of physiology, Section 11: Aging* (pp. 633-666). New York: Oxford Press.
14. Howley, E.T. (2001). Type of activity: Resistance, aerobic and leisure versus occupational physical activity. *Medicine and Science in Sports and Exercise, 33,* S364-S369.
15. Kraemer, W.J., Fleck, S.J., & Evans, W.J. (1996). Strength and power training: Physiological mechanisms of adaptations. *Exercise and Sport Sciences Reviews, 24,* 363-397.
16. Minor, M.A., & Kay, D.R. (1997). Arthritis. In *ACSM's exercise management for persons with chronic diseases and disabilities* (pp. 149-152). Champaign, IL: Human Kinetics.
17. Pate, R.R., Pratt, M., Blair, S.N., Haskell, W.L., Marcera, C.A., & Bouchard, C. (1995). Physical activity and public health: A recommendation from the Centers for Disease Control and Prevention and the American College of Sports Medicine. *Journal of the American Medical Association, 273,* 402-407.
18. Rikli, R.E., & Jones, C.J. (2001). *Senior fitness test manual*. Champaign, IL: Human Kinetics.
19. Rimmer, J.H. (1994). *Fitness and rehabilitation programs for special populations*. Dubuque, IA: Brown & Benchmark.
20. Rogers, M.A., & Evans, W.J. (1993). Changes in skeletal muscle with aging: Effects of exercise training. *Exercise and Sport Sciences Reviews, 21,* 65-102.
21. Shephard, R.J. (1997). *Aging, physical activity, and health*. Champaign, IL: Human Kinetics.
22. Skinner, J.S. (1993). Importance of aging for exercise testing and exercise prescription. In J.S. Skinner (Ed.), *Exercise testing and exercise prescription for special cases* (2nd ed., pp. 75-86). Philadelphia: Lea & Febiger.
23. Spirduso, W.W. (1995). *Physical dimensions of aging*. Champaign, IL: Human Kinetics.
24. Spirduso, W.W., & Cronin, D.L. (2001). Exercise dose-response effects on quality of life and independent living in older adults. *Medicine and Science in Sports and Exercise, 33,* S598-S608.
25. U.S. Department of Human and Health Services. (1996). *Physical activity and health: A report of the Surgeon General*. Washington, DC: Author.
26. U.S. Department of Health and Human Services. (2000). *A profile of older Americans: 2000*. Washington, DC: Author.
27. World Health Organization. (1997). *A summary of the physiological benefits of physical activity for older persons*. Geneva, Switzerland: Author.

seventeen

Exercise and Coronary Heart Disease

David R. Bassett, Jr.

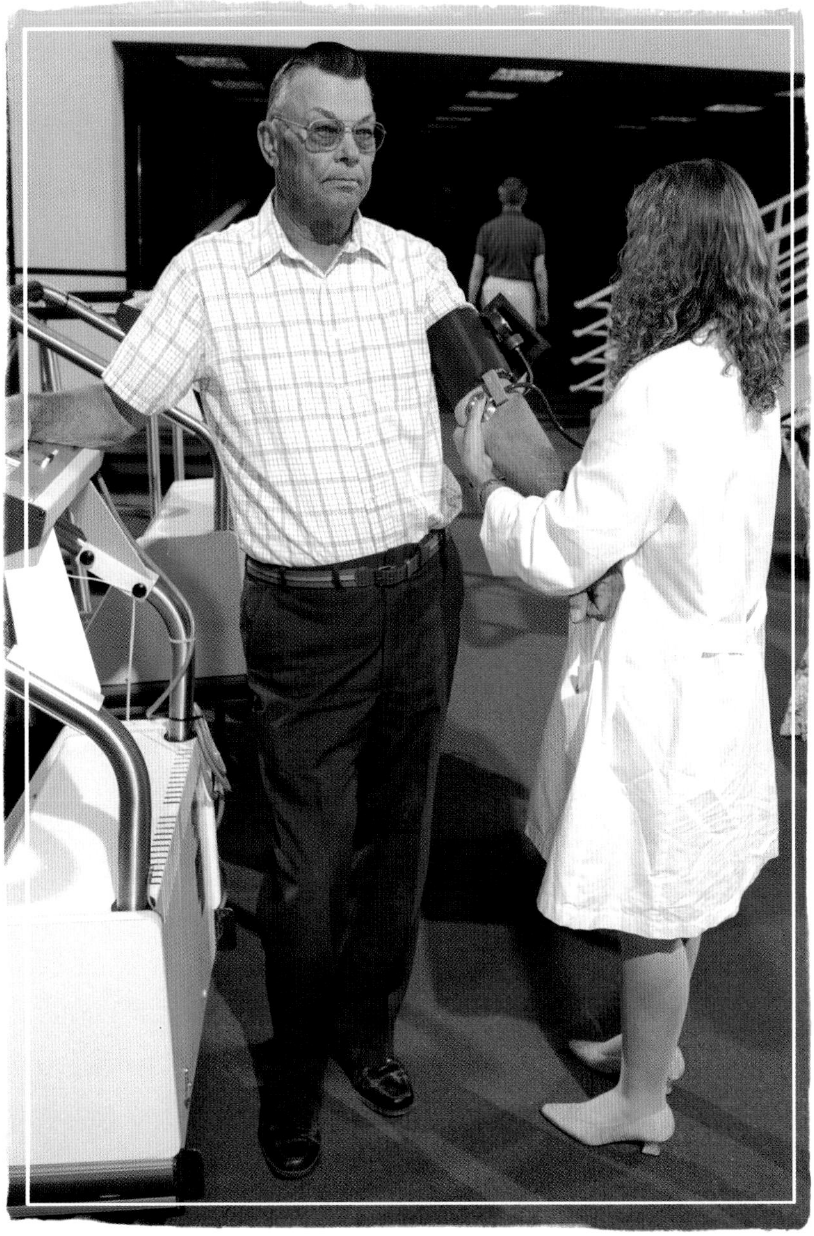

Objectives

The reader will be able to do the following:

1. Describe how the atherosclerotic process occurs and the resulting outcome if blood flow becomes obstructed in the arteries of the heart, brain, or periphery.
2. Quantify the magnitude of cardiovascular disease as a health problem in the United States and list the various subcategories of cardiovascular disease.
3. Identify the various patient populations found in cardiac rehabilitation programs.
4. Describe the physiological and mental health benefits of exercise for individuals with cardiovascular disease.
5. Define what is meant by secondary prevention of CHD.
6. Describe special tests that can be performed to diagnose the presence or absence of CHD, including those that use exercise and nonexercise challenges to stress the heart.
7. Describe how to prescribe aerobic exercise (frequency, intensity, and duration) in cardiac rehabilitation programs.
8. Discuss special considerations in prescribing exercise intensity for individuals who are taking β-blocker medications.

Coronary heart disease (CHD) is a major problem in the United States and in other industrialized nations. This chapter is intended to provide the HFI with a basic understanding of the development of CHD, the types of patients found in cardiac rehabilitation programs, the benefits of exercise for a cardiac population, and special considerations for exercise prescription in this group. It is not a comprehensive guide to the use of exercise in cardiac rehabilitation; a number of excellent texts provide more complete information on the topic (3, 5, 18).

Atherosclerosis

Atherosclerosis refers to an accumulation of lipid deposits in the large and medium-sized arteries, a process that provokes fibrosis and calcification. The atherosclerotic process begins early in life, as evidenced by studies of soldiers killed in the Korean War. Approximately three fourths of the 300 soldiers examined (mean age 22.1 years old) had some degree of blockages in their coronary arteries (7). It is believed that the atherosclerotic process is initiated when the endothelial cells lining the artery become damaged because of smoking, toxic agents, or high blood pressure (see the box titled Hypertension). When lipoproteins are deposited at the damaged site, plaque formation (or atherosclerosis) occurs. Eventually, these deposits impede blood flow in the affected arteries, sometimes to the point of complete occlusion (17).

Consequences of Atherosclerosis

Atherosclerosis can occur in various arteries throughout the body, with different results. Blockages in the coronary arteries will lead to **myocardial ischemia** (reduced blood flow to the heart) and in severe cases to **myocardial infarction (MI)**. If the blood vessels in the brain become occluded, a **stroke** will result. Blockages in the peripheral leg vessels can result in **claudication**, or intermittent muscle pain on exertion (16).

Cardiovascular Disease

In the United States, cardiovascular disease (CVD) is the leading cause of death, with 445,692 males and 503,927 females dying from CVD in 1998. CHD accounts for 48% of these deaths, with stroke (17%),

Hypertension

Hypertension, or high BP, greatly increases a person's risk of developing cardiovascular disease. It usually is defined as an SBP of ≥140 mmHg or a DBP ≥90 mmHg. It is estimated that more than 50 million people in the United States have hypertension (4). Typically, hypertension is controlled through the use of medications (see chapter 24), particularly if the patient's BP is very high (e.g., BP ≥160 mmHg systolic or 95 mmHg diastolic). For those who have only moderate hypertension, a variety of nonpharmacological approaches to reducing blood pressure are recommended. Dietary change includes a reduction in sodium intake, which has been shown to independently lower SBP and DBP by 5 and 3 mm Hg, respectively (11, 12). Obesity is linked to hypertension, and in general, research shows that a loss of 1 kg of body weight decreases SBP and DBP by 1.6 and 1.3 mmHg, respectively (11, 12). Last, participation in an endurance exercise program has been shown to decrease SBP and DBP by 6 to 10 mm Hg (1, 11, 12).

The standard ACSM exercise prescription for improving $\dot{V}O_2$max (see chapter 10) is also effective at reducing BP in previously hypertensive individuals (1, 11). In addition, endurance exercise at moderate intensities (40-70% $\dot{V}O_2$max) has been shown to reduce BP. Moderate-intensity exercise should be done frequently and for durations long enough to expend a large number of calories. Furthermore, for those with higher BPs who are taking medication, such an exercise program can be used along with changes in diet, smoking, and body weight to lower BP. In these cases, BP should be checked frequently to allow medications to be reduced as needed. The gradual establishment of appropriate diet and exercise habits improves the chance that a person will maintain an appropriate BP once it has been normalized.

hypertensive disease (5%), and congestive heart failure (5%) comprising most of the other leading causes (4). The rates of deaths attributable to coronary artery disease have declined in recent decades, but it remains a problem of huge proportions. According to the AHA, approximately 1,100,000 Americans will have a coronary attack this year. About 650,000 of these will be first heart attacks, with the rest representing recurrent attacks. Sixty percent of those suffering a heart attack will survive, and some of these individuals will be referred to cardiac rehabilitation programs (4).

1 In Review

Atherosclerosis is a disease that starts early in life and leads to blockages in the arteries of the heart, brain, or peripheral muscles. If a blockage occurs in a coronary artery, myocardial ischemia or infarction will result. There is a high prevalence of such health problems in the United States.

Populations in Cardiac Rehabilitation Programs

Cardiac rehabilitation programs include persons who have experienced angina pectoris, MI, **coronary artery bypass grafts** (CABGs), and angioplasty (8, 9). **Angina pectoris** refers to the chest pain attributable to ischemia of the ventricle resulting from an occlusion of one or more of the coronary arteries. The pain appears when the oxygen requirement of the heart (estimated by the double product SBP × HR) exceeds a value that coronary blood flow cannot meet. The ischemia can be transient and may subside once the oxygen demand of the heart returns to normal.

MI patients have actual heart damage (death of ventricular muscle fibers) caused by the occlusion of one or more of the coronary arteries. The degree to which left ventricular function is affected depends on the mass of the ventricle permanently damaged. Individuals who have suffered an MI usually take medications (β-blockers) to reduce the work of the heart and control the irritability of the heart tissue so that dangerous arrhythmias (irregular heartbeats) do not occur. Generally, these individuals experience a training effect similar to those who did not have an MI.

CABG patients have had surgery to bypass one or more blocked coronary arteries. In this procedure, a blood vessel is sewn into existing coronary arteries above and below the blockage, to reroute the blood flow (see figure 17.1). Those with chronic angina pectoris before CABG find a relief of symptoms, with 50 to 70% having no more pain. Generally, with an increased blood flow to the ventricle,

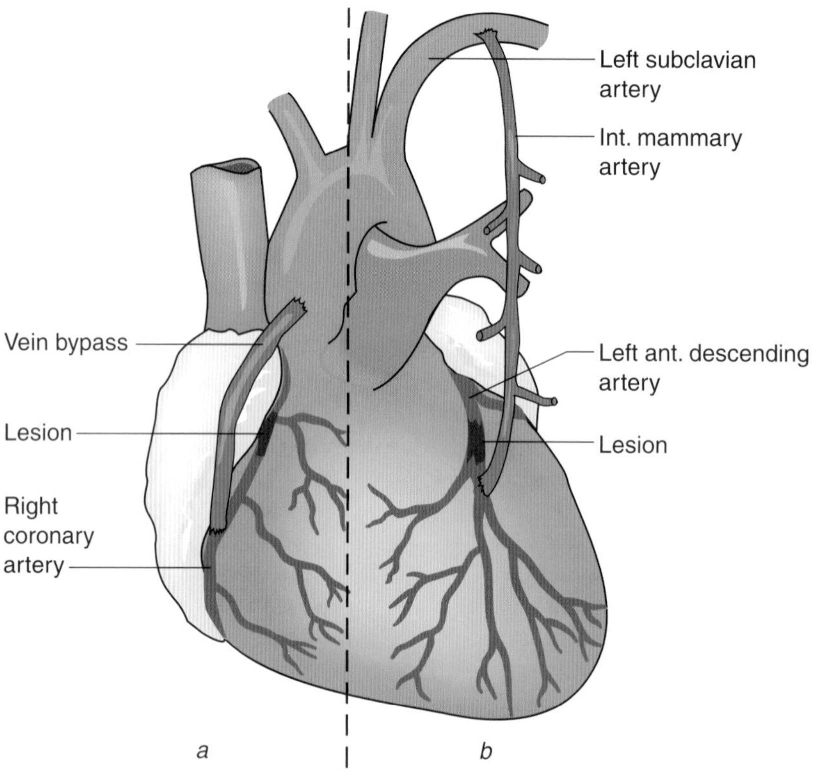

Figure 17.1 Coronary artery bypass surgery. Blood flow is rerouted around the site of obstruction by taking a blood vessel from another part of the body and sewing it to the affected coronary artery, distal to the site of the obstruction. Blood vessels typically used in the procedure are the saphenous (leg) vein and the mammary artery.

From Price SA, Wilson LM: Pathophysiology: Clinical Concepts of Disease Processes. New York: McGraw-Hill, 1978, with permission.

left ventricular function and the capacity for work improve (20). These patients benefit from systematic exercise training because most are deconditioned before surgery as a result of activity restrictions related to chest pain.

Some CHD patients undergo a special procedure, percutaneous transluminal coronary angioplasty (PTCA), to open occluded arteries. In this procedure, the chest is not opened; instead, a balloon-tipped catheter (a long slender tube) is inserted into the coronary artery, where the balloon is inflated to push the plaque back toward the arterial wall (see figure 17.2). These patients tend not to have as severe disease as those who undergo CABGs. For these patients, PTCA has some advantages, including the less invasive nature of the procedure, shorter hospital stay (1-2 days vs. 6-9 days), and lower cost (9). However, a problem with PTCA is that reocclusion of the coronary artery occurs in approximately one third to one half of these patients within 6 months of the procedure (10).

To help prevent reocclusion, **intracoronary stents** are often used to help keep the lumen of the coronary artery open. Stents are composed of a metal mesh that is inserted into the artery on a balloon catheter and positioned in the area of obstruction. The balloon is first inflated to increase the lumen size; then it is deflated and pulled back while the stent remains embedded in the artery. The main disadvantage of metal stents is that they increase the risk of blood clots; hence, anticoagulation therapy is needed to reduce this risk (5).

2 In Review

CHD is treated by CABG, angioplasty, or intracoronary stents. Patients who have undergone these procedures are candidates for a hospital-based cardiac rehabilitation program.

Evidence That Exercise Training Plays a Role

Fifty years ago, the most common advice given to patients who had suffered an MI was to take several

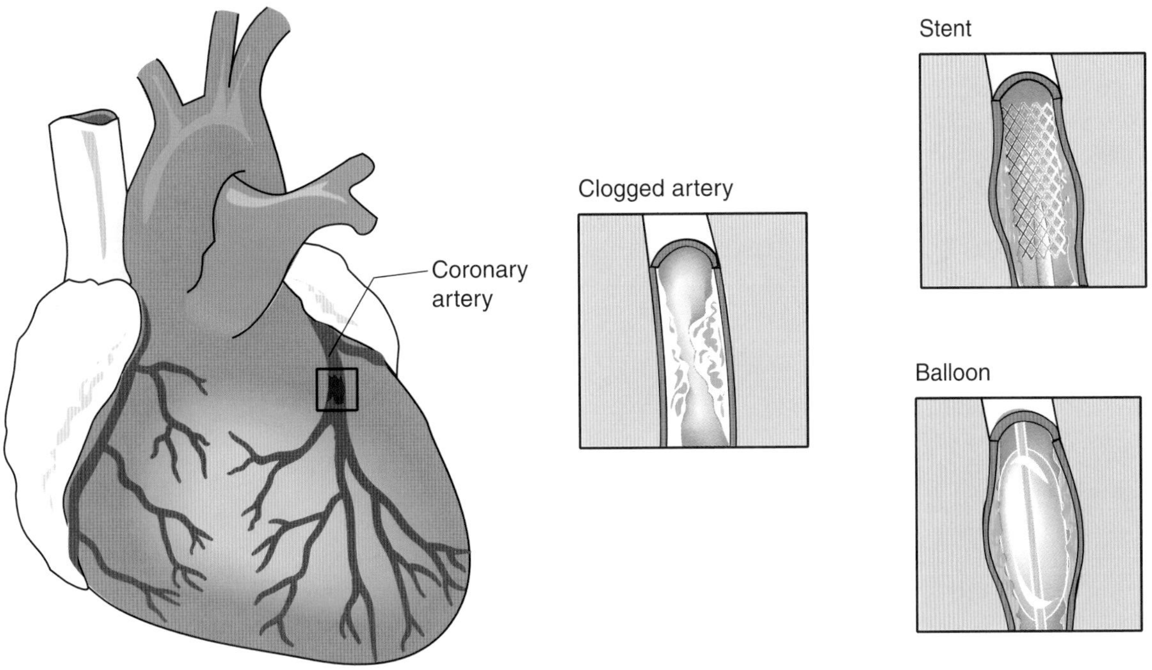

Figure 17.2 Percutaneous transluminal coronary angioplasty. A guide wire is used to position the balloon catheter at the site of obstruction inside the coronary artery. The balloon is inflated, increasing the lumen size and capacity for blood flow. The catheter then is deflated and removed. In some cases, a metal stent is placed inside the artery to keep it open.

weeks of complete bed rest (3). Today, however, exercise training is an ordinary part of the treatment of individuals with CHD. Cardiac rehabilitation programs use a multidisciplinary approach of education and exercise to help clients with heart disease return to normal function, within the limits of their disease (18).

There is no question that CHD patients have improved cardiovascular function as a result of exercise programs. This is evidenced by higher $\dot{V}O_2max$ values, higher work rates achieved without ischemia (as shown by angina pectoris or S-T segment changes), and an increased capacity for prolonged submaximal work (6, 15, 19). Moderate reductions in body fat, blood pressure, total cholesterol, serum triglycerides, and LDL-C have been shown to occur with regular exercise, along with increases in HDL-C. The improved lipid profile is a function of more than the exercise alone, given that weight loss and the saturated fat content of the diet can modify these variables.

A major focus of cardiac rehabilitation programs is to reduce the occurrence of subsequent MIs (3). This is referred to as **secondary prevention** of CHD. The Framingham Heart Study has shown that individuals who have suffered one heart attack are at increased risk of a second occurrence. Furthermore, the likelihood of recurrence clearly is associated with many of the same risk factors that caused atherosclerosis in the first place. Thus, cardiac rehabilitation personnel must be concerned with monitoring blood pressure, blood cholesterol levels, and smoking status in their patients. In general, research studies have shown that a cardiac rehabilitation program involving exercise results in a 20 to 25% reduction in all-cause and cardiovascular mortality after an MI. This is good news, because it indicates that such patients derive a substantial benefit from participating in cardiac rehabilitation. In addition, patients gain an improved sense of well-being (18).

One of the most exciting developments in cardiac rehabilitation in recent years is the demonstration that a "lifestyle modification" approach can reverse coronary artery disease. Ornish et al. (13) conducted a series of studies in which they showed that a program consisting of a strict vegetarian diet, yoga, meditation, smoking cessation, and physical activity reversed the atherosclerotic process. Patients in this study showed actual reversal of blockages in their coronary arteries, lending credibility to the idea that this condition can, in some cases, be treated with nonsurgical interventions.

3 In Review

Cardiac rehabilitation programs are designed to help people with heart disease regain their fitness and return to normal, everyday activities. The benefits of such programs include increased work capacity and reductions in cardiovascular risk factors. Cardiac rehabilitation programs generally reduce the risk of a second heart attack.

Special Diagnostic Tests to Detect CHD

Testing patients with CHD is much more involved than testing the apparently healthy person as described earlier. There are some classes of CHD patients for whom exercise or exercise testing is inappropriate and dangerous (2). In other persons, however, the benefits of a graded exercise test (GXT) outweigh the risks. Diagnostic exercise testing is nearly always performed in a hospital environment, with a physician present. A 12-lead electrocardiogram (ECG) is monitored at discrete intervals during the GXT, and three leads are displayed continuously on an oscilloscope. Blood pressure, rating of perceived exertion (RPE), and various signs and symptoms also are noted. Emergency equipment includes a defibrillator, supplemental oxygen, and emergency medications. Personnel trained and certified in advanced cardiac life support are on hand to provide assistance if needed.

Treadmill tests commonly used in diagnostic exercise testing are the Naughton, Balke, Bruce, and Ellestad protocols, named after their developers (2). These protocols are all GXTs that use increases in speed and/or grade at regular intervals to increase the exercise intensity. For those who are unable to perform treadmill exercise, a cycle test or arm ergometer test may be used. The criteria for terminating the GXT focus on various pathological signs (e.g., S-T segment depression on the ECG) or symptoms (e.g., angina pectoris) rather than on achieving some percentage of age-adjusted maximal heart rate. A subjective "angina scale" may be used to assess the severity of the symptoms (see table 17.1).

Other tests of heart function are obtained through radionuclide procedures, typically done in conjunction with either exercise or pharmacological (nonexercise) stress tests (5, 14). In the latter case, administration of pharmacologic agents provokes myocardial ischemia by (a) increased myocardial oxygen demand or (b) coronary vasodilation. For instance, thallium-201 (a radioactive substance) can be injected intravenously to assess myocardial perfusion. Thallium is taken up by well-perfused myocardium in a manner similar to potassium. Ischemic myocardium tends not to take up the thallium, thus allowing areas of the heart with poor blood flow to be identified. Another technique involves the use of a radioisotope that binds to the red blood cells (technetium-99m), which is useful for cardiac blood-pool imaging. This allows the end-systolic volume (ESV) and end-diastolic volume (EDV) to be measured, and the ejection fraction then can be computed as follows: ejection fraction = (EDV – ESV) / EDV. Ventricular wall motion abnormalities also can be identified (14).

The most definitive tests for CHD are coronary angiography and positron emission tomography (PET) scans. In angiography, a cardiac catheter is inserted into the femoral artery and pushed all the way up the aorta until it reaches the entrance to a coronary artery, and the curved tip of the catheter guide allows it to be inserted into the artery. A contrast dye is injected through the catheter into the coronary artery. By viewing an image of the coronary arteries on a screen, the cardiologist can measure the degree of occlusion (narrowing) that exists (see figure 17.3). PET scans involve infusion of [^{18}F]-deoxyglucose or [^{13}N]-ammonia. These substances allow the level of myocardial cell metabolism to be assessed. Metabolically active areas, indicative of good perfusion, can be distinguished from underperfused areas of the heart by color.

Table 17.1 Angina Rating Scale

1	Perceptible but mild
2	Moderate
3	Moderately severe
4	Severe

Note. This scale is used in rating the subjective pain associated with myocardial insufficiency. From *ACSM's Guidelines for Graded Exercise Testing and Prescription* (2).

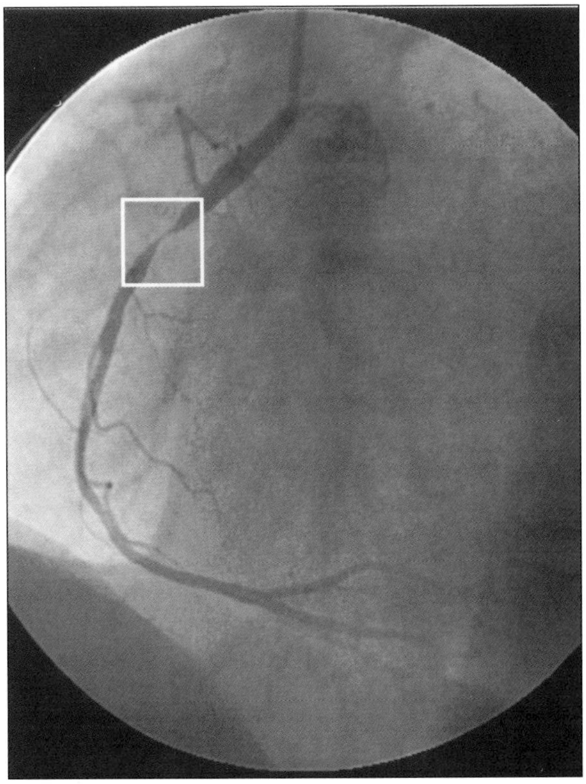

Figure 17.3 Coronary angiogram showing occlusion (narrowing) of a coronary artery. A catheter has been inserted into a coronary artery and radiographic contrast dye injected to allow the artery to be seen.

4 In Review

Special types of diagnostic tests can be done to determine whether a patient has CHD. GXTs on the treadmill (with close monitoring of the ECG and blood pressure) are a common method of detecting signs and symptoms of heart disease. Other types of radionuclide tests can provide more definitive confirmation of the presence or absence of heart disease.

Typical Exercise Prescription

The details of how to design and implement cardiac rehabilitation programs, from the first steps taken after the patient is confined to bed to the time he or she returns to work and beyond, are provided in the American Association for Cardiovascular and Pulmonary Rehabilitation guidelines (3). This section briefly introduces various aspects of such programs.

Cardiac rehabilitation programs are organized in progressive phases of programming to meet the needs of clients and their families. Phase I (the acute phase) begins when a patient arrives in the hospital stepdown unit, after leaving the intensive or coronary care unit (18). Within 1 to 3 days of the MI or revascularization procedure, the patient has already begun the rehabilitation process. Patients are exposed to orthostatic or gravitation stress by intermittently sitting and standing. Later, bedside activities and slow ambulation (i.e., walking) in the hallways are recommended (3).

Phases II and III refer to outpatient exercise programs conducted in a hospital environment. Rhythmic, large muscle group activities are recommended for physical conditioning; this includes treadmill exercise, cycle ergometry, combined arm and leg exercise, rowing, and stair climbing. Light- to moderate-resistance exercise training is accomplished through use of free weights (dumbbells) and elastic tubing (Theraband). Special care must be taken when prescribing upper body exercises to clients who have undergone CABG procedures, because of limitations related to the chest incision. See chapter 12 for more details on strength training in cardiac populations.

Recommendations for aerobic exercise programming in outpatient cardiac rehabilitation (phases II-III) are as follows (8, 9):

- Frequency: 3 to 4 days per week
- Intensity: 40 to 75% of $\dot{V}O_2$max or HRR
- Duration: 20 to 40 min per session
- 5 to 10 min of warm-up and cool-down exercises

Health professionals who work in cardiac rehabilitation must have knowledge of cardiovascular medications (for a description of these, see chapter 24). Special consideration must be given to patients who are on β-blockers, because the Karvonen formula for computing THR range is invalid if the client was not on β-blockers at the time of testing. For these individuals, a THR is sometimes computed by adding 20 to 30 beats · min^{-1} to the client's standing, resting HR. However, in view of the wide differences in physiological responses to β-blockade, another approach is to use RPE ratings around "somewhat hard," which correspond to 11 to 14 on the original Borg scale (3).

In phase II, clients are monitored carefully for vital signs (HR, BP, ventilation), and the ECG is monitored at a central observation station via telemetry (radio signals). A single-channel recording of 6 to 10 patients can be monitored simultaneously on a computer screen, and in the event of arrhythmias or S-T segment changes, a rhythm strip is printed out. Phase II programs are typically about 12 weeks in length and are covered by insurance reimbursement.

Phase III programs are hospital-based programs where clients are encouraged to continue their exercise regimens and are provided access to continuing health care and patient education. In these cases, the client's ECG usually is not monitored by telemetry but clients continue to follow an individualized exercise prescription and continue to attend patient education classes. Eventually, the client may enter the maintenance phase and move to a phase IV program in a nonhospital setting.

5 In Review

Cardiac rehabilitation programs are divided into four phases. Phase I is the acute phase, performed while the patient is still in the hospital. Phases II and III are conducted on an outpatient basis, whereas phase IV is the maintenance phase. Cardiac patients can benefit from a variety of aerobic and resistance training exercises, but working with this population requires special knowledge of their medical conditions.

Case Studies

You can check your answers by referring to appendix A.

17.1

John is a 46-year-old male. He is an insurance executive who is married with two children. John is active in his church and plays golf on the weekends. He went to see his cardiologist because he had recent fatigue with chest pain on exertion. He has never smoked but he consumes one to two alcoholic drinks per day. His medical history reveals a blood cholesterol level of 263 mg/dl, a triglyceride level of 195 mg/dl, and an HDL-C value of 45 mg/dl. Considering his sex, age, symptoms, and risk factors, what do you think is the likelihood he has CHD? What would be a reasonable next step to diagnose the presence or absence of CHD?

17.2

Jane is a 61-year-old retired female. On February 15 of this year, she underwent a left heart catheterization. The heart catheterization revealed significant occlusion in the left anterior descending artery and the circumflex artery. Therefore, a balloon angioplasty procedure was performed. Approximately 2 weeks later, she performed a GXT with the following results:

Protocol: Balke (3.3 mph)

Resting: HR= 72 bpm

BP = 130/72

End point: stage 3 for 1 min (approximately 7 METs)

HR = 126 bpm

BP = 160/90

Reason for termination: Fatigue

No S-T segment depression, no reported symptoms

Jane was taking atenolol (a β-blocker) at the time of her test, and her physician instructed her to continue taking this medication. She was referred to the cardiac rehabilitation center for supervised exercise and risk factor modification. List some types of exercise that would be appropriate for her.

Source List

1. American College of Sports Medicine. (1993). Position stand: Physical activity, physical fitness, and hypertension. *Medicine and Science in Sports and Exercise, 25(10)*, i-x.
2. American College of Sports Medicine. (2000). *ACSM's guidelines for graded exercise testing and prescription* (6th ed.). Baltimore: Lippincott Williams & Wilkins.
3. American Association for Cardiovascular and Pulmonary Rehabilitation. (1999). *Guidelines for cardiac rehabilitation and secondary prevention programs* (3rd ed.). Champaign, IL: Human Kinetics.
4. American Heart Association. (2001). *Heart and stroke statistical update.* Dallas, TX: American Heart Association.
5. Brubaker, P.H., Kaminsky, L.A., & Whaley, M.H. (2002). *Coronary artery disease: Essentials of prevention and rehabilitation programs* (pp. 83-110). Champaign, IL: Human Kinetics.
6. Clausen, J.P. (1977). Circulatory adjustments to dynamic exercise and physical training in normal subjects and in patients with coronary artery disease. In E.H. Sonnenblick & M. Lesch (Eds.), *Exercise and the heart* (pp. 39-75). New York: Grune & Stratton.
7. Enos, W., Holmes, R., & Beyer, J. (1953). Coronary disease among United States soldiers killed in action in Korea. *Journal of the American Medical Association, 152*, 1090-1093.
8. Franklin, B.A. (1997). Myocardial infarction. In J.L. Durstine (Ed.), *ACSM's exercise management for persons with chronic disease and disability* (pp. 19-25). Champaign, IL: Human Kinetics.
9. Franklin, B.A. (1997). Coronary artery bypass grafting and angioplasty. In J.L. Durstine (Ed.), *ACSM's exercise management for persons with chronic disease and disability* (pp. 26-31). Champaign, IL: Human Kinetics.
10. Grines, C.L. (1996) Aggressive intervention for myocardial infarction: Angioplasty, stents, and intra-aortic balloon pumping. *American Journal of Cardiology, 78*, 29-34.
11. Hagberg, J.M. (1990). Exercise, fitness, and hypertension. In C. Bouchard, R.J. Shephard, & T. Stephens (Eds.), *Physical activity, fitness, and health* (pp. 993-1005). Champaign, IL: Human Kinetics.
12. Kaplan, N.M. (1994). *Clinical hypertension* (6th ed.). Baltimore: Williams & Wilkins.
13. Ornish, D., Scherwitz, L.W., & Billings, J.H. (1998). Intensive lifestyle changes for reversal of coronary heart disease. *Journal of the American Medical Association, 280*, 2001-2007.
14. Paschkow, F.J., & Harvey, S.A. (2001). Diagnosis of coronary artery disease. In J.L. Roitman (Ed.), *ACSM's resource manual for guidelines for exercise testing and prescription* (4th ed., pp. 246-253). Baltimore: Lippincott Williams & Wilkins.
15. Pollock, M.L., & Wilmore, J.H. (1990). *Exercise in health and disease* (2nd ed.). Philadelphia: Saunders.
16. Regensteiner, J.G., & Hunt, W.G. (2001). Exercise in the management of peripheral arterial disease. In J.L. Roitman (Ed.), *ACSM's resource manual for guidelines for exercise testing and prescription* (4th ed., pp. 292-298). Baltimore: Lippincott Williams & Wilkins.
17. Squires, R.W. (1998). Coronary atherosclerosis. In J.L. Roitman (Ed.), *ACSM's resource manual for guidelines for exercise testing and prescription* (3rd ed., pp. 225-230). Baltimore: Lippincott Williams & Wilkins.
18. Temes, W.C. (1994). Cardiac rehabilitation. In E.A. Hillegass & H.S. Sadowsky (Eds.), *Essentials of cardiopulmonary physical therapy* (pp. 633-675). Philadelphia: Saunders.
19. Thompson, P.D. (1988). The benefits and risks of exercise training in patients with chronic coronary artery disease. *Journal of the American Medical Association, 259*, 1537-1540.
20. Wenger, N.K., & Hurst, J.W. (1984). Coronary bypass surgery as a rehabilitative procedure. In N.K. Wenger & H.K. Hellerstein (Eds.), *Rehabilitation of the coronary patient* (pp. 115-132). New York: Wiley.

eighteen

Exercise and Obesity

Dixie L. Thompson

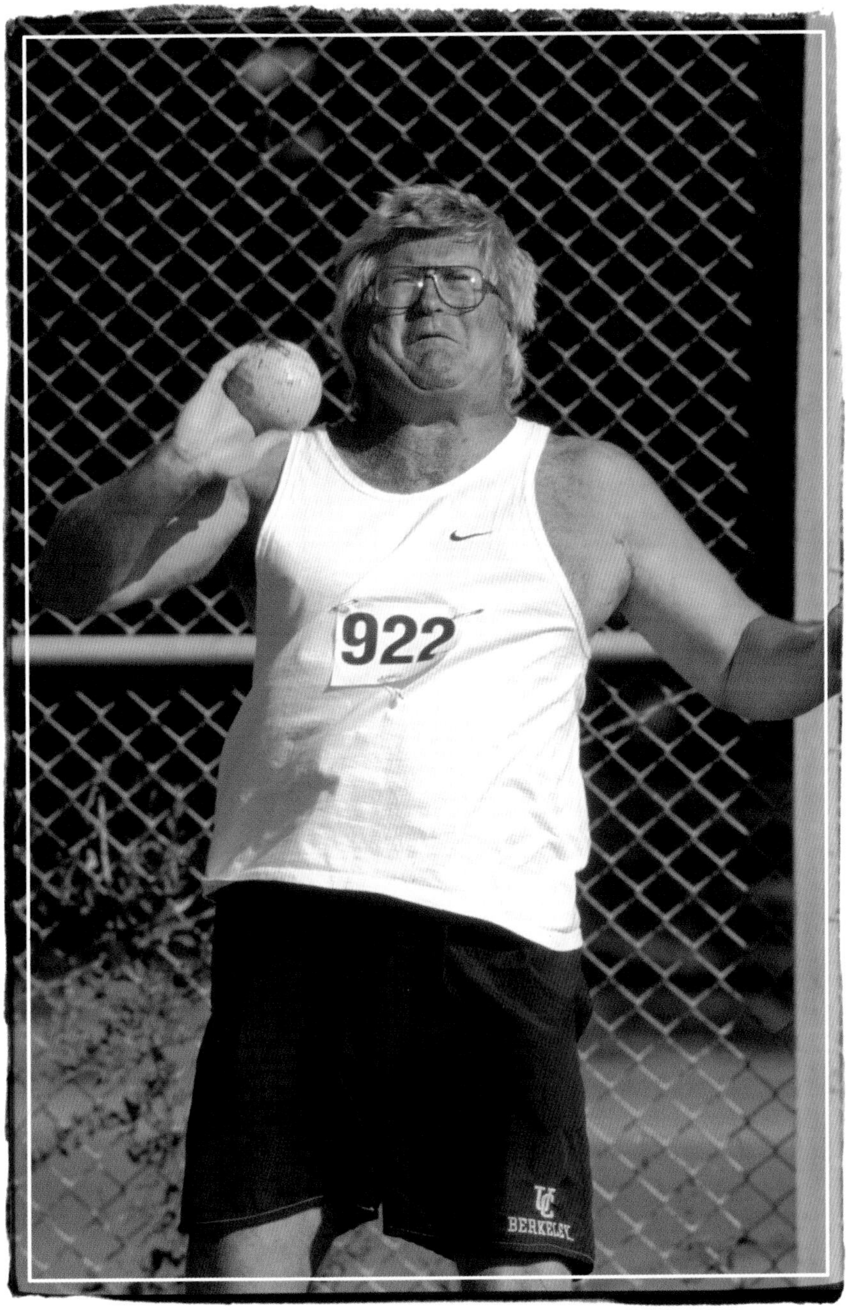

© Human Kinetics

Objectives

The reader will be able to do the following:

1. Define obesity and describe health risks of obesity.
2. Describe the role that exercise plays in preventing and treating obesity.
3. Explain the modifications to standard testing procedures necessary for obese clients.
4. Write an exercise prescription for someone who is obese.

Overview

Obesity is a condition defined by excessive body fat. Obesity can be documented by examining the relationship between height and weight (e.g., BMI) or by evaluating percent body fat (%BF). Because BMI requires simple measurements and, for the majority of adults, is closely related to body fatness, it has become the clinically preferred method of assessing obesity (see chapter 6). NIH guidelines classify a BMI of 30 kg/m^2 or higher as obese. Class I obesity ranges from 30.0 to 34.9 kg/m^2, class II obesity ranges from 35.0 to 39.9 kg/m^2, and class III (extreme) obesity is a BMI of 40 kg/m^2 or higher (14). Although there are no universally agreed on standards for classification of obesity from %BF, a %BF of greater than 38% for females and greater than 25% for males generally is considered in the obese range (5, 11).

Potential Causes

Although consumption of calories in excess of daily caloric need is an easily identified culprit in the etiology of obesity, this condition is much more complex than suggested by that simple explanation. Both biological (e.g., genetic predisposition attributable to lower than normal RMR) and psychological (e.g., poor body image) factors can contribute to the development of obesity and can pose significant obstacles when a person attempts to lose weight (7). Genetics is thought to contribute 25 to 40% of the variance in body weight. A number of biological factors have been identified as possible mechanisms through which the predisposition for obesity is established. These factors include the protein leptin, sympathetic nervous system activity, several neuropeptides, and some hormones (16). Suggested pathways through which these factors may work include lowering RMR, influencing eating behaviors, or slowing the rate of fat oxidation. Because of the media attention recently focused on the genetic roots of obesity, obese individuals can become discouraged from attempting to lose weight. Although biological factors clearly contribute to obesity, the imbalance between energy intake and expenditure is the ultimate reason for fat accumulation. Educating clients concerning the role of good nutrition and appropriate exercise in maintaining a healthy weight is an important aspect of the HFI's responsibilities.

The prevalence of obesity in the United States and in many countries around the world is increasing (10). In the 1990s, for example, there was a 50% increase in the prevalence of obesity among U.S. adults (12). A recent study estimated that 63% of U.S. men and 55% of U.S. women are either overweight or obese (13). Government estimates indicate that only about 42% of U.S. adults are at a healthy weight (BMI ≥ 18.5 and < 25 kg/m^2), and one of the *Healthy People 2010* objectives is to increase this level to 60% (19) (see figure 18.1). The prevalence of obesity is particularly high among African American and Mexican American women (14). Another disturbing trend is the increasing rates of obesity for children (17). Some have linked the rising prevalence of childhood obesity to an increase in inactive leisure-time pursuits such as television viewing (6, 15). Clearly, the rapid increase in obesity rates supports the contention that lifestyle choices (i.e., diet and physical activity), not genetics, are primarily responsible for the increasing prevalence of obesity.

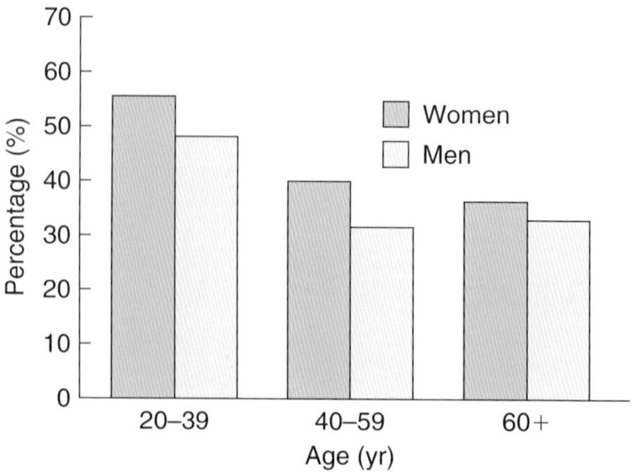

Figure 18.1 Percentage of U.S. adults at healthy body weight. Healthy body weight is body mass index ≥18.5 and <25 kg/m^2.

Complications

The increasing prevalence of obesity is important because of the negative health complications that accompany this condition. Obesity is linked with increased mortality and morbidity rates. Diseases and conditions associated with obesity include CHD, congestive heart failure, stroke, type 2 diabetes, hypertension, dyslipidemia, gallbladder disease, osteoarthritis, some cancers (e.g., breast, colon), sleep apnea, and respiratory problems (14). Women who are obese are more likely to experience menstrual irregularities and complications with pregnancy (14). Overall, approximately 300,000 deaths per year in the United States can be attributed to the complications of obesity (3). The direct cost of obesity in 1995 was approximately $51 billion (14), with the total economic cost near $100 billion (14). In 2000, the total economic cost of obesity increased to approximately $117 billion (18). Clearly, obesity results in major personal as well as financial strains. The serious impact of overweight and obesity is reflected by the issuance of *The Surgeon General's Call to Action to Prevent and Decrease Overweight and Obesity* (18). This report outlines the problem of overweight and obesity and calls for both public and private commitments to address this health concern (18).

1 In Review

Obesity is a complex condition with biological and lifestyle links. More than one half of U.S. adults are classified as either overweight or obese, and the prevalence is rising. Many comorbidities exist with obesity, including type 2 diabetes, CHD, stroke, and some cancers. The economic cost of obesity is more than $100 billion per year.

Role of Physical Activity in Prevention and Treatment of Obesity

The rapid increase in obesity prevalence appears more related to a decline in physical activity than an increase in energy intake (9). This relationship supports the contention that altering sedentary lifestyles will lower rates of obesity. Although the evidence is indirect, an overview of cross-sectional and prospective studies suggests that active people are less likely to be obese, and those who maintain an active lifestyle are least likely to become obese over time (4, 9). However, estimation of energy intake and expenditure on a population level is crude, the studies do not always agree, and much additional research is needed to clarify these issues.

A number of studies have used exercise as a means for treating obesity. Most of these trials were short-term, and many had design flaws that limit the conclusions that can be drawn. In general, well-controlled, randomized control trials typically have found modest weight reduction with the use of exercise as a treatment for obesity (8, 22). Slightly greater weight loss typically is seen when caloric restriction is combined with exercise (8, 22). There is also evidence that a combination of dietary restriction and exercise is better at helping maintain weight loss than is either method alone (8, 22). An examination of data from the National Weight Control Registry (NWCR) suggests that regular aerobic exercise is common among those who successfully maintain significant weight loss (23).

2 In Review

Active people are less likely to be overweight or obese. Exercise can be an important part of a weight loss program. Exercise is a key to maintaining weight loss.

Research Insight

The National Weight Control Registry was established in 1994 to provide insight into ways that people are successful at losing weight and then maintaining weight loss. Currently, more than 3000 people participate in the NWCR, with an average weight loss of 30 kg maintained for 5.5 years. About half of these participants used commercial weight loss programs, whereas the others lost weight without formal guidance. Several interesting facts have been gathered from these "successful losers": (1) 89% report using both caloric restriction and exercise in their weight loss programs; (2) the most common dietary approach taken by the participants involved choosing a diet low in total calories and low in fat (~24% of calories from fat); (3) most participants weighed themselves frequently to provide feedback on the success of their behaviors; (4) a typical exercise routine was 1 hr per day of moderate physical activity; and (5) walking was the most frequently reported exercise (77% of participants), and about 20% used resistance training. For more information on the NWCR, see Wing and Hill (23).

Special Medical Screening

A number of conditions frequently coexist with obesity (e.g., type 2 diabetes, hypertension). The high prevalence of these comorbid conditions requires that the HFI carefully screen obese individuals before performing exercise testing. Health histories and pretesting screenings should be designed to identify these conditions (see chapter 3). The presence of these conditions as well as the individual's overall physical condition will determine the types of exercise testing needed before exercise programming. Once the initial health history screening process is completed, the ACSM risk stratification categories can be used to guide decisions on the need for medical clearance and physician supervision of exercise tests.

Medications

Like any client, an obese person should provide documentation of medications. Because of the wide-ranging comorbidities that can exist with obesity, a variety of medications may be prescribed. It is also becoming common to prescribe medication for both weight loss and weight control (see the box below). Over-the-counter weight loss aids and herbal supplements are also taken frequently by those desiring weight loss. Although there are many of these products, one commonly found ingredient in over-the-counter weight loss products is ephedrine. This nonregulated stimulant has been linked with tachycardia, hypertension, and even heart attacks. It is beyond the scope of this chapter to review all products used to promote weight loss. The HFI should encourage clients to be wise consumers of such products by learning all the potential side effects and discussing the use of these substances with their physicians.

Testing

Typically, standard testing modes and protocols can be used when testing obese persons; however, the initial intensity as well as the incremental increases should reflect the individual's fitness / activity level (see chapter 5). This is particularly important because of the severe deconditioning that often exists with obesity. With severe obesity or when ambulation is problematic, it may be preferable to use cycle or arm ergometry for testing. However, if walking will be the exercise of choice for programming, treadmill testing will provide useful insight into the velocity that the client can be expected to maintain during walking. This can be helpful information when the HFI is attempting to design a workout with a targeted caloric expenditure.

For an obese individual, the physiological response to exercise typically will be similar to that of a normal weight individual, except that cardiorespiratory function often is reduced by the excessive weight. However, the existence of comorbidities, especially hypertension and type 2 diabetes, can alter the exercise or postexercise response.

3 In Review

The large number of comorbidities that accompany obesity necessitates careful screening of obese clients. Exercise testing of obese clients should be individualized, taking into account any special needs.

Exercise Prescription

ACSM guidelines state that obese individuals should be encouraged to exercise on most, if not all, days of the week for a minimum of 150 min per week (1, 2). Generally, the duration of the exercise should be 40 to 60 min each day, which may be done in one long bout or divided into two shorter bouts (1). Some

Prescription Medications for the Treatment of Obesity

Two commonly prescribed drugs used to treat obesity are orlistat (i.e., Zenical) and sibutramine (i.e., Meridia). Orlistat interferes with the absorption of fat in the digestive system. This drug commonly results in weight loss and improved blood lipid profile. Although an increase in BP occasionally is reported with the use of orlistat, more common side effects are oily discharge and fecal urgency. Sibutramine works through the brain neurotransmitters serotonin and norepinephrine. It increases metabolic rate, creates a sense of fullness, and elevates energy levels. Potential cardiovascular side effects include increased HR and BP.

evidence indicates that an even greater caloric expenditure (i.e., >2000 kcal per week or 200-300 min per week) may be most beneficial for long-term weight control (2). Participants initially may be unable to exercise this long, so an initial focus of programming is to build enough endurance to sustain aerobic activity to reach these duration goals. The initial intensity may be 40 to 50% of $\dot{V}O_2max$, with an eventual goal of sustaining activity between 50 and 70% of $\dot{V}O_2max$. A balance between intensity and duration should be used to achieve a target energy expenditure of 300 to 500 kcal each day for those attempting to lose weight (1).

Designing exercise programs for obese individuals requires some special considerations. One of the primary aims of any exercise program should be safety. For obese individuals, avoiding orthopedic injuries is a particular concern because of the additional loading to joints. Therefore, low-impact activities (water exercise, cycling, and walking) are preferable when individuals begin to exercise regularly. After some weight loss and conditioning occur, individuals may choose to participate in higher impact sports and activities. Another safety concern is thermoregulation (20). Because of excessive body fatness and the increased energy demands of activity, keeping the body cool during exercise can be problematic for obese individuals. Individuals should be encouraged to exercise at cool times of the day or in temperature-controlled environments. These exercisers should maintain adequate hydration by drinking lots of water.

Resistance training also may be an important component of one's overall exercise program. Although resistance training typically does not burn off a large number of calories, it can serve important functions for obese individuals (2). During weight loss, both lean and fat tissues are typically reduced. However, lean tissue may be maintained, or at least muscle loss can be minimized, by using resistance training during periods of caloric restriction. Maintaining muscle mass is important for both functional capacity and metabolic rate. Compared with fat, muscle is a metabolically active tissue, so maintaining lean mass is important in minimizing decreases in metabolic rate.

Rarely will obese individuals seek to begin exercise without also setting some goals related to weight loss (although exercise provides benefits even in the absence of weight loss; see box on this page). The HFI should assist the client in developing healthy weight loss goals. Appropriate weight loss goals are 0.5 to 1 kg per week. For example, reducing caloric intake by 500 kcal per day and expending an additional 300 kcal per day would lead to a caloric deficit that would approximate a 0.7-kg loss per week (7 × [500 + 300] = 5600 kcal per week). Typically, diets with fewer than 1200 kcal per day are not recommended without physician supervision. A well-planned, low-fat diet with a caloric deficit of 500 to 1000 kcal per day allows for gradual weight reduction without sacrificing nutritional needs (2). An appropriate distribution of macronutrients along with the necessary amounts of vitamins and minerals should be included in the dietary planning (see chapter 7). Diets that are low in fat, particularly saturated fat, not only effective for weight loss but are also associated with long-term weight maintenance. See chapter 11 for additional information on weight loss and weight management strategies. It is recommended that overweight and obese individuals reduce body weight by at least 5 to 10% to gain health benefits such as lower BP and a more favorable blood lipid profile (2). For some individuals, an even greater reduction in body weight may be optimal for health improvement (2).

4 In Review

Prudent weight loss goals for overweight and obese clients range from 0.5 to 1.0 kg per week. For obese individuals, the ACSM recommends exercise programs that create a daily caloric deficit of 300 to 500 kcal. Both aerobic exercise and resistance training can be used effectively by obese clients. For weight loss, exercise programs should be combined with a low-fat, reduced-calorie diet. When prescribing exercise for obese clients, place special emphasis on avoiding musculoskeletal injuries and heat injury.

Exercise Without Weight Loss

Even without weight loss, exercise provides a number of benefits for overweight individuals. The benefits of exercise (e.g., an improved blood lipid profile, lower BP, and better stress management) are much the same in overweight and normal weight individuals. Although the health benefits are optimal if both weight is reduced and fitness improved, participation in regular exercise results in significant protection against disease even when the individuals remain overweight. Data from the Cooper Clinic in Dallas have demonstrated that fitness protects against early death in overweight persons (21). Because of these findings, it is important to emphasize an active lifestyle, even if weight loss is not an outcome.

Case Study

You can check your answers by referring to appendix A.

18.1

Marsha is a 48-year-old female who comes to your fitness facility and expresses interest in purchasing a membership. She is responding to a series of advertisements that your facility is using to attract individuals interested in weight loss. Your screening reveals the following.

- Her height is 5 ft 5 in. and her weight is 220 lb.
- Her blood pressure is 152/88 mm Hg.
- She has never exercised regularly.
- It has been more than 3 years since she had a medical examination.
- There is a history of heart disease on her father's side of the family, and her mother developed type 2 diabetes after menopause.

a. What, if any, medical screening would you recommend before this client enrolls in your facility's programs?

b. What fitness testing would you suggest for this individual?

c. Assuming that no medical conditions are revealed with the screening and initial testing, describe a diet and exercise program that Marsha could use to achieve her weight loss and fitness goals.

Source List

1. American College of Sports Medicine. (2000). *ACSM's guidelines for exercise testing and prescription* (6th ed.). Philadelphia: Lippincott Williams & Wilkins.
2. American College of Sports Medicine. (2001). Appropriate intervention strategies for weight loss and prevention of weight regain for adults. *Medicine and Science in Sports and Exercise, 33*(12), 2145-2156.
3. Allison, D.B., Fontaine, K.R., Manson, J.E., Stevens, J., & VanItallie, T.B. (1999). Annual deaths attributable to obesity in the United States. *Journal of the American Medical Association, 282*(16), 1530-1538.
4. DiPietro, L. (1999). Physical activity in the prevention of obesity: Current evidence and research issues. *Medicine and Science in Sports and Exercise, 31*(11, Suppl.), S542-S546.
5. Going, S., & Davis, R. (2001). Body composition. In J.L. Roitman (Ed.), *ACSM's resource manual for guidelines for exercise testing and prescription* (4th ed., pp. 391-400). Baltimore: Lippincott Williams & Wilkins.
6. Gortmaker, S., Must, A., Sobel, A., Peterson, K., Colditz, G.A., & Dietz, W.H. (1996). Television viewing as a cause of increasing obesity among children in the United States. *Archives of Pediatric Adolescent Medicine, 150,* 356-362.
7. Grilo, C.M., & Brownell, K.D. (2001). Interventions for weight management. In J.L. Roitman (Ed.), *ACSM's resource manual for guidelines for exercise testing and prescription* (4th ed., pp. 584-591). Baltimore: Lippincott Williams & Wilkins.
8. Grundy, S.M., Blackburn, G., Higgins, M., Lauer, R., Perri, M.G., & Ryan, D. (1999). Physical activity in the prevention and treatment of obesity and its comorbidities: Roundtable consensus statement. *Medicine and Science in Sports and Exercise, 31*(11, Suppl.), S502-S508.
9. Jebb, S.A., & Moore, M.S. (1999). Contribution of a sedentary lifestyle and inactivity to the etiology of overweight and obesity: Current evidence and research issues. *Medicine and Science in Sports and Exercise, 31*(11, Suppl.), S534-S541.
10. Khan, L.K., & Bowman, B.A. (1999). Obesity: A major global public health problem. *Annual Review of Nutrition, 19,* xiii-xvii.
11. Lohman, T.G., Houtkooper, L., & Going, S.B. (1997). Body fat measurement goes high-tech: Not all are created equal. *ACSM's Health & Fitness Journal, 1,* 30-35.
12. Mokdad, A.H., Serdula, M.K., Dietz, W.H., Bowman, B.A., Marks, J.S., & Koplan, J.P. (1999). The spread of the obesity epidemic in the United States, 1991-1998. *Journal of the American Medical Association, 282*(16), 1519-1522.
13. Must, A., Spandano, J., Coakley, E.H., Field, A.E., Colditz, G., & Dietz, W.H. (1999). The disease burden associated with overweight and obesity. *Journal of the American Medical Association, 282*(16), 1523-1529.
14. National Heart, Lung, and Blood Institute. (1998). *Clinical guidelines on the identification, evaluation, and treatment of overweight and obesity in adults* (NIH Publication 98-4083). Bethesda, MD: National Institutes of Health, National Heart, Lung, and Blood Institute.
15. Robinson, T.N. (1998). Does television cause childhood obesity? *Journal of the American Medical Association, 279,* 959-960.
16. Salbe, A.D., & Ravussin, E. (2000). The determinants of obesity. In C. Bouchard (Ed.), *Physical activity and obesity* (pp. 69-102). Champaign, IL: Human Kinetics.
17. Seidell, J.C. (2000). The current epidemic of obesity. In C. Bouchard (Ed.), *Physical activity and obesity* (pp. 21-30). Champaign, IL: Human Kinetics.
18. U.S. Department of Health and Human Services. (2001). *The Surgeon General's call to action to prevent and decrease overweight and obesity.* Rockville, MD: U.S. Government Printing Office.
19. U.S. Department of Health and Human Services. (2000). *Healthy people 2010: Understanding and improving health* (2nd ed.). Washington, DC: U.S. Government Printing Office.
20. Wallace, J.P. (1997). Obesity. In J.L. Durstine (Ed.), *ACSM's exercise management for persons with chronic diseases and disabilities* (pp. 106-111). Champaign, IL: Human Kinetics.
21. Welk, G.J., & Blair, S.N. (2000). Physical activity protects against the health risks of obesity. *PCPFS Physical Activity and Fitness Research Digest, 3*(12), 1-7.
22. Wing, R.R. (1999). Physical activity in the treatment of the adulthood overweight and obesity: Current evidence and research issues. *Medicine and Science in Sports and Exercise, 31*(11, Suppl.), S547-S552.
23. Wing, R.R., & Hill, J.O. (2001). Successful weight loss maintenance. *Annual Review of Nutrition, 21,* 323-341.

nineteen

Exercise and Diabetes

Dixie L. Thompson

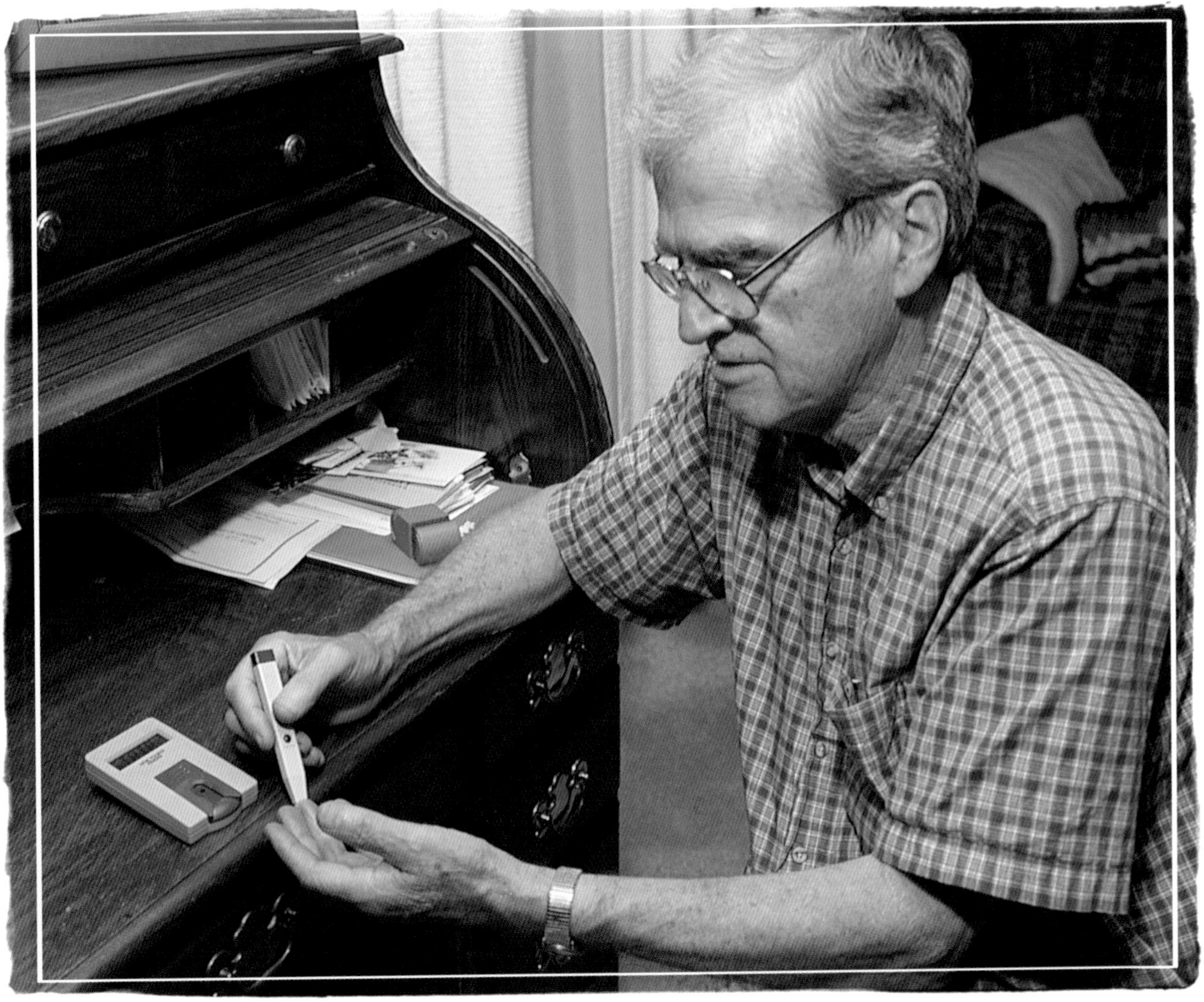

Objectives

The reader will be able to do the following:

1. Define diabetes mellitus, and describe the characteristics of type 1 and type 2 diabetes.
2. Describe the role that exercise plays in the prevention and treatment of type 2 diabetes.
3. Describe special considerations needed regarding exercise testing for diabetic clients.
4. Describe special considerations regarding exercise prescription for diabetic clients.

Overview

Diabetes mellitus is a term used to identify metabolic diseases characterized by **hyperglycemia** (i.e., elevated plasma glucose). The blood glucose levels used to identify someone with diabetes mellitus are outlined in the box titled Diagnosing Diabetes Mellitus. The cause of hyperglycemia varies depending on the type of diabetes present, with the most common forms being type 1 and type 2 diabetes. **Type 1 diabetes** is characterized by a deficiency of insulin often attributable to an autoimmune destruction of the insulin-producing β-cells of the pancreas. In **type 2 diabetes**, the insulin receptors become insensitive or resistant to insulin and, because glucose cannot move readily into the cells, hyperglycemia results. Although there are other forms of diabetes mellitus (e.g., gestational diabetes), type 1 and type 2 account for the vast majority of cases. Regardless of the type of diabetes, a number of complications may result. These complications typically affect the blood vessels and nerves and include vision impairment, kidney disease, peripheral vascular disease, atherosclerosis, and hypertension (2). The estimated economic burden of diabetes is $100 billion per year (11).

It is estimated that more than 15 million Americans suffer from diabetes, with approximately 90% of the cases being type 2 diabetes. This form of diabetes has both lifestyle and genetic roots. Many type 2 diabetics are relatively inactive and overweight or obese, particularly with excessive abdominal fat. Other risk factors include a family history of type 2 diabetes, older age, and belonging to an ethnic minority (prevalence is higher among Hispanic, Native, and African Americans compared with Caucasians). Type 2 diabetes frequently coexists with other conditions such as hypertension and dyslipidemia. Although type 2 diabetes can appear at any age, the highest rates are seen among people age 60 years and older (11). However, there is an increasing prevalence of type 2 diabetes among children, and this trend seems linked with increasing obesity rates (11). Type 2 diabetes usually develops over time, first appearing as impaired fasting glucose or **impaired glucose tolerance**. Impaired glucose tolerance is a condition in which the increase in blood glucose after ingestion of carbohydrate is higher than normal and remains elevated longer than normal. Examples of normal and abnormal blood glucose responses are shown in figure 19.1. A person with either impaired fasting glucose or impaired glucose tolerance is classified as having **prediabetes**. Without intervention, prediabetes generally evolves into type 2 diabetes.

Diagnosing Diabetes Mellitus

For a diagnosis of diabetes, one of the following must exist:

- Fasting plasma glucose ≥126 mg/dl (7.0 mM; fasting means no food intake within the past 8 or more hours)
- Symptoms of diabetes (e.g., unusual thirst, frequent urination, unexplained weight loss) and a casual plasma glucose of ≥200 mg/dl (11.1 mM; casual means that time of last food ingestion prior to testing was not controlled)
- A glucose value of ≥200 mg/dl 2 hr after the ingestion of 75 g of carbohydrate

Note. Normal fasting plasma glucose concentration is <110 mg/dl (6.1 mM). Fasting plasma glucose concentration ≥110 mg/dl but <126 mg/dl classifies the individual as having impaired fasting glucose.

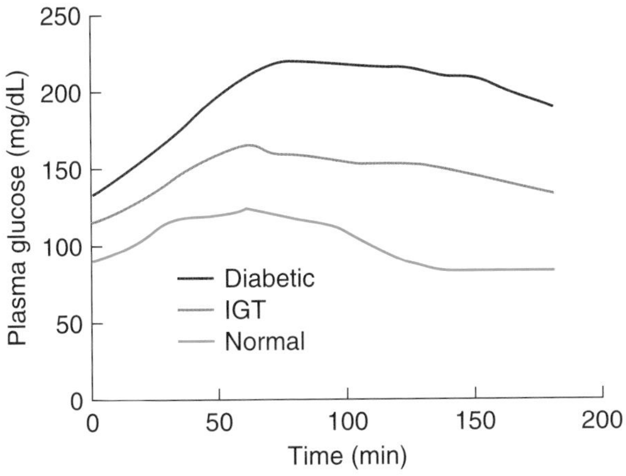

Figure 19.1 Comparison of glucose response to carbohydrate ingestion. IGT = impaired glucose tolerance.

Type 2 diabetes is characterized by **insulin resistance**, a condition in which the body's insulin receptors no longer respond normally to insulin. Because the insulin receptors do not respond normally, glucose entry into cells is impaired and hyperglycemia results. Plasma insulin levels of type 2 diabetics may be normal, suppressed, or elevated depending on the individual. Regardless, type 2 diabetes is considered a disease of relative insulin deficiency because the insulin available is inadequate to maintain normal glucose concentrations. Although some type 2 diabetics can control their disease through exercise and weight loss, others require medications such as oral hypoglycemic agents and possibly even insulin injections (4).

Type 1 diabetes is a disease that results from a lack of insulin. In this disease, the most common cause is autoimmune destruction of the insulin-producing β-cells of the pancreas leading to lack of insulin. Without insulin, the body's cells are unable to take in glucose. People with this disease require insulin injections. Unlike type 2 diabetes, type 1 diabetes often appears early in life and is more closely linked to genetic than lifestyle factors. See the box titled Medications to Control Diabetes Mellitus.

Medications to Control Diabetes Mellitus

All persons with type 1 diabetes require insulin injections. There are a number of types of insulin, and they vary by how rapidly they begin working, the peak time of action, and how long they continue to work.

Type of Insulin	Onset of action	Peak	Duration
Rapid acting	15 min	30-90 min	≤ 5 hr
Short acting	30 min	2-4 hr	4-8 hr
Intermediate acting	2-6 hr	4-14 hr	14-20 hr
Long acting	6-14 hr	10-16 hr	20-24 hr

Some people with type 2 diabetes also require insulin injections. More often, however, they take other types of prescription medications to lower blood glucose. A number of types of medications are used for this purpose.

Class of medication	Example	Mode of action
Sulfonylureas	PresTab	Stimulates insulin production
Biguanides	Glucophage	Reduces glucose release from liver
α-glucosidase inhibitors	Precose	Slows the absorption of carbohydrates
Thiazolidinediones	Avandia	Increases insulin sensitivity
Meglitinides	Prandin	Stimulates insulin production
D-phenylalanine derivatives	Starlix	Increases the rate of insulin production

For more information on medications used to treat diabetes mellitus, see the Web sites of the American Diabetes Association (3) and the National Institute of Diabetes and Digestive and Kidney Diseases (10).

1 In Review

Diabetes mellitus is a disease characterized by hyperglycemia. More than 15 million Americans have diabetes mellitus, and the economic cost is approximately $100 billion each year. Type 1 diabetes results from a lack of insulin production. Type 2 diabetes, the most common form of diabetes, is characterized by the cells becoming insensitive to insulin. Risk factors for type 2 diabetes include older age, a family history of type 2 diabetes, excess weight, and inactivity.

Exercise in the Prevention and Treatment of Type 2 Diabetes

Exercise can provide many benefits to individuals with either type 1 or type 2 diabetes. This is particularly true because of the strong link between diabetes and cardiovascular disease. However, because of the nature of type 1 diabetes, exercise cannot prevent nor is it essential for the treatment of this form of diabetes. On the other hand, exercise has been shown effective in the prevention and treatment of type 2 diabetes (see the box below).

Inactivity and obesity are common characteristics of persons with type 2 diabetes. Cross-sectional studies show that those who are regularly active are less likely to develop type 2 diabetes than their inactive counterparts (2, 9). Additionally, those who have impaired glucose tolerance are less likely to develop type 2 diabetes if they begin to exercise regularly (2, 9). Evidence also is mounting that type 2 diabetics will experience better glucose tolerance and improved insulin sensitivity through regular exercise (2, 7). There are a number of reasons that exercise can be beneficial in the treatment of type 2 diabetes (4, 5). These include the following:

- Lower fasting blood glucose concentrations
- Better glucose tolerance (less of a spike in glucose after eating)
- Improved insulin sensitivity (more glucose uptake with a given amount of insulin)
- Weight control (increased lean mass and reduced fat mass)
- Improved lipid profiles
- Reduction in blood pressure for those with hypertension
- Lower risk of cardiovascular disease
- Stress management (stress can affect glucose control via increased levels of catecholamines)

2 In Review

Exercise has been shown to be effective in preventing and treating type 2 diabetes. Exercise provides a number of benefits to the diabetic person.

Screening and Testing Diabetic Clients

Medical clearance should be required of all clients with diabetes mellitus to ensure that exercise can be performed safely. This is particularly an issue with type 1 diabetics, who may have difficulty controlling blood glucose levels. It is important that these patients discuss with their physicians how to modify their insulin dosage with exercise. Because exercise increases glucose uptake from peripheral tissues regardless of insulin levels, hypoglycemia may result if insulin intake is not adjusted (see next section for tips on avoiding hypoglycemia). It is also important to remember that diabetes is a primary risk factor for the development of cardiovascular disease, so diabetic clients should be screened carefully for signs and symptoms of disease (chapter 3).

Type 1 Diabetes and the Benefits of Exercise

Although exercise will not prevent or cure type 1 diabetes, exercise should be encouraged in this population for a number of reasons (5). Exercise improves insulin sensitivity and reduces disease risk for diabetic people, much like in the nondiabetic population. Because of the high rate of cardiovascular disease among diabetics, exercise can be an important part of promoting overall well-being. Exercise protects against coronary artery disease, dyslipidemia, hypertension, and obesity. Increased physical activity and improved physical fitness also promote psychological health and quality of life.

Additionally, type 2 diabetics frequently are overweight and hypertensive and have a poor blood lipid profile; therefore, these clients may be taking a number of medications that can influence the exercise response. For people who have suffered from diabetes for a number of years, peripheral neuropathy may be a problem. Damage to the sensory nerves in the feet can lead to ulcerations, and if there is damage to blood vessels, healing can be slow. Because of these and other issues, conducting a thorough medical history is particularly important with diabetic clients.

The type of testing performed before exercise programming depends on the individual. Diagnostic exercise stress testing, under the supervision of a physician, may be necessary for individuals with numerous risk factors. The choice of protocol will depend on the client's age and functional ability. Submaximal exercise testing can be used to estimate aerobic power (see chapter 5). However, the presence of autonomic neuropathy can cause unusual HR and BP responses during exercise. For more information on testing diabetic clients, see Albright (4).

3 In Review

Because of the increased risks associated with diabetes mellitus, physician clearance should be obtained before exercise testing. What tests are appropriate will depend on the client's needs.

Typical Exercise Prescription

The goals of exercise programming with diabetic clients (e.g., increasing aerobic power, reducing disease risk, increasing flexibility, increasing muscular strength and endurance) are similar to those of nondiseased individuals with the exception of improving glucose control.

Type 1 Diabetes

The type 1 diabetic must carefully consider modifying insulin dosage and carbohydrate ingestion before beginning an exercise program. Increasing the intake of carbohydrate and/or reducing insulin dosage is often needed to maintain proper glucose control and avoid hypoglycemia that can result from exercise. The adjustment in carbohydrate intake and insulin dosage will depend on the intensity and duration of activity. Glucose should be measured before initiation of an exercise session. If glucose is <100 mg/dl, carbohydrates should be ingested before beginning exercise. If glucose is >300 mg/dl or >240 mg/dl with urinary ketones, exercise should be delayed (1).

For the previously inactive type 1 diabetic client, progression should be slow with careful monitoring of blood glucose and symptoms of cardiovascular and metabolic distress. Initially, supervised exercise is recommended. After the person is able to maintain glucose control with exercise, unsupervised exercise is acceptable. However, it is always preferable that diabetic clients not exercise alone because of the need to have someone nearby in case of a hypoglycemic event. Symptoms of hypoglycemia include dizziness, nausea, headache, confusion, and irritability (6) (see the following box).

Regular aerobic exercise is recommended to maximize blood glucose control. Although resistance exercise is safe for most diabetic clients, those with advanced complications (e.g., kidney disease, vision impairment) should avoid heavy lifting where

Precautions for Avoiding Exercise-Induced Hypoglycemia

- Measure blood glucose immediately before and 15 min after exercise (also during exercise if the exercise lasts longer than 30 min).
- Consume carbohydrates if glucose is <100 mg/dl.
- Delay exercise if glucose is >240 mg/dl with ketone bodies or >300 mg/dl without ketones.
- Avoid exercising during times of peak insulin action.
- Reduce insulin dose (and inject into inactive areas) on days of planned exercise.
- Consume carbohydrates after exercise. Hypoglycemia can appear several hours after exercise, so monitoring after exercise is crucial.
- Avoid exercise late at night because hypoglycemia could occur while sleeping.
- Warm-up and cool-down may need to be extended with diabetic clients.

extreme BP elevation is possible. Because peripheral neuropathy can lead to ulcerations of the feet, good foot care is essential. Properly fitting and supportive shoes are particularly important for diabetic clients engaging in weight-bearing exercise. For more information, Neil Gordon's book, *Diabetes: Your Complete Exercise Guide*, provides guidelines for foot care that may be useful to diabetic clients (8). For those with advanced peripheral neuropathy, low-impact and potentially non-weight-bearing exercises are more appropriate.

Type 2 Diabetes

The ACSM recommends that individuals with type 2 diabetes engage in both endurance and resistance training, unless significant complications or limitations exist (2). At least 1000 kcal per week should be expended in aerobic activity. For those who are overweight or obese, the focus of the aerobic activity should be caloric expenditure and weight control. Although at least 3 nonconsecutive days of exercise per week are recommended, individuals may choose to engage in daily physical activity to maximize glucose control and caloric expenditure. Low to moderate exercise intensity (40-70% $\dot{V}O_2max$) is recommended, although higher intensity activity is not contraindicated in those who are conditioned and choose more vigorous exercise. Because of the possibility of autonomic neuropathy, the use of HR to monitor exercise intensity may be problematic. Therefore, RPE may be a better choice for individuals to self-monitor exercise intensity (see chapter 5). Exercise intensity and duration should be balanced to achieve caloric expenditure goals. Typically, exercise sessions of at least 10-15 min are suggested, with accumulated physical activity of 30-60 min per day. The mode of aerobic exercise should be based on the client's needs and abilities. Walking is the mode of choice for many diabetic clients, but for those with peripheral nerve damage, other modes (e.g., swimming, nonimpact exercise equipment) may be preferable.

Resistance training also is suggested for many individuals with type 2 diabetes (2). Resistance training maintains, or even increases, muscle mass and assists with glucose tolerance and insulin sensitivity. The program should be designed to focus on major muscle groups (8-10 exercises) and consist of at least 1 set of 10 to 15 repetitions (see chapter 12). This routine should be performed at least 2 days per week. Those without advanced complications can follow more aggressive programs. However, for those with eye or kidney damage as a result of diabetes, particular caution should be taken to avoid extreme BP elevations.

Because many clients with type 2 diabetes have a history of being relatively inactive and are often overweight, beginning and then maintaining an active lifestyle presents particular challenges. Creating a supportive environment is especially important for the success of these clients. It is particularly important early in the exercise program to provide information on the benefits of a lifetime commitment to exercise. It is also important to design a program that progresses slowly, is based on realistic goals, and incorporates the client's needs and desires. Additional information on increasing adherence to exercise can be found in chapter 22 and in the ACSM position stand on exercise and type 2 diabetes (2).

4 In Review

Exercise prescription for the diabetic client must take into account special needs caused by the disease. Careful monitoring of blood glucose levels is needed to help avoid hypoglycemic events. For individuals with type 2 diabetes, the ACSM recommends an exercise program that results in an expenditure of at least 1000 kcal per week. Resistance training can be used with diabetic clients as long as the client avoids damage to already weakened blood vessels.

Case Study

You can check your answers by referring to appendix A.

19.1

Dave is a 45-year-old man who, in response to doctor's orders, appears at your medical wellness facility for exercise programming. He recently sought the care of his physician after suffering from fatigue and headaches. Dave's physician ordered a series of tests (see table). Dave was placed on a cholesterol-lowering medication and a diuretic to lower his blood pressure. He was told to begin to exercise and lose weight to lower his blood glucose.

Dave will enroll in a 3-month weight loss and supervised exercise program at your facility. Determine a reasonable 3-month weight loss goal for Dave and design a caloric intake and exercise plan that will help him realize these goals.

Weight = 265 lb	Total cholesterol = 270 mg/dl	Fasting plasma glucose = 128 mg/dl
Height = 5 ft 9.5 in.	LDL-C = 190 mg/dl	Blood pressure = 148/94 mmHg
No smoking	HDL-C = 32 mg/dl	Estimated $\dot{V}O_2max$ = 22 ml · kg^{-1} · min^{-1}
High stress	Previously inactive	No ischemia with exercise stress test

Note. LDL-C = low-density lipoprotein cholesterol; HDL-C = high-density lipoprotein cholesterol.

Source List

1. American College of Sports Medicine. (2000). *ACSM's guidelines for exercise testing and prescription* (6th ed.). Philadelphia: Lippincott Williams & Wilkins.
2. American College of Sports Medicine. (2000). Exercise and type 2 diabetes. *Medicine and Science in Sports and Exercise, 32*(7), 1345-1360.A
3. American Diabetes Association. About Insulin. [Online]. Available: www.diabetes.org/main/application/commercewf?origin=*.jsp&event=link(C4_3) [July 10, 2002].
4. Albright, A.L. (1997). Diabetes. In J.L. Durstine (Ed.), *ACSM's exercise management for persons with chronic diseases and disabilities* (pp. 94-100). Champaign, IL: Human Kinetics.
5. Campaigne, B.N. (2001). Exercise and diabetes mellitus. In J.L. Roitman (Ed.), *ACSM's resource manual for guidelines for exercise testing and prescription* (4th ed., pp. 277-284). Baltimore: Lippincott Williams & Wilkins.
6. Cola, S.G. (2001). Understanding the effects of exercise and the onset of hypoglycemia. *ACSM's Health and Fitness Journal, 5*(3), 15-21.
7. Eriksson, J.G. (1999). Exercise and the treatment of type 2 diabetes mellitus: An update. *Sports Medicine, 27*(6), 381-391.
8. Gordon, N.F. (1993). *Diabetes: Your complete exercise guide.* Champaign, IL: Human Kinetics.
9. Kriska, A. (2000). Physical activity and the prevention of type 2 diabetes mellitus: How much for how long? *Sports Medicine, 29*(3), 147-151.
10. National Institute of Diabetes and Digestive and Kidney Diseases. (2002). Medicines for People With Diabetes. [Online], April 2002. Available: www.niddk.nih.gov/health/diabetes/pubs/med/index.htm [July 10, 2002].
11. U.S. Department of Health and Human Services. (2000). *Healthy people 2010: Understanding and improving health* (2nd ed.). Washington, DC: U.S. Government Printing Office.

twenty

Exercise, Asthma, and Pulmonary Disease

David R. Bassett, Jr.

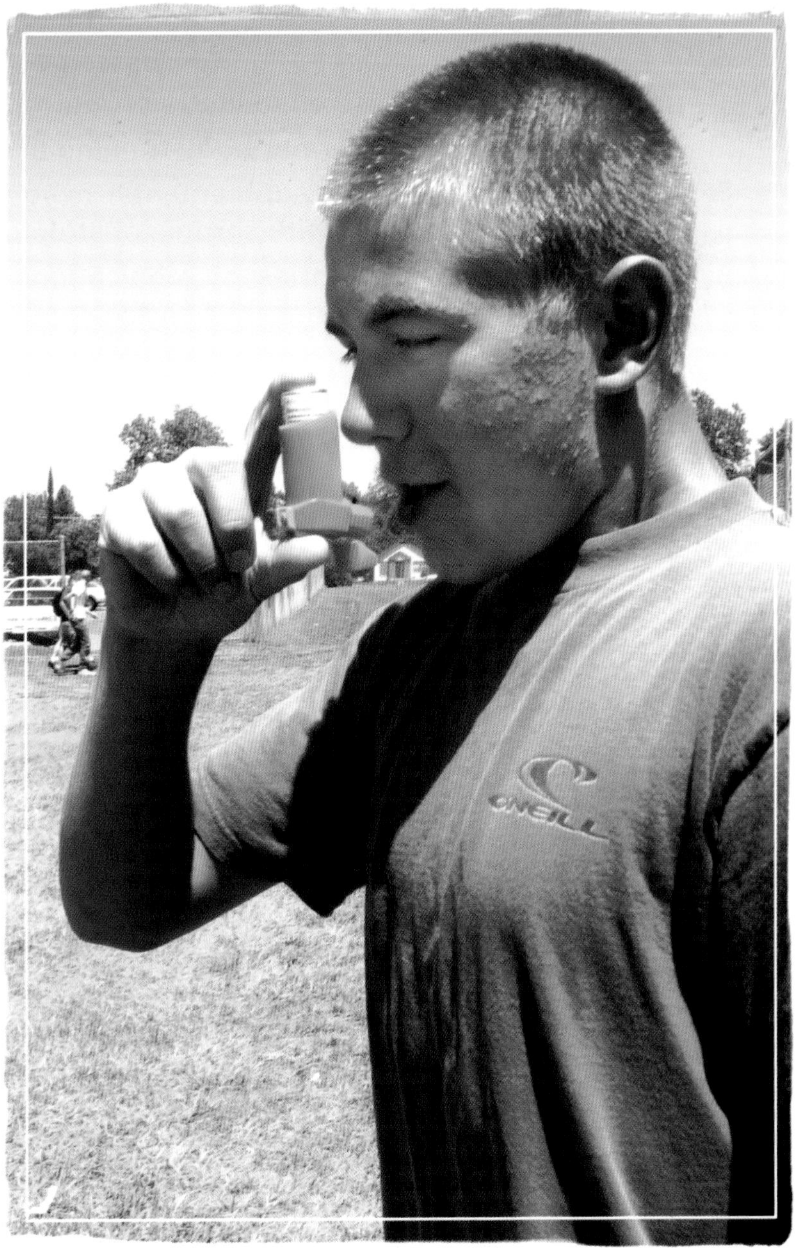

Objectives

The reader will be able to do the following:

1. Describe the differences between chronic obstructive lung diseases and restrictive lung diseases.
2. Define the underlying physiological problems associated with asthma, emphysema, bronchitis, and cystic fibrosis.
3. List physiological and mental health benefits of exercise for individuals with pulmonary disease.
4. Describe how pulmonary function testing can be used to diagnose chronic obstructive lung diseases versus restrictive lung diseases.
5. Describe how signs (e.g., dyspnea) and symptoms (e.g., hypoxemia) of pulmonary disease typically are monitored during a GXT.
6. Describe how to prescribe aerobic exercise (frequency, intensity, and duration) in pulmonary rehabilitation programs.
7. Identify the benefits of upper body training in pulmonary rehabilitation.
8. Describe the benefits of supplemental oxygen therapy and pursed lip breathing in individuals with chronic obstructive pulmonary disease.
9. List the common categories of medications used to treat pulmonary disease, some of the members of each category, and the probable impact of these medications on exercise performance.

Pulmonary diseases can be subdivided into two major categories. In chronic obstructive pulmonary diseases (COPDs), the airflow into and out of the lungs is impeded. In restrictive lung diseases, the expansion of the lungs is reduced because of conditions involving the chest cavity or parenchyma (lung tissue). Some forms of pulmonary disease are genetically inherited (e.g., cystic fibrosis), but in other cases a history of cigarette smoking, environmental pollutants, or occupational exposure to silica, coal dust, or asbestos is the primary contributing factor. The common factor in all pulmonary diseases is a disruption in the exchange of gases between the ambient air and the pulmonary capillary blood. As a result, $\dot{V}O_2$max is reduced, the work of breathing is increased, and the ability to perform exercise is limited.

Chronic Obstructive Pulmonary Diseases

COPDs cause a reduction in airflow that can dramatically affect one's ability to perform daily activities. Characteristics of COPDs include expiratory flow obstruction and shortness of breath on exertion. These diseases include chronic bronchitis, emphysema, and bronchial asthma. Each of these diseases obstructs airflow, but the underlying reason is different for each (3, 16):

Bronchial asthma is caused by bronchial smooth-muscle contraction and increased airway reactivity.

Chronic bronchitis results from persistent production of sputum attributable to a thickened bronchial wall with excess secretions.

Emphysema is caused by loss of elastic recoil of alveoli and bronchioles and enlargement of those pulmonary structures.

According to 1994 data from the National Center for Health Statistics, 14 million people have chronic bronchitis, and 2.2 million people have emphysema (15). Unfortunately, the mortality rates associated with COPDs have increased over the past 2 decades. It is important to recognize that chronic bronchitis and emphysema are not reversible. The patient with developing COPD perceives an inability to do normal activities without dyspnea, but, tragically, by the time this occurs the disease is already well advanced (3, 14).

Asthma

An estimated 14.6 million people in the United States suffer from asthma (15); 36% of these are children under 18 (5). It is a reversible condition that varies from wheezing and slight breathlessness to severe attacks that nearly result in suffocation. Causes of asthma include allergic reactions to antigens such as dust, pollen, smoke, and air pollution. Nonspecific factors such as emotional stress, exercise, and viral infections of the bronchi, sinuses, or tonsils can also result in asthma. People with exercise-induced asthma may have normal resting pulmonary function but suffer from bronchospasms during exercise. In some cases, no specific cause of the asthma can be identified (14). Treatment involves bronchodilators (often administered by inhalers) and other drugs that thin the secretions and help eject them (expectorants) (6).

Cystic Fibrosis

Cystic fibrosis, another type of COPD, is a recessively inherited genetic disorder. It is a fatal disease. Three decades ago, most cystic fibrosis patients died in childhood, but better treatments have prolonged life expectancy by 20 years (11). In Caucasian children, 1 in 2500 is born with the condition, although the disease is rare in Asians and African Americans (11). Thick mucous secretions by the exocrine glands affect many systems in the body. In fact, clinical diagnosis is based on excessive chloride concentration in the sweat. In the lungs, the mucous secretions plug the airways and cause inflammation of the airways and chronic bacterial infections. Treatment for cystic fibrosis consists of having the patient lie with his or her head facing downhill while percussion is used to enhance mucous drainage. In addition, aerobic exercise has been shown to be beneficial. The increased use of antibiotics is yet another reason that survival of cystic fibrosis patients has increased dramatically in recent years (12).

1 In Review

COPDs reduce the capacity for airflow during respiration. Two of these diseases, chronic bronchitis and emphysema, are irreversible. Bronchial asthma is an intermittent condition caused by restriction of airways; it can be relieved with medications. Cystic fibrosis is another form of COPD that is the result of a genetic defect.

Restrictive Lung Diseases

Restrictive lung diseases have many causes, including diseases of the rib cage and spine such as kyphoscoliosis and pectus excavatum (or "sunken chest"). Other causes include pulmonary edema, pulmonary embolisms, exposure to toxic substances (coal workers' pneumoconiosis, silicosis, asbestosis), chemotherapy, and radiation therapy. Often, these result in inflammation of the interstitium with development of fibrotic tissue. Various types of neuromuscular diseases (spinal cord injury, amyotrophic lateral sclerosis or Lou Gehrig's disease, Guillain-Barré syndrome, tetanus, and myasthenia gravis) can also cause restrictive lung disease. Obesity and pregnancy can restrict lung expansion because of the abdomen pushing up into the thoracic cavity. In general, people with restrictive lung diseases have reductions in residual volume (RV), inspiratory reserve volume (IRV), expiratory reserve volume (ERV), forced vital capacity (FVC), and maximal tidal volume (TV) (see figure 20.1). They experience an increased work of breathing because the respiratory muscles must work harder to inflate the lungs (8, 14).

2 In Review

Restrictive lung diseases have numerous causes, but the common factor among all of them is that the capacity to expand the lungs is reduced. Thus, reductions in lung volumes, assessed through pulmonary function testing, typically are seen in these individuals.

Evidence That Exercise Plays a Role

Pulmonary rehabilitation programs are often found alongside cardiac rehabilitation programs in many hospitals. Most pulmonary rehabilitation programs focus on the individual with COPD, although those with other types of pulmonary disease may also benefit from exercise (2, 7). Support for pulmonary rehabilitation programs is limited by the fact that patients typically show little or no improvement in $\dot{V}O_2$max, tests of lung function, and mortality rates. As a result, many insurance providers have been reluctant to pay for pulmonary rehabilitation because they view it as medical management rather

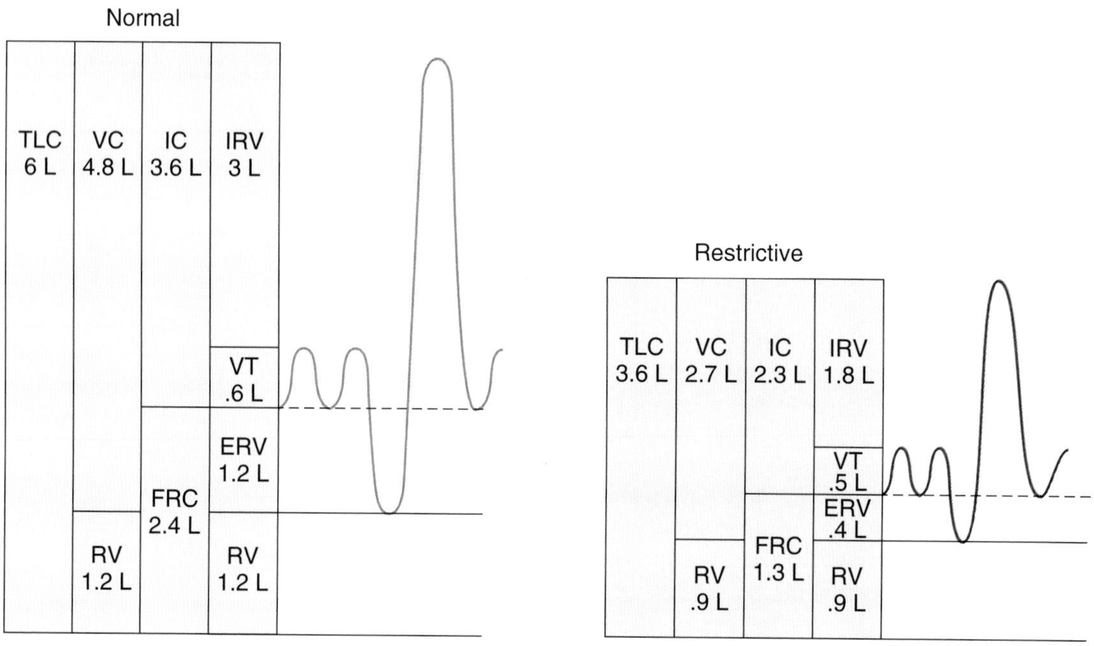

Figure 20.1 Lung volumes in a patient with restrictive lung disease versus a person with normal pulmonary function. Lung volumes are total lung capacity (TLC), vital capacity (VC), inspiratory capacity (IC), inspiratory reserve volume (IRV), tidal volume (TV), expiratory reserve volume (ERV), and residual volume (RV).

From Clough, P. (1994), Restrictive lung dysfunction. In E.A. Hillegass and H.S. Sadowsky (Eds.) *Essentials of Cardiopulmonary Physical Therapy* (pp. 189-255). Philadelphia: WB Saunders Co., with permission.

than a way to restore the patient to normal function, insofar as possible.

However, most pulmonary rehabilitation patients do exhibit improvements in functional outcomes, including symptom-limited GXT, symptoms of dyspnea, quality of life, and frequency of hospitalization (2). Thus, pulmonary rehabilitation should be viewed as a desirable part of the patient's medical treatment (9). The overall goals are to improve the patient's general health status, to optimize oxygen saturation, to improve the ease with which activities of daily living are accomplished, and to improve self-efficacy (2).

3 In Review

Patients with lung diseases can benefit from a pulmonary rehabilitation program. Although these patients usually demonstrate little improvement in $\dot{V}O_2$max and pulmonary function tests, they do exhibit improvements in their functional ability to carry out tasks and in other measures of quality of life.

Testing and Evaluation

In most instances, **pulmonary function testing** is carried out for diagnostic purposes and to assess the severity of the disease (13). Computerized spirometry systems are used to assess lung volumes and flow parameters. In COPD, the principal measure is forced expiratory volume (FEV_1), which reflects the maximum volume of air that can be moved in 1 s (see figure 20.2). Sometimes it is expressed as a ratio of FEV_1/VC, where VC (vital capacity) represents the volume of air that can be breathed out when going from maximal inhalation to maximal exhalation. Because of airway obstruction, individuals with COPD have a decreased ability to exhale quickly; if the FEV_1 is below 80% of the expected value, the test is considered abnormal (5). In restrictive lung disease, the lung volumes (e.g., RV, IRV, ERV, FVC, and maximal TV) are smaller than normal because lung expansion is limited. Individuals with restrictive lung disease compensate by taking faster, smaller breaths, which reduces the work that the respiratory muscles must perform to inflate the lung.

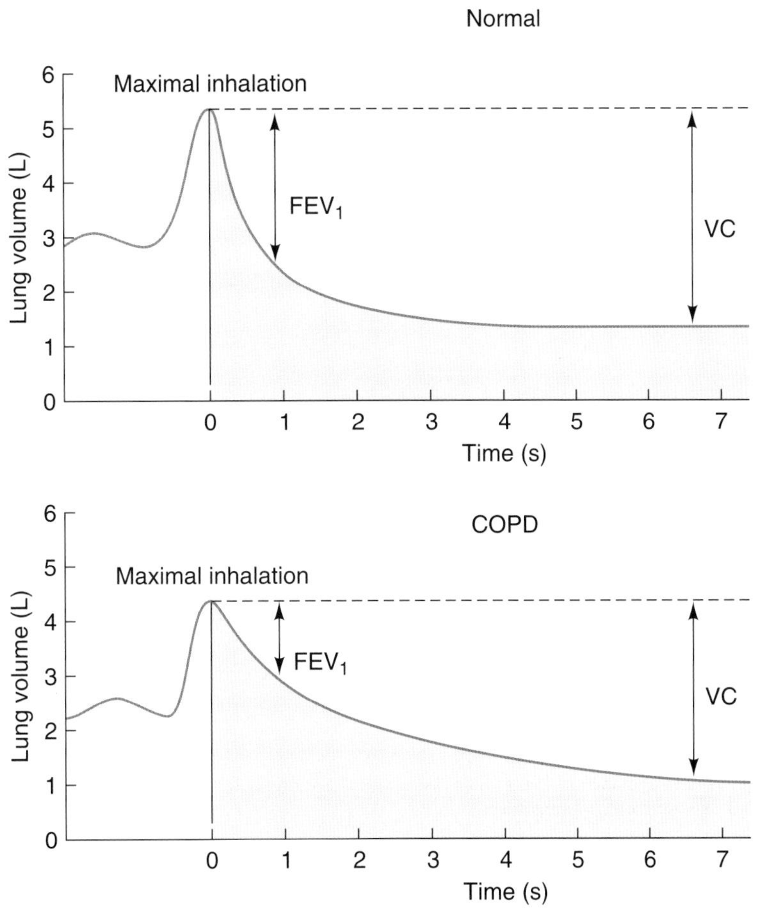

Figure 20.2 Pulmonary function test showing the volume versus time curves in a normal person and a patient with obstructive lung disease. FEV_1 = forced expiratory volume in the first second of exhalation; VC = vital capacity.

Exercise tests are often done to assess the patient's ability to exercise. The test may be a standard graded exercise test (GXT) on a treadmill or cycle ergometer or a simple 6- or 12-min walk test on a flat surface. In a pulmonary patient, exercise capacity is limited more by the lungs than the cardiovascular system. As a result, these patients typically suffer from **hypoxemia** (low arterial oxygen content) and **dyspnea** (shortness of breath). Measurements of maximal ventilation rates ($\dot{V}_E max$), obtained during the final minute of an exercise test, are also clinically useful. $\dot{V}_E max$ is typically about 60 to 70% of the maximal voluntary ventilation (MVV), although in COPD patients it may approach 80 to 100% of MVV. MVV can be measured via a special spirometry test, or it can be predicted from the following formula: $MVV = FEV_1 \times 40$.

In pulmonary patients, a device known as a **pulse oximeter** is used to assess the percent saturation of hemoglobin in the arterial blood (S_aO_2). This noninvasive device uses a probe that shines a light beam through the finger or earlobe to assess the color of the arterial blood (figure 20.3). Values for S_aO_2 below 90% indicate that client needs supplemental oxygen to increase the driving force for diffusion of oxygen into the lungs. Frequently, a "dyspnea rating scale" is used to evaluate symptoms during exercise testing (4, 17). Cardiovascular, pulmonary, metabolic, and power output measurements are obtained and used to evaluate the severity of disability (table 20.1).

4 In Review

In COPD, one of the main pulmonary function tests is the FEV_1. COPD patients demonstrate a reduced ability to exhale quickly because of obstruction of the airways. In restrictive lung diseases, many of the lung volumes are reduced because the ability to expand the lungs is compromised. Exercise testing of patients with lung diseases, with appropriate monitoring of signs (e.g., hypoxemia) and symptoms (dyspnea) to assess the severity of the patient's condition, is beneficial.

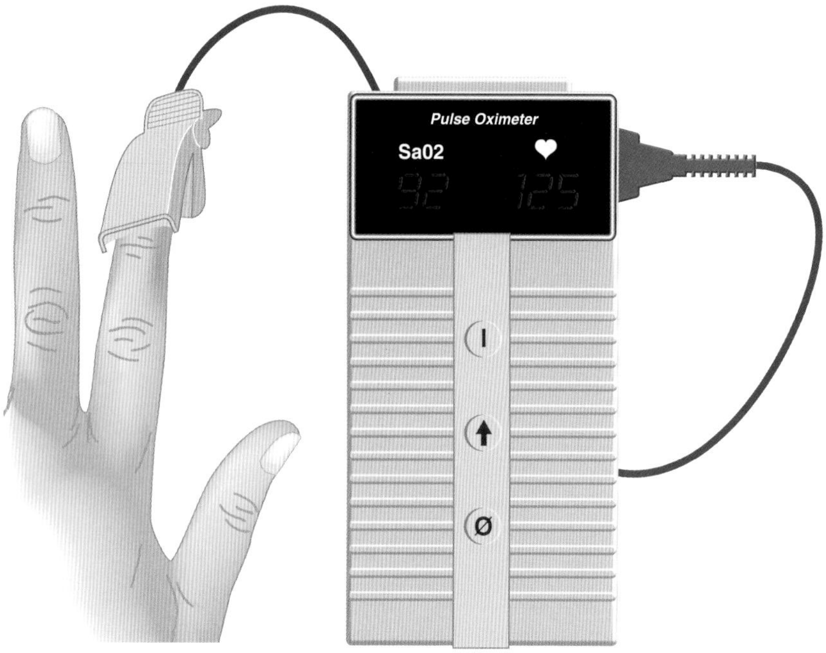

Figure 20.3 A portable pulse oximeter used to assess a pulmonary patient's arterial oxygenation. The number on the left of the display shows the percent saturation of hemoglobin in arterial blood (S_aO_2), whereas the number on the right shows the heart rate.

Typical Exercise Prescription in Pulmonary Diseases

The goal of a typical pulmonary rehabilitation program is the client's self-care, and to achieve that goal, physicians, nurses, respiratory therapists, exercise specialists, nutritionists, and psychologists are recruited to deal with the various manifestations of the disease process (2). The pulmonary patient receives education about the different ways to deal with the disease, including breathing exercises, ways to approach the activities of daily living at home, and how to handle work-related problems. The emphasis in most pulmonary rehabilitation programs is on the COPD patient, although patients with restrictive lung disease often participate as well (2, 14). The American Association of Cardiovascular and Pulmonary Rehabilitation has published a detailed description of exercise testing and prescription in its *Guidelines for Pulmonary Rehabilitation Programs* (1).

Table 20.1 Guide to Grading Chronic Obstructive Pulmonary Disease (Based on a 40-Year-Old Man)

Grade	Cause of dyspnea	FEV_1 (% pred)	$\dot{V}O_2max$ (ml · kg^{-1} · min^{-1})	Exercise $\dot{V}_Emax$ (L · min^{-1})	Blood gases
1	Fast walking and stair climbing	>60	>25	Not limiting	Normal P_aCO_2, S_aO_2
2	Walking at normal pace	<60	<25	>50	Normal P_aCO_2, S_aO_2 above 90% at rest and with exercise
3	Slow walking	<40	<15	<50	Normal P_aCO_2, S_aO_2 below 90% with exercise
4	Walking limited to less than one block	<40	<7	<30	Elevated P_aCO_2, S_aO_2 below 90% at rest and with exercise

Note. FEV_1 = forced expiratory volume in 1 s; $\dot{V}_Emax$ = maximal ventilation rate; P_aCO_2 = partial pressure of CO_2 in arterial blood; S_aO_2 = saturation of hemoglobin in the arterial blood.

Reprinted from Jones et al., 1987, Chronic obstructive respiratory disorders. In *Exercise testing and exercise prescription for special cases.* By permission of Lea & Febiger.

Aerobic training is usually accomplished with rhythmic, dynamic exercise that uses large muscle groups. As with healthy individuals and other clinical populations, the frequency is typically 3 to 5 times per week, with a duration of at least 30 min of exercise per session. However, the assignment of appropriate exercise intensities poses a particular problem. Pulmonary patients usually cannot achieve the same peak HRs as healthy individuals of the same age. Thus, computing a THR from a typical percentage of age-predicted HRmax often results in target intensities that are too high. On the other hand, using THR values computed from a typical percentage of measured HRmax underestimates the appropriate training intensity (1, 5).

Various methods can be used to estimate the appropriate exercise intensity for pulmonary patients. Generally, the method of assigning exercise intensity in the pulmonary rehabilitation program varies with the level of the disability (16). In patients with mild or moderate impairment, setting the intensity at the anaerobic threshold or the point where the person became noticeably dyspneic is appropriate. In clients with more severe disability, it is often necessary to let symptoms of dyspnea be the guiding factors (5). Intermittent exercise, interspersed with rest periods, may be all that the client can tolerate. If the impairment is severe, supplemental oxygen will be needed to maintain S_aO_2 above 90% (10).

Individuals with emphysema should be instructed in pursed lip breathing, which involves pressing the lips together and exhaling through a small opening in the center of the mouth. This slows the rate of respiration and prevents collapse of small airways, resulting in better oxygenation (2, 14). In some instances, a resistive breathing device may be recommended to specifically train the respiratory muscles at rest.

Upper body exercise also is recommended for pulmonary patients. This can be achieved through the use of exercise modalities that require a combination of arm and leg muscles, such as the Schwinn Airdyne or the rowing ergometer. Additionally, resistance training can be accomplished through the use of dumbbells, machines, or elastic bands. Increasing arm strength and endurance improves the client's ability to perform functional activities and decreases local muscle fatigue (2, 5).

5 In Review

Pulmonary rehabilitation programs involve many different types of health professionals. The primary goals are to educate patients about how to deal with their disease and help them to improve their exercise capacity. A health professional in pulmonary rehabilitation must understand the client's medical conditions and physiological limitations. Sensations of dyspnea and pulse oximeter readings are frequently used to determine the appropriate exercise intensity.

Medications for Pulmonary Diseases

Bronchodilators are used to relax smooth muscle surrounding airways in the lungs and relieve the symptoms of asthma, bronchitis, and related lung disorders (6). These medications can be taken orally or from an inhaler. The inhalers are generally used for acute asthma episodes, whereas long-term bronchodilation usually is obtained with oral preparations. Most of these drugs stimulate the β_2 receptors that relax bronchial smooth muscle and increase the airway lumen. Because of their β-adrenergic stimulating effect, these medications can increase HR and BP, although most of their effect is focused on the smooth muscle found in airways. Some of the inhaler brand names include Brethaire Inhaler, Alupent, Maxair, and others. A second class of drugs is the methylxanthines, which include Theobid, Aminophyllin, Theo-Dur, and many others. Side effects of this class include tachycardia, arrhythmias, central nervous system stimulation, and risk of seizures. A third class of bronchodilators is the anticholinergics (Atrovent).

Additional medicines are used to treat common respiratory disorders. These include **decongestants** to dry out the mucous membranes, **antihistamines** to provide relief from seasonal allergies (e.g., hay fever), anti-inflammatory agents, expectorants, and cough medications. Antibiotics are often given to fight off infections (6), which tend to occur if mucous secretions block off the airways.

Diuretics are important in treating a condition that afflicts about half of pulmonary patients with severe disease, known as *cor pulmonale*. Cor pulmonale is defined as pulmonary hypertension with right ventricular hypertrophy. Because right heart failure often follows, diuretics may be needed to enhance fluid excretion (9). There are three different types of diuretics: the thiazide diuretics (e.g., Esidrix), potassium-sparing diuretics (e.g., Aldactone), and loop diuretics (e.g., Lasix) (6).

6 In Review

Bronchodilators are the most common class of medications for patients with COPD. Decongestants, antihistamines, anti-inflammatory agents, and antibiotics are often prescribed to treat respiratory disorders. Diuretics are sometimes needed for patients with severe pulmonary disease if they develop heart failure.

Case Studies

You can check your answers by referring to appendix A.

20.1

A 38-year-old woman with asthma would like to enter your fitness program. What kinds of questions would you ask her during your screening interview?

20.2

A 50-year-old man with a history of smoking a pack of cigarettes per day for the past 25 years enters a hospital complaining of dyspnea. A chest x-ray shows that his lungs are hyperinflated, and spirometry tests show that his FEV_1 is only one half of the normal value. What type of pulmonary disease does he have, and what is the logical course of treatment?

20.3

A middle-aged patient with severe kyphoscoliosis is referred to a pulmonary rehabilitation program. He has restrictive pulmonary disease, demonstrating a vital capacity of only 1.5 L (compared with the normal value of 5.0 L). During a 6-min walk test, he manages to cover 865 ft, stopping once because of shortness of breath. His S_aO_2 at the end of the test has fallen to 87%. What type of exercise training would you recommend? What types of other therapies might assist this individual in completing his exercise sessions?

Source List

1. American Association of Cardiovascular and Pulmonary Rehabilitation. (1998). *Guidelines for pulmonary rehabilitation programs* (2nd ed.). Champaign, IL: Human Kinetics.
2. Barr, R.N. (1994). Pulmonary rehabilitation. In E.A. Hillegass & H.S. Sadowsky (Eds.), *Essentials of cardiopulmonary physical therapy* (pp. 677-701). Philadelphia: Saunders.
3. Berman, L.B., & Sutton, J.R. (1986). Exercise and the pulmonary patient. *Journal of Cardiopulmonary Rehabilitation, 6,* 52-61.
4. Borg, G.A. (1998.) *Borg's perceived exertion and pain scales.* Champaign, IL: Human Kinetics.
5. Brubaker, P.H., Kaminsky, L.A., & Whaley, M.H. (2002). *Coronary artery disease: Essentials of prevention and rehabilitation programs* (pp. 271-289). Champaign, IL: Human Kinetics.
6. Cahalin, L.P., & Sadowsky, H.S. (1994). Pulmonary medications. In E.A. Hillegass & H.S. Sadowsky (Eds.), *Essentials of cardiopulmonary physical therapy* (pp. 531-548). Philadelphia: Saunders.
7. Casaburi, R. (2001). Special considerations for exercise training in chronic lung disease. In J.L. Roitman (Ed.), *ACSM's resource manual for guidelines for exercise testing and prescription* (4th ed., pp. 346-352). Baltimore: Lippincott Williams & Wilkins.
8. Clough, P. (1994). Restrictive lung dysfunction. In E.A. Hillegass & H.S. Sadowsky (Eds.), *Essentials of cardiopulmonary physical therapy* (pp. 189-255). Philadelphia: Saunders.
9. Cooper, C.B. (1995) Determining the role of exercise in patients with chronic pulmonary disease. *Medicine and Science in Sports and Exercise, 27,* 147-157.
10. Davidson, A.C., Leach, R., George, R.J.D., & Geddes, D.M. (1988). Supplemental oxygen and exercise ability in chronic obstructive airways disease. *Thorax, 43,* 965-971.
11. Davis, P.B. (1991). Cystic fibrosis: A major cause of obstructive airway disease in the young. In N.S. Cheniack (Ed.), *Chronic obstructive pulmonary disease* (pp. 297-307). Philadelphia: Saunders.
12. Garritan, S.L. (1994). Chronic obstructive pulmonary disease. In E.A. Hillegass & H.S. Sadowsky (Eds.), *Essentials of cardiopulmonary physical therapy* (pp. 257-284). Philadelphia: Saunders.
13. Guyton, A.C., & Hall, J.E. (1996). *Textbook of medical physiology* (9th ed., pp. 537-595). Philadelphia: Saunders.
14. Hsia, C.W. (2001). Pathophysiology of lung disease. In J.L. Roitman (Ed.), *ACSM's resource manual for guidelines for exercise testing and prescription* (4th ed., pp. 327-337). Baltimore: Lippincott Williams & Wilkins.
15. Hurd, S. (2000). The impact of COPD on lung health worldwide. *Chest, 117,* 1S-4S.
16. Jones, N.L., Berman, L.B., Barkiewig, P.D., & Oldridge, N.B. (1987). Chronic obstructive respiratory disorders. In J.S. Skinner (Ed.), *Exercise testing and exercise prescription for special cases* (pp. 175-187). Philadelphia: Lea & Febiger.
17. Mahler, D.A., & Horowitz, M.B. (1994). Perception of breathlessness during exercise in patients with respiratory disease. *Medicine and Science in Sports and Exercise, 26,* 1078-1081.

twenty-one

Exercise and Women's Health

Dixie L. Thompson

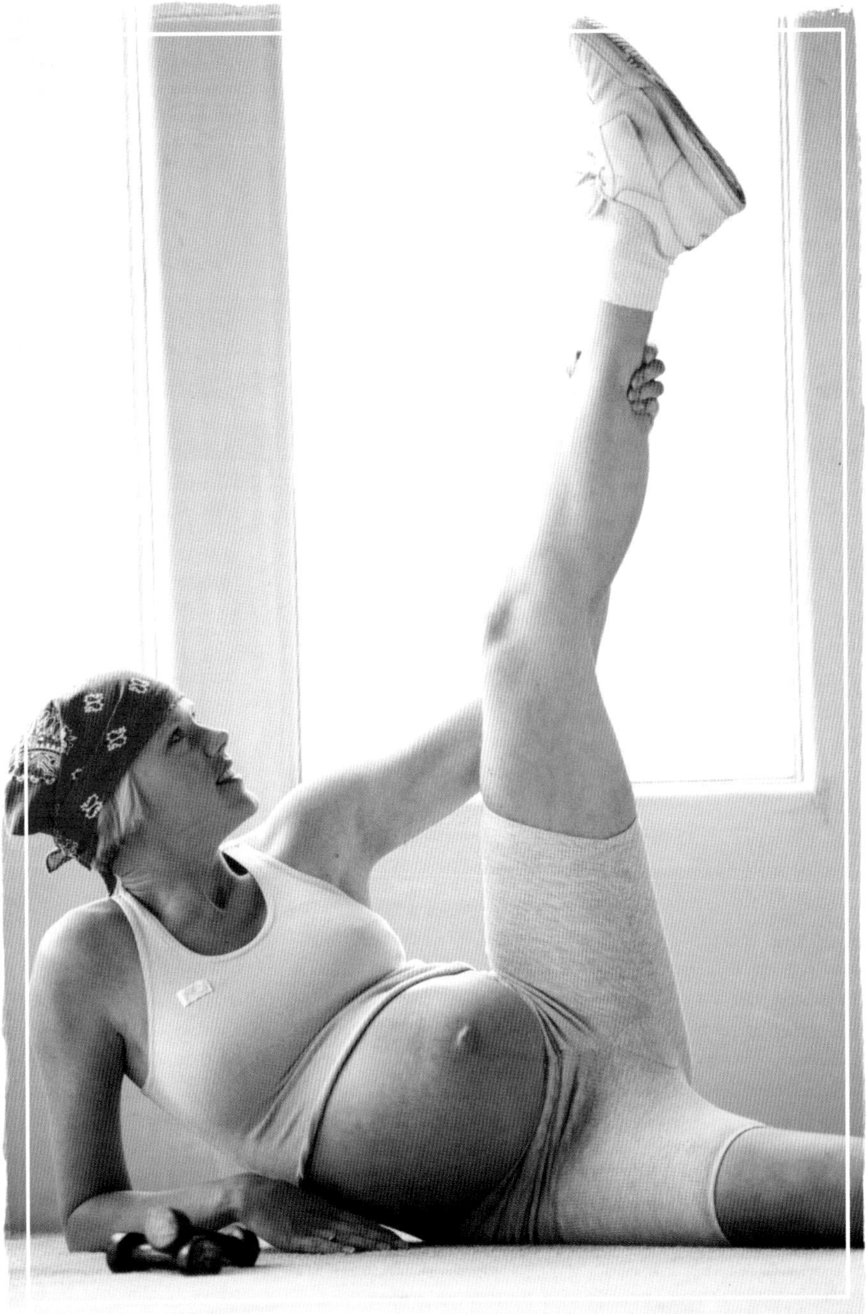

© ImageState/Caroline Wood

Objectives

The reader will be able to do the following:

1. Describe the risks and benefits of exercise during pregnancy, and suggest alterations in exercise that make exercise more comfortable and safe for pregnant women.
2. Define osteoporosis and risk factors for this disease and prescribe exercise to promote bone health.
3. Define the female athlete triad.

Women and men share most of the same obstacles to good health (e.g., cardiovascular disease, type 2 diabetes, obesity). The benefits that exercise provides to combat these diseases are similar for men and women, as are exercise guidelines. However, some conditions are faced exclusively, or primarily, by women. In this chapter, we examine three of these: pregnancy, osteoporosis, and the female athlete triad.

Pregnancy and Exercise

Pregnancy places enormous demands on a woman's body. Justified concern about the safety of the fetus and the mother leads to questions about whether exercise is wise during pregnancy. Fortunately, there is now substantial evidence that for healthy pregnant women, exercise is safe and provides benefits during this critical period (4). Although difficult to document, proposed benefits of exercise during pregnancy include increases in psychological well-being, less fatigue, and shorter and easier delivery (5, 17). However, some conditions require that exercise be approached cautiously. Pregnant women with cardiovascular, pulmonary, or metabolic disease as well as those with severe obesity or who are considerably underweight should seek physician guidance concerning exercise (9). The American College of Obstetricians and Gynecologists (1) lists the following as contraindications for exercise during pregnancy:

- Pregnancy-induced hypertension
- Premature rupture of membranes
- Preterm labor during prior or current pregnancy
- Incompetent cervix
- Persistent second or third trimester bleeding
- Intrauterine growth retardation

Potential Problems With Exercising During Pregnancy

Concerns about exercise during pregnancy have targeted four crucial areas: heat dissipation, oxygen delivery, supply of nutrition, and premature delivery. During the first trimester, the fetus is particularly vulnerable to developmental defects caused by excessive heat. Although the body's core temperature can increase with exercise, there are no known links between a greater prevalence of birth defects and exercise. An increase in the woman's blood volume provides adequate blood for heat dissipation, exercise, and nourishment of the fetus. Increases in ventilation and skin blood flow also help protect against excessive changes in body temperature (17). Additionally, the temperature at which sweating begins decreases as pregnancy progresses, providing an additional protective mechanism against increases in core temperature (9). Concern that vigorous exercise could compromise uterine blood flow is unsubstantiated. The increase in maternal blood volume coupled with a decrease in systemic vascular resistance results in an increase in cardiac output and provides adequate blood flow, and therefore oxygen, to the fetus (5, 17). The fact that fetal HR is only modestly, if at all, affected by exercise provides evidence that this type of physical activity does not produce significant fetal distress (5, 17). Because of the nutritional demands of pregnancy, an increase in caloric consumption is needed. It is important that the nutritional demands of exercise and fetal development be adequately met by the exercising woman. Evidence that the nutritional needs of the developing fetus are not compromised by exercise comes from studies showing very little difference between the weight of newborns from exercising versus nonexercising mothers (5, 17). Another major concern is that exercise may bring about premature delivery. For normal pregnancies, there is no evidence that gestational length is affected by exercise (5, 17). Care should be taken, however, to avoid activities (i.e., contact sports) in which injury could lead to fetal injury or premature delivery.

Exercise Prescription During Pregnancy

Moderate, and even vigorous, exercise can be performed safely by previously active pregnant women. It is suggested that women who were not previously active follow low- to moderate-intensity programs if they begin an exercise program while pregnant. The mode of exercise can be based on comfort and convenience. Some women find that non-weight-bearing exercises such as swimming and stationary cycling are more comfortable, especially as pregnancy advances. The return to activity after pregnancy should be gradual and "based on a woman's physical capability" (4, p. 231). The following precautions should be considered when prescribing exercise for a pregnant client (1, 4, 5, 9, 17).

1. Exercise in a supine position should be avoided after the first trimester. The enlarged uterus can apply pressure to the surrounding blood vessels and limit venous return.

2. Take precautions to avoid heat injury. Avoiding exercise in hot and humid environments, ensuring adequate hydration (before, during, and after exercise), and dressing appropriately for the heat are important tools for avoiding hyperthermia.

3. Limit exposure to falling and impact injury. Although total elimination of risk is impossible, participation in competitive contact sports (e.g., soccer, boxing) and activities where trauma risk is great (e.g., skydiving, water skiing) should be discouraged. As pregnancy advances, center of gravity and balance are altered; therefore, exercises that requires rapid change in direction may be more problematic than before pregnancy.

4. Be aware that joint laxity is increased during pregnancy. The release of relaxin is important in allowing the pelvis to undergo the changes needed during pregnancy and delivery. However, this hormone also leads to greater laxity in other joints. Following the precautions in item 3 will help avoid joint injury.

5. Resistance training can be used during pregnancy with the following precautions: (a) avoid the Valsalva maneuver during lifting, (b) keep the programs of low to moderate intensity (resistance should be low enough that at least 12-15 repetitions can be completed without fatigue), and (c) use slow and steady rather than ballistic movement patterns. For more information on resistance training during pregnancy, see chapter 12.

6. Avoid exercise where extremes in air pressure occur. Scuba diving and exercise at altitude, when unacclimatized, should be avoided.

7. Be aware of the body's warning signs (4, 5). Each woman should be encouraged to closely monitor her body for signs or symptoms that something may be wrong. If any of the following occur, exercise should be stopped and a physician consulted: vaginal bleeding, membrane rupture, chronic fatigue or pain, regular contractions 30 min after exercise ends, unexplained increases in HR or BP, and lack of fetal movement.

1 In Review

Exercise during pregnancy is safe and beneficial for most women. Protecting against traumatic impact, heat injury, musculoskeletal injury, and overexertion is key to planning safe exercise programs for pregnant women.

Osteoporosis

Osteoporosis is a disease characterized by fragile bones. Approximately 10 million Americans have osteoporosis and another 18 million have low bone mass (**osteopenia**) and are at risk for developing osteoporosis (14). Annually, osteoporosis accounts for $10 to 15 billion in direct medical costs (14). The most common sites for osteoporotic fractures are the hip, vertebrae, and wrist. Bone strength is determined by **bone mineral density** (BMD) and the structural integrity of the bone. BMD commonly is measured by using dual energy x-ray absorptiometry (DXA; see chapter 6) and provides a measure of the amount of bone mineral per unit area (g/cm^2). BMD, accounting for about 70% of bone strength, is highly correlated with a bone's resistance to fracture (14). Structural integrity is determined by the microarchitecture of the bone and is much more difficult to assess, requiring invasive testing of bone (2). Because of the low risk, ease, and availability of DXA testing, this has become the preferred method for diagnosis of osteoporosis. According to World Health Organization guidelines, osteoporosis is defined as a BMD 2.5 standard deviations below the mean for young white women. When BMD is in the osteoporotic range, fracture risk is high. Common pharmaceutical treatments for osteoporosis are selective estrogen receptor modulators, hormone replacement therapy (for women), and bisphosphonates. These interventions are effective in slowing bone loss. More information can be found on osteoporosis by visiting the Web site of the National Institute of Arthritis and Musculoskeletal and Skin Diseases (13).

Risk Factors for Osteoporosis

Osteoporosis can affect both males and females across all ages and ethnicities. However, older women, particularly of Caucasian and Asian descent, are especially vulnerable. Bone accumulates during childhood and generally peaks in the third decade of life. Although there is some decline in BMD during the middle adult years, the most rapid loss in women occurs in the years surrounding menopause. The decline in estrogen levels around the time of menopause is the reason for the rapid bone loss, which can be as great as 3 to 5% of bone mass per year (7). In men, the loss of bone is typically quite slow but steady from the time of peak accumulation until death. Men, in general, are less likely than women to suffer osteoporotic fractures because their peak BMD is higher than women, although some sources estimate that 25% of men over age 60 will suffer an osteoporotic fracture (7). Peak BMD is also generally higher in individuals of African descent when compared with those of European and Asian descent (see the box below) (14).

Sometimes osteoporosis results from the presence of another condition. Examples of conditions that can lead to osteoporosis are endocrine disorders, gastrointestinal diseases, nutritional deficiencies, and the long-term use of glucocorticoid medications. Because of the many factors that may lead to low bone density, people of all ages, including children, can develop osteoporosis. Low intake of calcium and vitamin D can limit the accumulation of bone during childhood, and it is estimated that only 25% of boys and 10% of girls achieve the recommended levels for calcium intake (14). The attainment of a lower than expected peak bone density increases the risk of osteoporosis in later life. The International Osteoporosis Foundation has developed a screening tool to assess risk for osteoporosis. This simple 10-question test, designed to help identify people at particularly high risk for osteoporosis, is found in the box on the following page.

Exercise in Prevention and Treatment of Osteoporosis

One of the primary means for preventing osteoporosis is maximizing bone accumulation during childhood and adolescence. In addition to adequate calcium and vitamin D intake, physical activity is important to the development of strong bones. Studies demonstrate that children who exercise regularly have higher bone mineral levels than their sedentary peers (7, 15). The research examining exercise as a tool to increase bone density among adults has produced mixed results. Although some studies have demonstrated gains in bone density with exercise, others have shown no impact. The wide variety among research protocols is one reason for the mixed results. Some common elements among studies that yielded the most profound effect on adult bone health are the use of moderate to vigorous activity, adequate calcium intake in conjunction with exercise (1000-1500 mg per day), and using movements that involve either impact loading or resistance training. For mature adults, exercise alone does not appear to be adequate to prevent age-related bone loss; however, exercise is an important tool in slowing this potentially devastating condition.

Risk Factors for Osteoporosis

- Female sex
- Increased age
- Estrogen deficiency
- Caucasian/Asian race
- Low weight or BMI
- Diet low in calcium
- Alcohol abuse
- Inactivity
- Muscle weakness
- Family history of osteoporosis
- Smoking
- History of prior fracture

Millennium One-Minute Osteoporosis Risk Test

1. Have either of your parents broken a hip after a minor bump or fall?
   ❑ yes ❑ no
2. Have you broken a bone after a minor bump or fall?
   ❑ yes ❑ no
3. Have you taken corticosteroid tablets (cortisone, prednisone) for more than 3 months?
   ❑ yes ❑ no
4. Have you lost more than 3 cm (just over 1 in.) in height?
   ❑ yes ❑ no
5. Do you regularly drink heavily (in excess of safe drinking limits)?
   ❑ yes ❑ no
6. Do you smoke more than 20 cigarettes a day?
   ❑ yes ❑ no
7. Do you suffer frequently from diarrhea (caused by problems such as celiac disease or Crohn's disease)?
   ❑ yes ❑ no

For women:

8. Did you undergo menopause before the age of 45?
   ❑ yes ❑ no
9. Have your periods stopped for 12 months or more (other than because of pregnancy)?
   ❑ yes ❑ no

For men:

10. Have you ever suffered from impotence, lack of libido, or other symptoms related to low testosterone levels?
    ❑ yes ❑ no

If you answered yes to one or more of these questions, it is possible that you are at increased risk for osteoporosis, and consultation with your physician is recommended.

International Osteoporosis Foundation: www.osteofound.org

Exercise Testing and Prescription for Bone Health

Exercise for children and adolescents is important for maximizing bone density. Regular participation in high-intensity loading activities should be encouraged. For nonosteoporotic adults, loading exercises and muscle-building activities are suggested for promoting bone health. An excellent example of this type of program is described by Metcalfe et al. (12). For individuals with osteoporosis, precautions should be taken with both exercise testing and prescription. For individuals with severe kyphosis that limits forward vision or balance, stationary cycling may be a better choice than treadmill walking (6). Testing muscular strength can be important in designing programs for osteoporotic clients; however, exercises that involve significant spinal flexion should be avoided because of the risk of compression fractures. Tests of balance and functionality can be useful in designing programs to reduce risk of falling. Improving functional muscle strength and balance is key to avoiding falls (15). Exercise prescription for the osteoporotic client must be individualized based on the severity of disease and the presence of other conditions. In general, exercise prescription should focus on aerobic activity, muscle strengthening exercises, and balance-improving activities. This combination is suggested because it incorporates three major components: cardiovascular health, bone health, and reduced risk of falling. For more details on exercise testing and prescription for osteoporotic clients, see Bloomfield (6) and Shaw et al. (15).

2 In Review

Osteoporosis, a disease characterized by fragile bones, affects millions of Americans. Although males and females of all ages can suffer from osteoporosis, it is most commonly seen in postmenopausal women. Healthy eating practices and an active lifestyle are keys to promoting bone health. Exercises that involve either impact loading or resistance training appear most beneficial for promoting bone development.

Female Athlete Triad

The female athlete triad (figure 21.1) is a condition that includes three major components: disordered eating, amenorrhea, and osteoporosis (3). This condition, if left untreated, can produce significant health consequences including glycogen depletion, anemia, and electrolyte imbalances (3). The precipitating factor in this triad is disordered eating. Anorexia nervosa and bulimia nervosa are two eating disorders commonly associated with the female athlete triad. Among athletes suffering from the female athlete triad, the range of unhealthy eating practices is varied. Some clearly present with eating disorders, whereas others limit calories without meeting the strict clinical definitions of an eating disorder (10). The unhealthy eating pattern with insufficient calories and nutritional density leads to amenorrhea. The estrogen deficiency seen in amenorrhea leads to osteopenia and potentially even osteoporosis. This loss of bone puts the athlete at great risk for stress fractures and for osteoporotic compression fractures.

In the general adult population, anorexia nervosa and bulimia nervosa occur at a rate of 0.5 to 1% and 2 to 4%, respectively (11). Although it is difficult to determine the percentage of athletes struggling with unhealthy eating practices, the prevalence seems at least as high as that for the general population (3). A recent meta-analysis found that some athletes are at particular risk for eating disorders (elite athletes, dancers, athletes in sports that emphasize thinness), whereas participating in other sports (non-elite status, sports without a thinness emphasis) may actually provide some protection from unhealthy eating (16). When left untreated, eating disorders will sometimes lead to death (see chapter 11).

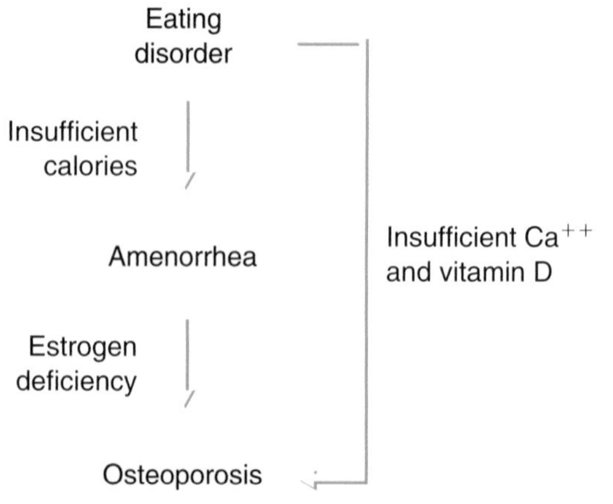

Figure 21.1 Female athlete triad.

Amenorrhea, lack of menses, is clinically divided into two categories. Primary amenorrhea is characterized by the absence of menarche (i.e., first menses) in girls age 16 or older. When there is a lack of menses for 3 or more consecutive months in females after menarche, it is classified as secondary amenorrhea. The cause of amenorrhea can be difficult to establish and involves a complex interaction between the hypothalamus, pituitary gland, and ovaries. Because of inadequate stimulation, the ovaries do not function normally, resulting in lower than normal estrogen and progesterone levels. The high prevalence of irregular menstruation has been observed in athletic women for a number of years, but the consequences on bone largely was ignored until Drinkwater et al.'s landmark study (8) in which the bones of young amenorrheic athletes were found to be comparable in density to those of postmenopausal women. To help protect against bone loss, many physicians now treat amenorrheic athletes by replacing the missing endogenous estrogen with oral contraceptives (10).

Recognition of the signs of disordered eating is necessary before successful intervention (see chapter 11). Often coaches and athletes are ill-informed about the female athlete triad. Therefore, education is an important first step in battling this condition. Successful intervention for the female athlete triad requires a multidisciplinary approach that includes input from medical, nutritional, and psychological professionals (3, 10).

3 In Review

The female athlete triad is a condition characterized by the presence of disordered eating, amenorrhea, and osteoporosis. Anorexia nervosa and bulimia nervosa are eating disorders frequently seen in the female athlete triad and can lead to significant health impairment, even death, if left untreated. Intervention for the female athlete triad should be multidisciplinary and should include psychological counseling.

Case Study

You can check your answers by referring to appendix A.

21.1

A 48-year-old woman with a family history of osteoporosis comes to your facility for information on exercise to promote bone health. Her doctor says she is in good health and does not have osteoporosis, but there are signs that her bones are weaker than when she was younger. What type of exercise would you recommend?

Source List

1. American College of Obstetricians and Gynecologists. (1994). *Exercise during pregnancy and the postpartum period* (Technical Bulletin 189). Washington, DC: Author.
2. American College of Sports Medicine. (1995). Position stand on osteoporosis and exercise. *Medicine and Science in Sports and Exercise, 27*(4), i-vii.
3. American College of Sports Medicine. (1997). Position stand on the female athlete triad. *Medicine and Science in Sports and Exercise, 29*(5), i-ix.
4. American College of Sports Medicine. (2000). *ACSM's guidelines for exercise testing and prescription* (6th ed.). Philadelphia: Lippincott Williams & Wilkins.
5. Artal, R., Sherman, C., & DiNubile, N.A. (1999). Exercise during pregnancy. *The Physician and Sportsmedicine, 27*(8), 51-60.
6. Bloomfield, S.A. (1997). Osteoporosis. In J.L. Durstine (Ed.), *ACSM's exercise management for persons with chronic diseases and disabilities* (pp. 161-166). Champaign, IL: Human Kinetics.
7. Bloomfield, S.A. (2001). Optimizing bone health: Impact of nutrition, exercise, and hormones. *Gatorade Sports Science Institute: Sports Science Exchange, 14*(3), 1-4.
8. Drinkwater, B.L., Nilson, K., Chesnut, C.H., Bremner, W.J., Shainholtz, S., & Southworth, M.B. (1984). Bone mineral content of amenorrheic and eumenorrheic athletes. *New England Journal of Medicine, 311*, 277-281.
9. Heffernan, A.E. (2000). Exercise and pregnancy in primary care. *The Nurse Practitioner, 25*(3), 42, 49, 53-56, 59-60.
10. Hobart, J.A., & Smucker, D.R. (2000). The female athlete triad. *American Family Physician, 61*, 3357-3364, 3367.
11. Johnson, M.D. (1994). Disordered eating. In R. Agostini (Ed.), *Medical and orthopedic issues of active and athletic women* (pp. 141-151). Philadelphia: Hanley & Belfus.
12. Metcalfe, L., Lohman, T., Going, S., Houtkooper, L., Ferriera, D., Flint-Wagner, H., Guido, T., Martin, J., Wright, J., & Cussler, E. (2001). Postmenopausal women and exercise for prevention of osteoporosis: The Bone, Estrogen, Strength Training (BEST) study. *ACSM's Health and Fitness Journal, 5*(3), 6-14.
13. National Institute of Arthritis and Musculoskeletal and Skin Diseases. (2000). Osteoporosis: Progress and Promise. [Online], August. Available: www.niams.nih.gov/hi/topics/osteoporosis/opbkgr.htm [July 10.2002].
14. National Institutes of Health. (2000). *Osteoporosis prevention, diagnosis, and therapy* (NIH Consensus Development Conference Statement, No. 17). Bethesda, MD: Author.
15. Shaw, J.M., Witzke, K.A., & Winters, K.M. (2001). Exercise for skeletal health and osteoporosis prevention. In J.L. Roitman (Ed.), *ACSM's resource manual for guidelines for exercise testing and prescription* (4th ed., pp. 299-307). Philadelphia: Lippincott Williams & Wilkins.
16. Smolak, L., Murnen, S.K., & Ruble, A.E. (2000). Female athletes and eating problems: A meta-analysis. *International Journal of Eating Disorders, 27*, 371-380.
17. Wang, T.W., & Apgar, B.S. (1998). Exercise during pregnancy. *American Family Physician, 57*(8), 1846-1852, 1857.

part five

Exercise Programming

Prior parts of the handbook have covered assessment and exercise prescription for components of physical fitness for individuals with a variety of characteristics and health conditions. This section includes other elements needed for a comprehensive and effective fitness program. We go over ways to help motivate individuals to adopt and maintain a healthy lifestyle in **chapter 22**. In **chapter 23,** we describe the relationship of physical activity to stress. In **chapter 24** we review analysis of the electrocardiogram and current medications used for cardiovascular problems. We summarize the prevention and treatment of injuries in **chapter 25**. Finally, in **chapter 26** we describe the processes used in program administration.

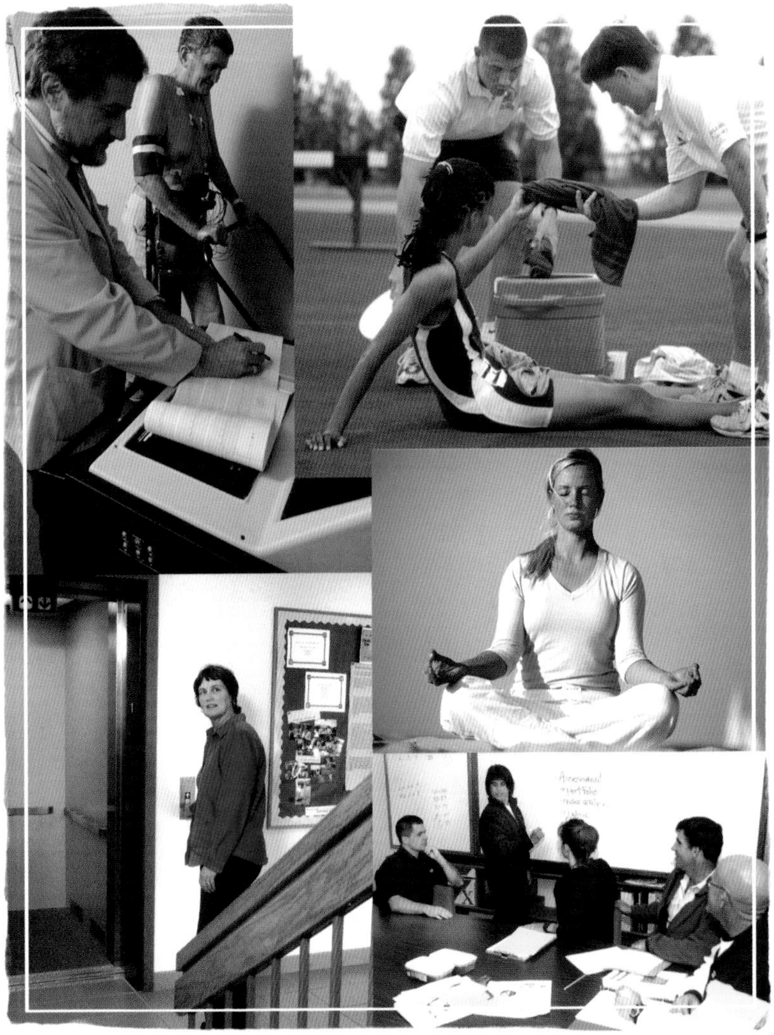

twenty-two

Behavior Modification

Janet Buckworth

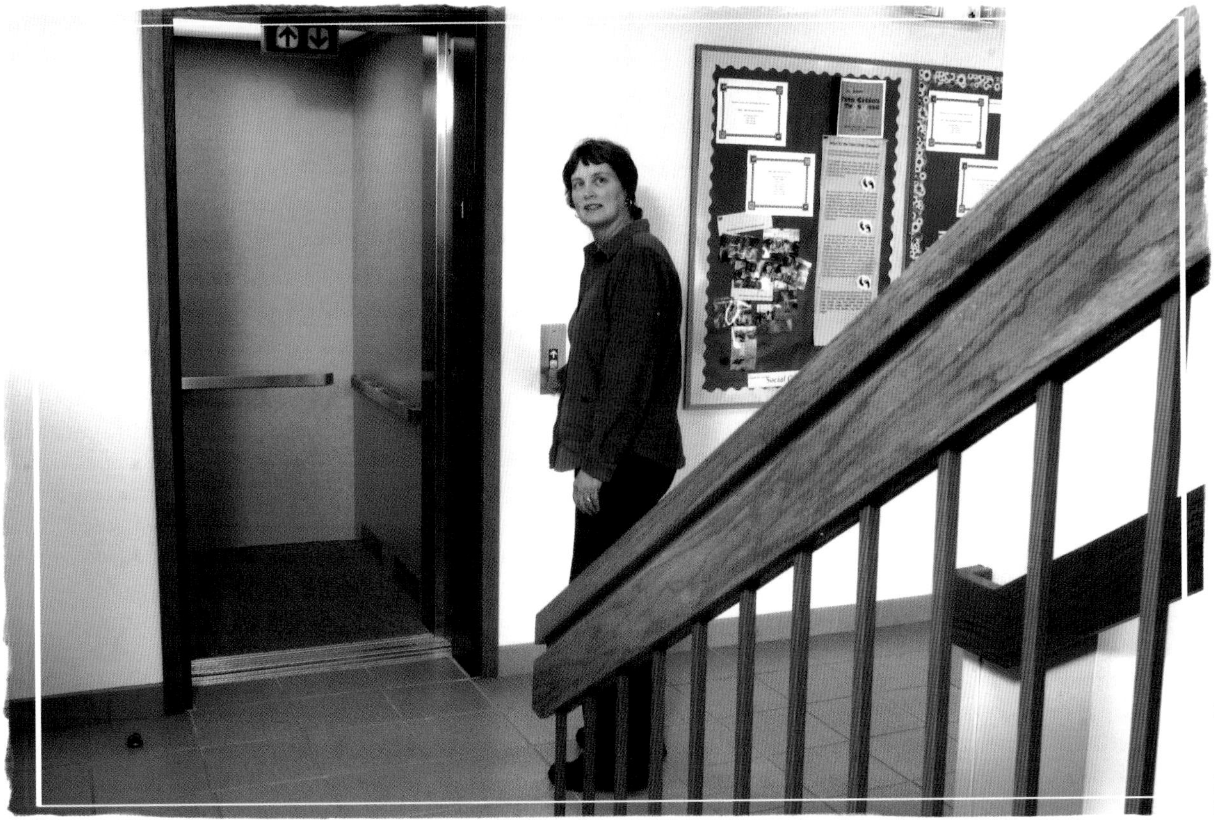

Objectives

The reader will be able to do the following:

1. Describe the transtheoretical model and stages involved in health behavior change.
2. Discuss the role of motivation in exercise adoption and adherence and identify behavioral strategies for enhancing motivation.
3. List and describe six strategies that HFIs and PFTs can use to monitor and support behavior change.
4. Describe ways that relapse prevention can be applied to exercise behavior.
5. Identify effective communication skills useful in motivating and fostering health behavior change.

Translating the desire to change a health behavior into action is a challenge for most people. Individuals may wish to be more active or to eat a healthier diet but may not have the knowledge, skills, or motivation to make the necessary behavior modifications and stick to them. To help people adopt and maintain a healthier lifestyle, the HFI and PFT should understand basic principles of behavior change and develop the skills to put those principles into practice.

This chapter begins with a brief description of theoretical models for explaining and predicting human behavior, with special attention to the transtheoretical model of behavior change, also known as the stages of change model. Methods and strategies are presented in the context of behavior change as a process, with suggestions for approaches to use based on exercise stages of change. For an excellent review of the transtheoretical model applied to exercise, refer to Prochaska and Marcus (19). Factors for the HFI to consider as he or she helps participants move through each stage of the model are discussed along with specific strategies for encouraging adoption of and adherence to exercise and other health behaviors. Additional strategies and suggestions for interventions can be found in Annesi's (1) text on enhancing motivation to exercise and in the chapter by Southard and Southard (22) in the ACSM resource manual. The last section in this chapter examines communication skills the HFI should possess to motivate participants and foster health behavior change.

Transtheoretical Model of Behavior Change

Several theories guide exercise behavior change strategies, such as behavior modification, social cognitive theory, and the transtheoretical model of behavior change (2). Behavior modification theory is based on the assumption that behavior is learned and can be changed by modifying the antecedents (prompts, cues) and consequences (rewards, punishments). A prompt could be a flyer listing the benefits of walking during lunch, and a reward could be a certificate presented to the aerobics participant with the best attendance. Social cognitive theory offers the view that behavior is influenced by the dynamic relationships among characteristics of the person, the environment, and the behavior itself. Someone training for a marathon would be more motivated than a novice fitness walker to exercise outside in the rain, but even the most dedicated marathoner will not run in a lightning storm. Although effective behavior change strategies have been developed with these and other theories, most theories of behavior treat change as an all-or-none event. In other words, participants go from being sedentary to being regularly active in response to an intervention. The transtheoretical model presents change as a dynamic process whereby attitudes, decisions, and actions evolve through different stages over a period of time. In the late 1970s and early 1980s, Prochaska and DiClemente (18) developed the transtheoretical model of behavior change by observing smokers trying to quit without professional intervention. They discovered that self-changers progressed through specific stages as they tried to decrease or eliminate their high-risk behavior. Although the model was developed based on stopping high-risk behaviors, it has been applied to promoting exercise (e.g., 7). This chapter describes the transtheoretical, or stages of change, model and ways this model can be used to help people think about, decide to begin, and continue an active lifestyle.

Concepts

The **transtheoretical model** is a general model of intentional behavior modification. Behavior change is described as a dynamic process that occurs through a series of interrelated stages that are mostly stable but open to change (20). This model emphasizes the individual's readiness to change and his or her history regarding the target behavior. For example, individuals who exercised successfully in the past would have more confidence in their ability to exercise again than would those who have been sedentary most of their lives. The problem with most interventions is that they are for people who are prepared to take action (19). According to the transtheoretical model, traditional participant recruitment strategies will not affect people who are not ready to change. Different strategies must be used to persuade people to consider change and then motivate them to take action. Other approaches will be more effective in supporting adherence to the new behavior.

Levels

The three levels of the transtheoretical model are described next (20). By evaluating the participant in respect to these factors (stage of change, beliefs, behavior change skills, and the level of change dimension), the HFI can design individually tailored and stage-specific interventions.

Level 1: Stages of Change

1. *Precontemplation*: In this stage, the individual is not seriously thinking about changing a health behavior in the next 6 months or denies the need to change.
2. *Contemplation*: The individual is seriously thinking about changing an unhealthy behavior within the next 6 months.
3. *Preparation*: This is a transitional stage in which the individual intends to take action within the next month. Some plans have been made, and the individual tries to determine what to do next.
4. *Action:* This stage is the 6-month period following the overt modification of an unhealthy behavior. Motivation and investment in behavior change are sufficient in this stage, but it is the least stable and busiest stage with the highest risk of relapse.
5. *Maintenance*: Maintenance begins after someone has successfully adhered to the healthy behavior for 6 months. The longer someone stays in maintenance, the less risk of relapse.

Level 2: Concepts Hypothesized to Influence Behavior Change

- *Processes of change* are strategies used to change behavior. They include strategies that use information gathered through experience (experiential / cognitive processes) and through the environment and actions (behavioral processes). Seeking out information about the best exercise for losing weight is a cognitive process, and creating reminders to register for a water aerobics class is a behavioral process.
- *Self-efficacy* is the confidence in one's ability to engage in a positive behavior or abstain from an undesired behavior. This expectation of success is an important factor in the decision to change and in maintaining the new behavior.
- *Decisional balance* refers to evaluating and monitoring potential gains (pros) and losses (cons) arising from any decision. Perceived gains increase and perceived losses decrease regarding the target behavior as one moves through the stages described previously.

Level 3: Level of Change Dimension

Identifying the context in which the problem behavior occurs helps the HFI determine what factors people must change to be successful. For example, one person may want to exercise but does not have access to facilities, and another person thinks he or she does not have the will power to stick with a program. The first person would be helped with a home exercise program, whereas the second would benefit from social support and rethinking discouraging thoughts.

Applying the Transtheoretical Model to Exercise

The transtheoretical model is applied to exercise by matching the appropriate intervention to an individual according to his or her physical activity history and readiness for change (20) (see figure 22.1). For example, the goal in working with people in the precontemplation stage is to get them to begin thinking about changing. The benefits of exercise should be strengthened and the costs reduced. Activities to help individuals develop a personal value for exercise and information about the role of exercise in a healthy lifestyle are useful in moving someone to the next stage (9).

Maintenance:	Social support, self-regulation skills, review and revision of goals, cross-training, periodic fitness testing, relapse prevention
Action:	Social support, stimulus control, self-reinforcement, self-efficacy enhancement, goal setting, self-monitoring, relapse prevention
Preparation:	Psychosocial and fitness assessment, evaluation of support/benefits and barriers/costs, personalized exercise prescription, goal setting, behavioral contracts, time management
Contemplation:	Market benefits of exercise, self- and environmental reevaluation, clear and specific guidelines for starting an exercise program, positive role models, identify social support for exercise
Precontemplation:	Exercise promotion media campaign, education about personal benefits of exercise, values clarification, health risk appraisals, fitness testing

Figure 22.1 Intervention strategies for various stages of change.

The goal with contemplators is to help them prepare to take action. Marketing and media campaigns that promote exercise, along with accurate, easy-to-understand information about how to start an exercise program, can help move contemplators into the action stage. Positive role models, perceived barriers and benefits, and psychosocial variables such as self-efficacy for exercise are other factors that will influence exercise adoption. The cognitive processes of change, such as consciousness raising and environmental reevaluation, are critical in these early stages of change.

Behavioral factors come into play more when a person moves from preparation to action and from action into maintenance. Working with a participant who is in the preparation stage must include a thorough assessment and a specific plan for change. The participant should set goals that are consistent with capabilities, values, resources, and needs. Exercise self-efficacy predicts adoption and maintenance; it can be increased with mastery experiences. Thus, initial goals should be set that will be challenging but that are certain of being met to foster increased exercise self-efficacy. The HFI and participant also should evaluate environmental and social supports and barriers and determine ways that barriers can be modified to promote the new behavior.

Participants in the action stage are at a high risk of relapse. Social support for exercise is critical in this stage. Another useful strategy is instruction in self-regulatory skills such as stimulus control, reinforcement management, and self-monitoring of progress. Relapse prevention, which is discussed later, is also critical.

Movement from the action stage to the maintenance stage follows a decrease in the risk of relapse and an increase in self-efficacy. The HFI can help the participant reevaluate rewards and goals and plan for ways to cope with potential lapses attributable to relocation, travel, inclement weather, or medical events. Social support and self-regulatory skills continue to be important.

1 In Review

The transtheoretical model addresses the dynamic nature of behavior change. Practitioners apply this model by selecting interventions based on characteristics of the individual, environment, and the stage of change. Interventions should match the stage the individual is in and the context in which the problem behavior occurs (see figure 22.1).

Promoting Exercise: Targeting Precontemplators and Contemplators

Understanding the knowledge, attitudes, and behavioral skills that foster adoption of a regular exercise program is important in helping people in the early stages of exercise behavior change. Remember, people in precontemplation are sedentary and have no plans to start exercising. They may be in this stage because they lack information about the long-term personal consequences of physical inactivity. They also may be demoralized from previous unsuccessful attempts to stick with an exercise program and may have low self-efficacy for exercise. People in the precontemplation stage can feel defensive about their lifestyle because of social pressures to be physically active. They have no personally compelling reasons to change, and the costs of exercising seem to outweigh the benefits.

Sedentary individuals move to the contemplation stage because of convincing, personal, and timely information (21). Contemplators are planning to become more physically active, but they are still ambivalent about changing. For them, the cons or costs of starting to exercise balance out the perceived benefits. Things that support the contemplator's desire and motivation to exercise can initiate the move to preparation. Specific factors related to the adoption of regular exercise are presented next, followed by a review of strategies to market exercise and increase motivation.

Factors Influencing Exercise Adoption

Identifying individual, social, and environmental factors related to exercise adoption can help the HFI select more effective behavior change interventions.

Individual Influences

Generally, individual characteristics that influence the initiation of exercise are demographics, activity history, past experiences, perception of health status, perceptions regarding access to facilities, time, enjoyment of exercise, aptitudes, beliefs, self-motivation, and self-efficacy (4). Higher education, higher income, male sex, and younger age are positively associated with exercise (4), and there is greater adherence for leisure-time physical activity than for high-intensity exercise (6).

Exercise history is an important factor in current level of physical activity. Past participation is linked with physical activity in supervised exercise programs and in treatment programs for patients with CHD and obesity (6). Past exercise experience also can influence expectations about exercise and self-efficacy, and high exercise self-efficacy is associated with increased exercise participation.

Motivation is another individual variable influencing exercise adoption. Motivation depends on expecting future benefits or outcomes from exercise, such as good health, improved appearance, social outlets, stress management, enjoyment, and competition (16). Self-motivation for exercise is the ability to continue an exercise program without the benefit of external reinforcement. Self-motivated participants have more intrinsic motivation to exercise and are probably good at goal setting, monitoring their progress, and self-reinforcement (21). Individuals with little self-motivation may need more external reinforcement and encouragement (e.g., group activities and social support) to adopt and adhere to exercise.

Perceived behavioral control has been found to be significantly correlated with intention to exercise (5). If participants believe they have more control over the exercise and have choices about when and how to exercise, they are more likely to begin a program. It follows that participants who set their own goals will have a greater chance of success than if goals are assigned to them (14).

Social Influences

Social support involves comfort, assistance, and/or information from individuals or groups. Social support for exercise from family and friends is usually associated with physical activity (4). Spouses appear to provide a consistent, positive influence on exercise participation; in one study, individuals who joined a fitness center with their spouse had better adherence and lower dropout than married individuals who joined without a spouse (23). Group factors may be particularly important for older adults and individuals who are motivated to exercise primarily for social reinforcement.

Environmental Influences

Research has shown that environmental prompts, social support, and convenience are factors in exercise adoption (4). Environments that have cues for exercise, easily accessible facilities, and few real or perceived barriers also make maintenance of exercise easier. Posters, e-mail messages, self-sticking notes, placement of exercise equipment in visible places, and bike/walking paths are examples of environmental cues.

Research Insight

Is it the quality or quantity of exercise prompts that influences adherence? Lombard, Lombard, and Winett (15) placed 135 volunteers who completed a structured exercise program into either a control group or one of four prompt condition groups. Prompts were delivered over the phone, and groups differed on frequency of prompts (one time per week vs. once every three weeks) and structure of prompts (high structure with feedback and goal setting vs. low structure with just "touching base"). Exercise adherence after 6 months was significantly better for participants who were prompted to exercise each week, regardless of how much or how little feedback they received.

The convenience of exercise is influenced by the sequence, or chain, of behaviors that must be completed for the person to exercise. For example, there is a greater potential for a break in the link if an individual must leave work, drive home, gather up exercise clothes, drive to a facility, park, sign in, and change clothes to exercise than if the individual walks first thing in the morning in the neighborhood. The longer and more complicated the behavior chain, the more potential barriers there are to exercise.

The primary reason given for not exercising is lack of time (4). Time can be a true determinant, a perceived determinant, an indication of poor time-management skills, or a rationalization for the lack of motivation to be active. Flexibility in an exercise program (e.g., classes offered at many different times of day and evening, a lunch-hour walking group) can help with actual time problems. The HFI can help identify how time is a barrier and then choose appropriate interventions, such as modification of an exercise schedule or referral to a time-management class.

Researchers and practitioners have recognized that the physical environment is a powerful influence on the level of physical activity in communities. For example, accessible, attractive, and safe places to walk, bike, or run can make physical activity more appealing and convenient. Certainly, workout facilities that are clean, are well ventilated, and have a good selection of equipment and adequate parking will be more enticing to novice exercisers than poorly maintained or managed fitness centers.

Research Insight

The impact of environment on physical activity was demonstrated in a sample of 449 Australian adults aged 60 and older. Environmental factors significantly associated with being physically active were finding footpaths safe for walking and access to local facilities (3).

Marketing and Motivational Strategies

Your goal as an HFI or PFT may be to help individuals who have not yet considered exercise to begin thinking about starting a fitness program (i.e., precontemplation stage). For example, the primary goal of a media campaign may be to capture the individual's attention and motivate him or her to contemplate beginning an exercise program or starting another health behavior. This might involve "point-of-decision" informational prompts such as catchy posters next to elevators encouraging people to take the stairs (10). Bulletin boards, pamphlets, flyers, and handouts with upbeat information about the benefits of exercise and practical suggestions for increasing physical activity can also be used to catch the attention of potential exercisers. Handing out passes for an aerobics class at local restaurants is a proactive form of recruitment. Fun runs / walks supporting a local charity may motivate people who primarily want to help the organization by participating in the event to begin thinking about exercise for its own sake. Health risk appraisals and fitness testing can also prompt contemplation and enhance motivation to become more active (10).

To increase participation in the early stages of behavior change, the HFI's role is to provide education about why individuals should be more active, describe how to exercise sensibly, and offer encouragement to follow through with a personal exercise program. Specific strategies to increase adoption and early adherence are recommended (8, 11, 12):

- Ask participants about their exercise history. They may need proper information to dispel myths (e.g., the myth of "no pain, no gain") and to develop positive attitudes about exercise.
- Help participants develop knowledge, attitudes, and skills to support the behavior change. In addition to providing information and self-management skills training, the HFI may use cognitive restructuring to identify discouraging thoughts and replace them with positive statements (see the box on the next page).

Cognitive Restructuring

Reframe Negative Statements Into Positive Statements

Negative statements

- I'm never going to get in shape.
- I'm fatter than everyone else in the class.
- I've tried to stay with exercise and each time I fail.
- It's just impossible to find time to exercise with my schedule.

Positive statements

- Change takes time. I didn't get out of shape overnight, and I am making progress bit by bit.
- Everyone has to start somewhere. Other people have worked long and hard to get where they are.
- Every time I begin a new exercise program, I get closer to sticking with it for good.
- I can take a little time for myself to exercise every day because I deserve it. I'm the one in control.

- Bolster the participant's exercise self-efficacy with success-producing learning experiences. Self-efficacy enhancement strategies include

  Mastery experiences (behavioral rehearsal with proper supervision and positive feedback). The HFI can make sure the participant has chosen activities that are appropriate for his or her fitness and skill level. Practical feedback will also help the participant be successful and thus feel more confident.

  Verbal persuasion or self-persuasion. The HFI can provide verbal encouragement and can teach the participant positive self-talk.

  Modeling. Modeling has been effective in increasing self-efficacy. The HFI can set up situations in which participants see someone like themselves succeed (e.g., post a newspaper story about seniors who now exercise regularly) or watch a peer who has trouble coping with the task succeed (e.g., the HFI can point out to a new participant that "Lynette also had difficulty jogging 3 miles when she first started the program, but after months of hard work, she can now reach her goal!").

  Interpretations of physiological and emotional responses. Novice exercisers may experience the increased HR, respiration, and muscle tension during exercise with anxiety or discomfort. The HFI can be sure that participants have information about the normal physiological responses to exercise and know how to interpret these responses.

- Clarify expectations and make sure they are reasonable and realistic. Use guidelines for goal setting to ensure initial successes.
- Identify potential barriers to behavior change and brainstorm with the participant about ways to overcome these barriers. Barriers can be personal (low exercise self-efficacy), physical (past injuries), interpersonal (peer pressure from sedentary friends to engage in competing behaviors), or environmental (inclement weather or lack of transportation to an exercise facility).
- Foster motivation to adopt and maintain an exercise program. Set up incentives to exercise. Incentives can be tangible (e.g., T-shirts, certificates, water bottles, recognition on a bulletin board) or intangible (e.g., a sense of competence, enjoyment). Tangible incentives are useful early in a program. Offer a variety of incentives and foster intrinsic motivation, like a sense of accomplishment or avoidance of obesity, for long-term adherence. Strategies to increase motivation are listed on the next page.

2 In Review

Individual, social, and environmental factors motivate people to move from precontemplation to contemplation of an exercise program. A variety of strategies can be used, from mass media campaigns to fitness testing, to motivate individuals to move from contemplation into the action stage. Six strategies to facilitate adopting and maintaining exercise are (1) asking participants about exercise history; (2) helping participants develop knowledge, attitudes, and skills to support the change; (3) bolstering self-efficacy; (4) setting clear and realistic goals; (5) identifying barriers to change; and (6) fostering motivation.

Motivational Strategies

- Provide positive behavioral feedback.
- Encourage group participation and group support to offer the opportunity for social reinforcement, camaraderie, and commitment.
- Recruit spouse and peers to support the behavioral change.
- Use upbeat, positive music. Make the program enjoyable.
- Provide a flexible routine to decrease boredom and increase enjoyment. Consider alternatives to traditional exercise modes such as games and backpacking to provide a variety of exercise options.
- Provide periodic exercise testing to give information about progress toward goals and the opportunity for positive reinforcement.
- Use behavioral change strategies, such as personal goal setting, contracting, and self-management, to foster personal control and perceived competency.
- Chart progress on record cards or graphs. Note and record progress daily to give immediate, positive feedback.
- Recognize goal achievement in newsletters and bulletin boards. Individual effort increases when individual effort is identifiable.
- Set up group or individual competitions.
- Offer lotteries based on individual or group accomplishment of a specific goal. Everyone can contribute money; set a winning criterion (such as the first one to walk 15 miles per week for 5 weeks wins), and the winner gets all the money. An alternative is to set a criterion (e.g., attending 20 of 24 aerobic classes) for participation in a random drawing.
- Organize teams to train for a charity-sponsored fun run/walk or road race.

Methods of Behavior Change

Various strategies have been discussed to illustrate behavior change principles and to describe ways to market and motivate exercise. Once a participant has started an exercise program (action stage), the HFI and PFT play an important role in monitoring and supporting the establishment and maintenance of behavior change.

Assessment

Regardless of the intervention, comprehensive fitness and psychosocial assessments are necessary to select and carry out the appropriate behavior change strategies for participants in the action stage. Reassessment should be conducted periodically to evaluate the effectiveness of the plan.

First, the problem must be identified and defined in behavioral terms. For example, being overfat is not the problem but rather the result of overeating and underexercising. The HFI can also help the participant decide what can be realistically changed and what cannot.

Next, examine past attempts at behavior change. Find out what worked, what did not, and why. This information will be useful in goal setting and identifying high-risk situations (see Relapse Prevention section).

It is also important to find out if initiation of the behavior change is voluntary or recommended by someone else. This will give you a sense of motivational level and commitment to change. If a participant is there because a doctor prescribed exercise, you may have to help the participant find personal reasons for exercising. There are many different reasons for beginning an exercise program, like health, enjoyment, weight loss, and anxiety reduction, but the initial motivation may not be why someone continues to exercise. Ask the participant what he or she expects to get out of exercise and be prepared to pique the person's interest by presenting additional short- and long-term benefits.

Another useful assessment tool is the decisional balance sheet. The participant lists all short- and long-term consequences, positive and negative, of both changing and not changing the behavior. The participant and the HFI then brainstorm ways to avoid or cope with the projected negative consequences of behavior change.

Self-Monitoring

Most people do not know exactly why they start and stop exercising unless they monitor their activity (11). Part of the assessment can be accomplished by self-monitoring, in which the participant records thoughts, feelings, and situations before, during, and after the target behavior. The participant can identify the internal and external cues and behavioral consequences that inhibit and prompt exercise. Barriers and supports also become evident with self-monitoring. The HFI can help the participant develop strategies to cope with the barriers and use the supports. The chain of behaviors encompassing exercise can also be evaluated and weak links identified. For example, if the participant discovers she always skips her 5:30 p.m. aerobics class when she oversleeps and doesn't have time to pack her workout clothes before she leaves for work, you can suggest that she pack her workout bag the night before. Immediate benefits and reinforcements tailored to individual preferences can also be established at critical links in the chain (e.g., if she remembers to pack her workout bag the night before, she can push the snooze button for an extra 10 min of sleep the next morning). Electronic notebooks, computer programs, calendars, graphs, and charts can be used for self-monitoring as part of the initial assessment and as a way to record progress.

Research Insight

Members of the Women's Cardiovascular Health Network joined forces to find out what strategies work best to change tobacco use, diet, or physical inactivity in women. Krummel and her colleagues (13) reviewed research reports for 65 population-based studies that described interventions to improve women's cardiovascular health, published from 1980 to 1998. The specific program components that seem to be effective include personalized advice on changing these health behaviors, multiple staff contacts with skills training, and daily self-monitoring.

Goal Setting

We set goals to accomplish a specific task in a specific period of time. Goals can be as simple and time limited as getting to the intersection before the traffic light turns yellow to the complicated and encompassing aim of earning an advanced degree. **Goal setting** provides a plan of action that focuses and directs activity and emphasizes a clear link between behavior and outcome.

Effective goal setting has several characteristics. Goals should be behavioral, specific, and measurable. Plans are easier to make if the goal is stated in behavioral terms. For example, a goal of "walking 4 days per week for 30 to 45 min" is easier to implement than a goal to "get in shape." Specific, measurable goals make it easier to monitor progress, make adjustments, and know when the goal has been accomplished. Goals also must be reasonable and realistic. A goal might be achievable, but personal and situational constraints can make it unrealistic. Losing 2 lb a week through diet and exercise is reasonable for many people, but it is almost impossible for the working mother of three who has minimal time for exercise and cooking. Unrealistic goals set the participant up to fail, which can damage self-efficacy and adherence to the behavior change program.

By using information from the assessment and self-monitoring, the HFI can help the participant set positive, realistic, behavioral goals based on the participant's age, sex, fitness, health, interests, exercise history, skills, and schedule. Both short-term and long-term goals should be included. Short-term goals mobilize effort and direct present actions, but both short- and long-term goals lead to a more effective plan of action (14) (see the box on the following page).

Reinforcement

Social **reinforcement** and self-reinforcement are crucial in the action phase, especially because the longer someone has been inactive, the longer it takes until exercise itself becomes reinforcing (11). Immediate consequences of exercise can be pain and fatigue, so external, immediate, positive rewards are necessary for beginners. Monitoring progress is rewarding and can involve charting miles walked after each session or asking for feedback from instructors after a difficult exercise class. Positive reinforcement from others can enhance self-esteem, especially when it is feedback from people whom the participant considers to be powerful. Praise is more effective if it is immediate and behaviorally specific (11). "Looking good!" is not as effective as, "Sally, you did a great job getting through all the leg lifts today," especially if Sally has been struggling with leg lifts.

Self-reinforcement should involve rewards that are important to the participant. Using special spa soaps and creams only after an aerobic workout and getting tickets to the big game after logging a certain

Characteristics of Effective Goals

1. Behavioral
2. Flexible (jog or cycle 5 times per week)
3. Specific (walk 3 miles without stopping)
4. Measurable
5. Reasonable (Is it possible?)
6. Realistic (Does it stand a good chance of happening?)
7. Challenging (but realistic!)
8. Meaningful (Is this important to the participant?)
9. Rewards for specific accomplishments
10. Time-frame (short and long-term goals)

---

number of miles are rewards that are personalized and administered by the participant.

Social support can be tangible, such as transportation to exercise class, or verbal. It can come from the class instructor, exercise partners, and family members. Significant others must be involved in the exercise plan and educated about the differences between support and nagging. Constructive verbal feedback, praise, encouragement, and positive attention will help a family member stick with exercise, whereas punishing comments, jokes about the person's efforts, or discouraging social comparisons can hinder adherence. Support focuses on what has been accomplished ("You're being consistent in your walking to lose weight. I'm proud of you."), whereas nagging harps on what has not been accomplished ("You should walk faster to lose weight. Why can't you pick up the pace?").

Friends in an exercise program can provide both social support and cues to exercise. They can be positive role models and part of a buddy system to support the exercise effort. Some participants are more likely to stick with a program if they know someone else is counting on them to be there to work out (10).

Behavioral Contracts

Behavioral contracts are written, signed, public agreements to engage in specific goal-directed behaviors, and they have been used effectively to increase exercise adherence (6). Contracts should include clear, realistic objectives and deadlines. Developing a contract engages the participant involved in the behavioral change program in a way that is motivating, challenging, and public. The public nature of contracts is especially important because public goals are more likely to be met than private or semiprivate goals (14).

Contracts can be set by individuals or groups. The benefits of a group contract are the feeling participants can have about not wanting to let others down and the desire to be part of a group. Individual contracts, however, can be tailored to the participant's specific situation and goals.

Consequences of meeting and not meeting the contracted goals should be clear and relevant to the participant. Material reinforcers are good initially but should be faded as natural reinforcers, such as social reinforcement and inherent benefits of exercise, are promoted. Contingency reinforcement can be set up so that the participant agrees to do a low-preference activity (e.g., squats) before a high-preference activity (e.g., sauna). Form 22.1 shows a sample contract for a middle-aged man starting a walking program.

3 In Review

Assessment is an important first step in the action stage of behavior change. Self-monitoring is useful in determining the antecedents and consequences of the target behavior as well as the potential costs and barriers to behavior change.

Strategies such as goal setting and behavioral contracts must be tailored to the individual participant and should be reevaluated regularly during the maintenance stage. Some of the variables that influence exercise maintenance are enjoyment, convenience, exercise intensity, program flexibility, social support, incentives, rewards, and skills like self-regulation and self-reinforcement.

form
22.1

Behavioral Contract

Goal: To walk 3 mi without stopping **Time frame:** By May 15

Benefits of meeting goal: Improve my blood pressure; feel better; manage stress; lose weight; keep up with son's scout troop on weekend camping trips

To reach my goal, I will:

1. Monitor my speed at the high school track during two walks on the weekend.
2. Walk at least 3 days a week during my lunch hour with Bob or Mary.

Goal supporting activities:

1. Keep a spare pair of walking shoes at work.
2. Watch sports on Saturday and Sunday only after I have completed my walks.
3. Reward myself with 30 min on the Internet each time I walk at least 30 min during my lunch hour.
4. Let my wife know about my plan and have her encourage me to walk on the weekends.
5. Purchase a new computer monitor when I reach my overall goal.

Barriers and countermeasures:

1. Luncheon meetings: I will walk for 30 min before I leave work on days I have a meeting during lunch.
2. Rain: I will walk the stairs for at least 30 min during lunch when it rains.

Signed: ______________________________ Date: ____________________

HFI: ________________________________ Date: ____________________

This contract will be evaluated every 2 weeks:

Date: ____________________

Revisions:

Date: ____________________

Revisions:

From Edward T. Howley and B. Don Franks, 2003, *Health Fitness Instructor's Handbook,* 4th ed. (Champaign, IL: Human Kinetics).

Relapse Prevention

The relapse prevention model is based on relapse in alcohol problems, smoking, and drug abuse, in which the goal is to decrease a high-frequency, undesired behavior. This model is best applied to voluntary behavior. Although exercise is voluntary, the goal is to increase a low-frequency, desired behavior. Even so, the concepts and techniques of relapse prevention can be used with exercise adherence (12).

Relapse occurs when people who have been exercising regularly or engaging in other positive health behaviors stop the healthy behavior and go back to the old, unhealthy behavior. It is important to understand the concepts of relapse applied to exercise, because relapse is inevitable for many people. The HFI must help participants understand that relapse does not mean failure; together, they can devise strategies to cope with temporary setbacks in the behavior change program.

Defining High-Risk Situations

Relapse begins with a **high-risk situation** that challenges an individual's perceived ability to maintain the desired behavioral change. A wedding reception with all her favorite foods can be a high-risk situation for a dieter, and weekend guests can challenge a jogger's motivation to keep up with his afternoon runs. Someone is predisposed to high-risk situations if he or she has a lifestyle imbalance in which "shoulds" exceed "wants." This leads to feelings of deprivation and desires for indulgence. Rationalization, denial, and apparently irrelevant decisions can then occur (12).

Successful coping in a high-risk situation leads to increased self-efficacy and decreased probability of relapse. Not coping or an inadequate coping response leads to decreased self-efficacy and positive expectations about not maintaining the behavior change (e.g., being able to eat like "normal people," having more time to spend with friends). If this leads to an actual "slip," the abstinence violation effect (or for exercise, the "adherence" violation effect) occurs in which the participant perceives he or she has failed. All-or-none thinking, such as the belief that you cannot skip a weekend of jogging and still be a jogger, makes the participant more susceptible to this effect. Feelings of failure lead to self-blame, lowered self-esteem, guilt, perceived loss of control, increased probability of relapse, and possibly giving up (12).

Fostering Coping Strategies for Exercise

Relapse prevention, as described by Marlatt and Gordon (17), is a method used to identify and deal with high-risk situations. The strategy begins by educating the individual about the relapse process and enlisting his or her help as an active participant in preventing a relapse (12).

Next are specific strategies to prevent exercise relapse:

1. Identify situations with a high risk of relapse. High-risk situations are behaviors that are incompatible with exercise, such as eating, drinking, overworking, or smoking. High-risk situations can also involve relocation, medical events, travel, and inclement weather. Personal high-risk situations can be determined from information gathered during assessment and self-monitoring. The HFI should help the participant recognize aspects of the exercise behavior itself, the time of day, place, people, moods, thoughts, and particular situations that can threaten exercise adherence.
2. Revise plans to avoid or cope with high-risk situations. Flexible, short-term goals can be adapted to uncontrollable situational demands. Resetting goals temporarily can decrease the sense of noncompliance and increase a sense of control. ("While my weekend guests are here, I will jog one day in the morning before they get up instead of trying to jog on both Saturday and Sunday afternoons.")
3. Improve coping responses by referring participants to classes covering techniques such as time management, relaxation training, assertiveness training, stress management, and confidence building.
4. Provide realistic expectations of potential outcomes from not exercising so the behavioral consequences of relapse are placed in proper perspective.
5. Encourage the participant to expect and plan for relapse. He or she should plan for some alternate modes of exercise, times of day, places, and so forth. If the individual is likely to skip a day of exercise if all the treadmills are in use, suggest that he or she use the cycle or stairclimber on those days.
6. Minimize the tendency to interpret a temporary relapse as a total failure. Use cognitive restructuring to change the definition of a missed exercise class from "the end of my exercise program" to "a temporary lapse that most people who exercise experience."
7. Correct a lifestyle imbalance in which "shoulds" outweigh "wants." Make exercise a "want" instead of a "should." Use positive reinforcement and other strategies to make exercise fun.

4 In Review

Because missing regular exercise is inevitable for many people, the HFI must be prepared to help the participant prevent lapses in an exercise routine from ending the exercise program. Strategies such as being flexible in setting goals, realizing that the occasional relapse is just temporary, and building one's self-confidence can help the participant deal successfully with a potential relapse.

Health Fitness Counseling

The HFI and PFT are called on to provide counseling during assessment, exercise prescription, and ongoing monitoring of exercise participants. Good communication skills are the foundation of effective counseling. For additional information, the reader is referred to the excellent chapter on health counseling skills by Southard and Southard (22) in the ACSM resource manual.

Communication Skills

To be able to communicate well, the HFI must be able to listen effectively and respond empathetically. Listening involves being able to accurately discriminate the feeling and meaning of the speaker's message. Listening is more complicated than simply hearing words. Communication occurs at different levels. There is the actual, objective meaning of the words, or the content of the message; however, tone of voice, loudness or softness of speech, speed, and nonverbal behavior can change the meaning of a statement. A participant who smiles and says, "My program is going really well," is not saying the same thing as the person who mumbles the same words and looks down at his or her shoes. To enhance our understanding of the message, we must be able to attend to the verbal and nonverbal as well as overt and covert messages. The HFI should pay attention to facial expressions, body language, and tone of voice in addition to listening to the actual words and should not always assume that what people say is what they mean.

The context of the message, determined by the social and cultural implications of the situation, can create "noise" that will interfere with sending and receiving the message. Noise is also created by the ideas, experiences, expectations, and prejudices of the speaker and listener. Barriers to communication occur not only in the context of the message but also in the way a listener responds. Ordering or commanding, threatening, criticizing, interpreting, interrupting, interrogating, and diverting, often by humor, are responses that shut off understanding and make the speaker feel you do not care.

Do not assume you understand what a person is saying. We react to a communicated message according to our own perceptions of the nature of the message. Use responsive listening to clarify communications and confirm with the speaker that you comprehend his or her message. Reflect back what you have heard, and ask questions and make statements that respond to the feeling and meaning of the message. Responsive listening lets the person know you understand what he or she has expressed, helps build a relationship, encourages the participant to keep talking, and clarifies what the person means. Responsive listening is illustrated in the following exchange:

Participant: I'm the only one in this class who can't get the new step routines. (The HFI should observe the tone of voice, eye contact, and posture.)

HFI: You think the other members of the class catch on before you do. That must be really frustrating. (The HFI paraphrased the participant's statement and interpreted probable underlying feelings. Other feelings could be discouragement or a sense of futility or failure. Responding with an offer to teach the participant the steps might not have addressed an underlying lack of confidence. Responsive listening keeps the communications open so the participant can express what kind of help he or she wants.)

Characteristics of an Effective Helper

The role of the HFI as counselor is to help the client achieve his or her health-related goals. It is easier to provide this help when the HFI responds to the client with empathy, respect, concreteness, genuineness, and confrontation:

- **Empathy** is an expression of a sensitive understanding of the personal meaning of events and experiences to the participant. This is different from sympathy, which is an attempt to experience another person's feeling. Empathy is also not the same as knowing what the problem is. You may know that John has 25% body fat because he eats fast food every day and does not exercise. Empathy means you have a sense of what it must be like for him to be overweight and inactive, and you are able to communicate your understanding in a non-judgmental manner. Even if you are not sure you are empathetic, when the participant perceives that you are trying to understand, he or she will be encouraged to communicate more of the problem. The additional information will help you empathize more and give you clues to the underlying nature of the problems and how to come up with a more realistic intervention plan. Your effort to understand also communicates to the participant that you value him or her as an individual.

- **Respect** is a feeling of positive regard for the participant. You display warm acceptance of the participant's experiences and place no conditions on your acceptance and warmth. This means not making judgments. It is often hard for the HFI to respect a person whose behavior (smoking, sedentary lifestyle, high-fat diet) shows a lack of self-respect for his or her body. We must prize the person but not necessarily the behavior. When we respect another person, we help that person develop self-respect.
- **Concreteness** is the ability to help the participant be specific about feelings and goals he or she is trying to communicate. Reflective listening enables the participant to become more precise in communicating what he or she experiences and wants to accomplish, which aids in setting goals.
- **Genuineness** is being real in a relationship with another person. In a helping relationship, the counselor is honest and open with the client. Some self-disclosure is appropriate and can help develop trust, but the goal of the relationship is to help the client, not deal with the HFI's personal issues.
- **Confrontation** involves telling the other person that you see things differently from how they are being presented to you. You point out incongruities that are observable facts about which the participant may not be consciously aware. Confrontation should be used only after you have an established relationship and should be directed toward behavior and not the person.

Other qualities important in effective health counseling are listed in the box below.

Ethical Considerations

There is an ethical dilemma in promoting health behavior change in people who don't want to change. The HFI and PFT, along with other health promotion professionals, must weigh the importance of persuading people to behave in ways conducive to good health versus the clients' right to do as they please with their own health as long as it does not impinge on the rights of others. "Informed consent" theoretically gives participants a free choice after they have been given all the information needed to make a decision. If an unhealthy lifestyle is based on ignorance or incorrect information, we should provide the necessary information for an informed choice, not aggravate feelings of guilt or failure. But if an individual has chosen an unhealthy lifestyle as

Qualities of an Effective Health Behavior Counselor

- Knowledgeable
- Supportive
- Model of healthy behavior
- Trustworthy
- Enthusiastic
- Innovative
- Patient
- Sensitive
- Flexible
- Self-aware
- Able to access material resources and services
- Able to generate expectations of success
- Committed to providing timely, specific feedback
- Capable of providing clear, reasonable instructions and plans
- Aware of his or her limitations

a matter of choice and free will, we must accept the "informed refusal," although healthcare providers seem to have some difficulty doing this. Thus, an awareness of our own value preferences is essential in helping others set goals. We must consider whose values are to be served by the intervention, ours or the clients', and we must respect their choices, even if we disagree with them.

Confidentiality is another critical ethical concern for the HFI. In addition to the client information that is clearly confidential, the HFI may become aware of other information the participant wants to keep private. Trustworthiness is an important characteristic of an effective helper and reflects an ethical stand. A participant will trust someone who keeps information confidential, treats him or her with respect, and keeps the relationship professional.

It is also important to recognize your limitations and know when to refer your client to a professional therapist. It is the role of the HFI to help people change health behavior, but marital problems, eating disorders, and affective disorders, such as depression, are a few of the areas that should be handled by someone trained to work with these issues. We must know our limits and help connect participants with the best resources for handling their unique problems.

5 In Review

Listening to the actual words and the nonverbal message in context is the foundation of good communication skills. To communicate effectively, the HFI should practice reflective listening and empathetic responding. Characteristics of an effective helper include empathy, respect, concreteness, genuineness, and confrontation.

Case Studies

You can check your answers by referring to appendix A.

22.1

Dana was given a 3-month membership to your facility by her boyfriend, Mike, who attends aerobics classes regularly. They are going on a backpacking trip in Colorado this summer, and Mike thought you could help get her ready for the physical strain of the trip. She is a self-proclaimed "couch potato." Dana started aerobics classes with Mike last year but got so sore she stopped after 1 week. Yesterday, you completed her fitness assessment; Dana is in good health, has 20% body fat, and is slightly below average in aerobic fitness. She said her goal is to be prepared for the trip, and she wants to try aerobics again. However, she confides she is afraid she will disappoint Mike because she is "really out of shape" and doesn't enjoy aerobics. What stage of behavior change is she in, and what strategies could you use to help her?

22.2

Jack is a middle-aged college English professor who joined the walking club in your facility after you conducted his fitness and psychosocial assessment 3 months ago. His long-term goal was to "walk around the world" (in terms of total miles walked), and his progress has been marked on the walkers' promotional map at the front entrance. His office is two blocks from your facility, and Jack usually walks on your indoor track before he goes home for the day. You notice his mileage has decreased over the past 2 weeks, and another walker tells you that Jack said, "I won't make it out of the state thanks to term papers and final exams." What stage of behavior change is he in, and what strategies could you use with him?

Source List

1. Annesi, J.J. (1996). *Enhancing exercise motivation.* Los Angeles: Leisure Publications.
2. Biddle, S.J.H., & Nigg, C.R. (2000). Theories of exercise behavior. *International Journal of Sport Psychology, 31,* 290-304.
3. Booth, M.L., Owen, N., Bauman, A., Clavisi, O., & Leslie, E. (2000). Social-cognitive and perceived environmental influences associated with physical activity in older Australians. *Preventive Medicine, 31,* 15-22.
4. Buckworth, J. (2000). Exercise determinants and interventions. *International Journal of Sport Psychology, 31,* 305-320.
5. Courneya, K.S., & McAuley, E. (1995). Cognitive mediators of the social influence-exercise adherence relationship: A test of the theory of planned behavior. *Journal of Behavioral Medicine, 18,* 499-515.
6. Dishman, R.K., & Buckworth, J. (1996). Increasing physical activity: A quantitative synthesis. *Medicine and Science in Sports and Exercise, 28,* 706-719.
7. Dunn, A.L., Marcus, B.H., Kampert, J.B., Garcia, M.E., Kohl, H.W., & Blair, S.N. (1999). Comparison of lifestyle and structured interventions to increase physical activity and cardiorespiratory fitness: A randomized trail. *Journal of the American Medical Association, 281,* 327-334.
8. Franklin, B.A. (1988). Program factors that influence exercise adherence: Practical adherence skills for the clinical staff. In R.K. Dishman (Ed.), *Exercise adherence* (pp. 237-258). Champaign, IL: Human Kinetics.
9. Gorely, T., & Gordon, S. (1995). An examination of the transtheoretical model of exercise behavior in older adults. *Journal of Sport and Exercise Psychology, 17,* 312-324.
10. King, A.C. (1994). Community and public health approaches to the promotion of physical activity. *Medicine and Science in Sports and Exercise, 26,* 1405-1412.
11. King, A.C., & Martin, J.E. (1993). Exercise adherence and maintenance. In J.L. Durstine, A.C. King, P.L. Painter, J.L. Roitman, & L.D. Zwiren (Eds.), *Resource manual for guidelines for exercise testing and prescription* (pp. 443-454). Philadelphia: Lea & Febiger.
12. Knapp, D.N. (1988). Behavioral management techniques and exercise promotion. In R.K. Dishman (Ed.), *Exercise adherence* (pp. 203-236). Champaign, IL: Human Kinetics.
13. Krummel, D.A., Koffman, D.M., Bronner, Y., Davis, J., Greenlund, K., Tessaro, I., Upson, D., & Wilbur, J. (2001). Cardiovascular health interventions in women: What works? *Journal of Women's Health & Gender-Based Medicine, 10,* 117-136.
14. Kyllo, L.B., & Landers, D.M. (1995). Goal setting in sport and exercise: A research synthesis to resolve the controversy. *Journal of Sport and Exercise Psychology, 17,* 117-137.
15. Lombard, D.N., Lombard, T.N., & Winett, R.A. (1995). Walking to meet health guidelines: The effects of prompting frequency and prompt structure. *Health Psychology, 14,* 164-170.
16. Markland, D., & Hardy, L. (1993). The exercise motivation inventory: Preliminary development and validity of a measure of individuals' reasons for participation in regular physical exercise. *Personality and Individual Differences, 15,* 289-296.
17. Marlatt, G.A., & Gordon, J.R. (1985). *Relapse prevention: Maintenance strategies in addictive behavior change.* New York: Guilford Press.
18. Prochaska, J.O., & DiClemente, C.C. (1983). Stages and processes of self-change of smoking: Toward an integrative model of change. *Journal of Consulting and Clinical Psychology, 51,* 390-395.
19. Prochaska, J.O., & Marcus, B.H. (1994). The transtheoretical model: Applications to exercise. In R.K. Dishman (Ed.), *Advances in exercise adherence* (pp. 161-180). Champaign, IL: Human Kinetics.
20. Prochaska, J.O., & Velicer, W.F. (1997). The transtheoretical model of behavior change. *American Journal of Health Promotion, 12,* 38-48.
21. Sonstroem, R.J. (1988). Psychological models. In R.K. Dishman (Ed.), *Exercise adherence: Its impact on public health* (pp. 125-153) Champaign, IL: Human Kinetics.
22. Southard, D.R., & Southard, B.H. (1998). Health counseling skills. In J.L. Roitman, M. Kelsey, T.P. LaFountaine, D.R. Southard, M.A. Williams, & T. Tork (Eds.), *ACSM's resource manual for guidelines for exercise testing and prescription* (3rd ed., pp. 523-526). Baltimore: Lippincott Williams & Wilkins.
23. Wallace, J.P., Raglin, J.S., & Jastremski, C.A. (1995). Twelve month adherence of adults who joined a fitness program with a spouse vs. without a spouse. *Journal of Sports Medicine and Physical Fitness, 35,* 206-213.

twenty-three

Exercise and Stress

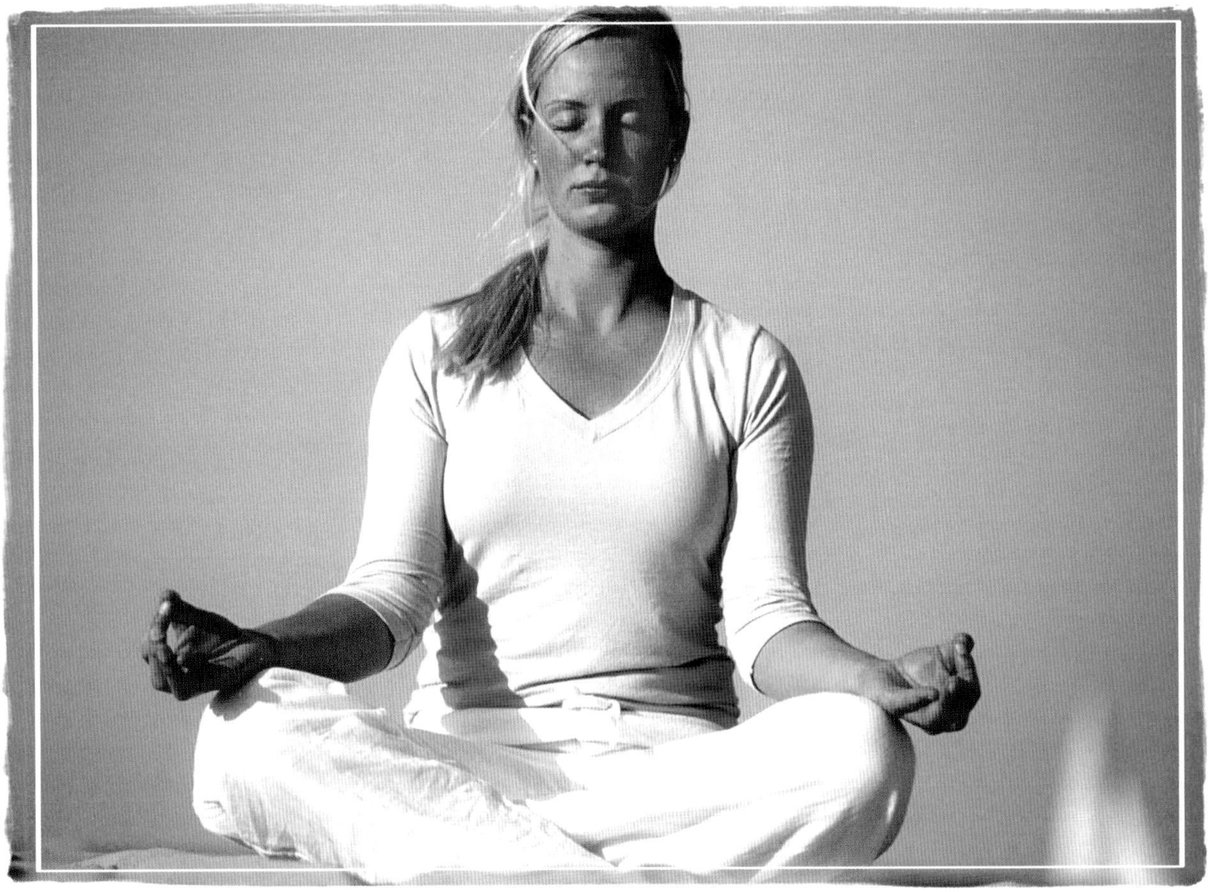

© Sport The Library/H. Schneider

Objectives

The reader will be able to do the following:

1. Describe the components of stress.
2. Explain how physical activity may affect stress.
3. Describe the positive and negative aspects of stress and how aging may affect responses to stressors.
4. List ways to minimize unhealthy stress levels.
5. Identify techniques that can be used in an exercise program to teach muscular relaxation.

This book emphasizes physical fitness, yet physical, mental, psychological, social, and spiritual aspects of life are all intertwined. This chapter deals with stress, an area that bridges the psychological and physiological aspects of fitness (3).

Stress Continua

A person's perception of a stimulus or situation largely determines how stressful the situation is for that person. No agreement exists on definitions of stress terms. For our purposes, a **stressor** is defined as any stimulus or condition that causes physiological arousal beyond what is necessary to accomplish the activity. This excessive arousal is called **stress**.

Stress has three major components (see figure 23.1). A complete description of a stressful event includes the amount by which the stress response exceeds the functional demand, how pleasant it is to the individual, and whether it causes development or deterioration. The following sections expand on each of these bases for understanding stress.

Functional-to-Severe Stress Continuum

The physiological response at any one time lies on a continuum from what is essential to provide the energy for that task to an extreme physiological response beyond what is needed. Physiological responses to stress include increased HR, BP, and catecholamine levels.

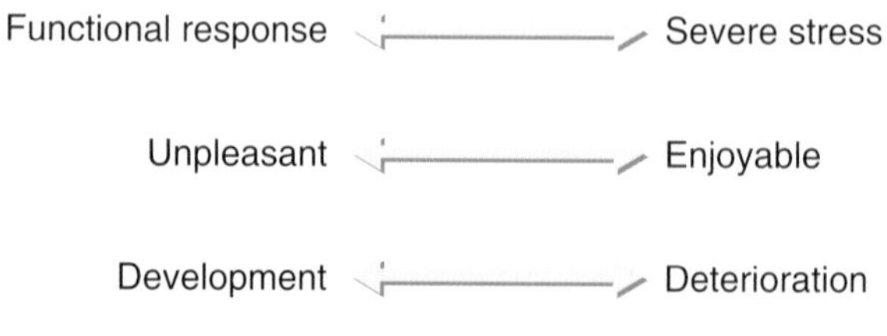

Figure 23.1 Stress continua.

Table 23.1 illustrates how typical resting and submaximal HRs include not only the HR needed to provide energy for the body but also the increased HR caused by chronic stressors (e.g., excess fat) and acute stressors (e.g., emotional states). The same principle applies to psychological attention needed for various tasks. For example, watching television, moving in a crowd, and responding to a conflict with a significant other require different levels of psychological attention. A psychological stress response would include a higher level of attention than needed for the situation. Individuals who overreact to stressors have a higher risk of a number of health problems (6, 8).

Unpleasant-to-Enjoyable Stress Continuum

Another aspect of stress is how the stressor is perceived by the individual on a continuum between unpleasant and enjoyable. A person might have similar stress responses to an exciting music concert and to taking a major examination, but she or he may perceive the concert as being more enjoyable.

Development-to-Deterioration Continuum

The third aspect of stress is what happens to an individual as a result of a stressful experience on a continuum from development to deterioration. What happens to the person under stress is, of course, the main criterion for determining whether the stressful event was positive or negative. The positive stressor results in a healthier, stronger person. The negative stressor leads to a weaker individual. The end result of stress is somewhat independent of the

Table 23.1 Stress Components of Heart Rate (beats · min^{-1})

Component of heart rate (HR)	Activity: Sitting	Climbing stairs	Running
HR needed to do task	30	50	100
Additional HR attributable to chronic stress			
Poor aerobic fitness	+15	+20	+40
Excess fat	+5	+15	+20
Additional HR attributable to acute stress			
Not relaxed	+10	+5	0
Emotional state	+15	+10	0
Total HR	75	100	160

Note. This HR model shows the contribution of the HR necessary to do various tasks plus the additional HR response caused by chronic and acute stressors. The actual HR values will vary with the individual depending on body size, fitness level, and type and severity of stressors.

other two aspects of stress previously discussed. For example, a very stressful event (i.e., causing a large stress response beyond what is essential physically) could inspire a person to achieve great things, or it might destroy a person's initiative. On the other hand, conditions that cause small stress responses might lead to steady development or gradually wear down a person's desire to excel. In addition, a person might grow and develop from stressors that are both pleasant (e.g., positive reinforcement) and unpleasant (e.g., deadline to have a project done). Either pleasant or unpleasant stressors might tempt a person to avoid dealing with important areas of life. For these reasons, the HFI should be cautious in identifying a specific stressor as being healthy or unhealthy based on the degree of physiological and psychological stress response or how much the individual liked the situation. A better criterion is to determine whether the experience led the person toward higher levels of mental, social, or physical health.

1 In Review

Excessive response (stress) to a situation (stressor) is described in terms of level of arousal (the functional-to-severe stress continuum), degree of unpleasantness (the unpleasant-to-enjoyable stress continuum), and, most important, whether it results in a positive or negative shift in health status (the development-to-deterioration stress continuum).

Physical Activity and Stress

One of the advantages of separating functional stimuli from stressors is that they interact with physical activity differently. Separating the effects of immediate and long-term physical activity on stress responses is also helpful in terms of understanding physical activity and stress.

Response to Acute Exercise and Functional (Environmental) Stimuli

The physiological response to acute physical activity and functional stimuli is additive. Numerous environmental stimuli such as exercise, heat, altitude, and pollution cause a functional increase in physiological response (see chapter 10). If more than one of these stimuli are present, the physiological response is greater than if only one stimulus is present. Thus, when people exercise in hot, humid, or polluted conditions or at high altitude, they must do less exercise to achieve the same physiological response (e.g., THR). The one exception is exercising in the cold, because the heat by-product of exercise helps one cope with the cold.

Response to Acute Exercise and Psychological Stressors

The physiological response to acute exercise and psychological stressors varies with the intensity of exercise, but generally it is not additive. Nonfunctional stimuli appear to affect the physiological response at rest and during light exercise but have little effect on the response to moderate or hard exercise. Nonfunctional stimuli also affect a person's decision about when to stop during a maximal task. Thus, if a person is very angry or happy, the HR and BP at rest and during light exercise may be elevated, and the person may decide to continue exercising longer or quit early. If the person is sad or relaxed, the HR and BP during light work may be depressed, and the decision to stop exercising may come earlier or later than usual. Thus, emotional state, such as anxiety about taking a GXT, may affect some of the physiological and psychological measurements taken early in the test as well as the length of time until voluntary exhaustion.

Physical Activity for Stress Reduction

Many professionals have justified exercise programs partly on the basis of stress reduction. Although the claims have often exceeded the evidence, there is some basis for a relationship between stress reduction and acute (immediate) and chronic (long-range) exercise.

Acute Activity and Stress Reduction

Acute exercise results in a positive mood change and has been shown to reduce state anxiety and muscle tension (8). Five factors are related to single bouts of exercise helping to reduce stress:

1. Distraction
2. Perception of personal control
3. Feeling good
4. Interaction with others
5. Physiological changes

As with many other activities, exercise can serve as a temporary distraction from stressors. Stepping away from a problem and then coming back to it later is often helpful. This technique is healthy as long as exercise does not become an avenue of escape from the problem. The ultimate reduction of stress must come from coping with the stressor. One part of the coping strategy, however, can be the distraction of physical activity.

One of the primary concepts in a person's ability to cope with stressors is the perception of personal control. In some cases, exercise enhances this feeling of control. For example, increased practice and skill acquisition decrease stress when a person is playing a game in the presence of others. One of the benefits of a postcardiac program is that it reduces the fear that any exertion will cause another heart attack and leaves the individual feeling more in control of his or her everyday life.

Stress is also reduced by the simple response of a positive mood change. Subjective reports indicate that feeling good after exercise lasts as long as 6 hr postexercise. Exercise is related to reduction in depression, anxiety, and tension (8).

Another way acute exercise may reduce stress is by providing a time to have either more or less interaction with others. Stress can be reduced when the exercise session provides a time to be alone for people who experience daily stress from constant contact with other people (e.g., the working parent who must spend almost every waking moment in the presence of others, such as children, spouse, employees, employer, and colleagues, all demanding time and attention). That person can use a walk/jog program as a time to be alone with her or his own thoughts. At the other extreme is the person who has little contact with other people during the typical day and for whom loneliness is a potential stressor. Doing activities and having time to talk with other people in an exercise program can aid that person. The HFI should be aware of individuals' needs in terms of amount of social interaction during exercise sessions.

The physiological changes that take place as a result of exercise also can affect levels of stress. For example, endorphins (i.e., endogenous, morphine-like chemicals) are increased as a result of exercise, a response that is associated with a reduced perception of pain. The increased arousal (sympathetic nervous system) may cause some individuals to feel good. After exercise, people often feel more relaxed (parasympathetic nervous system), with reduced muscle tension.

Chronic Activity and Stress Reduction

The long-term effects of a regular exercise program also provide basis for stress reduction. Reduced arousal before, during, and after exposure to stressors; quicker recovery from stressors; and improved emotional reactions to some stressors are related to habitual exercise.

Regular acute bouts of exercise provide substantial time when people are less affected by stressors—one additional benefit of physical conditioning. This includes positive mood changes and reduction in tension. Several studies have found that regular physical activity reduces anxiety and depression in individuals who start with high levels of these traits (5).

Increased cardiorespiratory fitness and decreased body fat cause individuals to be less stressed throughout the day. Furthermore, these changes reduce the risk of CHD, hypertension, glucose intolerance, and sudden death.

With increased fitness levels, physical activity itself becomes less of a stressor. For example, numerous studies have shown that a fit person can do the same amount of external work with lower HR, BP, and catecholamines. Thus, the functional response to the work (the energy necessary to accomplish the task) remains the same, but the stress response is reduced.

Some researchers believe, with some support, that increased adaptation to physical activity provides a basis for better adaptation to other stressors. Others believe, with some support, that increased adaptation is specific to different stimuli and stressors. Additional research into this question is needed before definitive claims can be made.

2 In Review

Exercise and physical stimuli, such as heat or altitude, interact to increase cardiorespiratory response at all levels of exercise intensity. Psychological stressors affect physiological and psychological responses at rest and during light work, as well as time to voluntary exhaustion, but have little influence on physiological response to strenuous work. Single bouts of activity may reduce stress through distraction, increased perception of control, positive mood shift, interaction with others, and physiological changes in the body. Chronic exercise (conditioning) may reduce stress through repeated acute activities, reduction of chronic stressors (e.g., poor aerobic fitness, excessive fat), lessened stress of exercise, reduction of anxiety and depression, and perhaps some cross-adaptation to stressors.

Relationship Between Stress and Health

Stress is important for both positive and negative aspects of health. No discussion of the highest quality of life possible or of serious health problems would be complete without including the relevance of stress.

Positive and Negative Stress

People often think of stress as primarily a negative influence on their lives, but it has many positive features. The presence of a great variety of stimuli and stressors provides the interesting experiences essential to a full life. People develop, learn, grow, and strive for their optimal potential through encountering stress. Even peak experiences, those special emotional moments of the good life that are remembered forever, are usually stressful. Without stress, life would be bland indeed.

The inability to cope with stress is considered a risk factor for many major health problems (e.g., CHD, hypertension, cancer, ulcers, low back pain, and headaches). Although inability to cope with stress probably is not sufficient to cause any of these problems if no predispositions exist, stress seems to manifest itself wherever the weak link is found. So for some people, stress results in an MI; for others, it results in hypertension, ulcers, low back pain, or headaches.

An inability to cope with one stressor can transfer to other stressors. Many people, because of stressors in other areas of their lives, find themselves getting upset (stressed) over something that normally would not bother them. Two aspects of the inability to cope are perception of and reaction to a potential stressor. Although the positive transfer of adaptation from one stressor to other stressors is an open question, there is little doubt about negative transfer: An inability to cope in one area leads to coping problems in other areas of life.

The health problems caused by lack of exercise can also be sources of stress, and negative physiological and psychological changes (stressors) have also been related to excessive exercise, for example, exercising more than 5 days per week, longer than 30 min per workout, or at intensities higher than THR (2). Health problems related to lack of or excess exercise include increased injury risk, soreness, obsession, impatience, strain on relationships, neglect of work, and withdrawal symptoms when one cannot exercise (2, 7).

Aging, Stress, and Health

It is difficult to separate the effects of aging itself from things that typically happen as a person gets older. Certain experiences are more likely to have happened (more often) as a person becomes older. Positive aspects of aging include increased opportunities to deal with a variety of stressors. From this, many people develop a varied repertoire of coping behaviors.

On the negative side, the longer a person lives, the more likely it is that he or she will develop a serious health problem (although not living longer does not appear to be an attractive alternative). Some of the special life events that appear to cause stress (e.g., death of a loved one) obviously become more frequent with age. Parents are often affected dramatically when all of their children leave home; retirement is also associated with a severe change of lifestyle. Lifestyle patterns developed over decades undergo major modifications, sometimes with additional financial difficulties. Evidence shows that people are more likely to have a number of health problems after a series of stressful life events.

Older people often become less active, causing more deterioration in fitness and performance than would occur naturally simply because of increased age. Careful warm-up, safety precautions, cool-down, and gradual progression in activity become even more important in older populations because of the higher risk of health problems and injury and decreased fitness and performance skills. The good news is that an active lifestyle can slow the physical deterioration of aging. It's never too late to start, and previously sedentary, elderly individuals show remarkable fitness improvements as a result of initiating fitness programs.

3 In Review

Stress is a factor in positive health. Stressors are involved in having varied experiences, coping with life's special moments, and accomplishing one's goals. Inability to cope with stress is related to major health problems as a secondary risk factor and can cause problems in other areas of one's life. Both too little and too much exercise can be related to stress. In addition, aging provides experiences that may cause more stress as the individual deals with the death of loved ones and changes in living conditions and relationships. Older individuals are often better able to cope with stressors because they have learned coping mechanisms over a lifetime of experience with stress. Physical activity can slow down typical aging deterioration.

Recommendations for Maintaining Healthy Stress Levels

People can do many things to maximize the positive aspects of stress while minimizing the negative aspects. In a fitness program, the HFI can help participants learn to fill their lives with healthy stress.

Seek Exposure to a Variety of Stimuli and Stressors

Exposure to a wide range of experiences helps a person become better educated in coping with and being less stressed by new situations. A good fitness program provides a variety of experiences, including cooperative, problem-solving, competitive, individual, partner, and team activities. This variety enriches the participant by improving fitness and improving the ability to cope with different physical and social experiences.

Develop a Range of Coping Abilities

People should observe the different strategies that seem to enhance coping with a potentially stressful situation. Facing the problem, looking at alternatives, talking about the problem with close friends, seeking professional or technical advice when needed, and stepping back or away from the problem for a brief time are all behaviors that people use to cope with stress. People should ask themselves which coping behaviors are better suited for particular situations. Do some behaviors help but feel uncomfortable to the individual? In terms of fitness, the varieties of activities in a good program require different coping strategies. The HFI should be sensitive to participants who need help just coping with physical activity itself. After easing these people into exercise, the HFI can use a variety of fitness activities (see chapter 14) and the behavior modification suggestions to help them develop coping abilities (see chapter 22).

Using the mind/body connection helps many individuals cope. Three examples are to use humor and laughter, adopt a positive attitude toward whatever happens, and do specific activities (e.g., yoga and many of the relaxation strategies mentioned later in the chapter) that integrate mental and physical exercises to enhance relaxation.

Maintain Social Support

Coping with stressors often is aided by positive connections between an individual and her or his social surroundings: family; close friends and relatives; and places of worship, clubs, unions, and other social groups. The support for one's health is related to a special kind of relationship to other individuals in these types of social settings (9).

Develop Optimal Fitness

Developing physical, mental, and social fitness characteristics causes potential stressors to be less threatening. For the person who can do hard physical work, physical stressors are not dreaded. For people who are accustomed to the mental processes that lead to problem solving, having a difficult problem is less stressful. Social fitness can be enhanced by doing such things as establishing meaningful relationships with other people, therein developing a support group that helps one respond positively to stressful situations.

Gain Control of As Much of Life As Possible

Perception of control repeatedly looms as a major element in coping with stress. Therefore, whatever a person can do to help gain control of her or his life diminishes the stress of potentially stressful conditions. Some ways to take control of one's life are to adopt healthy behaviors, gain competence in important areas, be assertive in resisting unreasonable demands, and learn to relax.

One of the by-products of exercising, eating nutritious foods, and refraining from use of harmful drugs is the feeling that one is taking responsibility for one's own life. Not only do the healthy behaviors reduce stress, but the fact that one has "taken charge" also reduces stress levels. Chapter 22 recommends ways to increase healthy behaviors.

People should give attention to the relationships, tasks, and other things that are important to them, so that they increase their skills in those areas and gain confidence that they can be successful in what they find important. In the fitness program, the HFI helps people improve skills in the activities in which they are interested.

People must learn to recognize unreasonable demands, whether imposed by themselves or by someone else, and to work with others (e.g., boss, spouse) to try to accomplish common goals in a reasonable way within an appropriate time frame; this is essential to good health. The HFI must be careful not to place unrealistic goals or demands for future activities and fitness gains on the participant. The HFI also can help individuals set goals that will not be sources of stress.

Techniques can be learned to help people relax (see next section). Benson (1) and others have demonstrated the benefits of the *relaxation response*, including increased parasympathetic dominance resulting in decreased HR, BP, and muscle tension. The HFI should include relaxation techniques as part of the program, perhaps including a short relaxation period after the cool-down.

4 In Review

Coping with stress can be aided by exposing oneself to many stimuli, developing a social network, and increasing levels of fitness. The concept of gaining control of one's life is important in learning to cope with stress. Gaining control includes exhibiting healthy behaviors, getting rid of unhealthy habits, increasing competence in important areas, becoming assertive related to unreasonable demands, and learning how to relax.

Teaching People to Relax

HFIs can use different methods to increase relaxation, including the following:

- Biofeedback-assisted relaxation
- Autogenic training
- Breathing strategies
- Quieting-reflex training
- Cognitive restructuring
- Sensory awareness
- Progressive relaxation

Biofeedback includes focusing on something (e.g., HR, muscle tension) and learning how to decrease it through relaxation. Autogenic training involves learning to relax by concentrating on respiration and feeling heaviness and warmth in different parts of the body, such as the solar plexus and forehead. Participants are asked to say phrases to themselves such as, "my left leg feels heavy" or "my right arm feels warm." Imagery is often evoked to help participants visualize or imagine the feeling of heaviness and warmth (e.g., "Imagine that your leg is a 25-lb bag of sand that is flowing from your pelvis out through your toes. As the sand flows out of you, imagine each muscle in your leg relaxing."). Attention to respiration can help one relax. The participant is asked to use primarily the abdomen (rather than the chest) in breathing and to relax during exhalation. Quieting-reflex training involves a combination of other methods, such as self-talk (encouraging an alert mind and a calm body), relaxed breathing, conscious relaxation during exhalation, and imagining a wave of warmth and heaviness. Cognitive restructuring helps the participant become more positive about her- or himself through self-talk. Sensory awareness can be used with other relaxation techniques by helping the person realize that the sensation of pressure from contact with objects (e.g., a ball, the floor, the wall) has diminished during the relaxation.

Progressive relaxation, a very effective technique introduced by Jacobsen (4), is aimed at having people recognize the feelings produced by tension. The HFI should have participants get into comfortable positions with their eyes closed. We recommend that the technique be done with the participants lying on mats, but they can do this technique while sitting. The procedure is to have people tense a specific area of the body, hold for about 20 s, then relax; then tense a larger segment, hold, relax; and so forth. The HFI talks in a calm voice, asking people to feel the tension during the hold period and to feel the tension leave the area during the relax period. The following tense/hold/relax sequence can be used:

Right toes
Left toes
Right foot
Left foot
Right leg below the knee
Left leg below the knee
Right leg below the hip
Left leg below the hip
Both legs below the hips
Abdomen and buttocks
Right fingers
Left fingers
Right arm below the elbow
Left arm below the elbow
Right arm below the shoulder
Left arm below the shoulder
Both arms below the shoulders
Chest
Neck
Jaw
Forehead
Entire head
Entire body

Extend the final whole-body relaxation period; have people feel the tension leaving their bodies, feel their breathing, and then be silent for several minutes.

5 In Review

Techniques the HFI can use in an exercise program to facilitate a participant's skill development in muscle relaxation include biofeedback-assisted relaxation, autogenic training, breathing strategies, quieting-reflex training, cognitive restructuring, sensory awareness, and progressive relaxation.

Case Study

You can check your answers by referring to appendix A.

23.1

Linda, a single parent with three young children, has an executive position dealing with personnel in the local government. She joined the fitness center several months ago and seemed to enjoy the walking and jogging programs. After she had advanced in her jogging to 3 miles per day, 4 days per week, you suggested that she might enjoy participating in the coed games group 2 days per week. She tried it for a couple of weeks and then quit coming to the center. You decide to call her and ask if she would like to come in to talk about why she is no longer active in the program. What do you think might be the problem? How would you proceed with the conversation?

Source List

1. Benson, H. (1975). *The relaxation response.* New York: Morrow.
2. Brown, D.R. (1990). Exercise, fitness, and mental health. In C. Bouchard, R.J. Shephard, T. Stephens, J.R. Sutton, & B.D. McPherson (Eds.), *Exercise, fitness, and health: A consensus of current knowledge* (pp. 607-626). Champaign, IL: Human Kinetics.
3. Franks, B.D. (1994). What is stress? *Quest, 46*(1), 1-7.
4. Jacobsen, E. (1938). *Progressive relaxation.* Chicago: University of Chicago Press.
5. Landers, D.M. (1999). The influence of exercise on mental health. In C.B. Corbin & R.P. Pangrazi (Eds.), *Toward a better understanding of physical fitness and activity* (pp. 137-142). Scottsdale, AZ: Holcomb Hathaway.
6. Plowman, S.A. (1994). Stress, hyperreactivity, and health. *Quest, 46*(1), 78-99.
7. Sime, W.E. (1990). Discussion: Exercise, fitness, and mental health. In C. Bouchard, R.J. Shephard, T. Stephens, J.R. Sutton, & B.D. McPherson (Eds.), *Exercise, fitness, and health: A consensus of current knowledge* (pp. 627-633). Champaign, IL: Human Kinetics.
8. Sime, W.E., Eliot, R.S., & Solberg, E.E. (1998). Stress and heart disease. In J.L. Roitman (Ed.), *ACSM's resource manual for guidelines for exercise testing and prescription* (3rd ed., pp. 43-49). Philadelphia: Lippincott Williams & Wilkins.
9. Sime, W.E., & Hellweg, K. (1998), Stress and coping. In J.L. Roitman (Ed.), *ACSM's resource manual for guidelines for exercise testing and prescription* (3rd ed., pp. 527-534). Philadelphia: Lippincott Williams & Wilkins.

twenty-four

Exercise Related to ECG and Medications

Daniel Martin and David R. Bassett, Jr.

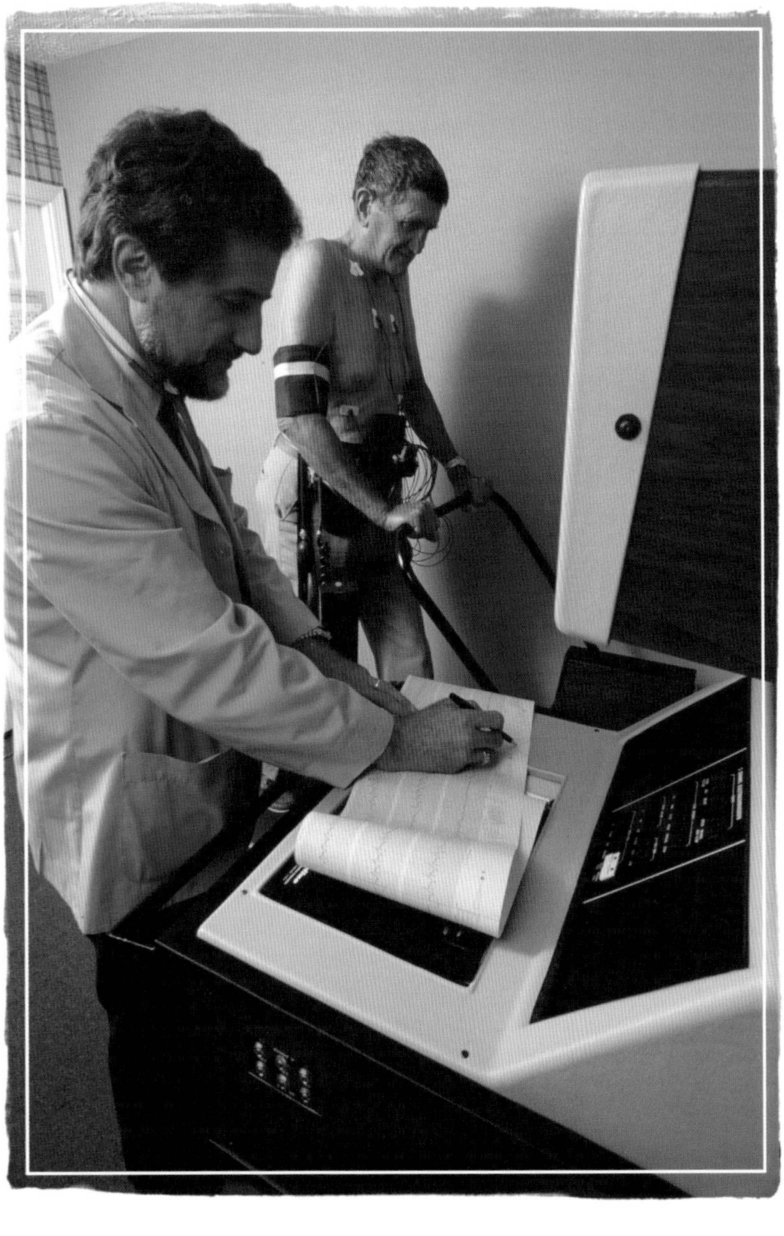

© Bachmann/The Image Finders

Objectives

The reader will be able to do the following:

1. Describe the basic anatomy of the heart.
2. Describe the basic electrophysiology of the heart.
3. Define the ECG and identify the standard settings for paper speed and amplitude.
4. Identify the basic electrocardiographic complexes and calculate HR from ECG rhythm strips.
5. Describe the various types of atrioventricular conduction defects and their probable impact on a subject's exercise response.
6. Identify the normal and abnormal cardiac rhythms and their significance and predict the probable impact of the abnormal rhythms on exercise performance.
7. Describe electrocardiographic signs and biochemical markers of a heart attack.
8. List the common categories of prescription medications used to treat cardiovascular and related diseases, some of the members of each category, and the probable impact of these medications on exercise performance.

The purposes of this chapter are to provide the HFI with background information on the heart, the basics of electrocardiogram (ECG) analysis, cardiovascular medications, and how these factors affect exercise testing and prescription in the basically healthy population. This chapter is not intended to be a complete guide to ECG interpretation and cardiovascular medications; there are several excellent texts on these topics (4, 7, 9, 10).

Understanding the Structure of the Heart

The heart is a muscular organ composed of four chambers: the right atrium, the right ventricle, the left atrium, and the left ventricle (see figure 24.1). The flow of blood through the heart is directed by pressure differences and valves between the chambers. Venous blood from the body enters the right atrium via the inferior and superior vena cava. From the right atrium, blood passes through the **tricuspid valve** into the right ventricle. The right ventricle pumps blood through the **pulmonary valve** into the pulmonary arteries to the lungs. In the lungs, blood gives up carbon dioxide and picks up oxygen. The oxygen-rich blood is returned to the heart via the pulmonary veins emptying into the left atrium. From the left atrium, blood passes through the **mitral valve** into the left ventricle. The left ventricle pumps oxygenated blood past the **aortic valve**, into the aorta and coronary arteries and to the rest of the body. The left ventricle, which generates more pressure than the right ventricle, is thicker.

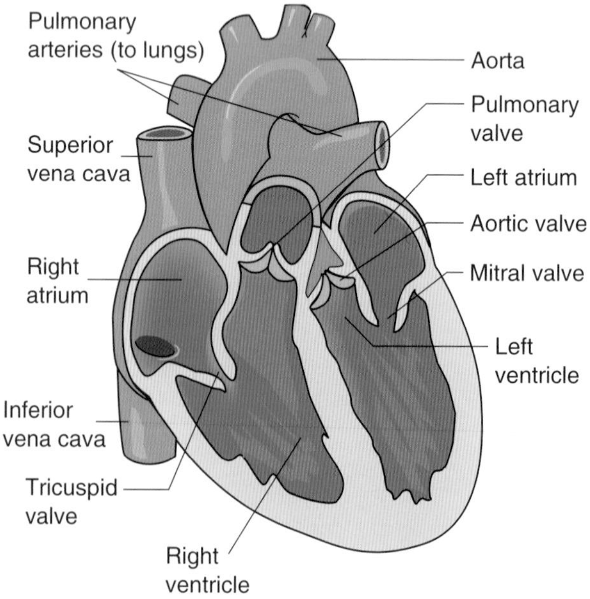

Figure 24.1 The chambers and valves of the heart.
Reprinted from Donnelly 1990.

Coronary Arteries

The heart muscle, or **myocardium**, does not receive a significant amount of oxygen directly from blood in the atria or ventricles. Oxygenated blood is supplied to the myocardium via the **coronary arteries**, which lie on the surface of the heart. There are two coronary artery systems (the right and left coronary arteries), which branch off the aorta at the coronary sinus. The left main coronary artery follows a course between the left atria and pulmonary artery and branches off into the left anterior descending, or interventricular, and left circumflex arteries (figure 24.2). The left anterior descending artery follows a path along the anterior surface of the heart and lies over the interventricular septum, which separates the right and left ventricles. The left circumflex artery follows the groove between the left atrium and left ventricle on the anterior and lateral surface of the heart. The right coronary artery follows the groove that separates the atria and ventricles around the posterior surface of the heart and forms the posterior descending artery, or posterior interventricular artery. Numerous smaller arteries branch off each of the major arteries and form smaller and smaller arteries, finally forming the capillaries in the muscle cells, where gas exchange occurs. A major obstruction in any of these coronary arteries reduces blood flow to the myocardium (**myocardial ischemia**) and decreases the ability of the heart to pump blood. If the coronary arteries become blocked and the heart muscle does not receive oxygen, then a portion of the heart muscle might die, which is known as a myocardial infarction (MI), or heart attack.

Coronary Veins

Venous drainage of the right ventricle occurs via the anterior cardiac vein, which normally has two or three major branches and eventually empties into the right atrium. The venous drainage of the left ventricle is provided primarily by the anterior interventricular vein, which roughly follows the same path as the left anterior descending artery, eventually forming the coronary sinus and emptying into the right atrium.

Oxygen Use by the Heart

The myocardium is very well adapted to use oxygen to generate adenosine triphosphate (ATP). Approximately 40% of the volume of a myocardial muscle cell is composed of mitochondria, the cellular organelle responsible for producing ATP with oxygen. The oxygen consumption of the heart in a resting person is about 8 to 10 ml · min^{-1} per 100 g of myocardium; in comparison, the total resting oxygen consumption for the body is about 0.35 ml · min^{-1} per 100 g of body mass (5). Myocardial oxygen consumption can increase six- to sevenfold during heavy exercise, whereas in young people the total body oxygen consumption can easily increase 12 to 15 times. Heart muscle has a limited capacity to

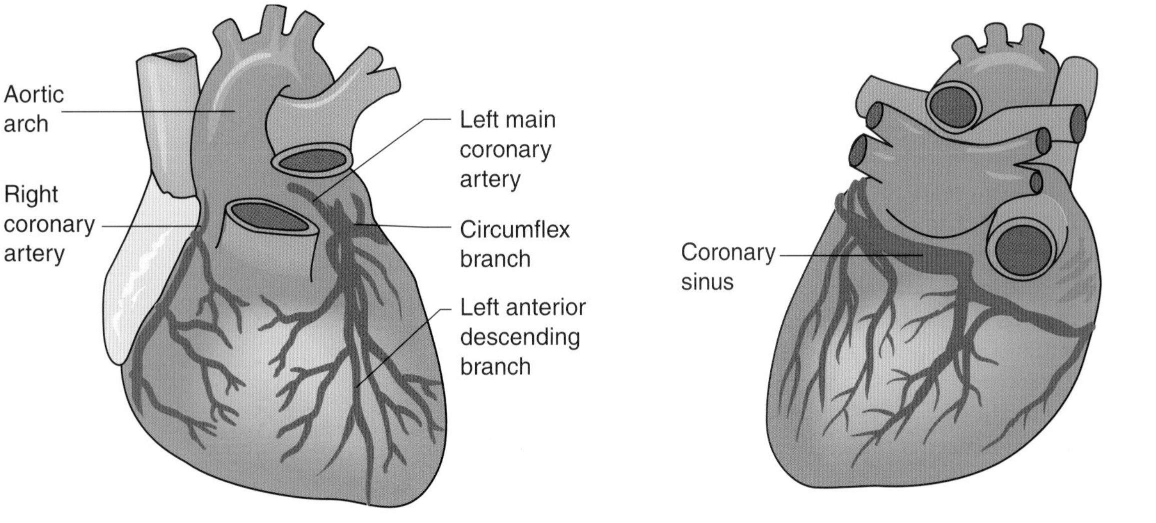

Figure 24.2 Coronary blood vessels.

Reprinted from Donnelly 1990.

produce energy via anaerobic pathways and depends on the delivery of oxygen to the mitochondria to produce ATP. At rest, the whole body extracts only about 25% of the oxygen present in each 100 ml of arterial blood, and the body can meet its need for oxygen by simply extracting more from the blood. In contrast, the heart extracts about 75% of the oxygen available in the arterial blood. Consequently, the heart muscle's oxygen needs must be met by increasing the delivery of blood via the coronary arteries. An adequate oxygen supply to the heart is needed not only to allow the heart to pump blood but also to maintain normal electrical activity, which is covered in the next section.

1 In Review

The heart is a muscular organ composed of four chambers: the right atrium, the right ventricle, the left atrium, and the left ventricle. The coronary arteries supply the heart muscle (myocardium) with blood, and the heart meets the increasing oxygen demands by increasing blood flow.

Electrophysiology of the Heart

At rest, the insides of the myocardial cells are negatively charged and the exterior of the cells is positively charged. When the cells are depolarized (stimulated), the insides of the cells become positively charged and the exteriors of the cells become negatively charged. If a recording electrode is placed so that the wave of depolarization spreads toward the electrode, the ECG records a positive (upward) deflection. If the wave of depolarization spreads away from the recording electrode, a negative (downward) deflection will occur. When the myocardial muscle cell is completely polarized or depolarized, the ECG will not record any electrical potential but rather a flat line, known as the isoelectric line. After depolarization, the myocardial cell undergoes repolarization to return its electrical state to what it was at rest. The steps leading from rest (complete polarization) to complete stimulation (complete depolarization) back to rest (repolarization) are shown in figure 24.3.

Conduction System of the Heart

The **sino-atrial (SA) node** is the normal pacemaker of the heart and is located in the right atrium near the superior vena cava (figure 24.4). Depolarization spreads from the SA node across the atria and results in the P wave. There are three conduction tracts within the atria that conduct depolarization to the **atrioventricular (AV) node**. Impulses travel from the SA node through the atrial muscle and conduction tracts and enter the AV node, where the speed of conduction is slowed to allow the atrial contraction to empty blood into the ventricles before the start of ventricular contraction. The **bundle of His** is the conduction pathway that connects the AV node with **bundle branches** in the ventricles. The right bundle branch splits off the bundle of His and forms ever-smaller branches that serve the right ventricle. The left bundle splits into two major branches that serve the thicker left ventricle. **Purkinje fibers** are the terminal branches of the bundle branches and form the link between the specialized conductive tissue and the muscle fibers. Small electrical junctions between adjacent cardiac muscle cells, known as **intercalated discs**, allow the electrical impulses to be passed from cell to cell. The intercalated discs allow for simultaneous contraction of the ventricular muscle fibers, which is needed for effective pumping action of the heart.

2 In Review

The electrical impulse originates in the SA node, located in the right atrium. From there the electrical impulse spreads to the AV node, the bundle of His, left and right bundle branches, and Purkinje fibers. Waves of depolarization then spread from cell to cell throughout the ventricular muscle. Any restriction in the blood flow to the myocardium could upset the electrical activity of the heart or damage the myocardium itself.

1 Completely polarized

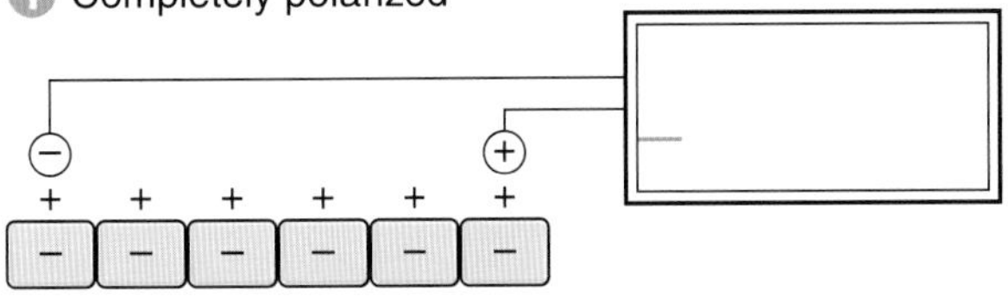

The myocardial cells shown on the left are at rest and are completely polarized. Because both of the recording electrodes are surrounded by positive charges, there is no voltage difference between them and the electrocardiogram shown on the right records the isoelectric line (0 mV).

2 Partially depolarized

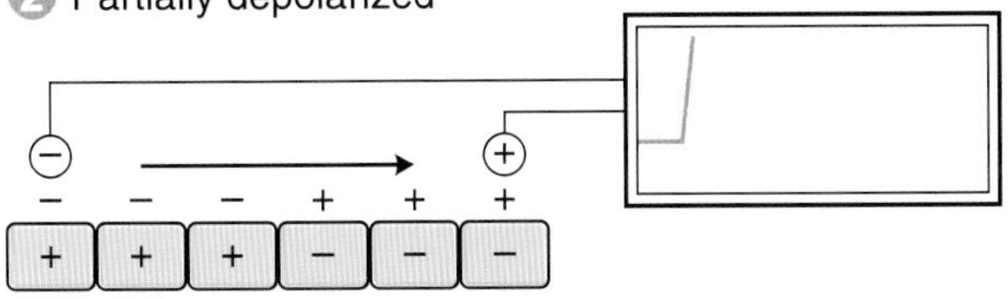

The process of depolarization (positive charges inside the cell and negative charges outside) is spreading from left to right. Because the electrode on the right is surrounded by positive charges, the ECG records a positive deflection. The amplitude of the deflection is proportional to the mass of the myocardium undergoing depolarization.

3 Completely depolarized

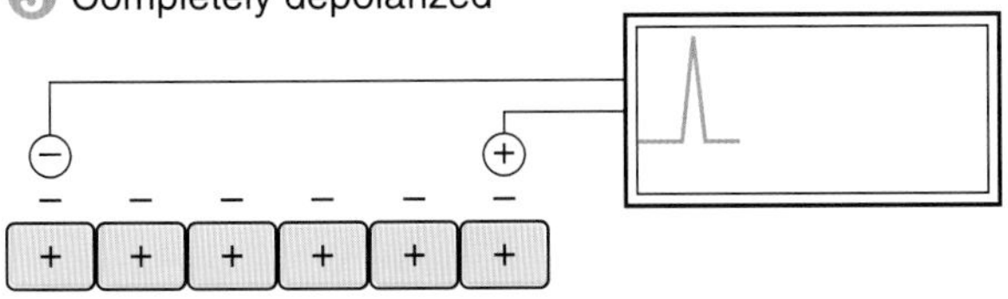

Depolarization is now complete, and both electrodes are surrounded by negative charges. Because there is no voltage difference between electrodes, the ECG is now recording 0 mV, or the isoelectric potential.

4 Partially repolarized

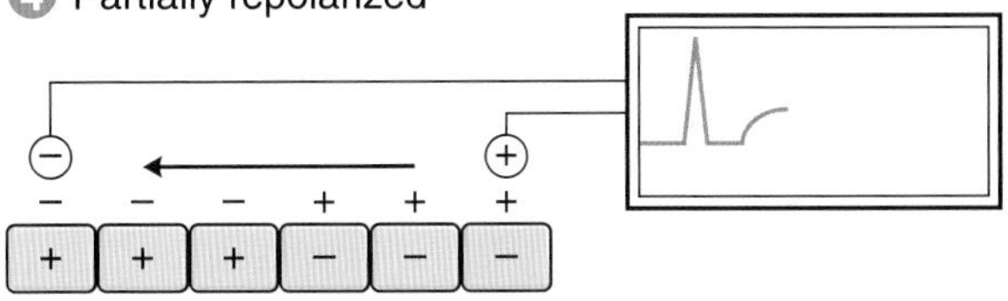

Repolarization has started from the right and is moving to the left. The ECG shows a positive (upward) deflection, because the right hand electrode is surrounded by positive charges. Note that repolarization occurs in the opposite direction from depolarization in the human heart, and this is the reason the depolarization and repolarization complexes are both normally positive. If repolarization had started on the left and moved to the right, the ECG deflection would have been negative.

5 Completely repolarized

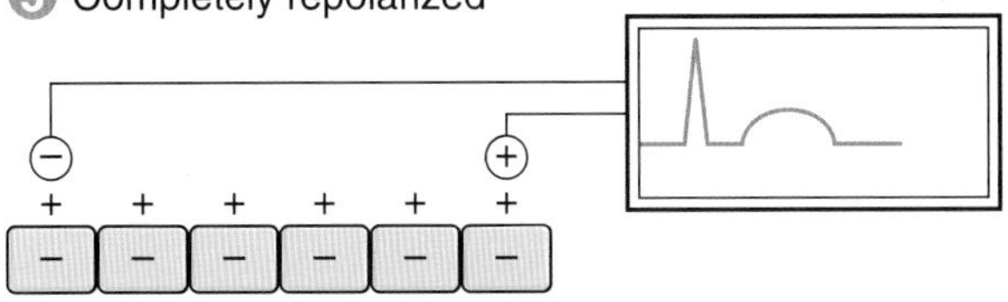

The muscle cells are now completely repolarized, or in the resting state, and the ECG records the isoelectric line. The myocardial cells are now ready to be depolarized again.

Figure 24.3 Steps in an electrocardiographic cycle.

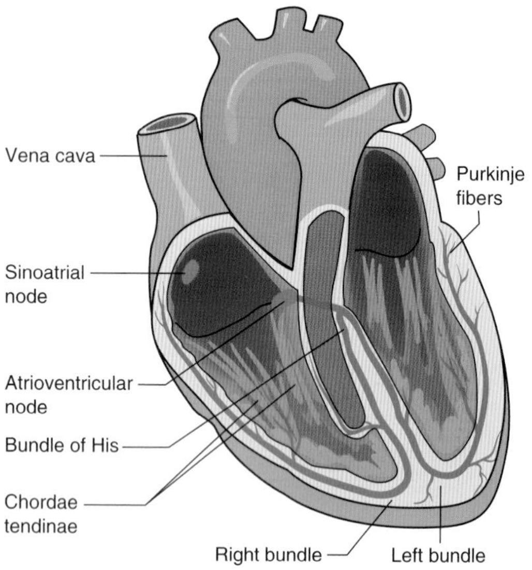

Figure 24.4 The electrical conduction system of the heart. These are the normal pathways used to ensure the rhythmic contraction and relaxation of the chambers of the heart.

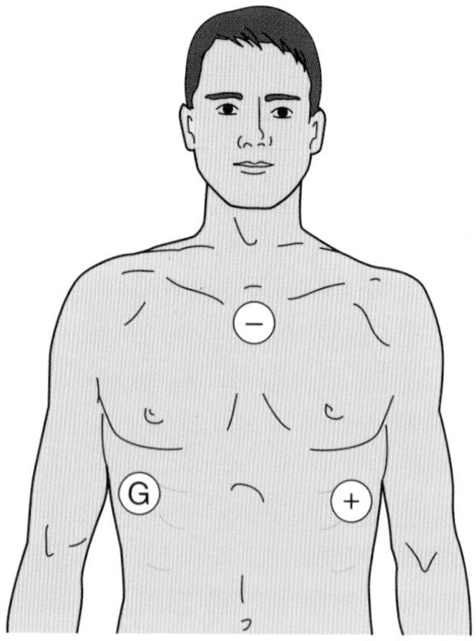

Figure 24.5 Lead placement for CM5: (–) negative electrode, (+) electrode, (G) ground.

Adapted from Ellestad 1994.

Basic Information for Interpreting the ECG

This section on analysis of the ECG may appear to be beyond what an HFI should know about the topic. In fact, the physician is the person to judge whether an ECG response is normal. However, the HFI must be aware of the basic information related to ECG interpretation to facilitate communication with the physician, program director, and exercise specialist.

A systematic approach to ECG evaluation allows the examiner to determine the HR, rhythm, and conduction pathways and to search for signs of ischemia or infarction. Physicians normally evaluate a 12-lead ECG, but for our purposes a single ECG lead will be adequate. A commonly used single ECG lead for exercise testing is the CM5 (see figure 24.5), which looks very similar to lead V5 on a 12-lead ECG.

Defining the ECG

The **ECG** is a graphic recording of the heart's electrical activity. As waves of depolarization travel through the heart, electrical currents spread to the tissues surrounding the heart and then travel throughout the body. If recording electrodes are placed on the surface of the skin, small voltage differences can be detected between various regions of the body. Thus, the ECG is a sensitive voltmeter that records the electrical activity of the heart.

Time and Voltage

ECG paper is marked in a standard manner to allow measurement of time intervals and voltages. Time is measured on the horizontal axis, and the paper normally moves at 25 mm · s^{-1}. Most ECG machines can be set to run at 50 or 25 mm · s^{-1}, so one must know the paper speed when measuring the duration of ECG complexes. ECG paper is marked with a repeating grid (see figure 24.6). Major grid lines are 5 mm apart, and at a paper speed of 25 mm · s^{-1}, 5 mm corresponds to 0.20 s. Minor lines are 1 mm apart, and at a paper speed of 25 mm · s^{-1}, 1 mm equals 0.04 s. Voltage is measured on the vertical axis, and the calibration of the machine must be known to evaluate the ECG. The standard calibration factor is normally 0.1 mV per millimeter of deflection. Most ECG machines can be adjusted to reduce this factor by 50% or to double it. It is very important to know the voltage calibration before evaluating an ECG. All ECG measurements in this chapter refer to a paper speed of 25 mm · s^{-1} and a voltage calibration of 0.1 mV · mm^{-1}.

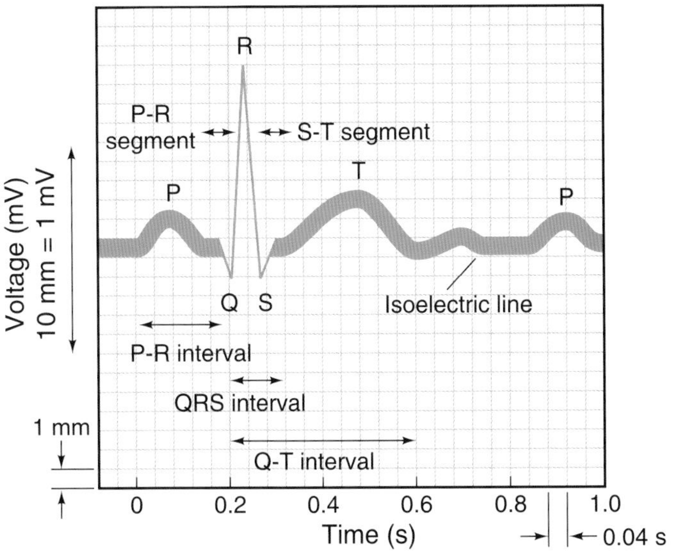

Figure 24.6 ECG complex with time and voltage scales.

Adapted from Goldman, *Principles of clinical electrocardiography,* 11th ed., Appleton & Lange, 1982.

3 In Review

The pattern of electrical activity across the heart is called the electrocardiogram (ECG). The ECG is recorded with an electrocardiograph, and it provides information about the rhythm of the heart. The ECG paper speed normally is set at 25 mm · s^{-1}, and at this speed each 1-mm mark represents 0.04 s. The standard calibration factor is normally 0.1 mV per millimeter of deflection.

Basic Electrocardiographic Complexes

The **P wave** is the graphic representation of atrial depolarization. The normal P wave is less than 0.12 s in duration and has an amplitude of 0.25 mV or less. The Ta wave is the result of atrial repolarization. It is not normally seen, because it occurs during ventricular depolarization, and the larger electrical forces generated by the ventricles "hide" the Ta wave. The **Q wave** is the first downward deflection after the P wave; the Q wave signals the start of ventricular depolarization. The **R wave** is a positive deflection after the Q wave, and it is the result of ventricular depolarization. If there is more than one R wave in a single complex, the second occurrence is called R′.

The **S wave** is a negative deflection preceded by Q or R waves, and it is also the result of ventricular depolarization. The **T wave** follows the **QRS complex**, and it represents ventricular repolarization.

Electrocardiograph Intervals

The **R-R interval** is the time between successive R waves. An approximate HR (beats · min^{-1}) can be determined by dividing 1500 (60 s at 25 mm · s^{-1}) by the number of millimeters between adjacent R waves (figure 24.7a). A second method of determining HR is to begin with an R wave that falls on a thick black line. As you move to the right, count off the next six black lines as 300, 150, 100, 75, 60, and 50 (memorize these numbers). If the next R wave falls on one of these lines, the corresponding number indicates the HR. If the next R wave falls in between two thick black lines, you can estimate the HR by interpolation (figure 24.7b). A third method of determining HR is commonly used when the HR is irregular. With this method, you count the number of complete R-R intervals in a 6-s ECG strip and multiply by 10 (figure 24.7*c*).

The P-P interval represents the time between two successive atrial depolarizations. The **P-R interval** is measured from the start of the P wave to the beginning of the QRS complex. The interval is called P-R even if the first deflection after the P wave is a Q wave. The P-R interval represents the time from the start of atrial depolarization, delay through the AV node, and the start of ventricular depolarization. The upper limit for the normal P-R interval is 0.20 s or 5 small blocks.

The width of the QRS complex represents the time for depolarization of the ventricles. A normal QRS complex lasts less than 0.10 s, or 2.5 small blocks on the ECG paper. The **Q-T interval** is measured from the start of the QRS complex to the end of the T wave and corresponds to the duration of ventricular systole.

Segments and Junctions

The **P-R segment** is measured from the end of the P wave to the beginning of the QRS complex. This segment forms the isoelectric line, or baseline, from which S-T segment deviations are measured. The RS-T segment or **J point** is the point at which the S wave ends and the S-T segment begins. The **S-T segment** is formed by the isoelectric line between the QRS complex and the T wave. This segment will be examined closely during an exercise test for depression or elevation, which may indicate the development of myocardial ischemia or perhaps MI. S-T segment deviation usually is measured 60 or 80 ms after the J point.

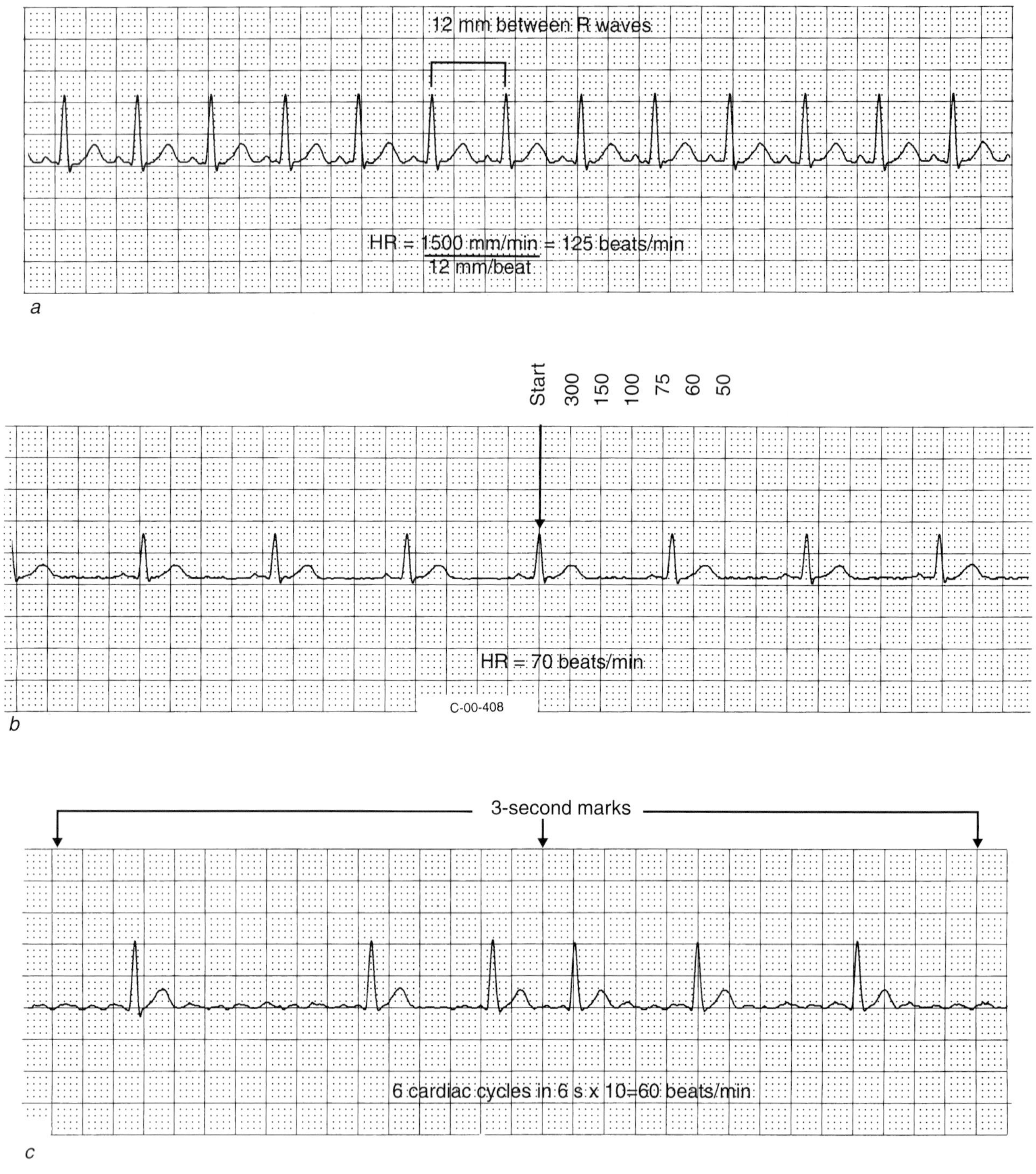

Figure 24.7 Three methods of determining heart rate from the electrocardiogram.

4 In Review

The P wave signifies atrial depolarization, the QRS complex signifies ventricular depolarization, and the T wave signifies ventricular repolarization. If the rhythm is regular, HR can be determined by dividing 1500 by the number of millimeters between successive R waves. HR also can be determined by starting with an R wave that falls on a thick black line and counting off the next six black lines as 300, 150, 100, 75, 60, and 50 and determining at which corresponding number the next R wave occurs. If the rhythm is irregular, HR can be determined by counting the number of R-R intervals in a 6-s ECG strip and multiplying by 10.

Heart Rhythms

The ECG provides vital information about heart rhythms. Abnormalities in the electrical activity of the heart can be diagnosed by examining the ECG.

Sinus Rhythm

Sinus rhythm is the normal rhythm of the heart (see figure 24.8). The HR is 60 to 100 beats · min^{-1} and the pacemaker is the sinus node.

Sinus Bradycardia

The pacemaker is the sinus node, and the rate in **sinus bradycardia** is 60 beats · min^{-1} or less (see figure 24.9). This is a normal rhythm, and it is often seen in conditioned subjects and patients taking β-blockers.

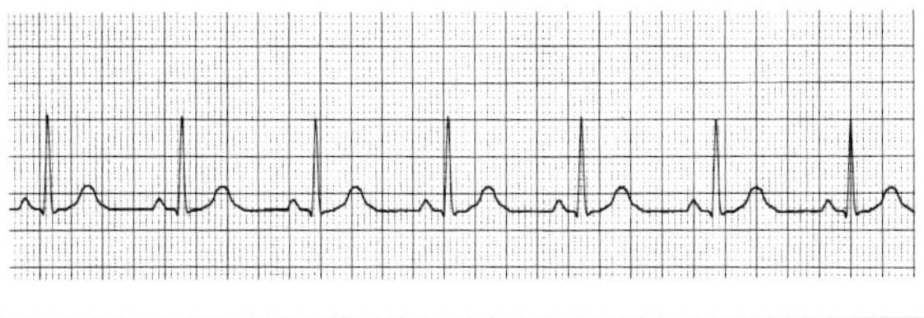

Figure 24.8 Normal sinus rhythm. In this example, the heart rate is 71 beats · min^{-1}.

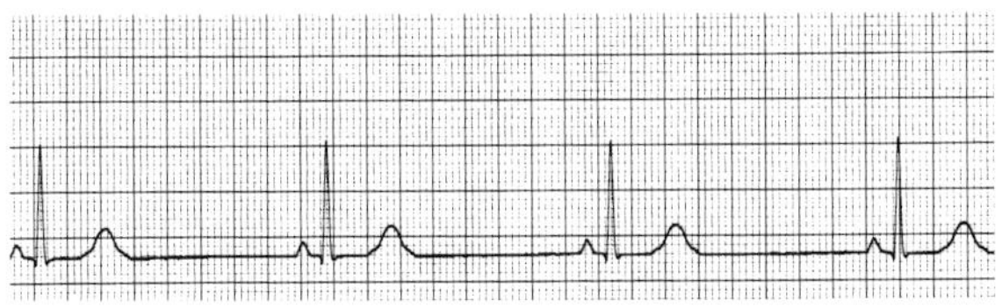

Figure 24.9 Sinus bradycardia. In this example, the heart rate is 35 beats · min^{-1}.

Sinus Tachycardia

Sinus tachycardia (HR more than 100 beats · min^{-1}) is normally seen during moderate and heavy exercise (see figure 24.10). Thus, exercise-induced sinus tachycardia is a perfectly normal condition. Resting sinus tachycardia may be seen in deconditioned people or in apprehensive patients before exercise testing. In these heart rhythms, the SA node is still functioning as the pacemaker.

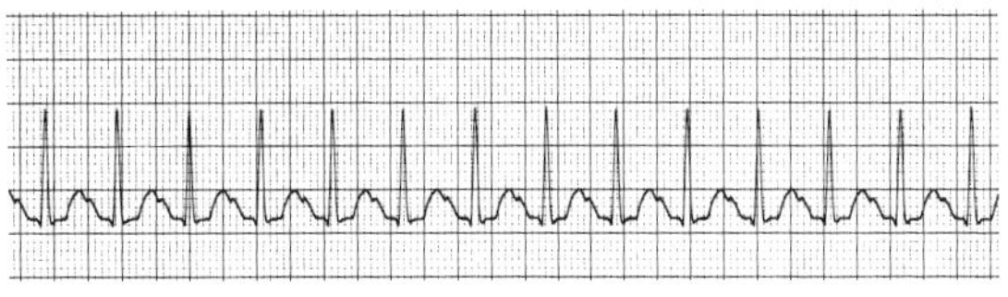

Figure 24.10 Sinus tachycardia. In this example, the heart rate is 143 beats · min^{-1}.

5 In Review

If the SA node is pacing the heart and the HR is between 60 and 100 beats · min^{-1}, the heart is in normal sinus rhythm. Bradycardia is defined as an HR less than 60 beats · min^{-1}. Tachycardia is an HR greater than 100 beats · min^{-1} (normally seen during moderate and heavy exercise).

Atrioventricular Conduction Disturbances

Atrioventricular conduction disturbances refer to a blockage of the electrical impulse at the AV node. The blockage may be either partial or complete.

First-Degree AV Block

When the P-R interval exceeds 0.20 s and all P waves result in ventricular depolarization, a **first-degree AV block** exists (see figure 24.11). Causes of a first-degree AV block can include medications such as digitalis and quinidine, infections, or vagal stimulation.

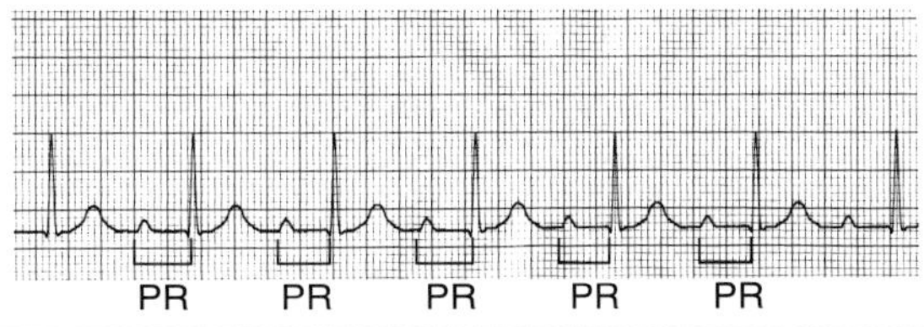

Figure 24.11 First-degree atrioventricular block. Note the prolonged P-R interval (0.28 s in this example).

Second-Degree AV Block

The main distinguishing feature of **second-degree AV block** is that some but not all P waves result in ventricular depolarization. There are two types of second-degree AV blocks: Mobitz type I and Mobitz type II. **Mobitz type I,** or Wenckebach, **AV block** is a form of second-degree AV block characterized by a progressively lengthening P-R interval until an atrial depolarization fails to initiate a ventricular depolarization and the QRS complex is skipped (see figure 24.12). This type of conduction disturbance is seen most commonly after an MI. The site of the block is within the AV node and is probably the result of reversible ischemia.

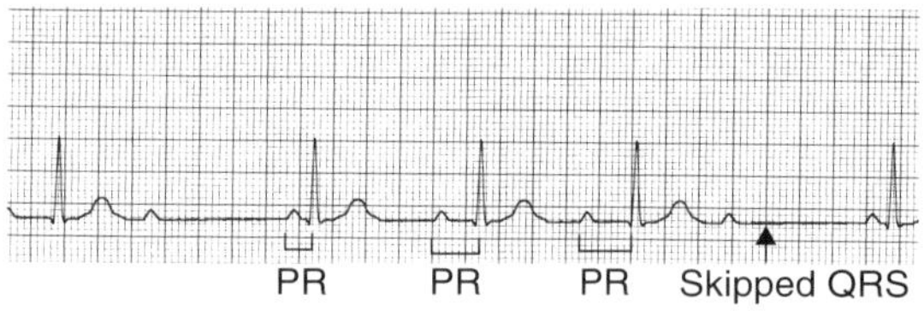

Figure 24.12 Mobitz type I (Wenckebach) atrioventricular block. There is a gradually lengthening P-R interval until finally a QRS complex is skipped.

Mobitz type II AV block is the more serious of the second-degree AV blocks, and it is characterized by atrial depolarization occasionally not resulting in ventricular depolarization with constant P-R intervals (i.e., no lengthening; see figure 24.13). The site of the block is beyond the bundle of His, and it is usually the result of irreversible ischemia of the interventricular conduction system.

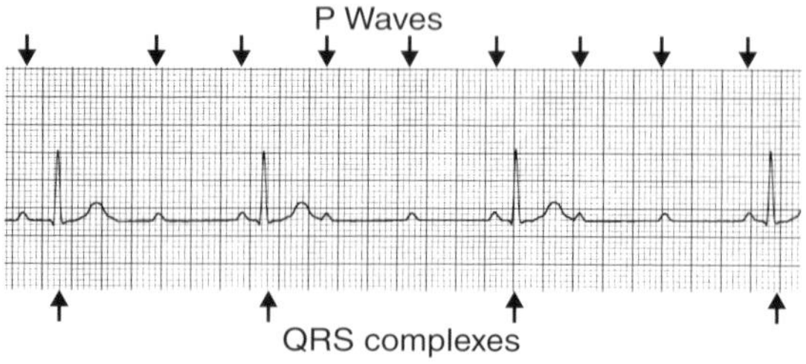

Figure 24.13 Mobitz type II atrioventricular block. Occasionally, and without lengthening of the P-R interval, QRS complexes are skipped.

Third-Degree AV Block

Third-degree AV block is present when the ventricles contract independently of the atria (see figure 24.14). The P-R interval varies and follows no regular pattern. The ventricular pacemaker may be either the AV node, the bundle of His, Purkinje fibers, or the ventricular muscle, and it will almost always result in a slow ventricular rate of less than 50 beats $\cdot$ min^{-1}.

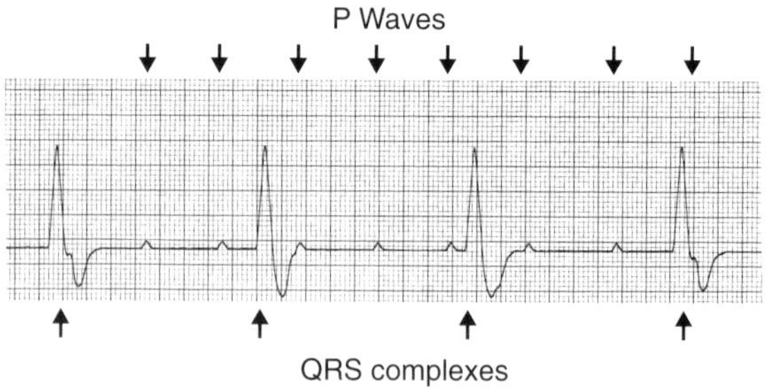

Figure 24.14 Third-degree atrioventricular block. There is no relationship between the atrial rate (e.g., 94 beats $\cdot$ min^{-1}) and the ventricular rate (e.g., 36 beats $\cdot$ min^{-1}), indicating complete blockage of the atrioventricular node.

Arrhythmias

An arrhythmia is an irregular heart beat. Arrhythmias often arise when the myocardium becomes hyperexcitable because of a lack of blood flow or the use of stimulants.

Sinus Arrhythmia

Sinus arrhythmia is a sinus rhythm in which the R-R interval varies by more than 10% beat to beat. There is a P wave before each QRS complex, but the QRS complexes are unevenly spaced. Sinus arrhythmia often is seen in highly trained subjects and occasionally in patients taking β-adrenergic receptor blocking medications. The rhythm may be associated with respiration because HR increases with inspiration and decreases with expiration.

Premature Atrial Contraction

In **premature atrial contractions,** the rhythm is irregular and the R-R interval is short between a normal sinus beat and the premature beat (see figure 24.15). The origin of the premature beat is somewhere other than the sinus node and is known as an **ectopic**

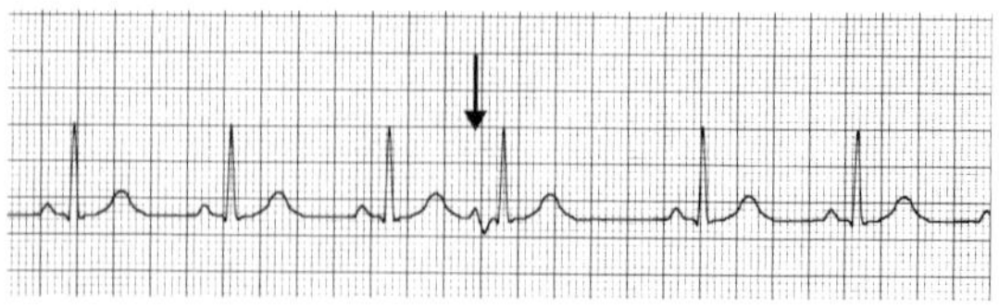

Figure 24.15 Premature atrial contraction. The arrow indicates a premature, diphasic P wave coming from an ectopic focus in the atria.

focus (an irritable spot on the myocardium that depolarizes on its own). An ectopic focus often is caused by stimulants (e.g., caffeine), antihistamines, diet pills, cold medications (e.g., ephedrine), and nicotine. Premature atrial contractions may be seen before exercise testing in apprehensive subjects.

Atrial Flutter

During **atrial flutter**, the atrial rate may be from 200 to 350 with a ventricular response of 60 to 160 beats $\cdot$ min^{-1}. The atrial rhythm is usually irregular, whereas the ventricular rhythm is either regular or irregular. The pacemaker site during atrial flutter is not the SA node but an ectopic focus, and as a result normal P waves are not present. F waves, resembling a sawtooth pattern, may be seen (see figure 24.16). The causes of atrial flutter include increased sympathetic drive, hypoxia, and congestive heart failure.

Atrial Fibrillation

During **atrial fibrillation**, the atrial rate is 400 to 700, and the ventricular rate is usually 60 to 160 beats $\cdot$ min^{-1} and is irregular. Multiple pacemaker sites are present in the atria, and P waves cannot be discerned (see figure 24.17). The significance of atrial fibrillation in an exercise testing and training setting lies in its effect on ventricular function. During atrial fibrillation, the atria and ventricles do not work together in a coordinated fashion, and the ability of the left ventricle to maintain an adequate cardiac output may be impaired. The causes of atrial fibrillation are essentially the same as those for atrial flutter.

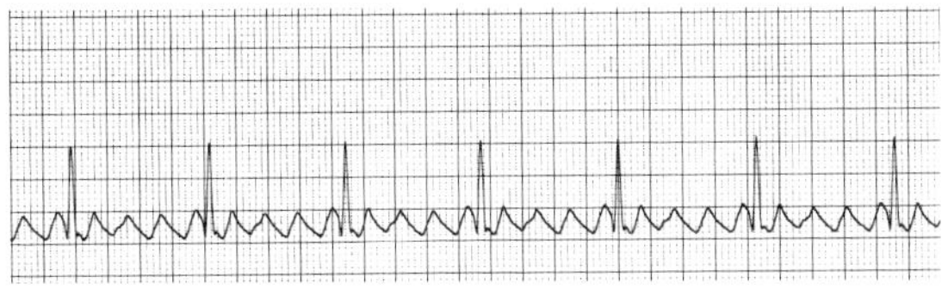

Figure 24.16 Atrial flutter. In atrial flutter, the atrial rate is 200 to 350 beats $\cdot$ min^{-1} (300 beats $\cdot$ min^{-1} in this example), but the ventricular rate is much slower.

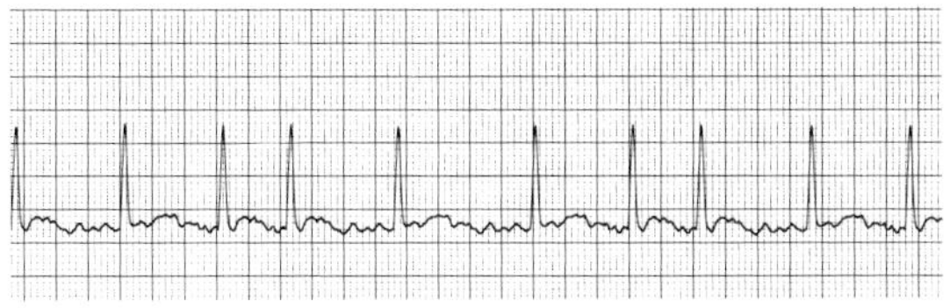

Figure 24.17 Atrial fibrillation. A jagged baseline and irregularly spaced QRS complexes are seen with atrial fibrillation.

Premature Junctional Contraction

A **premature junctional contraction (PJC)** results when an ectopic pacemaker in the AV junctional area depolarizes the ventricles. Inverted P waves frequently are seen with PJCs as the atrial depolarization proceeds in an abnormal direction (see figure 24.18). This characteristic of PJCs may allow them to be distinguished from premature atrial contractions, which frequently have diphasic P waves. If a distinction cannot be made between these two conditions, the more general term *premature supraventricular contraction* may be used to indicate an ectopic focus above the ventricles.

If the nodal tissue is still in the refractory phase after a PJC, then normally conducted waves of depolarization initiated from the sinus node will not be conducted into the ventricles and a compensatory pause will develop. PJCs usually result in a QRS complex of normal duration, or they may slightly prolong the QRS complex. PJCs may be caused by catecholamine-type medications, increased parasympathetic tone on the AV node, or damage to the AV node. PJCs are of little consequence, unless they occur very frequently (more than four to six PJCs per minute) or compromise ventricular function (9).

Although the supraventricular arrhythmias may cause concern among exercise leaders and patients, Ellestad (10) found that the long-term prognosis of CAD patients with exercise-induced supraventricular arrhythmias does not seem to be compromised. The significance of the supraventricular arrhythmias lies in the uncoupling of coordination between the atria and ventricles and the resulting effect on the ability of the ventricles to maintain an adequate cardiac output. Recurrent atrial fibrillation may have little effect on the exercise response of an individual with good left ventricular function, but it may cause significant symptoms in a person with poor ventricular function.

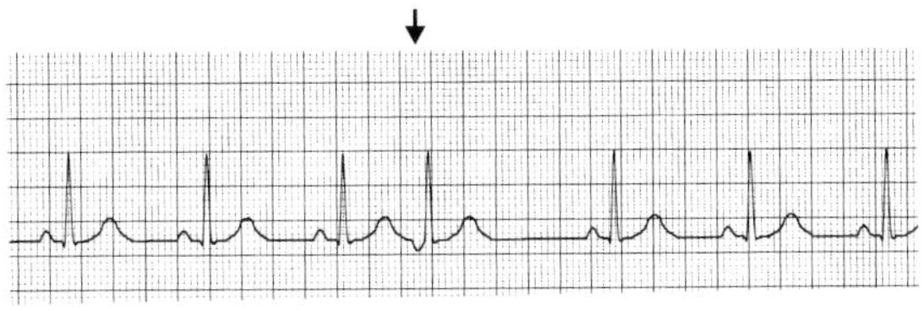

Figure 24.18 Premature junctional contraction. The arrow indicates a premature, inverted P wave coming from the AV node.

Premature Ventricular Contractions

Premature ventricular contractions (PVCs) are the result of an ectopic focus in the His-Purkinje system, which initiates a ventricular contraction. PVCs have a QRS complex that is wide (>0.12 s) and irregularly shaped (see figure 24.19). PVCs often result in the ventricles being in the refractory phase of depolarization when the normal sinus depolarization wave reaches the ventricle and a compensatory pause develops. PVCs are among the most common arrhythmias seen with exercise testing and training in CAD patients. If PVCs have the same shape, they originate from the same site (ectopic focus) and are called *unifocal*. Multiple-shape PVCs that originate from multiple sites in the ventricles are called *multifocal* and are much more serious than unifocal PVCs. The rhythm of normal contractions alternating with PVCs is called *bigeminy*; if every third contraction is a PVC, the rhythm is called *trigeminy*. Three or more consecutive PVCs are known as **ventricular tachycardia**. If a single PVC falls on the descending portion of the T wave, the "vulnerable time," the ventricles may be thrown into fibrillation. Premature ventricular contractions have an adverse effect on the prognosis of CAD patients; generally, the more complex the PVC, the more serious the problem. Ellestad (10) showed that the combination of S-T segment depression and PVCs increases the incidence of future cardiac events.

If a PVC occurs during pulse counting, patients may report that the heart "skipped a beat" and may undercount his or her HR. They should be instructed not to increase the exercise intensity in an attempt to keep the HR in the target zone as a result of skipped beats. They should immediately reduce the exercise intensity and report the appearance or increase in number of skipped beats to the exercise leader and physician.

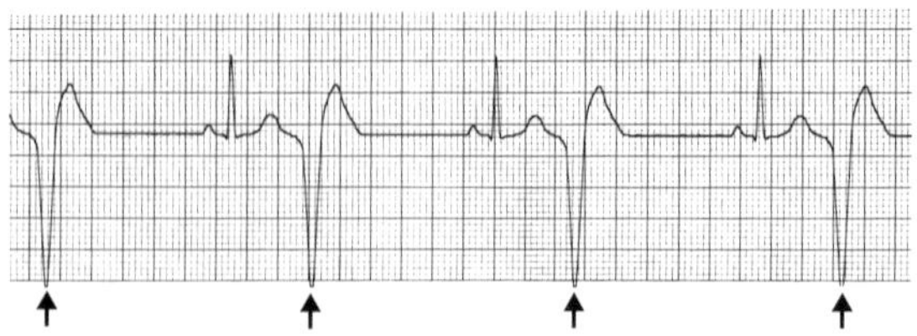

Figure 24.19 Premature ventricular contractions. The arrows indicate premature ventricular contractions coming from a single ectopic focus in the ventricles (unifocal premature ventricular contractions).

Ventricular Tachycardia

Ventricular tachycardia is present whenever three or more consecutive PVCs occur (see figure 24.20). This situation is an extremely dangerous arrhythmia that may lead to ventricular fibrillation. The rate is usually 100 to 220 beats · min^{-1}, and the heart may be unable to maintain adequate cardiac output during ventricular tachycardia. Ventricular tachycardia may be caused by the same factors that initiate PVCs; it requires immediate medical attention.

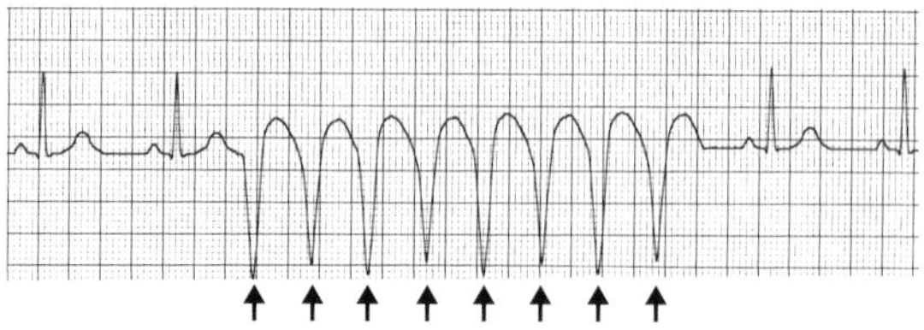

Figure 24.20 Ventricular tachycardia. A succession of three or more premature ventricular contractions in a row is seen in ventricular tachycardia.

Ventricular Fibrillation

Ventricular fibrillation is a life-threatening rhythm, and it requires immediate cardiopulmonary resuscitation until a defibrillator can be used to restore a coordinated ventricular contraction; otherwise, death will result. A fibrillating heart contracts in an unorganized, quivering manner, and the heart is unable to maintain significant cardiac output. P waves and QRS complexes are not discernible; instead the electrical pattern is a fibrillatory wave (see figure 24.21).

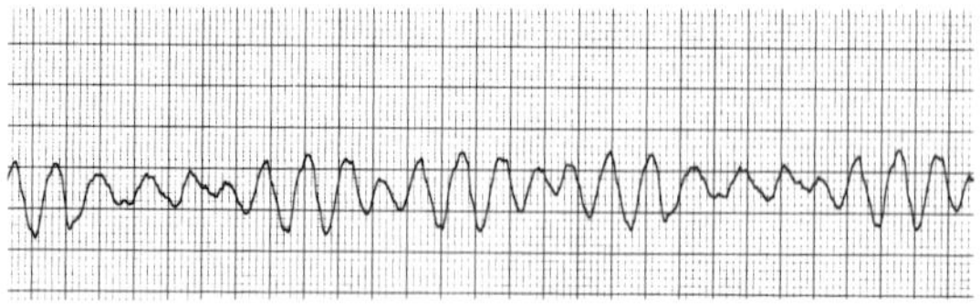

Figure 24.21 Ventricular fibrillation. When there are no discernible P waves or QRS complexes, the heart contracts in a disorganized, quivering manner.

6 In Review

The ECG can be used to detect various conduction disturbances in the electrical conducting system of the heart such as first-, second-, or third-degree AV block. The ECG also can be used to detect arrhythmias (abnormal heart rhythms) including sinus arrhythmia, premature beats, tachycardia, flutter, and fibrillation. Abnormal rhythms may limit exercise performance by decreasing cardiac output. In the case of severe arrhythmias, the HFI should terminate the exercise session and obtain immediate medical assistance.

Automated External Defibrillators

Defibrillators are devices used to treat ventricular fibrillation. They work by sending a momentary electrical shock to the heart, often causing the heart to return to its normal rhythm. Recent advances in technology have permitted the development of portable, battery-powered devices called automated external defibrillators (AEDs). The operator applies two surface electrodes to the person's chest. These electrodes are connected to the AED, which has computer software that is capable of determining the person's heart rhythm. If ventricular fibrillation is detected, the AED gives a command to stand clear and then signals the operator to deliver a shock by pushing a button. Police, fitness instructors, flight attendants, and even laypersons are being trained to use AEDs, by organizations such as the AHA and the American Red Cross. Research studies have shown that the use of AEDs hastens response time and greatly improves one's chances of survival (3).

Myocardial Ischemia

Myocardial ischemia is a lack of oxygen in the myocardium attributable to inadequate blood flow. Obstruction of the coronary arteries is the most common cause of myocardial ischemia. A coronary artery is significantly obstructed if more than 50% of the diameter is occluded. A 50% reduction in diameter is equal to a loss of 75% of the arterial lumen (12). An obstructed coronary artery may be able to supply an adequate blood flow at rest, but it will probably be unable to provide enough blood and oxygen during periods of increased demand such as during exercise. Ischemia often, but not always, results in angina pectoris.

Angina pectoris is defined as pain/discomfort caused by temporary, reversible ischemia of the myocardium that does not result in death or infarction of heart muscle. The pain often is located in the center of the chest, but pain may occur in the neck, jaw, or shoulders or may radiate into the arms and hands. Angina pectoris tends to be reproducible; patients often report they get anginal symptoms at roughly the same level of exertion. During exercise, a patient experiencing anginal discomfort may deny pain, but on further questioning, the individual will admit to the sensation of burning, tightness, pressure, or heaviness in the chest or arms. Patients frequently confuse angina pectoris with musculoskeletal pain and with the discomfort resulting from the sternal incision of coronary artery bypass surgery. Anginal pain generally is not altered by movements of the trunk or arms, whereas musculoskeletal pain may be decreased or increased by trunk or arm movement. Discomfort is probably not angina if the pain changes in quality or intensity when you press on the affected area (12).

Myocardial ischemia may cause **S-T segment depression** on the ECG during an exercise test. S-T segment depression usually occurs at a relatively constant double product. The double product equals the HR times SBP, and it is a good estimate of the amount of work the heart is doing. Three types of S-T segment depression are recognized: up-sloping, horizontal, and down-sloping (figure 24.22). Ellestad (10) and coworkers have shown the prognostic implications of up-sloping and horizontal S-T segment depression to be roughly similar. Down-sloping S-T segment depression, however, has a more adverse impact on survival.

S-T segment elevation also may occur during exercise testing. S-T segment elevation during an exercise test usually indicates the development of an **aneurysm**, or a weakened area of noncontracting myocardium or scar tissue.

Myocardial Infarction

If the myocardium is deprived of oxygen for a sufficient length of time, a portion of the myocardium dies; this is known as a myocardial infarction, or MI. Pain is the hallmark symptom of an MI. It is often very similar to anginal pain, only more severe, and may be described as a heavy feeling, a squeezing in the chest, or a burning sensation. Other symptoms that may accompany an MI are nausea, sweating, and shortness of breath.

S-T segment elevation is often the first ECG sign of an acute MI. Later, pronounced Q waves and T wave inversion may appear in certain leads. Over

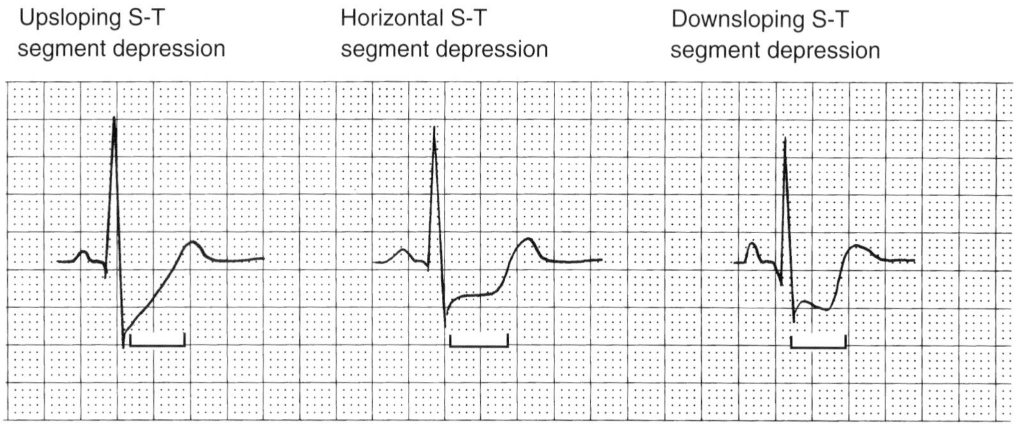

Figure 24.22 S-T segment depression.

time, the S-T segment changes subside and the T wave returns to normal (see figure 24.23) (18). Other clinical signs of an acute MI include elevations in cardiac muscle enzymes (serum lactate dehydrogenase and creatine phosphokinase), which leak into the blood after the myocardium is damaged (12).

Information from the Framingham Heart Study indicates that up to 25% of MIs may be "silent infarctions," meaning that the infarction does not cause sufficient symptoms for the victim to seek medical attention (13). These silent infarctions may be recognized later during routine ECG examinations by the presence of significant Q waves in certain leads.

CAD patients should be instructed how to differentiate anginal attacks from possible MIs. If an

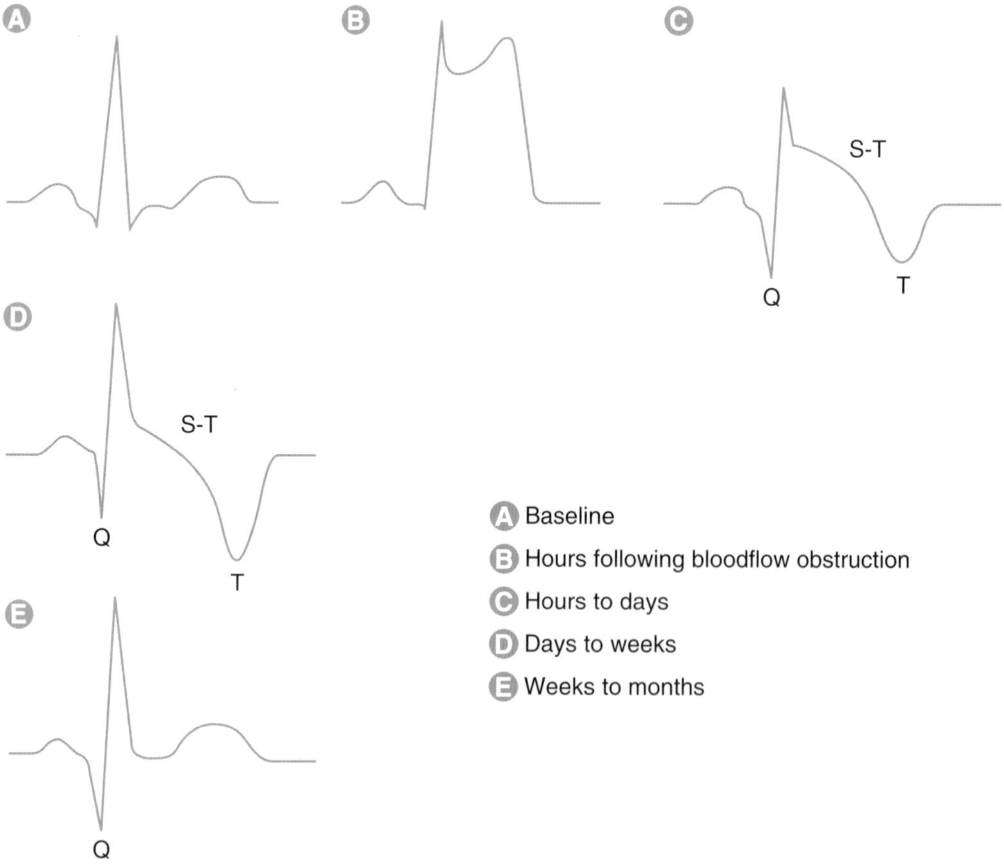

Figure 24.23 Evolution of ECG changes after obstruction of a coronary artery.

Reprinted from Stein, 2000, *Rapid analysis of electrocardiograms: A self-study program*, 3rd ed. By permission of Lea & Febiger.

anginal attack occurs, the patient should stop the activity, if any, that precipitated the discomfort and take a nitroglycerin (NTG) tablet under the tongue. If the anginal discomfort persists after 5 min, a second sublingual NTG tablet is taken. This procedure is repeated, if needed, for a total of three NTG tablets. If the pain persists 5 min after the third NTG tablet, the patient should seek immediate medical attention (4).

7 In Review

An inadequate blood flow to the myocardium often results in symptoms of chest pain (angina pectoris), but this is not always the case. The presence of S-T segment depression or elevation on the ECG can indicate inadequate blood flow (ischemia). The presence of significant Q waves on the ECG can indicate that a portion of the heart muscle has died (MI).

Cardiovascular Medications

A wide variety of medications are used to treat people with heart disease. Some medications control blood pressure, whereas others control heart rate or rhythm; still others affect the force of contraction of the ventricles. Other drugs likely to be encountered by the HFI include medications to control blood glucose concentrations, medications for patients with hyperlipidemia to control abnormal blood lipid levels, and bronchodilators for individuals with asthma. The HFI will not prescribe medications or deal on a day-to-day basis with patients taking these medications, but he or she eventually will encounter participants taking some of these medications. The purpose of this section is to summarize the major classes of drugs, describe how they affect the exercise HR response, and indicate possible side effects.

β-Adrenergic Blockers

β-adrenergic blocking medications (β-blockers) are commonly prescribed for patients with CAD, for those with hypertension, and occasionally for patients with migraine headaches. All of these medications compete with epinephrine and norepinephrine for the limited number of **β-adrenergic receptors**. β-blockers are generally used to reduce the HR and vigor of myocardial contraction, thus reducing the oxygen requirement of the heart. Because of the effect these medications have on submaximal and maximal HR, β-blockers have a profound impact on exercise prescription. Subjects should be tested on β-blockers if they will be training while taking these medications. All β-blockers lower HR at rest and particularly during exercise, as seen in figure 24.24.

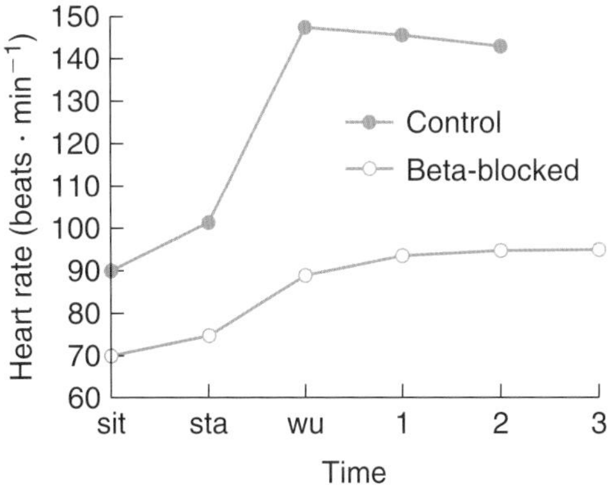

Figure 24.24 The heart rate before and after β-blockade (two days of 40 mg of Inderal per day) in a very apprehensive patient during treadmill testing; sit = sitting, sta = standing, wu = warm-up at 1.0 mph, 0% grade. Minutes 1 and 2 are 2.0 mph, 0% grade. Minute 3 is 2.0 mph and 3.5% grade.

Two types of β-adrenergic receptors are recognized: β_1 and β_2. β_1 receptors are found mainly in the heart, and β_2 receptors are located primarily in the smooth muscle in the lungs, arterioles, intestine, uterus, and bladder. Some β-blockers selectively block the β_1 receptors in the heart. The β_1-selective (cardioselective) blockers include Sectral, Tenormin, Brevibloc, and Lopressor. Other β-blockers are less selective and act on the β_1 and β_2 receptors. The less specific (nonselective) β-blockers include Inderal, Corgard, Visken, and Blocadren. An undesirable side effect of the nonselective β-blockers is contraction of the smooth muscle surrounding the airways in the lungs and reduction of the airway lumen, which increases the work of breathing. This can result in labored breathing, shortness of breath, and other asthma-like symptoms.

Indications for the use of β-blockers include hypertension, angina pectoris, and supraventricular arrhythmias. In addition, as previously mentioned, some β-blockers are used to treat migraine headaches. As a general rule, nonselective β-blocking medications are not recommended for use in patients with asthma, bronchitis, or similar lung problems. β-blocking medications may also blunt some of the symptoms of hypoglycemia in insulin-dependent diabetics, an undesirable side effect (4).

The use of Inderal and presumably other β-blocking medications does not invalidate the THR method of prescribing exercise intensity. Hossack, Bruce, and Clark (11) showed that the regression equations relating %HRmax to %$\dot{V}O_2$max are similar in β-adrenergic blocked and nonblocked CAD patients. Thus, it is assumed that the THR method of exercise prescription is valid if the patient's measured HRmax is determined while he or she is on β-blocking medications.

Because β-blockers lower HRmax, the use of these medications invalidates estimating THR based on taking 70 to 85% of age-adjusted, predicted HRmax (predicted HRmax = 220 – age). For example, a 40-year-old individual has a predicted HRmax of about 180, with an estimated 70 to 85% THR of 126 to 153 beats · min^{-1}. If this individual were given a β-blocker, HRmax could easily be reduced to 150 beats · min^{-1}. If the estimated THR of 126 to 153 beats · min^{-1} were used for training, this individual could be training at HRmax. Measurement of HRmax is required to calculate an appropriate THR for anyone taking β-blockers, and testing should be repeated after any change in β-blocking medicines.

There has been some question as to whether the use of β-blocking medicines reduces or blocks the effectiveness of endurance training. In general, work capacity and endurance training effects are impaired to a greater extent after nonselective β-blockade than selective β_1-blockade (19). Ades and coworkers (1) examined the effects of endurance training in 30 hypertensive adults taking either placebo, metoprolol (a β_1-selective blocker) or propranolol (a nonselective β-blocker). $\dot{V}O_2$max increased 24% in the placebo group and 8% in the metoprolol group but did not increase in the propranolol group. Pavia and coworkers (17) found that chronic use of β_1-selective blocker (metoprolol) in postmyocardial patients did not interfere with the typical endurance training effects. They observed similar increases in $\dot{V}O_2$peak in patients taking metoprolol and those who were not on β-blockers.

Nitrates

The **nitrates** exist in several forms including patches, ointments, long-acting tablets, and sublingual tablets, and they are used to prevent or stop attacks of angina pectoris. This class of compounds is produced from amyl nitrate (a volatile agent), which is rendered nonexplosive by adding an inert chemical such as lactose. The physiological mechanism of action is relaxation of vascular smooth muscle. Nitrate preparations relax venous smooth muscle, which reduces venous return and the quantity of blood the heart has to pump. Arterial smooth muscle is also relaxed, although to a lesser degree than venous smooth muscle, thus reducing the peripheral vascular resistance against which the heart has to pump. Both of these actions help reduce the work and oxygen requirement of the heart. Many patients use NTG on a 24-hr basis with ointment or patches. Longer-acting tablet forms of NTG (Isordil, Sorbitrate, Dilatrate) may be taken before activities that are likely to provoke anginal attacks, whereas sublingual tablets (Nitrostat) are used to treat acute anginal episodes. Headaches, dizziness, and hypotension are the main side effects of NTG use (4). β-adrenergic blocking medications may potentiate the hypotensive actions of NTG.

Calcium Channel Blockers (Calcium Antagonists)

The **calcium channel blockers** currently include verapamil (Isoptin), nifedipine (Procardia), and diltiazem (Cardizem). These drugs interfere with the slow calcium currents during depolarization in cardiac and vascular smooth muscle. Verapamil is used primarily to treat atrial and ventricular arrhythmias, whereas nifedipine and diltiazem are used to treat exertional angina and variant angina pectoris, or angina pectoris attacks that occur at rest (4).

The effects of calcium channel blockers on exercise prescription and training have been studied. Chang and Hossack (6) showed that the regression equations relating %HRmax and %$\dot{V}O_2$max are the same in patients taking diltiazem and nonmedicated patients. Isoptin and Procardia are assumed not to alter the relationship between %HRmax and %$\dot{V}O_2$max. Calcium antagonists are not thought to affect endurance training adversely in healthy subjects or CAD patients (15). MacGowan and coworkers (16) showed that verapamil does not diminish training responses in healthy, young subjects.

Antiarrhythmic Medications

Some of the more commonly used **antiarrhythmics** include Pronestyl, Norpace, Cardioquin, Quinaglute, Tambocor, Sectral, Cordarone, Tonocard, and the digitalis preparations. The β-blocking medications also are used to treat some types of arrhythmias. With the exception of the β-blockers, these medications will have little influence on the HR response to exercise; in fact, the reduction in arrhythmias may improve work capacity.

Digitalis Preparations

The **digitalis** medications are used to increase the vigor of myocardial contractions (contractility) and treat atrial flutter and fibrillation (4). In individuals with poor ventricular function, the increased contractility resulting from digitalis preparations may increase work capacity. Digitalis medications are marketed under several trade names including Lanoxin, Lanoxicaps, Purodigin, and Crystodigin. Cardiac side effects of the digitalis group include premature ventricular contractions, Wenckebach AV block, and atrial tachycardia. Digitalis drugs can cause false-positive tests due to S-T segment depression during exercise testing (9). The side effects of the digitalis drugs can be potentiated by quinidine sulfate.

Antihypertensives

The **antihypertensives** can be broken down into five groups according to the mechanism of action. Drugs in the first group, *diuretics*, work by increasing the excretion of electrolytes and water. Drugs in this group include Lasix, Diamox, Diuril, Esidrix, Enduron, Hydrodiuril, and many others. This group is often used as the first treatment for hypertension. Side effects of these medications include hypokalemia, or low blood levels of potassium. Hypokalemia can induce arrhythmias and is a potentially serious problem. Diuretic-induced hypokalemia often can be prevented by increasing consumption of citrus fruits, which are high in potassium. If dietary sources of potassium prove to be ineffective, a prescription potassium supplement (K-Tab, Kay Ceil, or Slo-K) can be used (4). Alternatively, a potassium-sparing diuretic (Midamor, Aldactone, Dyrenium) can be prescribed.

The second group of antihypertensive medications are the *antiadrenergic agents*. These include drugs with the principal action at the central nervous system level, such as clonidine (Catapres) and methyldopa (Aldomet), which reduce sympathetic outflow from the brain. This group also includes drugs that act principally on α-adrenergic receptors to reduce peripheral vascular resistance, such as prazosin (Minipress). In addition, this group includes those drugs that block β-adrenergic receptors (see previous section) to reduce cardiac output, renin release, and sympathetic outflow from the brain.

The diuretics and the β-blockers have the important metabolic side effect of elevating triglyceride and cholesterol levels and impairing glucose and insulin metabolism. Thus, although they effectively lower BP and reduce the incidence of stroke and of severe kidney disease, they have a less-than-predicted effect on reducing the incidence of heart attacks.

The third group of antihypertensive medications are the *vasodilators*. These medications decrease BP by relaxing vascular smooth muscle. Some of the brand names in this category are Apresoline, Vasodilan, and Loniten. Side effects associated with these medications include hypotension, dizziness, and tachycardia. The active chemical in Loniten is also marketed under the name Rogaine in the form of a topical solution for use as a hair growth stimulant in male pattern baldness. Rogaine has little or no antihypertensive effect.

The fourth group of antihypertensive medications work through the renin-angiotensin system. These drugs lower BP by inhibiting angiotensin-converting enzyme (ACE), which converts angiotensin I to angiotensin II. They are called *ACE inhibitors* for that reason. Some of the brand names in this category are Vasotec, Zestril, and Capoten. The ACE inhibitors are expensive, and they may produce a dry cough in 5 to 10% of patients. They have the advantages of decreasing left ventricular hypertrophy, decreasing proteinuria in diabetic patients, and maintaining blood lipid levels.

The fifth group of antihypertensive medications are the *calcium antagonists* (calcium channel blockers; see previous page). As with the ACE inhibitors, drugs in this class do not have adverse effects on lipid, glucose, and insulin metabolism.

Lipid-Lowering Medications

The lipid-lowering medications (Questran and Colestid; Pravachol, Zocor, and Lescol; Lopid and Atromid-S; and nicotinic acid) are used to lower cholesterol and triglycerides in individuals who are unable to adequately control lipids through diet and exercise. These lipid-lowering medications are unlikely to have any substantial effects on exercise testing or training. Patients taking these medications need to be closely followed by their physician because of potential toxic effects on the liver by some of these drugs. Some lipid-lowering agents (Lopid, Atromid-S) can potentiate the effects of anticoagulants and make participants in exercise programs more susceptible to bruising.

Anticoagulants

The **anticoagulants** are used to delay the clotting process. Oral anticoagulants include Dicumarol and Coumadin. These medications are unlikely to have any direct effect on exercise testing or training, but they do increase the risk of bruising. Aspirin and some other medications (e.g., nonsteroidal anti-inflammatory drugs such as Motrin, Advil, and Nuprin) can potentiate the action of anticoagulants and increase the risk of bruising with minimal trauma.

Nicotine Gums and Patches

Nicotine gums and patches are used as smoking substitutes for individuals who are trying to stop smoking. With **nicotine gum** the nicotine is absorbed through the oral mucosa, providing sufficient plasma nicotine concentrations to curb the craving to smoke. Nicotine gums are marketed under the names Bantron and Nicorette. With transdermal nicotine patches, the nicotine is absorbed through the skin. Nicotine may affect the exercise response, particularly if a person still smokes and chews nicotine gum concurrently. Nicotine may increase heart rate and blood pressure as well as the incidence of cardiac arrhythmias (2).

Bronchodilators

The **bronchodilators** are used to relax smooth muscle surrounding airways in the lungs and relieve the symptoms of asthma, bronchitis, and related lung disorders. These medications can be taken orally or from an inhaler. The inhalers are generally used for acute asthma episodes, whereas long-term bronchodilation is usually obtained with oral preparations. Most of these drugs stimulate the β_2 receptors that relax bronchial smooth muscle and increase the airway lumen. Because of their β-adrenergic stimulating effect, these medications can increase HR and BP, although most of their effect is focused on the smooth muscle found in airways. Some of the inhaler brand names include Brethaire Inhaler, Ventolin, Alupent, Maxair, and others. The oral bronchodilators include Theobid, Aminophyllin, Theo-Dur, and many others (4).

Oral Antiglycemic Agents

A substantial number of obese participants in fitness programs have hyperglycemia, or elevated levels of blood glucose. In this condition the pancreas is able to produce insulin, but it is unable to produce sufficient quantities to maintain normal blood glucose control. This condition is called non-insulin-dependent diabetes mellitus; often this condition can be controlled with **oral antiglycemic agents**. The oral antiglycemic medications work by stimulating the pancreas to secrete more insulin, which facilitates tissue uptake of glucose. The stimulating action of the oral antiglycemic medications requires a functioning pancreas. Brand names of the oral antiglycemic agents include Diabeta, Diabinese, Glucotrol, Micronase, Orinase, and Tolinase. These drugs are in the sulfonylurea class (4). Recently, a new type of oral antiglycemic drug has become available (Glucophage, in the metformin class). Metformin's principal effect is to reduce insulin resistance, thereby lowering blood sugar. A serious side effect of these drugs is hypoglycemia or low blood sugar. Hypoglycemia is potentially dangerous, and the HFI should be cognizant of any changes in alertness and orientation in patients taking any medication that can lower plasma glucose concentrations.

Insulin-dependent diabetes mellitus is a more serious disorder of carbohydrate metabolism. Insulin-dependent diabetes mellitus is characterized by an absence of insulin and requires frequent insulin injections. Insulin cannot be taken orally because it is a protein and would be inactivated by the digestive process. When working with an insulin-dependent diabetic who is taking insulin, the HFI should be aware of the possibility of hypoglycemia. Signs of hypoglycemia include bizarre behavior and slurred speech. When individuals with insulin-dependent diabetes mellitus are exercising, it is a good idea to have a source of sugar readily available in the event of a hypoglycemic episode. See chapter 19 for additional details on the diabetic.

Depressants

Tranquilizers are sometimes prescribed to reduce anxiety. Minor tranquilizers may lower HR and BP by controlling anxiety, but otherwise the exercise response is not affected. With major tranquilizers, HR may be increased while BP is either reduced or unchanged (2). **Alcohol** is a depressant that can affect the exercise test by impairing motor coordination, balance, and reaction times. Chronic alcohol consumption tends to elevate resting and exercise BP. The acute effects of alcohol ingestion on the exercise response have been examined. During brief maximal exercise, small to moderate doses of alcohol exert no significant effect on oxygen uptake, stroke volume, ejection fraction, cardiac output, arteriovenous oxygen difference, and peak lactate concentration (20). However, with higher doses (blood alcohol content = 0.20 mg/dl), myocardial function may be impaired, as shown by a 6% decrease in ejection fraction (14). Alcohol intake can provoke arrhythmias at rest and during exercise.

8 In Review

Medications are prescribed for a variety of reasons: high BP, abnormal heart rhythms, elevated blood lipids, asthma, and other medical concerns. Appendix D summarizes the common categories of prescription medicines for cardiovascular and related diseases, some of the members of each category, and the impact on exercise performance.

Case Studies

You can check your answers by referring to appendix A.

24.1

The following ECG tracing (see Case Study figure 24.1) was obtained on a 38-year-old female before undergoing a GXT on the treadmill.

a. Determine the HR (beats · min^{-1}) and the durations of the P-R interval, QRS complex, and Q-T interval (seconds).

b. What condition does she have?

c. What factors might be responsible for this condition?

24.2

A 21-year-old male college student, taking a cold medication containing ephedrine, showed the following ECG tracing at rest (see Case Study figure 24.2).

a. What type of arrhythmia does he have?

b. What is the ventricular rate?

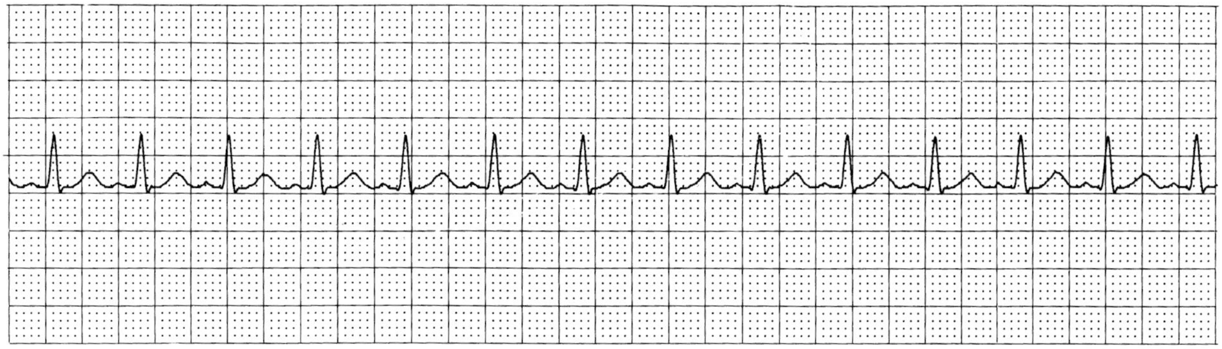

Case Study Figure 24.1

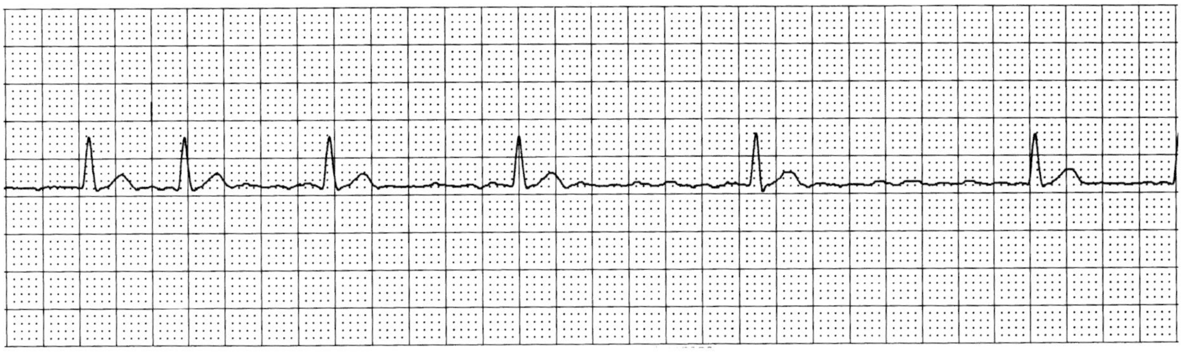

Case Study Figure 24.2

24.3

A 57-year-old participant in your exercise program showed the following ECG tracing (see Case Study figure 24.3) while she was exercising at 3.5 miles per hour (6% grade) on the treadmill.

a. What ECG abnormality is shown here?
b. What action should be taken?

24.4

A 55-year-old, apparently healthy male is referred to your facility for an exercise program and brings with him the results of his most recent exercise test. You notice that the participant was taking Coumadin and Inderal when he took his exercise test. Since the test, his physician has stopped the Inderal. What impact, if any, would this change in medication make on the exercise prescription? (See appendix D.)

24.5

A participant in your exercise program has been taking a β-blocking medication for several years without experiencing any significant side effects. He was recently given a prescription for Isordil and now reports that he often becomes dizzy upon standing suddenly. Could this be related to his medication? If so, why? (See appendix D.)

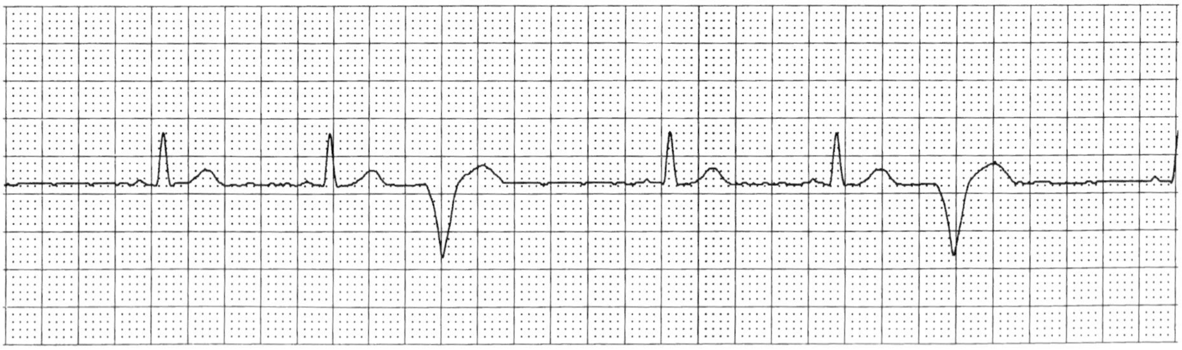

Case Study Figure 24.3

Source List

1. Ades, P.A., Gunter, P.G., Meyer, W.L., Gibson, T.C., Maddalena, J., & Orfeo, T. (1990). Cardiac and skeletal muscle adaptations to training in systemic hypertension and effect of beta blockade (metoprolol or propranolol). *American Journal of Cardiology, 166*(5), 591-596.
2. American College of Sports Medicine. (2000). *Guidelines for exercise testing and prescription* (6th ed.). Baltimore: Lippincott Williams & Wilkins.
3. American College of Sports Medicine and American Heart Association. (2002). Joint position statement: Automated external defibrillators in health/fitness facilities. *Medicine and Science in Sports and Exercise,*34(3), 561-564.
4. American Hospital Formulary Service. (2001). *Drug information 2001.* Bethesda, MD: American Society of Hospital Pharmacists.
5. Berne, R.M., & Levy, M.N. (2001). *Cardiovascular physiology* (8th ed.). St. Louis: Mosby.
6. Chang, K., & Hossack, K.F. (1982). Effect of diltiazem on heart rate responses and respiratory variables during exercise: Implications for exercise prescription and cardiac rehabilitation. *Journal of Cardiac Rehabilitation, 2,* 326-332.
7. Conover, M.B. (1996). *Understanding electrocardiography* (7th ed.). St. Louis: Mosby.
8. Donnelly, J.E. (1990). *Living anatomy* (2nd ed.). Champaign, IL: Human Kinetics.
9. Dubin, D. (2000). *Rapid interpretation of EKGs* (6th ed.). Tampa, FL: Cover.
10. Ellestad, M. (1994). *Stress testing: Principles and practice.* Philadelphia: Davis.
11. Hossack, K.F., Bruce, R.A., & Clark, L.J. (1980). Influence of propranolol on exercise prescription of training heart rates. *Cardiology, 65,* 47-58.
12. Hurst, J.W. (1994). *Diagnostic atlas of the heart.* Philadelphia: Lippincott-Raven.
13. Kannel, W.B., & Abbot, R.D. (1984). Incidence and prognosis of unrecognized myocardial infarction. *New England Journal of Medicine, 311,* 1144-1147.
14. Kelbaek, H., Gjorup, T., Floistrup, S., Hartling, O., Christensen, N., & Godtfredsen, J. (1985). Acute effects of alcohol on left ventricular function in healthy subjects at rest and during upright exercise. *American Journal of Cardiology, 55,* 164-167.
15. Kinderman, W. (1987). Calcium antagonists and exercise performance. *Sports Medicine, 4*(3), 177-193.
16. MacGowan, G.A., O'Callaghan, D., & Horgan, J.H. (1992). The effects of verapamil on training in patients with ischemic heart disease. *Chest, 101*(2), 411-415.
17. Pavia, L., Orlando, G., Myers, J., Maestri, M., & Rusconi, C. (1995). The effect of beta-blockade therapy on the response to exercise training in postmyocardial infarction patients. *Clinical Cardiology, 18*(12), 716-720.
18. Stein, E. (2000). *Rapid analysis of electrocardiograms: A self-study program* (3rd ed.). Philadelphia: Lea & Febiger.
19. Tesch, P.A. (1985). Exercise performance and beta-blockade. *Sports Medicine, 2*(6), 389-412.
20. Williams, M.H. (1991). Alcohol, marijuana and beta blockers. In D.R. Lamb & M.H. Williams (Eds.), *Perspectives in exercise science and sports medicine: Vol. 4. Ergogenics: Enhancement of performance in exercise and sport* (331-372). Dubuque, IA: Brown & Benchmark.

twenty-five

Injury Prevention and Treatment

Sue Carver

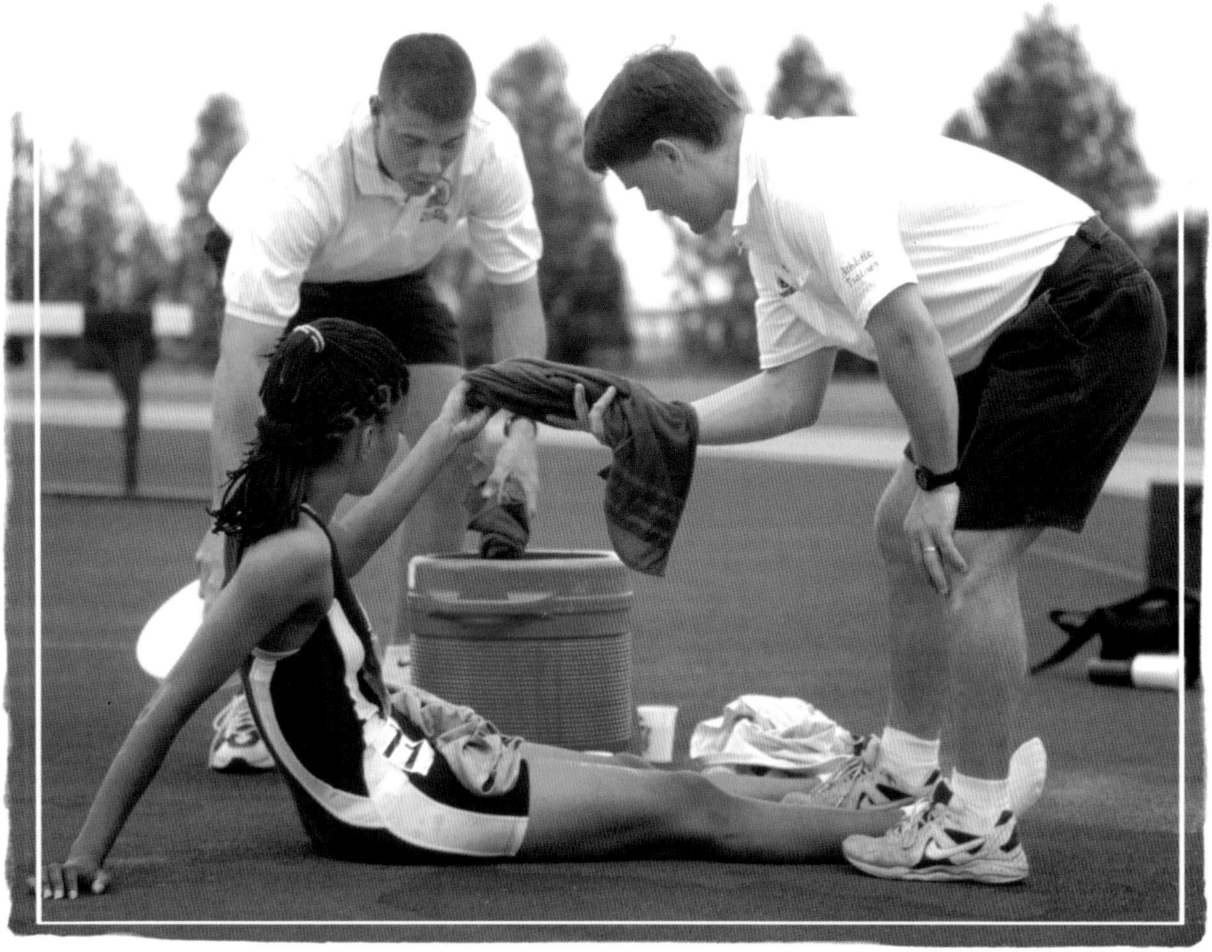

© Human Kinetics

Objectives

The reader will be able to do the following:

1. Describe ways to minimize injury risk and prevent the transmission of bloodborne pathogens.
2. Describe the signs and symptoms of soft-tissue injuries (sprains, strains, contusions, and heel bruises), how to initially treat injuries, and when to use heat in long-term treatment.
3. Identify signs, symptoms, and proper treatment measures for bone injuries, wounds, and common skin irritations.
4. Describe the causes of heat-related disorders, how to prevent heat illness, and how to treat a heat-related emergency; and provide guidelines for fluid replacement before and after exercise.
5. Explain the causes of cold-related disorders and how to prevent frostnip, superficial and deep frostbite, and hypothermia; and how to treat a cold-related emergency.
6. Distinguish between the signs and symptoms of diabetic coma and those of insulin shock; describe the proper treatment for each.
7. Identify common cardiovascular and pulmonary complications resulting from participation in exercise.
8. Identify the signs, symptoms, and management of common orthopedic problems; classify injuries as mild, moderate, and severe; and recommend appropriate modification of exercise programs when injury occurs.
9. Describe procedures to check vital signs.
10. Describe artificial respiration and cardiopulmonary techniques for adults.

The HFI must be prepared to safely handle an emergency medical situation. This chapter will discuss injury prevention, injury recognition, and common treatment approaches as well as planning for and handling a medical emergency.

Preventing Injuries

Certain inherent risks are associated with participation in physical activity. The HFI should be aware of those risks and take steps to control factors that increase the risk of injury. Advanced planning, training in injury recognition and emergency care, adequate equipment and facilities, and counseling in the selection of activities all help to reduce the possibility of injury. The following is a brief discussion of the factors contributing to injury and steps that can be taken to reduce injury risk (2-7, 9-14, 16, 18, 22, 23).

Controlling Injury Risk

Injury risk in competitive athletic events is controlled by game rules. In exercise programs where games are used for aerobic activity, injury risk may be reduced by controlling the tempo of the activity or by modifying existing rules to enhance participant safety (e.g., limiting body contact, using a softer ball).

The HFI should encourage participants to seek professional advice regarding the selection and fitting of proper equipment. The equipment most commonly used, and most widely abused, is footwear. Inadequate protection of the foot is a major contributor to a variety of leg and low back problems. Improperly maintained exercise equipment and facilities also contribute to higher overall injury risk.

In this age of concern over bloodborne pathogens such as the **human immunodeficiency virus (HIV)** and **hepatitis B virus (HBV)**, precautions should be taken to protect both the participant and the HFI. Open cuts should be covered, and clothing that is blood-saturated should be changed. Necessary supplies should be available to care safely for an open wound, including latex gloves, biohazard containers, antiseptic solution, dressings, disinfectant, and a sharps container if applicable. Participants should be instructed to report all wounds immediately. The HFI should be instructed in **universal precaution** guidelines for management of acute blood exposure as well as appropriate cleaning and disposal policies for contaminated areas.

Factors Contributing to Injury

Activity implies movement, and with increased movement comes a corresponding increase in the risk of injury. In fitness programs, the frequency of injuries increases when the frequency of the exercise sessions increases and when the intensity of the exercise is maintained at the high end of the THR zone (figure 25.1). The risk of injury is also heightened by increased speed of movement, as found in competitive activities; in activities requiring quick changes in direction (e.g., fitness games); and in activities that focus on smaller muscle groups. Environmental conditions such as extreme heat or cold can also increase the risk associated with physical activity. Lack of proper adaptation to the environment, as well as lack of education in prevention, recognition, and treatment of problems associated with these extreme environments, can lead to devastating results.

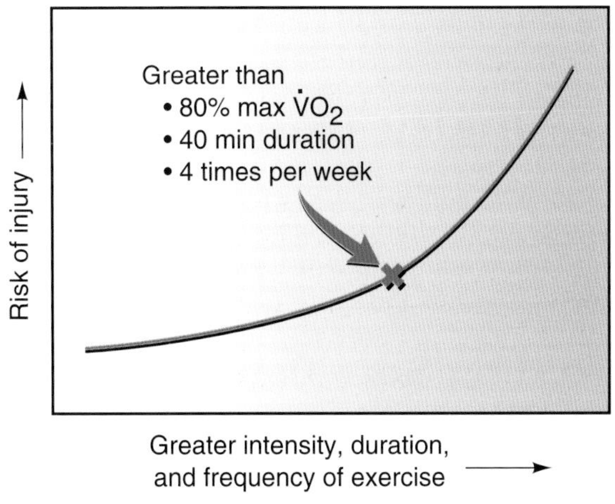

Figure 25.1 Increased risk of injury with too much activity.

Age, sex, and body structure influence the risk of injury. In general, very young and very old people are at the greatest risk, and older individuals usually require longer periods of time for recovery. Because of body structure and strength differences, females are often more susceptible to injury in coed activities and games requiring quick changes of direction and/or body contact. For either males or females, a lack or an imbalance of muscle strength, a lack of joint flexibility, and poor CRF increase the chance of injury. Obese individuals may not only have low CRF, but the excess weight places additional stress on weight-bearing joints. Individuals with specific medical problems such as asthma, diabetes, or known allergic reactions may need special attention to avoid potentially serious complications.

Reducing Injury Risk

Screening participants before any physical activity program can help to reduce injury risk. The screening should highlight the major areas that increase health risk. Proper screening assists the participant in recognizing problems and alerts the HFI to potential problems that could occur in an exercise session (e.g., asthma attack, diabetic shock). Proper planning for emergency situations contributes to a low overall risk. Individuals who cannot be properly supervised or given adequate care as a result of their physical problems should be referred to a program or facility that can provide the needed services. Policies to handle such referrals and all major emergency situations should be written and communicated to all HFIs in a fitness center.

A major factor involved in reducing the risk associated with physical activity is the design and implementation of an individual's exercise program. The program can focus attention on problems encountered in the preliminary tests, which might include the following:

- Flexibility measures
- Assessment of body fat composition
- Evaluation of muscular strength, power, and endurance
- Posture assessment
- Cardiovascular fitness evaluation

The manner in which the HFI conducts the exercise program has a major bearing on the risk of injury to the participant. To highlight this point, figure 25.2 contrasts the "train, don't strain" fitness goal with the "no pain, no gain" performance goal. Educating participants about the proper intensity

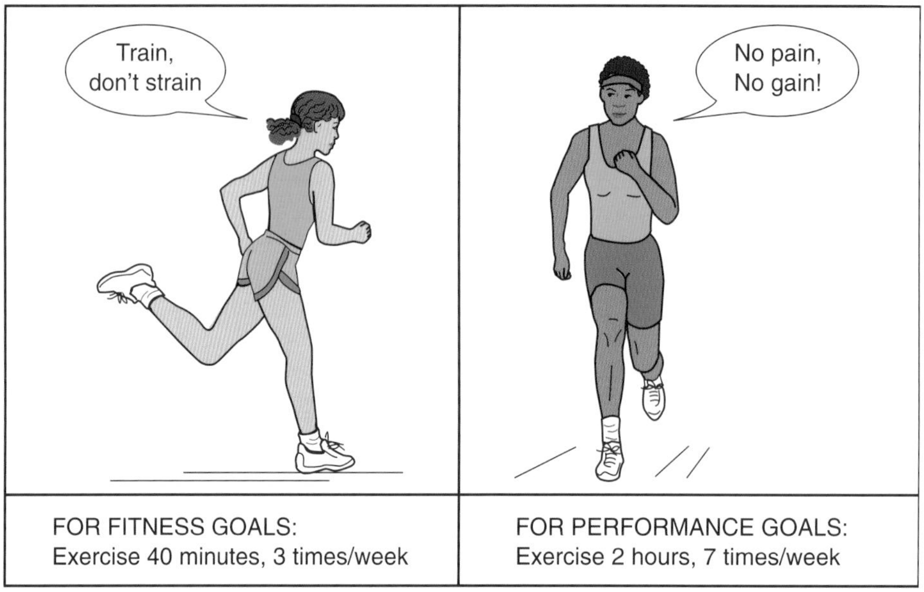
Train,
don't strain
No pain,
No gain!
FOR FITNESS GOALS:
Exercise 40 minutes, 3 times/week
FOR PERFORMANCE GOALS:
Exercise 2 hours, 7 times/week

Figure 25.2 Fitness programs versus performance training.

of the exercise session (i.e., to stay in the THR zone) and how to recognize the signs and symptoms of overuse is important in reducing injury risk. The HFI should emphasize that the entire program and each individual session are graduated so the participant will avoid doing too much too soon. This precaution is especially true for individuals who have not been involved in a regular exercise program and who tend to overestimate their abilities. Overexertion can lead to chronic overuse injuries, extreme muscle soreness, and undue fatigue.

In educating participants about the signs and symptoms of overuse, the HFI should distinguish between simple muscle soreness and injury. Muscle soreness tends to peak 24 to 48 hr postexercise and dissipates with use and time. The signs and symptoms of injury include the following:

- Exquisite point tenderness
- Pain that persists even when the body part is at rest
- Joint pain
- Pain that does not go away after warming up
- Swelling or discoloration
- Increased pain in weight-bearing activities or with active movement
- Changes in normal bodily functions

1 In Review

The HFI should be aware of inherent risks associated with activity and take steps to minimize risk by advanced planning, using proper equipment and facilities, educating participants regarding injury recognition and care, evaluating participants to determine fitness needs and/or special health problems that may need monitoring, and giving clear guidelines for graduating activity. The HFI should follow universal precaution guidelines and use appropriate gloves, biohazard containers, sharps containers, and disinfectant to reduce the spread of bloodborne pathogens.

Injury Treatment

The treatment of an injury depends on the type and severity of the injury. This section describes approaches to take with injuries that are common to fitness programs and sports (2-7, 9-12, 15-21, 24-28).

Treating Soft-Tissue Injuries

Sprains (overstretching or tearing of ligamentous tissue) and strains (overstretching or tearing of muscle or tendon) are common injuries associated with adult fitness programs. Most significant injuries to joint structures or to soft tissue require *protection, rest,* and the immediate application of *ice, compression,* and *elevation* (known by the acronym "PRICE"). Figure 25.3 reinforces the PRICE concept. Usually, a wet wrap is applied first to give compression. Start distal to the injury and wrap toward the heart. Compression should be firm but not tight. If a joint structure is involved, surround the entire area with ice and secure with another elastic wrap. If the injury involves a contusion (bruise) or strain to a muscle belly, put the muscle on mild stretch before applying ice. If possible, elevate the injured part above heart level to minimize the effect of gravity and reduce bleeding into tissues. With any injury, shock is a possibility, and the HFI should be prepared to handle this situation.

In most cases, the participant should be instructed to continue applying ice anywhere from 24 to 72 hr, depending on the severity of the injury. Ice causes vasoconstriction of the blood vessels, thus helping to control bleeding into tissues. Ice also reduces the sensation of pain. Standard treatment times with ice are 15 to 20 min, with reapplication hourly or when pain is experienced. In the acute phase, when ice is not being used, the compression bandage should be in place to minimize swelling. Using ice or compression at bedtime is not necessary unless pain interferes with sleep. If this occurs, applying ice frequently (every 1-2 hr) may help to control the pain. Physician referral is recommended in moderate to severe cases.

An injured participant may want to apply heat sooner than is warranted. Heat usually is applied in the later stages of an acute injury, when the risk of bleeding into tissues is minimal. In contrast, the application of heat is a common treatment for chronic inflammatory conditions as well as generalized muscle soreness. Heat causes a vasodilation of the blood vessels and reduces muscle spasm. Standard treatment time for a moist heat pack is 15 to 20 min. When in doubt about which mode of treatment to use, ice is the safer choice. Table 25.1 outlines common soft-tissue injuries, signs and symptoms, and immediate care.

2 In Review

When soft tissues are injured, proper assessment and initial treatment can reduce the possibility of further trauma and can aid in the healing process (see table 25.1 for details). Protection, rest, ice, compression, and elevation (PRICE) are the important steps for immediate care of most musculoskeletal and joint injuries. Heat is often used in chronic inflammatory conditions or with general muscle soreness and should be applied only in the later stages of an acute injury when the risk of bleeding into tissues is minimal.

Treating Fractures

Fractures, or injury to bone, should be suspected if there is exquisite point tenderness over a bone, visual or palpable deformity, or referred pain to an

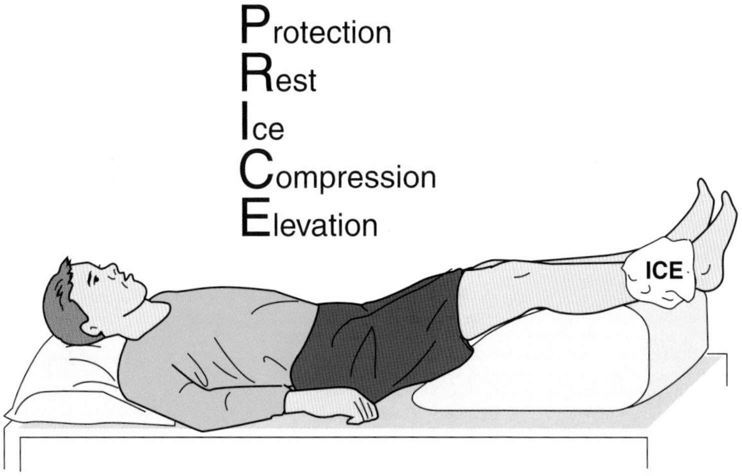

Figure 25.3 The PRICE method for treating sprains and strains.

Table 25.1 Soft-Tissue Injuries and Their Treatment

Injury	Signs and symptoms	Immediate care
Sprain—stretching or tearing of ligamentous tissue **Strain**—overstretching or tearing of a muscle or tendon **Contusion**—impact force that results in bleeding into the underlying tissues; a bruise	1st degree—mild injury resulting in overstretching or minor tearing of tissue. Range of motion is limited. Point tenderness is minimal. No swelling. 2nd degree—moderate injury resulting in partial tearing of tissue. Function is limited. Point tenderness and probable muscle spasm. Range of motion is painful. Swelling and/or discoloration is probable if immediate first-aid care is not given. 3rd degree—severe tearing or rupture of tissue. Exquisite point tenderness. Immediate loss of function. Swelling and muscle spasm likely to be present with discoloration appearing later. Possible palpable deformity.	Protection, rest, ice, compression, and elevation Usual treatment time: 15–20 min ice bag 5–7 min ice cup or ice slush How often: Moderate and severe—every hour, or when pain is experienced Less severe—as symptoms necessitate Continue with ice treatments at least 24–72 hr, depending on the severity of the injury. Refer to a physician if function is impaired. Mild to moderate strains—gradual stretching to the point of discomfort is recommended.
Heel bruise (stone bruise)—sudden abnormal force to heel area that results in trauma to underlying tissues		PRICE Pad for comfort when weight bearing is resumed

(9–12, 15, 18–25, 27, 28)

area of bone with percussion or vibrational stress. X-rays should be taken if a fracture is suspected. If deformity is present, do not push the bone back into place. Splint and refer to a physician. Table 25.2 gives additional procedures to follow when treating a fracture.

Treating Wounds and Other Skin Disorders

Wounds are another group of common injuries associated with activity programs. The major concern with an open wound is bleeding. Once bleeding is controlled, steps can be taken to give further care. This may consist of protecting the wound from infection, covering the wound with a bandage, treating the participant for shock, or referring the participant immediately to a physician for suturing. In minor cases, a thorough cleansing and application of a sterile dressing may be all that is needed. The HFI should use safety measures to prevent risk from exposure to blood. Internal bleeding is a very serious condition. The HFI should treat for shock and obtain medical assistance immediately.

Shearing and pressure forces attributable to poorly fitting shoes and socks, poorly conditioned or sensitive skin, and incorrect foot biomechanics can lead to friction and compression injuries of the foot. Hand calluses and other skin irritations can develop from friction during activities that require frequent gripping of an object (e.g., a tennis racket or a bat) or rubbing of body parts against each other or another object (e.g., as is frequently the case in gymnastics or wrestling).

Table 25.3 outlines and provides guidelines for immediate care of wounds. Table 25.4 discusses care of common skin irritations. The HFI should use universal precautions in treating an open wound. Latex gloves should be worn when handling potentially infectious materials. Proper disposal of infectious materials and decontamination of infected areas should be routine policy.

3 **In Review**

The steps to follow in dealing with simple and compound fractures, wounds (and excessive bleeding), and other skin disorders are listed in tables 25.2, 25.3, and 25.4, respectively.

Table 25.2 Fractures and Their Treatment

Injury	Signs and symptoms	Immediate care
Fracture—disruption of bone with or without loss of continuity or external exposure, ranging from periosteal irritation to complete separation of bony parts **Simple**—bone fracture without external exposure **Compound**—bone fracture with external exposure	Acute: Direct trauma to bone resulting in disruption of continuity and immediate disability. Deformity or bony deviation. Swelling. Pain. Palpable tenderness. Referred pain or indirect point tenderness. Crepitus. False joint. Discoloration—usually becoming apparent later.	Acute: Control bleeding—elevation, pressure points, direct pressure. Treat for shock. If an open fracture, control bleeding and apply a sterile dressing, prevent further disruption and infection; do not move bones back into place. Control swelling with pressure and ice, if wound is closed. Splint above and below the joint and apply traction if necessary. Protect body part from further injury. Refer to physician.
	Chronic: Low-grade inflammatory process causing proliferation of fibroblasts and generalized connective-tissue scarring. Pain progressively worsens until present all of the time. Direct point tenderness.	Chronic: Rest. Heat. Refer to physician.

(1, 5, 6, 19, 21, 22)

Environmental Concerns

The environment can play an important role in the development of serious problems related to maintaining normal body temperature during exercise. This section examines the factors related to an increased risk of heat- and cold-related injuries.

Heat-Related Problems

Heat illness can strike anyone. Poor physical condition, although a contributing factor, is not the primary cause. Even the most highly conditioned athlete can suffer a heat-related disorder. The exercise load and the environment can place large heat loads on an individual. Excessive heat loads stimulate a high production of sweat because evaporation of sweat is the major mechanism for cooling the body. As a result, large amounts of water may be lost during physical activity, causing an increase in the core body temperature (hyperthermia). If too much water is lost, circulatory collapse and death can occur. The following information outlines methods of recognizing dehydration (excessive loss of body fluids) and presents measures to prevent heat illness.

A water loss up to 3% of body weight is considered safe. A 3 to 5% loss is considered borderline, and more than a 5% loss is considered serious. Water loss can be monitored by weighing participants before and after activity. Individuals who are outside the 3% range from one workout to the next may have an increased risk of heat injury and should be monitored carefully if allowed to participate.

The practical experience of the military and athletic teams working in the heat and humidity has led to the development of guidelines to prevent heat injury. Applying these guidelines to adult fitness programs will enhance participants' enjoyment and safety. Participants should follow these guidelines for preventing heat injury:

- Acclimatize to heat and humidity by training over a period of 7 to 10 days.
- Hydrate before activity and frequently during activity.
- Decrease the intensity of exercise if the temperature or humidity is high; use THR as a guide.

Table 25.3 Treatment of Wounds

Injury	Signs and symptoms	Immediate care
Incision—cutting of skin resulting in an open wound with cleanly cut edges and exposure of underlying tissues	Smooth edges may bleed freely. Signs of infection (see laceration)	Clean wound with soap and water, moving away from injury site. Minor cuts can be closed with a butterfly bandage or steri-strip. Apply a sterile dressing. Refer to a physician if wound needs suturing (e.g., facial cuts and large or deep wounds) or signs of infection are present.
Laceration—tearing of skin resulting in an open wound with jagged edges and exposure of underlying tissues	Jagged edges may bleed freely. Signs of infection: redness; swelling; increase in skin temperature; tender, swollen, and painful lymph glands; mild fever; and headache	Soak in antiseptic solution such as hydrogen peroxide to loosen foreign material. Clean with antiseptic soap and water using sterile technique and moving away from the injury site. Apply a sterile dressing. Instruct to seek medical attention if signs of infection are recognized. Usually refer to a physician; a tetanus shot or sutures may be needed. If injury is extensive, control bleeding, cover with thick sterile bandages, and treat for shock. Refer to a physician.
Puncture—direct penetration of tissues by a pointed object	Small opening may bleed freely. Signs of infection (see laceration)	If object is embedded deeply: Protect body part and refer to physician for removal and care. Treat for shock. Clean around wound, moving away from injury site. Allow wound to bleed freely to minimize risk of infection. Apply a sterile dressing. Puncture wounds are usually referred to a physician. A tetanus shot may be needed. Instruct individual to seek medical attention if signs of infection are present.

Table 25.3 *(continued)*

Injury	Signs and symptoms	Immediate care
Abrasion—scraping of tissues resulting in removal of the outermost layers of skin and the exposure of numerous capillaries	Superficial, reddish, irregular surface Oozing or weeping from underlying capillaries May contain dirt, debris, or bacteria embedded in tissue	Debride and flush with antiseptic solution such as hydrogen peroxide. Follow with soap-and-water cleansing. Apply a petroleum-based antiseptic agent to keep wound moist. This allows healing to take place from the deeper layers. Cover with non-adherent gauze. Instruct to seek medical help if signs of infection are recognized.
Excessive bleeding—internal or external bleeding that results in massive loss of circulating blood volumes; often results in shock and can lead to death	External hemorrhage 1. Arterial Color: bright red Flow: spurts, bleeding usually profuse 2. Venous Color: dark red Flow: steady, oozing	Elevate affected part above heart. Put direct pressure over the wound, using a sterile compress if possible. Apply a pressure dressing. Use pressure points. Treat for shock. Refer to a physician.
Internal bleeding—bleeding within the deep structures of the body (chest, abdominal, or pelvic cavity) and bleeding of any of the organs contained within these cavities	Internal hemorrhage—bleeding into chest, abdominal, or pelvic cavity and bleeding of any of the organs contained within these cavities. Generally, there are no external signs. However, any time an individual coughs up blood or finds blood in the urine or feces, internal hemorrhage must be suspected. The following signs are also indicative of internal bleeding: Restlessness Thirst Faintness Anxiety Cold, clammy skin Dizziness Pulse—rapid, weak, and irregular Blood pressure—significant fall	Treat for shock. Refer to hospital immediately. Don't give water or food.

(continued)

Table 25.3 *(continued)*

Injury	Signs and symptoms	Immediate care
Shock caused by bleeding	Restlessness Anxiety Pulse—weak, rapid Skin temperature—cold clammy, profuse sweating Skin color—pale, later cyanotic Respiration—shallow, labored Eyes—dull Pupils—dilated Thirsty Nausea and possible vomiting Blood pressure—marked fall	Maintain an open airway. Control bleeding. Elevate lower extremities approximately 12 in. (exceptions: heart problems, head injury, or breathing difficulty—place in comfortable position, usually semi-reclining, unless spinal injury is suspected, in which case do not move). Splint any fractures. Maintain normal body temperature. Avoid further trauma. Monitor vital signs and record at regular intervals—every 5 min or so. Do not feed or give any liquids.

(5-7, 9, 10, 13, 14, 18, 19, 25, 27)

- Monitor weight loss by weighing before and after workouts. Consume fluids if more than 3% of body weight is lost during activity. Minimize participation until weight is within the 3% range.
- Consume a diet high in carbohydrates; carbohydrates contain a high water content and help to maintain fluid balance.
- Wear appropriate clothing for hot or humid weather conditions. Expose as much skin surface as possible.

Further precautions include wearing light-colored clothing because it does not absorb as much heat as darker clothing. Cotton materials absorb sweat and allow evaporation to occur. Certain synthetic clothing and materials with paint screens do not absorb sweat and should be avoided.

Participants should be educated to recognize symptoms of overexertion: nausea or vomiting, extreme breathlessness, dizziness, unusual fatigue, muscle cramping, and headache. Symptoms related to heat illness include hair standing on end on chest or upper arms, body chills, headache or throbbing pressure, nausea or vomiting, labored breathing, dry lips or extreme cotton mouth, faintness (heat syncope) or muscle cramping (heat cramps), and cessation of sweating. Heat rash can also be a symptom and is attributable to inflamed sweat glands and usually occurs in children who have sweated profusely. If these symptoms are present, the risk for developing heat exhaustion or heat stroke rises dramatically. The participant should stop the activity and get into the shade. In addition, the participant should be instructed to ask for help if he or she is disoriented or if the symptoms are severe. The HFI should provide fluids and encourage the individual to drink.

Individuals who experience heat stroke may sustain permanent damage to the thermoregulatory system. People who do not have efficient cooling mechanisms may be highly susceptible to heat injury. Individuals who use medications such as antihistamines or diuretics, use high quantities of salt in their diet or consume **salt tablets**, or drink alcohol in large quantities (particularly before activity) will have a higher risk of heat injury. Furthermore, people who participate in physical activity while experiencing fever could elevate their body temperature to dangerous levels. Table 25.5 outlines the various stages of heat illness, the signs and symptoms associated with each, and guidelines for immediate care.

Be aware of environmental factors such as relative humidity and temperature. The relative humidity can be calculated by measuring dry-bulb and wet-bulb atmospheric temperatures (see chapter 10) using a sling psychrometer. As mentioned earlier, the evaporation of sweat is a primary means to lose heat during exercise. This fluid loss must be replaced to minimize health risk and maximize safe

Table 25.4 Skin Irritations and Treatment

Skin irritation	Signs and symptoms	Immediate care
Blister—a collection of serum just below the superficial layer of skin	Defined area of fluid accumulation under skin Feels hot Painful to touch	Prevent by engaging in heavy activity slowly and toughening skin by use of astringents: tannic acid or salt water soaks. Stop activity if friction area develops, apply ice, and cover irritation with a friction-proofing material or donut pad. Prevent contamination of torn blister; clean with soap and water. Refer to physician if signs of infection are present.
Callus—markedly thickened area of skin, usually over an area of pressure	Visible and excessive callus formation: May be painful May have cracks or fissures May become infected May develop blisters	Prevent excessive callus formation by using an emery callus file. Take measures to reduce friction by wearing properly fitted shoes and socks, using powder or lubricant, and correcting abnormal biomechanical foot faults with orthotics. Protect susceptible areas by using special protective devices such as gloves, tape, or pad. Prevent infection by keeping callus trimmed down and using a lubricant to prevent cracks and tears in callus.
Corns		
Hard corn—thickening of skin located on toes	Local pain Inflammation and thickening of soft tissue Generally seen on top of toes and associated with hammer toe deformity	Prevent by wearing properly fitted shoes or fitting with orthotics if cause is due to abnormal foot biomechanics.
Soft corn—circular area of thickened white macerated skin between toes and proximal head of phalanges	Pain and inflammation	Prevent with properly fitted shoes, and control moisture accumulation by keeping skin dry in between toes. Separate toes with cotton or lamb's wool.

(continued)

Table 25.4 *(continued)*

Injury	Signs and symptoms	Immediate care
Ingrown toenail—leading side edge of toenail grows into soft tissue	Severe inflammation, pain, and infection	Apply hot antiseptic soaks for 20 min, 2–3 times a day, at 110–120 °F. When toenail is pliable, insert wisp of cotton under leading edge of toenail and lift from soft tissue beneath. Refer to physician or podiatrist if signs of infection are present.
Intertrigo—chafing due to excessive rubbing of body parts in combination with perspiration	Pain, inflammation, burning, itching, moistness, cracking, lesion	Cleanse frequently. Use medicated drying powder.
Plantar wart—viral infection on foot, leading to a localized overgrowth of skin; can be confused with callus	Distinct edge with central core Sometimes appears to be growing inward; small black dot in center surrounded by clearer callus area Excessive thickening of skin	Donut to take pressure off of wart. Keep callus area around wart filed down (do not file down wart). See physician or podiatrist for cure and/or removal.

(9, 10, 13-19, 25, 27)

and enjoyable participation in an exercise program. For most individuals who participate in CRF programs, thirst is an adequate indicator of when to hydrate. Generally, replacing fluids as they are used is the best way to meet the demands of the body. When extreme sweating or dry atmospheric conditions are present, however, the thirst mechanism may not be able to keep up with the need for fluid intake.

Normal daily intake of fluid for the sedentary individual is between 60 and 80 oz (1.8-2.4 L). The actual fluid requirement depends on too many factors to establish a single recommendation for maintaining hydration. However, drinking 8 to 10 oz (240-300 ml) of fluid before heavy exercise, in addition to drinking frequently during activity, helps to prevent heat illness.

Salt and other minerals may be lost during prolonged exercise, particularly during hot and humid weather. Even so, the use of salt tablets is not recommended unless accompanied by a large intake of water. Water with 0.1 to 0.2% salt solution may be given to individuals with high water loss. Increasing the use of salt at mealtimes and consuming a high intake of water throughout the day, however, generally meet the body's need for sodium and fluid replacement.

Most **electrolyte** drinks are diluted solutions of glucose, salt, and other minerals, with added artificial flavoring. Some brands also contain as much as 200 to 300 kcal per quart of solution. Other than sodium, the minerals provided by an electrolyte solution do not provide much benefit. When sweating is profuse, large amounts of electrolyte solution may serve the same function as a diluted salt solution. In cases of mild to moderate sweating, the normal intake of salt in food provides adequate sodium replacement. The main advantage of using a flavored solution is that the individual might drink more than if ingesting plain water or a salt solution. However, considering the prices of commercially prepared electrolyte solutions, plain water or homemade solutions, such as the one presented next, are much more economical.

Homemade Electrolyte Solution

1 qt water

1/3 tsp salt

Some sugar for flavoring (0.5-1.5 tbsp)

Fluids at a temperature of 5 to 15° C (41-59° F) are absorbed faster than fluids at other temperatures.

Table 25.5 Heat-Related Problems and Their Treatment

Heat illness	Signs and symptoms	Immediate care
Heat cramps—spasmodic muscular contraction caused by exertion in extreme heat	Muscle cramping (calf is very common)	Isolated cramps: Pressure to the cramp and release, stretch muscle slowly and gently, apply gentle massage, and ice.
	Multiple cramping (very serious)	Multiple cramps: Danger of heat stroke; treat as heat exhaustion.
Heat exhaustion—collapse with or without loss of consciousness, suffered in conditions of heat and high humidity, largely resulting from the loss of fluid and salt by sweating	Profuse sweating Cold, clammy skin Normal temperature or slightly elevated Pale Dizzy Weak, rapid pulse Shallow breathing Nausea Headache Loss of consciousness	Move individual out of the sun to a well-ventilated area. Place in shock position (feet elevated 12–18 in.); prevent heat loss or gain. Gently massage the extremities. Apply gentle range-of-motion movement to the extremities. Force consumption of fluids. Reassure the individual. Monitor body temperature and other vital signs. Refer to a physician.
Heat stroke—final stage of heat exhaustion in which the thermoregulatory system shuts down to conserve depleted fluid levels	Generally no perspiration Dry skin Very hot Temperature as high as 106 °F Skin color bright red or flushed (dark-pigmented individuals will have ashen skin) Rapid, strong pulse Labored breathing	Treat as an extreme medical emergency. Transport to hospital quickly. Remove as much clothing as possible without exposing the individual. Cool quickly, starting at the head and continuing down the body; use any means possible (fan, hose down, pack in ice). Wrap in cold, wet sheets for transport. Treat for shock; if breathing is labored, place in a semi-reclining position.
Heat syncope—fainting or excessive loss of strength because of excessive heat	Headache Nausea	Normal intake of fluids

(9, 10, 25-27, 29)

4 In Review

Inefficient body cooling mechanisms, certain medications, high intake of salt or alcohol, and exercising with a fever or in high heat and humidity may cause heat-related disorders. Heat illness is potentially deadly, and the HFI must be aware of ways to prevent it and must be able to recognize the signs of heat illness and act on them (see table 25.5). Proper hydration, evaluated through a weight chart, is a good first step in prevention. Provide water before, during, and after activity to prevent dehydration.

5 In Review

Exercising in cold, rainy weather or when the windchill factor is high, as well as exercising in cold water, may lead to cold-related disorders. Precautionary measures such as avoiding exposure to extreme cold, wearing removable layers, warming up before activity, remaining constantly active, and understanding the effect of windchill on air temperature can help prevent cold-related problems. See table 25.6 for specifics on how to treat cold-related problems.

Cold-Related Problems

Exercising in cold, windy weather can produce some problems if certain precautions are not taken. Considerable heat loss can occur through convective heat loss from the skin and evaporation of skin moisture. Hypothermia occurs when body heat is lost at a faster rate than it is produced and core body temperature drops below 35° C (95° F). Peripheral blood vessels in cold areas constrict, which conserves body heat but increases risk of frostbite. Exercising in cold, rainy weather can compound the problem by increasing the rate of evaporation. Windchill is another factor that must be taken into account. A high windchill factor can result in severe loss of body heat even when air temperature is above freezing. Additionally, exercising in cold water results in even faster loss of body temperature than exercising in the same air temperature. Cold-related problems are preventable if participants follow these precautions:

- Avoid exercising outdoors in extreme cold and wind.
- Layer clothing and remove layers as needed to avoid sweating.
- Warm up before exercise and avoid periods of inactivity.
- Stay dry.
- Cover face, nose, ears, fingers, and head (a great deal of heat loss occurs when the head is exposed).
- Avoid swimming or exercising in cold water, particularly when the surrounding air temperature is low.

Table 25.6 describes how to recognize and treat cold-related problems.

Medical Concerns

Some individuals have controlled medical conditions that might be aggravated by exercise. In addition, it is important to recognize major cardiovascular and respiratory problems. This section summarizes information on some common medical concerns.

Diabetic Reactions

The HFI should be familiar with the signs and symptoms of diabetic coma and insulin shock (see table 25.7). When an emergency situation arises with a diabetic and the individual is conscious, he or she is usually able to indicate what the problem is. If the individual cannot tell you this, then ask when food was last eaten and whether insulin was taken that day. If the person has eaten but has not taken insulin, then the individual is probably going into a diabetic coma, a condition in which there is too little insulin to fully metabolize the carbohydrates consumed (hyperglycemia). If the individual has taken insulin but has not eaten, then he or she probably is suffering from insulin shock, a condition in which there is too much insulin or not enough carbohydrate to balance the insulin intake (hypoglycemia).

If the individual lapses into unconsciousness, check for a medical-alert identification tag. This may help to identify the problem. If you don't know whether the individual is suffering from diabetic coma or insulin shock, give sugar. Brain damage or death can occur quickly if insulin shock is left untreated; it is a far more critical state than diabetic coma. If the problem is insulin shock, the individual should respond quickly, within 1 to 2 min; then transport the individual to a hospital as quickly as possible. If the individual is in a diabetic coma, there is little chance of seriously worsening the condition

Table 25.6 Cold-Related Problems and Their Treatment

Cold-related problems	Signs and symptoms	Immediate care
Deep frostbite—freezing of deep tissue, including muscle and bone	Hard, cold, numb, pale, or white area Permanent damage to tissue may be sustained	Refer to a physician. Rapid rewarming is necessary.
Frostnip—freezing of tips of extremities such as ears, nose, or fingers, involving only the surface of the skin	Skin firm and cold Burning, itching, local redness Skin may peel or blister in a day or two	Rewarm by applying firm pressure over the affected area, blowing warm air over the area, submerging in warm water 100 to 105 °F, and holding frostnipped area against body.
Superficial frostbite—freezing of layers of skin and subcutaneous tissue	Pale, waxy, and cold skin Purple coloring Following rewarming there may be swelling and superficial blisters Stinging, burning, and aching may be present for several days or weeks	Remove from cold. Rewarm area.
Hypothermia—core body temperature drops below 95 °F	Shivering Impairment of neuromuscular function Decreased ability to make decisions Muscle rigidity Hypotension Shock Death	Treat as a medical emergency. Remove from cold. Treat for shock. Immediately transport to hospital.

(9, 10, 25-27)

by giving sugar. Several hours of fluid and insulin therapy will be needed, under a physician's direction. Table 25.7 outlines the diabetic reactions, signs and symptoms, and immediate care of each.

6 In Review

Diabetic coma is related to hyperglycemia, and insulin shock is attributable to hypoglycemia. Table 25.7 describes how to deal with these conditions.

Cardiovascular and Pulmonary Complications

Cardiovascular complications can occur with injury because of decreased circulating blood volumes as may occur with bleeding, hyperthermia or hypothermia, shock, or heart attack. The HFI should be able to recognize and deal with potential complications such as **tachycardia** (excessively rapid heartbeat), **bradycardia** (abnormally slow heartbeat), **hypertension** (high blood pressure), and **hypotension** (low blood pressure).

Pulmonary complications may be observed more readily. **Apnea**, or temporary cessation of breathing, can be caused by an obstructed airway, allergic reaction, drowning, or intrathoracic injury. **Dyspnea**, or labored breathing, can be caused by hyperventilation, asthma, and chest or lung injury. **Tachypnea**, excessively rapid breathing, may be a sign of overexertion, shock, or hyperventilation. The HFI should feel comfortable assessing circulation and respiration and have the knowledge and skills to perform appropriate emergency procedures.

Table 25.7 Diabetic Reactions and Their Treatment

Diabetes	Signs and symptoms	Immediate care
Diabetic coma/hyperglycemia— loss of consciousness caused by too little insulin	May complain of a headache Confused Disoriented Stuporous Nauseated Coma Skin color—flushed Lips—cherry red Body temperature—decreased; skin—dry Breath odor—sweet, fruity Vomiting common Abdominal pain frequently present	Call for medical assistance. Little can be done unless insulin is at hand. If medical assistance is not quickly available, 1. treat as shock; 2. administer fluids in large amounts by mouth, if individual is conscious; 3. maintain an open airway; 4. turn the head to the side to prevent aspirating vomitus if individual is nauseated; and 5. do not give sugar, carbohydrates, or fats in any form. Recovery—gradual improvement over 6–12 hr. Fluid and insulin therapy should be directed by a physician.
Insulin shock/hypoglycemia— anxiety, excitement, perspiration, delirium, or coma caused by too much insulin or not enough carbohydrates to balance insulin intake	Skin color—pale (dark-pigmented individuals will appear ashen) Skin temperature—moist and clammy; cold sweat Pulse—normal or rapid Breathing—normal or shallow and slow No odor of acetone on breath Intense hunger Possible double vision	Administer sugar as quickly as possible (e.g., orange juice, candy). If individual is unconscious, place sugar granules under the tongue. If individual is unconscious or recovery is slow, call for medical assistance. Recovery—generally quick; 1 or 2 min. Refer to a physician if still unconscious or recovery is slow.

(1, 18)

Most common respiratory disorders include hyperventilation, asthma, and **airway obstruction**. Hyperventilation can occur with heavy exhalation or rapid breathing, resulting in breathing out too much carbon dioxide (CO_2) and thereby reducing CO_2 levels in the blood. Low CO_2 levels may cause a feeling of dizziness, faintness, chest pains, and tingling in the feet and hands. Reassuring the individual in a calm manner, encouraging a slower breathing rate, and helping the person breathe into a paper bag or into hands cupped over the nose and mouth will help restore CO_2 levels.

Asthma is a condition in which the smooth muscles of the bronchial tubes go into spasm; edema and inflammation of the mucous lining are triggered by exercise, changes in barometric pressure or temperature, virus, emotional upset, and noxious odors. The affected individual may appear anxious, pale, and sweaty; may cough or wheeze; and may seem to be short of breath. Hyperventilation may occur resulting in dizziness, and, because of mucous secretions, the individual may frequently try to clear the throat.

The HFI should be prepared to handle an asthma attack. Generally, people with asthma know how to care for themselves and will carry medication. Individuals with exercise-induced asthma are often given medication to take before activity. Encourage individuals with asthma to drink water, and promote relaxation and breathing exercises. Remove any known irritants from the environment if possible. If bronchial spasm is excessive, seek medical attention.

Airway obstruction can occur by a foreign object or by the tongue blocking the airway. If breathing is labored but the individual is coughing forcefully, stay with the person and encourage continued coughing. If, however, the person is unsuccessful in expelling the object or the airway becomes totally blocked, have someone call for an ambulance and begin abdominal thrusts (**Heimlich maneuver**). In an unconscious victim, visually checking the airway passage or performing a finger sweep or Heimlich maneuver may dislodge a known obstruction. Generally, moving the lower jaw forward or tilting the head and lifting the chin will open an airway blocked by the tongue. **Rescue breathing** should be performed if the person has stopped breathing and repositioning the head does not change the status.

Respiratory shock, a condition in which the lungs are unable to supply enough oxygen to the circulating blood, can result in a medical emergency. Signs and symptoms include paleness of skin or cyanosis; weak, rapid pulse; rapid, shallow breathing rate; decrease in BP; changes in personality including disinterest, irritability, restlessness, and excitement; extreme thirst; and in severe cases, urinary retention and fecal incontinence.

Treatment includes maintaining body heat and elevating feet and legs 12 to 18 in. If head or neck injury is suspected, protect the involved area and raise the head and shoulders. Keep the participant warm, reassure, and seek medical attention. Employ **cardiopulmonary resuscitation (CPR)** techniques (see pages 413 and 418).

7 In Review

Common cardiovascular complications from exercise include excessively rapid or abnormally slow heartbeat and high or low BP. Pulmonary complications include temporary cessation of breathing, labored breathing, or airway obstruction.

Common Orthopedic Problems

Many injuries that are commonly referred to an orthopedic physician for diagnosis and treatment result from overuse or irritation of a chronic musculoskeletal problem. In most instances, the injuries do not incapacitate the participant immediately. It may be weeks or months after the onset of pain before the participant seeks medical consultation. By this time, the **inflammation** is severe and generally prevents normal function of the part involved. In many cases, a severe injury can be avoided if proper care is initiated early. Table 25.8 outlines common orthopedic problems, their causes, signs and symptoms, and general treatment guidelines.

Shin Splints

Shin splint is a catch-all expression used to describe a variety of conditions of the lower leg. It is often used to define any pain located between the knee and the ankle (usually anterior medial and lateral). A diagnosis of shin splints should be limited to conditions involving inflammation of the musculotendinous unit caused by overexertion of muscles during weight-bearing activity. A more specific diagnosis is preferred over the general term "shin splints." In any event, the physician must rule out the following conditions: stress fracture, metabolic or vascular disorder, **compartment syndrome**, and muscular strain. The physical complaints often accompanying shin splint pain include the following:

- A dull ache in the lower leg region after workouts
- Decreased performance and work output because of pain
- Soft-tissue pain
- Mild swelling along the area of inflammation
- Slight temperature elevation at the site of inflammation
- Pain on moving the foot up and down

The individual with shin splints usually has no history of trauma. The symptoms start gradually and progress if activity is not reduced. The following is the usual symptomatic treatment:

- Rest in the acute stage; reduce weight-bearing activity.
- In mild cases brought on by overuse, decrease or modify activity for a few days (e.g., choose swimming or bicycle workouts instead of running).
- Apply heat or ice before activity; use ice after activity. Heat treatments may consist of moist heat packs for 15 to 20 min or whirlpool treatments. The temperature of the whirlpool water should be approximately 100 to 106° F. Treatment time is usually 15 to 20 min. Ice application may consist of ice-bag treatments for 15 to 20 min or ice massage/ice slush treatments for 5 to 7 min.

Table 25.8 Common Orthopedic Problems and Their Treatment

Injury	Common causes	Signs and symptoms	Treatment
Inflammatory reactions: **Bursitis**—inflammation of bursa (sac between a muscle and bone that is filled with fluid, facilitates motion, pads and helps to prevent abnormal function) **Capsulitis**—inflammation of the joint capsule **Epicondylitis**—inflammation of muscles or tendons attached to the epicondyles of the humerous **Myositis**—inflammation of voluntary muscle **Plantar fasciitis**—inflammation of connective tissue that spans the bottom of the foot **Tendinitis**—inflammation of a tendon (a band of tough, inelastic, fibrous tissue that connects muscle to bone) **Tenosynovitis**—inflammation of a tendinous sheath **Synovitis**—inflammation of the synovial membrane (a highly vascularized tissue that lines articular surfaces)	Overuse Improper joint mechanics Improper technique Pathology Trauma Infection	Redness Swelling Pain Increased skin temperature over the area of inflammation Tenderness Involuntary muscle guarding	Ice and rest in the acute stages. If chronic, heat is generally used before exercise or activity, followed by ice after activity. Massage. Perform muscle stretching exercises. Correct the cause of problem. If correction of the cause and symptomatic treatment does not relieve symptoms, referral to a physician is recommended; anti-inflammatory medication is usually prescribed. If disease process or infection is suspected, refer to a physician immediately.

Table 25.8 *(continued)*

Injury	Common causes	Signs and symptoms	Treatment
Tennis elbow—inflammation of the musculotendinous unit of the elbow extensors where they attach on the outer aspect of the elbow (lateral epicondylitis)	Faulty backhand mechanics—faults may include leading with the elbow, using an improper grip, dropping the racket head, or using a top-spin backhand with a whipping motion Improper grip size—usually too small Racket strung too tightly Improper hitting—hitting off center, particularly if using wet, heavy balls Overuse of forearm supinators, wrist extensors, and finger extensors	Pain directly over the outer aspect of the elbow in region of the common extensor origin Swelling Increased skin temperature over the area of inflammation Pain on extension of the middle finger against resistance with the elbow extended Pain on racket gripping and extension of the wrist	Ice and rest in the acute stages. If chronic, heat is generally used before exercise or activity, followed by ice after activity. Apply deep friction massage at the elbow. Perform strengthening and stretching exercises for the wrist extensors. Correct the cause of problem: 1. Use proper techniques. 2. Use proper grip size (when racket is gripped, there should be room for one finger to fit in the gap between the thumb and fingers). 3. Racket should be strung at the proper tension (usually between 50 and 55 lb). 4. Avoid stiff rackets that vibrate easily. Keep elbow warm, particularly in cold weather. Use a counterforce brace, a circular band that is placed just below the elbow (serves to reduce the stress at the origin of the extensors). If correction of cause and symptomatic treatment does not relieve symptoms, referral to a physician is recommended; anti-inflammatory medication is usually prescribed.

(continued)

Table 25.8 *(continued)*

Injury	Common causes	Signs and symptoms	Treatment
Mechanical low-back pain— low-back pain that results from poor body mechanics, inflexibility of certain muscle groups, or muscular weakness	Tight low back musculature Tight hamstrings Poor posture or postural habits Weak trunk musculature, particularly abdominals Differences in leg length because of a structural or functional problem Structural abnormality Obesity	Generalized low back pain, usually aggravated by activity that accentuates the curve in the low back (e.g., hill running) Muscle spasm Palpable tenderness that is limited to musculature and not located directly over the spine May see a difference in pelvic height or other signs that would indicate a possible leg-length discrepancy Muscle tightness, particularly of the hamstrings, hip flexors, and low back	Any individual with acute onset of low back pain or any signs of nerve impingement should be referred to a physician for evaluation and X ray. It is necessary to rule out structural abnormalities such as spondylolisthesis, ruptured disc, fractures, neoplasms, or possible segmental instability prior to instituting a general exercise program. Further diagnostic procedures may be warranted. Symptomatic treatment consists of ice application and referral to physician in acute cases. Chronic cases are generally treated with moist heat to reduce muscle spasm and ice after activity. Correct the causes of low back pain: 1. Stretch tight muscles. 2. Strengthen weak muscles. 3. Do a thorough warm-up prior to activity and proper cool-down following activity. 4. Correct leg-length differences. 5. Emphasize correct postural positions. 6. If possible, correct or compensate for structural abnormalities (e.g., orthotics for a biomechanical problem).

(9-11, 20)

Treatment should begin at the first sign of pain. If pain is extreme, the participant should see a doctor. Determination and treatment of the cause, in addition to symptomatic treatment, are necessary to prevent recurrence of the problem. Table 25.9 cites the major causes for shin splints as well as the signs and symptoms and steps that can be taken to prevent the onset or recurrence of lower leg pain.

Exercise Modification

Most orthopedic injuries can be classified as mild, moderate, or severe. When in doubt, conservative treatment is recommended. Any injury that results in acute pain or affects performance, and any injury in which the individual hears or feels a pop at the time of injury, should be referred to a physician. If conservative measures fail to improve the condition within a reasonable period of time (2-4 weeks), physician consultation is again recommended.

Other conditions may call for modifying the exercise program. The participant may be obese or arthritic or may have a history of musculoskeletal problems. Pool work often is used with such individuals. Warm water is very therapeutic, body weight is supported, and the water generally allows for a greater range of movement. In any case, the activity should be suited to the condition. Any individual who requires exercise modification should be monitored closely. Table 25.10 summarizes the general guidelines used to classify injuries and offers suggestions for modifying activity.

8 In Review

Table 25.8 summarizes information on how to deal with common orthopedic injuries including inflammatory reactions, tennis elbow, stress fractures, and mechanical low back pain. Procedures for treating shin splints are described in table 25.9. A summary of how to classify an injury as mild, moderate, or severe and how to modify an exercise program to accommodate the problem is presented in Table 25.10.

CPR and Emergency Procedures

All HFIs should be well versed in CPR techniques. (Courses are generally available through the local [AHA] or American Red Cross.) In an emergency situation there is little time to think. Most reactions occur automatically. Having a plan of action and routinely running through practice drills helps to ensure that proper procedures are followed in an emergency situation (1-7, 9-12).

Basic Emergency Plan

First, be prepared. Have a cell phone, or make sure a phone is available for use during the exercise class, and know where the phone is located. If a phone is not available, have an alternative emergency plan in mind. The HFI should identify the **emergency medical system (EMS)** and services that are to be used (e.g., ambulance, hospital, doctor) and have a phone list located in a convenient place. Decide who is to phone for medical help in an emergency situation, and make sure that he or she knows how to direct help to the location of the injured individual. All necessary medical information (e.g., release forms, medical history forms) should be readily available, and all emergency equipment and supplies should be easily accessible (e.g., stretcher, emergency kit and supplies, automated external defibrillator [AED], splints, ice, inhaler, money for phone call, blanket, spine board). The equipment should be checked periodically to ensure that it is in proper working order, and the supplies should be up to date. And, of course, know where the fire alarms and fire exits are located.

Remain calm to reassure the injured person and help prevent the onset of shock. Clear thinking allows for sound judgment and proper execution of rehearsed plans. In most instances, speed is not necessary. Cases of extreme breathing difficulty, stoppage of breathing or circulation, choking, severe bleeding, shock, head or neck injury, heat illness, and internal injury are exceptions to this and require urgent action. Otherwise, careful evaluation and a deliberate plan of action are desirable. The HFI should have a system for evaluating and dealing with a life-threatening situation. All procedures should be conducted in a calm, professional manner.

Determine the history of the injury from direct observation of what happened, the injured person's account of what happened, or a witness's account of the injury. If the injured person is unconscious or semiconscious and no cause is determined, check for a medical-alert identification tag.

Check vital signs—HR, breathing, BP, and bleeding—to determine the seriousness of the situation. The outcome of this evaluation will identify a course of action.

Table 25.9 Shin-Splint Syndrome

Injury	Common causes	Signs and symptoms	Treatment
Shin splints—inflammatory reaction of the musculotendinous unit, caused by overexertion of muscles during weight-bearing activity. The following conditions must be ruled out: stress fracture, metabolic or vascular disorder, compartment syndrome, and muscular strain.	Prominent callus in metatarsal region Fallen metatarsal arch Weak longitudinal arch Muscular imbalance Poor leg, ankle, and foot flexibility Improper running surface Improper running shoes Overuse Biomechanical problems or structural abnormalities Improper running or skills technique Training in poor weather	Lower longitudinal arch on one side in comparison to the opposite side Tenderness in arch area Abnormal wear patterns of shoes	Keep callus filed down. Wear a metatarsal arch pad. Conduct strengthening exercises for toe flexors. Wear longitudinal arch tape for support. Wear arch supports. Conduct strengthening exercises for the dorsiflexors and inverters. Exercise to increase range of motion. Avoid hard surfaces. Avoid changing from one surface to another. Select a shoe with good shock-absorbency qualities; be sure that the shoe is properly fitted. Be flexible about changing the training program if there are signs that a great deal of physical stress is occurring. Encourage year-round conditioning. Always warm up properly. Refer to podiatrist or other professional specializing in foot care; orthotics may be indicated. Design a special training program to allow for individual differences (e.g., increase intensity of work-outs reduce duration). Correct technique. Perform specific stretching or strengthening exercises as well as technique work. Use common sense when training in cold or foul weather. Dress properly to maintain warmth. Warm up and cool down properly.

Table 25.9 *(continued)*

Injury	Common causes	Signs and symptoms	Treatment
Stress fracture—a bone defect that occurs because of overstress to weight-bearing bones which causes an accelerated rate of remodeling. Inability of the bone to meet the demands of the stress results in a loss of continuity in the bone and periosteal irritation. Tibial stress fractures—more common in individuals with high-arched feet Fibula stress fractures—more common in pronators	Overuse or abrupt change in training program Change in running surface Change in running gait	Referred pain to the fracture site when a percussion test is used (e.g., hitting the heel may cause pain at the site of a tibial stress fracture) Pain usually localized to one spot and exquisitely tender to palpation Pain generally present all of the time but increases with weight-bearing activity; no lessening of pain after warm-up	Refer to physician. X-ray films should be obtained. Usually no crack is detected in the bone. A cloudy area becomes visible when the callus begins to form. Often this does not show up until 2–6 weeks after onset of pain. Early detection can usually be made through a bone scan or thermogram. If a stress fracture is suspected but not diagnosed, treat as a stress fracture. Running and other high-stress, weight-bearing activities should not be allowed until the fracture has healed and the bone is no longer tender to palpation. Tibial stress fractures usually take 8–10 weeks to heal; fibula stress fractures take approximately 6 weeks. When acute symptoms have subsided, bicycling and swimming activities can usually be initiated to maintain cardiovascular levels. This should be cleared with the supervising physician. If a specific cause is attributed to the development of a stress fracture, steps should be taken to correct the cause.

(2, 5, 6, 9-13, 15, 18-26)

Table 25.10 Injury Classification Criteria and Exercise Modifications

Criteria	Modifications
Mild injury Performance is not affected. Pain is experienced only after athletic activity. Generally, no tenderness is felt on palpation. No or minimal swelling is present. No discoloration is apparent.	Reduce activity level, modify activity to take stress off of the injured part, treat symptomatically, and gradually return to full activity.
Moderate injury Performance is mildly affected or not affected at all. Pain is experienced before and after athletic activity. Mild tenderness is felt on palpation. Mild swelling may be present. Some discoloration may be present.	Rest the injured part, modify activity to take stress off of the injured part, treat symptomatically, and gradually return to full activity.
Severe injury Pain is experienced before, during, and after activity. Performance is definitely affected because of pain. Movement is limited because of pain. Moderate-to-severe point tenderness is felt on palpation. Swelling is most likely present. Discoloration may be present.	Rest completely and see a physician.

(9)

Checking Vital Signs

The following paragraphs describe vital signs and how to monitor each. Important vital signs to check include the pulse, color, body temperature, mobility, and BP of the injured person.

Check HR. Use light finger pressure over an artery to monitor pulse rate. The most common sites are the carotid, brachial, radial, and femoral pulses. If there is no pulse and the individual is unconscious, begin CPR.

Assess color. For light-pigmented individuals, if skin, fingernail beds, lips, sclera of eyes, and mucous membranes are red, heat stroke, high blood pressure, or carbon monoxide poisoning are possible. If the person is pale or ashen, changes in skin color could be attributable to shock, fright, insufficient circulation, heat exhaustion, insulin shock, or a heart attack. If the person is bluish, the poor oxygenation of the blood could be attributable to an airway obstruction, respiratory insufficiency, heart failure, or some poisonings. For dark-pigmented individuals, assess nail beds, inside of lips, mouth, and tongue. Pink is the normal color for these; a bluish cast suggests shock. A grayish cast suggests shock from **hemorrhage**. A red flush at the tips of the ears suggests fever.

Take body temperature. Normal body temperature is 98.6° F. Record temperature with a thermometer placed under the tongue (for 3 min); in the axilla, or armpit (10 min); or in the rectum (1 min). Cool, clammy, damp skin suggests shock or heat exhaustion; cool, dry skin indicates exposure to cold air; and hot, dry skin suggests fever or heat stroke.

Check mobility. Inability to move (paralysis) suggests injury or illness of the spinal cord or brain.

Take BP. BP usually is taken at the brachial artery with a BP cuff and sphygmomanometer. The following will aid in determining the problem:

- Normal BP—in men, SBP, the pressure during the contraction phase of the heart, is equal to 100 plus the age of the individual up to 140 to 150 mmHg; DBP, the pressure during the relaxation phase of the heart, is equal to 65 to 90 mmHg. In women, both readings are generally 8 to 10 mmHg lower.
- Severe hemorrhage, heart attack—marked decrease (20-30 mmHg) in BP.
- Damage or rupture of vessels in the arterial circuit—BP is abnormally high (>150/>90).
- Brain damage—increase in SBP with a stable or falling DBP.
- Heart ailment—decrease in SBP with an increase DBP.

Questions to Determine a Course of Action

Ask the following questions to help determine a course of action for treating injured participants.

Is the individual conscious? If not, a head, neck, or back injury is possible. If you are unsure as to why the individual is unconscious, check for a medical-alert identification tag. Assess airway, breathing, and circulation. Do not use ammonia capsules to arouse; the individual may suddenly move the head backward in response, causing additional injury. If breathing has stopped and the individual is in a prone position, he or she should be log-rolled as carefully as possible, keeping the head, neck, and spine in the same relative position, to begin CPR techniques.

If the individual is unconscious but breathing, protect from further injury. Do not move unless the individual's life is in danger. Wait for medical assistance to arrive. Systematically evaluate the entire body and perform necessary first-aid procedures.

Is the individual breathing? If not, establish an airway and administer artificial respiration. Summon medical help. The following information will aid in determining the problem:

- Normal respiration—20 breaths · min^{-1}
- Respiration in well-trained individuals—6 to 8 breaths · min^{-1}
- Shock—rapid, shallow respiration
- Airway obstruction, heart disease, pulmonary disease—deep, gasping, labored breathing
- Lung damage—frothy sputum with blood at the nose and mouth, accompanied by coughing
- Diabetic acidosis—alcoholic or sweet, fruity odor to breath
- Cessation of breathing—lack of movement of abdomen and chest as well as airflow at nose and mouth

Is the individual bleeding profusely? If so, control bleeding by elevating the body part; putting direct pressure over the wound or at **pressure points**; and, as a last resort, putting on a tourniquet. A tourniquet should only be used in life-threatening situations in which choosing to risk a limb is a reasonable action to save a life. Treat for shock.

Is there evidence of a head injury? This can be determined through a history of a blow to the head or a fall onto the head, deformity of the skull, loss of consciousness, clear or straw-colored fluid coming from the nose or ears, unequal pupil size, dizziness, loss of memory, and nausea. Prevent any unnecessary movement. If it is necessary to move the individual, use a stretcher with the individual's head elevated. If the individual is unconscious, assume there is also a neck injury. Summon medical help immediately. The following information will aid in determining the problem:

- Drug abuse or nervous system disorder—constricted pupils
- Unconscious, cardiac arrest—dilated pupils
- Head injury—pupils unequal size
- Disease, poisoning, drug overdose, injury—pupils do not react to light
- Death—pupils widely dilated and unresponsive to light

Is there evidence of a neck or back injury? The history of the injury may give a clue. Other indications of a possible neck or back injury include pain directly over the spine, burning or tingling in the extremities, and loss of muscle function or strength in the extremities. When in doubt, assume there is a neck or back injury. The following information will aid in determining the problem:

- Probable injury of spinal cord—numbness or tingling in the extremities
- Occlusion of a main artery—severe pain in the extremity, with loss of cutaneous sensation
- Hysteria, violent shock, excessive drug or alcohol use—no pain

9 In Review

When an exercise participant is injured, check for consciousness, breathing, bleeding, and head, neck, or back injuries. Take a pulse, temperature, and BP reading according to the guidelines in the previous section.

Rescue Breathing, CPR, and Use of the Automated External Defibrillator

Cardiac arrest is the single leading cause of death in the United States, leading to more than 350,000 deaths each year. An abnormal, chaotic heart rhythm known as ventricular fibrillation (see chapter 24) keeps the heart from filling with blood. CPR, started early enough, can keep oxygen flowing to the brain but cannot correct or restore a normal heartbeat. Shocking the heart with an electrical impulse often restores a normal sinus rhythm. The sooner the shock is delivered, the greater the chance of survival. Recent technology has emerged with a piece of equipment called the automated external defibrillator (AED), which allows for rescuers with limited experience and training to defibrillate a heart. The AED has significantly increased the survival rate of individuals suffering from myocardial infarction (MI). A participant may stop breathing and not suffer from cardiac arrest. Rescue breathing (RB) will help restore breathing, but pulse should also be checked to ensure that the heart is pumping blood throughout the body. A pulse may be faint or undetectable and the rescuer may believe that a participant requires CPR and/or the AED. If no pulse is found, CPR should be started until the AED is available. The design of the AED allows for the rescuer to prepare to shock but has a safety device to ensure that a shock is not delivered unless needed. The HFI should be prepared to use any of the previously mentioned techniques to restore breathing and/or blood flow in a potentially fatal situation involving a participant. The following outlines current steps for RB, CPR, and the use of the AED taught by the American Red Cross. The HFI should review current recommended techniques (8).

If the HFI believes that a participant has stopped breathing, RB should be initiated. If the HFI finds that breathing has stopped and there is no pulse, the AED (if readily available) should be used or CPR should be started immediately. Although the steps for RB and CPR techniques are for adults only, the HFI should review current recommended techniques for all age categories: adults, children, and infants. The following is a list of steps to use in rescuing an unconscious victim:

1. Check the scene for safety and to help determine probable cause for collapse.

2. Check the victim for injuries and responsiveness as well as any additional clues as to the cause.

3. Determine responsiveness by gently shaking or tapping the individual and asking if he or she is okay.

4. If you are alone and the person is unresponsive, immediately call for help, get any needed supplies if close by, and determine whether the victim should be moved before you begin the rescue attempt. If there are other people around, instruct someone to call for help and another to get needed supplies, and cautiously move the victim if safety dictates. Then begin the rescue attempt following basic precautions for preventing disease transmission.

5. Look, listen, and feel for breathing. If the victim is not breathing, and if necessary, move the victim to a face-up position while supporting the head and neck. Reposition the neck by using a head tilt/chin lift or jaw thrust maneuver and reassess. If the person is still not breathing, pinch the victim's nose shut, cover his or her mouth with yours, and give two slow breaths. Then assess circulation by sliding the index and middle finger of one hand into the groove at the side of the victim's neck closest toward you. Take no more than 10 s to check the carotid pulse.

6. If there is a pulse but the person is still not breathing, initiate RB at a rate of one breath every 5 s. Recheck for signs of circulation and breathing in 1 min, or 12 cycles, and then every 2 to 3 minutes thereafter.

7. If there is no breathing but circulation is still present, continue RB.

8. If there is no breathing or pulse, begin using the AED and CPR; if the AED is not readily available, begin CPR and continue until the AED arrives.

9. If CPR is initiated, place two fingers above the ziphoid process at the lower end of the sternal notch, place the heel of one hand above the two fingers in the middle of the sternum, and place the second hand on top. Interlace fingers and lift off of the chest wall. With your shoulders positioned over your hands, compress the chest 1.5 to 2 in. Give 15 compressions and 2 rescue breaths at a rate of 80 per minute for an adult. Continue for 4 cycles or 1 min and recheck for signs of circulation. If there is no circulation, continue CPR, checking circulation every few minutes. If the AED is ready to use, recheck the pulse, and if you find no pulse, follow the steps as outlined next.

10. Turn on the AED. Do not use the AED
    - near or with alcohol or any other form of flammable material,
    - in a moving vehicle,
    - if victim is lying on a conductive surface or in water, or
    - on an individual weighing less than 55 lb or less than 8 years of age.

Do not use cellular phones within 6 ft of the AED.

To use the defibrillator:

a. Wipe the victim's chest dry.

b. Remove any metal on or around victim, including bra with underwire and/or clothing with metal hooks.

c. Remove any patches on chest with gloved hand.
d. Attach the pads as instructed, one to the upper right chest and the other on the victim's lower left side.
e. Plug the electrode into the AED. Follow the instructions as the computerized voice runs you through the various steps in using the AED.
f. Be ready to analyze the victim's heart rhythm.
g. Make sure no one is touching the victim; advise to stand clear; push analyze button.
h. The AED will analyze the rhythm and will instruct to shock or to begin CPR.
i. If a shock is advised, anyone near the scene should be instructed to stand back; deliver the shock by pushing the shock button.
j. The AED will then analyze the rhythm again.
k. If the AED advises no shock is needed, check the pulse again; if there is no pulse, begin CPR until the AED reanalyzes.

If a second rescuer is available and the initial rescuer gets tired, the second rescuer can prepare the AED for use, if available, or can take over CPR at the end of a cycle of 15 compressions.

10 In Review

Steps to take when dealing with a breathing emergency or heart attack should be learned and maintained at a high level. The HFI should update his or her training regularly to keep informed about the latest technology for dealing with these emergency situations.

Case Studies

You can check your answers by referring to appendix A.

25.1

You are instructing an aerobics class when a participant collapses. On approaching the individual, you note that breathing is shallow and slow and that the skin color is pale, moist, and clammy. The individual is conscious but not alert. The individual reports double vision and an intense hunger. The individual is wearing a medical-alert tag.

a. What illness do you suspect?
b. What questions would you ask?
c. What action should you take?

25.2

You are leading an aerobics class and a participant collapses. You observe that the participant's skin is dry and red, breathing is labored, and pulse is rapid and strong. No trauma was experienced.

a. What heat-related illness should be suspected?
b. What is the immediate care?
c. What emergency planning should be in effect?

Source List

1. American Academy of Orthopedic Surgeons. (1977). *Emergency care and transportation of the sick and injured* (2nd ed.). Menasha, WI: Banta.
2. American Medical Association. (1966). *Standard nomenclature of athletic injuries*. Chicago: Author.
3. American Red Cross. (1993). *Adult CPR*. St. Louis: Mosby.
4. American Red Cross. (1993). *Community CPR*. St. Louis: Mosby.
5. American Red Cross. (1993). *Community first aid and safety*. St. Louis: Mosby.
6. American Red Cross. (1993). *Emergency response*. St. Louis: Mosby.
7. American Red Cross. (1993). *Preventing disease transmission*. St. Louis: Mosby.
8. American Red Cross. (2001). *First aid/CPR/AED program: Participant's booklet*. San Bruno, CA: Author.
9. Arnheim, D.D. (1987). *Essentials of athletic training*. St. Louis: Times Mirror/Mosby.
10. Arnheim, D.D. (1989). *Modern principles of athletic training*. St. Louis: Times Mirror/Mosby.
11. Arnheim, D.D., & Prentice, W.E. (1993). *Principles of athletic training*. St. Louis: Mosby.
12. Bloomfield, J., Fricker, P.A., & Fitch, K.P. (Eds.). (1992). *Textbook of science and medicine in sport*. Champaign, IL: Human Kinetics.
13. Booher, J.M., & Thibadeau, G.A. (1994). *Athletic injury assessment* (3rd ed.). St. Louis: Mosby.
14. Department of Labor, Occupational Safety and Health Administration. (1991). Occupational exposure to bloodborne pathogens: Final rule. *Federal Register* [Online], *56*(235), 1-36. Available: osha.gov/Publications/Osha3127.pdf [July 10, 2002].
15. Fahey, T.D. (1986). *Athletic training*. Mountain View, CA: Mayfield.
16. Franks, B.D., & Howley, E.T. (1989). *Fitness facts: The healthy living handbook*. Champaign, IL: Human Kinetics.
17. Franks, B.D., & Howley, E.T. (1989). *Fitness leaders' handbook*. Champaign, IL: Human Kinetics.
18. Henderson, J. (1973). *Emergency medical guide* (3rd ed.). St. Louis: Mosby.
19. Klafs, C.E., & Arnheim, D.D. (1977). *Modern principles of athletic training*. St. Louis: Mosby.
20. Morris, A.F. (1984). *Sports medicine: Prevention of athletic injuries*. Dubuque, IA: Brown.
21. Nieman, D.C. (1990). *Fitness and sports medicine: An introduction*. Palo Alto, CA: Bull.
22. Pfeiffer, R.P., & Pfeiffer, B.C. (1995). *Concepts of athletic training*. Boston: Jones & Bartlett.
23. Rankin, J.M., & Ingersoll, C.H. (1995). *Athletic training management: Concepts and applications*. St. Louis: Mosby.
24. Reid, D. (1992). *Sports injury assessment and rehabilitation*. New York: Churchill Livingstone.
25. Ritter, M.A., & Albohm, M.J. (1987). *Your inquiry: A commonsense guide to sports injuries*. Indianapolis: Benchmark Press.
26. Scribner, K., & Burke, E. (Eds.). (1978). *Relevant topics in athletic training*. New York: Mouvement.
27. Thygerson, A.L. (1987). *First aid and emergency care workbook*. Boston: Jones & Bartlett.
28. Torg, J.S., Welsh, P.R., & Shepard, R.J. (1990). *Current therapy in sports medicine*. St. Louis: Mosby.
29. Williams, M.H. (1988). *Nutrition for fitness and sport*. Dubuque, IA: Brown.

twenty-six

Program Administration/ Management

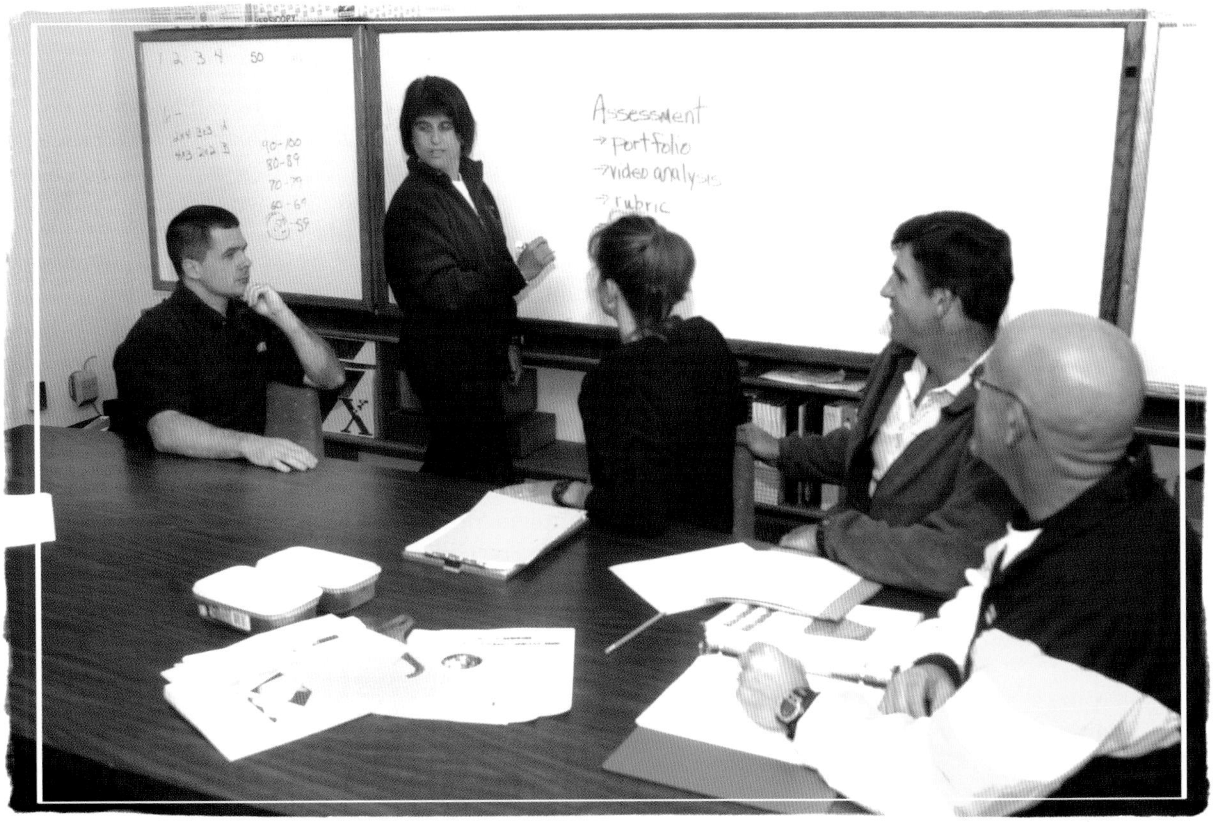

© Human Kinetics

Objectives

The reader will be able to do the following:

1. Describe the importance of long-range planning.
2. Describe the personnel and working environment recommended for a fitness program.
3. Identify the elements of a comprehensive fitness program.
4. Describe the potential legal issues related to fitness programs.
5. Explain the elements of the budget.
6. Describe the equipment recommended for a fitness program.
7. Describe the importance of keeping records of all aspects of a fitness program.
8. Describe the importance of evaluation.

In small fitness programs the HFI may be in charge of administering the program, but in most cases a program director has the major administrative responsibilities. The person in charge of the program may want to consider qualifying for the ACSM Health Fitness Director certification. However, all staff should understand the types of decisions that are made and the processes that are used by the program executive.

Setting Long-Range Goals

The key concept to administration is planning. Many different programs and management styles can be successful when carefully planned; almost nothing works well over the long term without planning. This chapter presents the items that need to be considered in establishing a long-range plan for a fitness center and makes suggestions for dealing with responsibilities that administrators normally have in any type of program. See Minor (6) for an extensive discussion of program management.

The program director is normally responsible for long-range planning in these areas:

- Deciding what specific classes will be offered, when, where, and for whom
- Hiring and evaluating personnel
- Preparing and executing a budget
- Maintaining communications
- Maintaining quality control

Any organization—private, public, for profit, or nonprofit—needs to carefully consider what it wants to accomplish. The long-range plan includes what goals should be accomplished, what is needed to accomplish these goals, how the organization will move from where it is to where it wants to be, and what processes should be followed to implement the program. The program director facilitates establishment of the long-range plan by working with the governing body in defining the areas that should be addressed, seeking input from appropriate individuals and groups, and providing working drafts for reactions and revisions. The program director implements the plan, including periodic evaluation. The HFI's role is to provide details concerning possible fitness programs that are consistent with the aims of the fitness center and will be popular with current and potential participants. The HFI works with the fitness director in determining appropriate equipment, facilities, scheduling, personnel, and supplies.

1 In Review

Long-range planning is the only way to set goals and to develop a plan for reaching them. No program can be successful without plans for program offerings, hiring and evaluating personnel, budgeting, communication, and quality control.

Managing Personnel

The most important aspect of any program is the quality of the staff. The processes of recruiting, hiring, supporting, and evaluating personnel to help achieve the organization's goals are essential, time consuming, and often sensitive.

Finding Qualified Staff

The first question to consider is what types of people are needed to carry out the planned program. Fitness programs need staff personnel who can present and supervise the fitness activities. A typical fitness center needs the following personnel:

Full time

- Program director
- HFI
- Educational coordinator
- Secretary

Part time

- Medical adviser
- Fitness leaders
- Nutritionist
- Psychologist
- Physical therapist
- Equipment technician

What characteristics are desired for the staff? The qualifications include education, personal qualities, and professional competence. Administrative responsibilities involved in a fitness program include managing, planning, supervising, educating, leading exercise, motivating, counseling, promoting, assessing, and evaluating.

During the search for specific personnel, decisions are made concerning which of these general responsibilities, and what specific tasks, will be assigned to each person. A realistic list of required and preferred qualifications is developed for each staff member. For example, an education requirement is established for each position. Requiring more education than is needed, or failing to require enough, causes problems. For fitness programs, the appropriate ACSM certification can be useful in establishing minimum qualifications. Use the certification that matches the position (see the box on the following page).

Cultivating a Good Working Environment

One of the traits of a successful administrator is the quality of **communication** with staff, program participants, and the public. Open and honest communication is essential so that staff personnel know what is expected and how they are being evaluated. The staff personnel need to feel appreciated and encouraged to find better ways of accomplishing the goals. Many advances in organizations come from staff personnel who are encouraged to help find better ways to improve the program content and procedures.

The fitness center should provide a good working environment and accurately describe the working conditions to prospective staff members. The physical environment should be safe, clean, and cheerful, with functioning equipment, available supplies, and quick repairs when needed. The professional environment is one in which the expectations for each staff member are clearly described and supervision is ample to assist professional growth and ensure quality performance. The psychological environment ensures that employees are valued and that their input is solicited and welcomed. Employees are communicated with openly and honestly, and they believe that they have support for problems that might arise.

2 In Review

Full- and part-time personnel are needed who are qualified to administer a fitness program, lead exercise, test fitness components, and deal with specific aspects of fitness, including counseling participants. The working environment should be clean, safe, cheerful, well-stocked, and in good repair.

Evaluating Personnel

A clear job description that is mutually understood provides the basis for periodic evaluations. The main purpose of the evaluation is to assist the staff member in improving her or his job performance. However, the evaluation also is used to determine whether employees are retained in the position and, if so, what merit raises should be awarded. Evaluation of the HFI includes the following:

Sample Job Description

Generic Fitness Center
Health Fitness Instructor

Qualifications

BS in kinesiology or related field
ACSM Health Fitness Instructor Certification
Experience instructing and leading exercise in adult fitness setting
Ability to relate to people with diverse backgrounds

Responsibilities

Administer physical fitness tests
Lead physical fitness exercise sessions
Work with program director in the following ways:
Scheduling fitness programs and staff
Adding variety to fitness classes
Training new staff members

Application Process

Send a letter of application, vita, and the names, addresses, and phone numbers of three references to

Dr. Drawde Yolwob, Director
Generic Fitness Center
Yarbrogh, MI 22222
To ensure consideration for the position, applications should be received by March 1, 2002.

Title and Starting Date

The health fitness instructor will begin September 1, 2002. The 12-month position includes 2 weeks of vacation and an excellent benefits package. The salary will be within the range of $32,500 to $38,000, depending on qualifications.

Affirmative Action

The Generic Fitness Center encourages minority, female, and physically challenged candidates to apply for this position.

- Content of the fitness program
- Manner in which the program is conducted
- Rapport with fitness participants, other staff, and the fitness director
- Response to emergency and unusual situations
- Accuracy in collecting and recording test data
- Prompt and professional manner of carrying out other assigned responsibilities

The Sample Evaluation Checklist (form 26.1) presents questions that can be asked in an annual evaluation conference.

Developing a Successful Program

The ACSM guidelines (1) list five aspects of interaction between the fitness program and the participant: screening, testing, counseling, exercise prescription, and delivery of the fitness program.

Participant Screening

All participants should be screened before they are placed in appropriate fitness programs. Chapter 3 deals with criteria for admission to various programs. For example, people with known or suspected health

form
26.1

Sample Evaluation Checklist
Generic Fitness Center

Evaluation of a Health Fitness Instructor ______________________________
(Name)

Attainment of Current Goals

Did the HFI

Adhere to Center procedures? ______________________________

Make proper screening decisions? ______________________________

Administer tests efficiently, with accurate results and good records? ______________

Provide appropriate content for the exercise sessions? ______________________

Conduct the sessions with enthusiasm? ______________________________

Provide a variety of fitness activities? ______________________________

Relate well with the clients? ______________________________

Provide comprehensive training and supervision of new staff members? __________

Understand and carry out emergency procedures? ______________________

Make suggestions for improvement in all aspects of the Center's activities and procedures? ______________________________

____

Make efforts to improve in identified areas of weakness? ______________________

Accomplish things not listed as specific goals for this year? ______________________

Evaluation of Past Activities

What responsibilities were carried out (be specific)

Very well? ______________________________

Adequately, but could be improved? ______________________________

Below expectations that must be corrected? ______________________________

From Edward T. Howley and B. Don Franks, 2003, *Health Fitness Instructor's Handbook,* 4th ed. (Champaign, IL: Human Kinetics).

(continued)

form 26.1 *(continued)*

Future Goals

What responsibilities should be

Continued? ______________________________

Added? ______________________________

Deleted or handled by someone else? ______________________________

What additional knowledge, skills, and so forth are needed? ______________________________

____

How will they be obtained? ______________________________

____

How can the evaluation process be improved? ______________________________

____

From Edward T. Howley and B. Don Franks, 2003, *Health Fitness Instructor's Handbook,* 4th ed. (Champaign, IL: Human Kinetics).

problems are not allowed in fitness programs aimed to increase the positive health of apparently healthy people. The administrator ensures that the testing criteria for exclusion or referral are applied consistently and that the personnel leading activities are able to recognize signs and symptoms of problems that require special attention.

Part of a thorough screening process includes following the informed consent procedures established to protect participants. Informed consent has several elements:

- Clear description of program and procedures
- Clear description of potential benefits and risks of the program
- Statement that the individual is participating voluntarily and has the right to withdraw at any time
- Statement that each individual's data are confidential

The first component of informed consent is to clearly describe the fitness program and all of the procedures that will be used. This description should be in writing, and each individual should read and receive a copy. In addition, each person should be given an opportunity to ask questions. The second element of this procedure, included in the written description of the program, is a list of the possible benefits and risks of such a program. The fitness benefits are extensive; however, the risk of certain kinds of injuries (e.g., ankle, knee) is increased, and heart attacks occasionally occur during or after exercise. Third, after reading the description of the potential benefits and risks, the person signs the form indicating that he or she is participating voluntarily, with the provision that the individual can stop tests and all other activities at any time without penalty or coercion to continue.

Fourth, each individual's data are confidential unless the individual gives permission to release them. People normally agree to have their test scores used in fitness reports and research, but these reports should be presented in such a manner that an individual's test score remains confidential. An exception to this guideline is using test scores to recognize people in newsletters or news releases—in these cases, permission should be obtained (and usually is granted) from the person before publishing the individual scores. A Sample Consent Form (form 26.2) that might be used in a fitness program is shown here. Specific procedures should be modified to fit the particular fitness testing and program.

Testing

Fitness participants should be tested to decide whether they can begin the program immediately, can enter the program only with medical clearance, or should be excluded (see chapter 3). For people in the program, testing is important to determine the extent to which their individual objectives are being met. The test results can motivate participants to

form
26.2

Sample Consent Form Generic Fitness Center

Informed Consent for Physical Fitness Test

In order to more safely carry on an exercise program, I hereby consent, voluntarily, to exercise tests. I shall perform a graded exercise test by riding a cycle ergometer or walking/running on a treadmill. Exercise will begin at a low level and be advanced in stages. The test may be stopped at any time because of signs of fatigue. I understand that I may stop the test at any time because of my feelings of fatigue or discomfort or for any other personal reason.

I understand that the risks of this testing procedure may include disorders of heart beats, abnormal blood pressure response, and, very rarely, a heart attack. I further understand that selection and supervision of my test is a matter of professional judgment.

I also understand that skinfold measurements will be taken at (number) sites to determine percent body fat and that I will complete a sit-and-reach test and a curl-up test to evaluate factors related to low-back function.

I desire such testing so that better advice regarding my proposed exercise program may be given to me, but I understand that the testing does not entirely eliminate risk in the proposed exercise program.

I understand that information from my tests may be used for reports and research publications. I understand that my identity will not be revealed.

I understand that I can withdraw my consent or discontinue participation in any aspect of the fitness testing or program at any time without penalty or prejudice toward me.

I have read the statements above and have had all of my questions answered to my satisfaction.

______________________	______________________
Date	Signature of Participant
______________________	______________________
Date	Signature of Witness
______________________	______________________
Date	Signature of Test Administrator

(Copy for participant and for program records.)

continue and can provide the basis for activity modification. Fitness testing procedures are included in chapters 3, 5, 6, 8, and 9.

Counseling and Exercise Prescription

Consumers need basic information concerning what the fitness program can (and cannot) do for them, periodic progress reports, and educational information to enhance their positive health knowledge and status. Minilectures during warm-up, bulletin boards, and newsletters have all been used to help educate participants. Electronic communication (e.g., e-mail, Web site) can be used to communicate with current and potential participants. The information should be accurate, brief, and to the point.

The HFI assists individual participants in setting goals and evaluating their progress toward those goals. Counseling about lifestyle changes and specific exercise recommendations are included in these goal-setting sessions.

Fitness programs have a responsibility to educate the public concerning positive health—its definition and recommendations for its achievement. Communicate the beneficial effects of fitness programs on health, with corresponding benefits for the family, community, and work performance, via the mass media and with interested groups such as local industry.

3 In Review

The fitness program must provide clear and helpful information to fitness participants and the public. Participants need to know what the program can and cannot do for them and how they are progressing in their fitness goals. The public should be educated about the benefits of positive health and how to achieve it.

Program Delivery

Although the general types of experiences offered by the organization are determined before staff selection, the staff can assist in fine-tuning the specific classes that will be offered to take advantage of the strengths of each staff member and provide the activities needed by each participant. Chapters 10 through 14 include suggestions and examples of activities to be included in the fitness program. Chapters 15 through 21 provide suggestions for modifications needed for individuals with different characteristics or health conditions.

Scheduling of personnel and facilities requires attention to the types of programs being offered, the desires of consumers for specific times, and the optimal work performance from staff. Priorities are established to ensure that the more important objectives receive the needed staff and facilities. Making the facilities available to other groups, although that is usually a lower priority, enhances public relations. Guidelines should be established to ensure that the top-priority activities have adequate time. For example, the main exercise room might be scheduled for classes first, and then other peak times could be set aside for members to use it on their own. Community groups could reserve it only during specific nonpeak times of the day. A form like the Sample Form for Use of Facility by Outside Group (form 26.3) could be used to lease the facilities to local groups.

Safety and Legal Concerns

The main concern for the fitness program is that it be conducted safely for everyone in the program. Fortunately, the same kinds of things that make the program safe also help protect the program legally. Chapter 25 includes detailed procedures to prevent and deal with injuries and emergencies, including CPR procedures, which are essential for all staff members who will work with fitness participants.

Liability

The program and its staff have a responsibility to perform the procedures as described in a professional manner, watch for any danger signs that might indicate a problem, and take appropriate actions to stop the activity before problems occur. The ACSM guidelines (1) indicate that a risk management orientation not only helps prevent legal actions but also adds value to the program for the following reasons:

- A risk management orientation emphasizes client satisfaction.
- It documents participant outcomes.
- It aims to reduce injuries.

Sample Form for Use of Facility by Outside Group Generic Fitness Center

Use of facility

Name of group: ____________________

Person responsible for the group: ____________________

Name: ____________________

Phone: ____________________

Purpose for use of building: ____________________

Estimated number of participants: ____________________

Age range of participants: ____________________

Room(s) desired: ____________________

Date(s) & Time(s)	Date	Time
First choice:	________	________
Second choice:	________	________
Third choice:	________	________

On behalf of the group desiring to lease a part of the Generic Fitness Center, I have read and agree to follow the regulations for the building. Our group understands that the security deposit may be used for any damage that occurs as a result of our group's activities. In addition, we will reimburse the Generic Fitness Center for any damages that exceed the deposit. We will not hold the Center liable for any accidents or injuries that occur during our use of the facility.

____
Signed

____
Witness

____
Date

From Edward T. Howley and B. Don Franks, 2003, *Health Fitness Instructor's Handbook,* 4th ed. (Champaign, IL: Human Kinetics).

Herbert and Herbert (4) suggested common potential **liability** problems. These include failure to do any of the following:

- Monitor and/or stop a GXT, using professional judgment
- Evaluate participants' physical capabilities or impairments that need special attention
- Recommend a safe exercise intensity
- Instruct participants adequately on safe activities and proper use of equipment
- Supervise exercise and advise individuals regarding restrictions or modifications needed during unsupervised exercise
- Assign participants to levels of monitoring, supervision, and emergency medical support commensurate with health status
- Perform in a nonnegligent manner
- Refrain from giving advice construed to represent diagnosis of a medical condition
- Refer participants to medical or other professionals based on appropriate signs or symptoms
- Maintain proper and confidential records

If problems do occur, take the appropriate actions to deal with minor problems and get immediate help for major problems. Professional organizations (e.g., the American Association for Health, Physical Education, Recreation and Dance, ACSM) have arrangements with insurance carriers to provide liability insurance for individuals. Staff members should be encouraged to have this type of insurance. In addition, the organization should include liability for the program and facilities in its insurance coverage.

No amount of informed-consent procedures can justify **negligence**. Participants and facilities must be supervised. Staff personnel should be trained in appropriate emergency procedures, which need to be followed. Failure to do so, or failure to act in a manner fitting for a fitness professional, constitutes negligence. If injury or death occur as a result of the negligence, then the leader and program are legally liable. The trend to seek official recognition of fitness professionals, although having many positive aspects, also may increase the possibility of malpractice legal actions for fitness programs (1). Although getting the participant's consent does not prevent legal actions or protect against negligence, it does indicate that the program is concerned with the participant and has acted in good faith.

Concern for safety includes regular inspection of equipment and facilities and periodic reviews of procedures that the staff use both in testing and in classes. Records showing when the review, training, and practice were carried out should be kept in the central office. Participants should be strongly encouraged to wear helmets for cycling, skating, and other similar activities and eye protectors for racquetball and similar sports.

Emergency Procedures

Written **emergency procedures** should be established, and staff members should be trained to carry them out. Local emergency services to be used should be contacted to help establish the procedure to be followed. For example, in a hospital program, the fitness participants can use the emergency facilities and procedures provided for all patients. However, in a program outside a medical facility, it will be important to have separate emergency procedures and equipment to deal with minor injuries as well as life-threatening emergencies. The Sample Emergency Procedures form (form 26.4) can be modified for a specific situation.

4 In Review

A comprehensive fitness program includes screening, individual program development, fitness program implementation, and maintenance. Decisions need to be consistent concerning screening of potential participants. Scheduling of the facilities, activities, and appropriate testing is an important aspect of the administration of a fitness program. Participants should be given good information and advice, facilities and programs must be supervised, and unusual events should be responded to professionally.

Developing a Budget

The **budget** is one aspect of long-range planning. Careful inventory, assessment of needs, and a balance among personnel, equipment, facilities, and other expenses provide the maximum service for the minimum cost. A suggested budget process includes the steps outlined in form 26.5. The Sample Monthly Budget Report (form 26.6) is adapted from Musser (8). More detailed examples of a fitness budget are presented by Ancharski (2) and Patton et al. (9).

Sample Emergency Procedures Generic Fitness Center

Cardiac Emergency

1. Do NOT move the victim, except to try to get him or her into a lying position.
2. Check for breathing and pulse; if absent, begin CPR immediately.
3. Call, or have someone call, the Emergency Room at

   ______________________________ Hospital ________________, ext. _________
4. Read the statement above the phone to the contact person:

(Statement to be posted by all phones:)

This is ________________________ at the ____________________ Fitness Center. We have a cardiac emergency. Please send an ambulance to the ____________________ Street entrance of the ____________________ building, at ______________________________ .

5. Send someone to get Dr. ________________________, whose schedule is posted by the phone [this is for centers that have medical personnel on the site].
6. Continue CPR until medical personnel arrive, then follow their instructions.

Other Serious Accidents or Injuries

For any of the following:

Airway problems of any type

Unconsciousness

Head Injury

Bleeding from ear, nose, or mouth

Neck or back injuries

Limb injury with obvious deformity

Severe chest pains

1. Do NOT move the person, except to try to get her or him into a lying position, with feet elevated (unless you suspect back injuries).
2. Contact ambulance and medical personnel—same as cardiac emergencies.
3. Treat for shock.
4. Control bleeding.

(continued)

form 26.4 *(continued)*

Other Injuries or Accidents

1. Do not allow a sick or injured person to sit, stand, or walk until you are sure that his or her condition warrants it.

2. Do not encourage a person who is "feeling bad" to begin or continue working out.

3. Check on people who have questionable symptoms in the locker room.

4. For less serious injuries, a first-aid kit is available at ____________________.

As soon as the situation is under control, inform ____________________ about the accident, complete accident report, and turn in to ____________________ within 24 hr.

Your suggestions for improving these instructions and the emergency procedures are welcome—talk to ______________________________.

From Edward T. Howley and B. Don Franks, 2003, *Health Fitness Instructor's Handbook,* 4th ed. (Champaign, IL: Human Kinetics).

Using Third-Party Payments

Insurance companies have always invested in health by providing health education, supporting research, and paying for treatment of health problems (e.g., cardiac rehabilitation programs). More recently, they have offered incentives for healthy behaviors such as lower premiums for nonsmokers and cash paybacks for people who do not use their medical insurance for a set period of time. A logical extension of these policies is for the insurance companies to pay for preventive programs and incentives for individuals who are physically active. With increasing evidence of the health benefits of fitness programs that emphasize a variety of healthy behaviors, the program director should approach insurance companies with proposals for third-party payment for some of the services and for premium incentives for people engaging in healthy behaviors.

Budgeting for Personnel and Facilities

The biggest part of the budget involves salary and benefits for the staff. Relatively high base salaries and benefits, with regular increments based on evaluations, will enable the program to employ qualified people. An attractive salary and benefits package results in higher job satisfaction, higher quality performance, and a lower turnover rate. Administrators attempting to economize in terms of staff salaries, benefits, and raises often find out that it is false economy.

ACSM guidelines for fitness facilities are described by Peterson and Tharrett (10). Other regular and ongoing expenses are for insurance, maintenance, and repair of facilities. People are often tempted to ignore regular maintenance and repair, but keeping the facilities in good shape is more efficient than incurring major expenses as a result of not having done so. Building new facilities or expanding existing facilities is usually handled in a separate fund-raising campaign and is not part of the normal budget process.

5 In Review

Financial management is a major part of long-range planning. The budget should be based on realistic estimates of income and expenditures, with the flexibility to adjust for unexpected developments. Salary and benefits for personnel and facility maintenance and repair are the biggest parts of the budget.

Acquiring Equipment and Supplies

Equipment should be available so participants may accomplish their goals; this equipment should be kept in good condition. However, programs often go beyond what is needed in terms of equipment. For a beginning program, exercise tests can be done without the most expensive treadmill. Many program administrators use nice-looking equipment to

form
26.5

Sample Budget Process
Generic Fitness Center

1. What are the purposes of your program?
2. Describe the current program.
3. What are your current expenditures?
   A. Personnel
   B. Facilities
      (1) Loan repayment
      (2) Insurance
      (3) Maintenance and repairs
      (4) Utilities
      (5) Taxes
   C. Supplies
   D. Other
4. What is your current income?
   A. Membership
   B. Insurance
   C. Gifts
   D. Investments
   E. Other
5. A. What changes should be made in your program (e.g., classes, workshops, personnel, facilities, equipment, renovation, repair) over the next 5 years?
   B. For each of these changes, indicate the change in cost and potential income.
   C. Can the changes be phased in logical steps?
6. A. What are the potential sources of increased revenue?
   B. What is needed to achieve this increased revenue?
   C. How much will it cost to secure the additional funding?
   D. What will be the net increase for each potential source of money?
7. What is a reasonable estimate for income for each year over the next 5 years?
8. What aspects of the program can be supported with this income for each year?
9. If the income exceeds expectations, what additional aspects of the program should be added?
10. If the income falls short of expectations, what aspects of the program can be reduced or eliminated?

From Edward T. Howley and B. Don Franks, 2003, *Health Fitness Instructor's Handbook,* 4th ed. (Champaign, IL: Human Kinetics).

form
26.6

Sample Monthly Budget Report

Item	For June Budgeted	For June Actual	Year-to-date Budgeted	Year-to-date Actual
Revenues				
Membership	________	________	________	________
Cardiac rehab	________	________	________	________
Fitness tests	________	________	________	________
Wellness programs	________	________	________	________
Other	________	________	________	________
Total	________	________	________	________
Expenses				
Salaries				
Administrative	________	________	________	________
Professional	________	________	________	________
Clerical	________	________	________	________
Commissions	________	________	________	________
Materials				
GXT	________	________	________	________
Wellness	________	________	________	________
Office	________	________	________	________
Towels	________	________	________	________
Other	________	________	________	________
Overhead				
Telephone	________	________	________	________
Maintenance	________	________	________	________
Heat/air cond.	________	________	________	________
Rent	________	________	________	________
Contracts	________	________	________	________
Other	________	________	________	________
Total	________	________	________	________
Balance	________	________	________	________
Compared with 1 year ago	________	________	________	________

Adapted from Musser 1988.

sell their programs, when the fitness benefits might be accomplished better with activities requiring less expensive equipment supervised by qualified personnel. Some testing equipment is needed, but once again, inexpensive items are often satisfactory for the essential fitness tests.

Testing and exercise equipment will vary with the specific program options. Table 26.1 presents some recommendations for acquiring equipment, listing both the minimum requirements and more advanced possibilities.

Ordering Supplies

The supplies for facility must be kept in stock, with a procedure for identifying what is needed. Normally, one person is designated to be in charge of checking supplies on a regular basis. Other staff members report potential shortages to this one person. Guidelines for ordering equipment and supplies include the following:

- Order early.
- Order on the basis of accurate inventory and estimate of needs—including replacement of old equipment, new equipment, and supplies for all programs.
- Buy from suppliers who have a good record of service.
- Each year, ask all personnel involved in the process to make suggestions to improve the system.

Table 26.1 Suggestions for Testing and Exercise Equipment

Area	Minimum	Advanced
Testing equipment		
Health status	Forms	Computer
Cardiorespiratory	Walking/running track	Cycle ergometer
	Bench	Treadmill
	RPE scale	Oxygen analysis
		ECG
		Blood pressure
		Lipid assays
Relative leanness	Scale	Underwater tank
	Tape measure	
	Skinfold calipers	
Abdominal strength/endurance	Mat	
Midtrunk flexibility	Sit-and-reach box	
Upper-body strength/endurance	Modified pull-up bar	Weights, machines
Exercise equipment		
Cardiorespiratory	Walking/running track	Cycle ergometer
Relative leanness	Bench	Treadmill
		Pool
		Stair climbing
		Rowing machine
		Skiing machine
Abdominal strength/endurance	Mat	
Midtrunk flexibility	Mat	
Upper body strength/endurance	Mat	Free weights
	Modified pull-up bar	Isokinetic machines
		Pull-up bars
		Dip bars

Note. RPE = rating of perceived exertion; ECG = electrocardiogram.

Adapted from Howley 1988.

6 In Review

Testing and exercise equipment as well as emergency equipment should be carefully selected to provide essential items economically. Table 26.1 lists suggestions for testing and exercise equipment. A process needs to be established to keep needed supplies in stock.

Keeping Records

Careful, systematic collection of personal and testing information, properly recorded and filed, provides the basis for much of the communication with the board, staff, and participants. This information can also be used to evaluate the effectiveness of various programs and the extent to which the long-range goals are being met. The program director should keep records of staff training, including a demonstration of competence in emergency and safety procedures.

Forms like the Sample Accident/Injury Form (form 26.7) can be used to keep a record of all accidents and injuries. Be sure to follow up to determine the status of the individual's recovery. The completed form provides a check on whether staff personnel used appropriate emergency procedures; it is essential to have this record when questions are raised about a particular incident.

What information is needed? How is it obtained? What forms are used? Where is the information stored? How is it retrieved? When is it used? Who evaluates particular programs? Address these questions before the program begins. After a reasonable amount of time working with the procedure, re-evaluate it to determine whether modifications would improve it. Software programs are increasingly used for these tasks. It is essential to get professional assistance in setting up computer resources so that they can be used effectively.

7 In Review

The fitness program administrator should keep complete and accurate records of all aspects of the fitness program, including screening, testing, and accidents so that the effectiveness of the program can be evaluated and the handling of emergencies can be documented.

Evaluating the Program

Evaluation has been mentioned throughout this chapter. Evaluation is used for the following:

- Health and fitness outcomes
- Changes in behavior and attitudes toward physical activity and other healthy behaviors
- Processes used in the program
- Cost of the program related to both fitness outcomes and financial benefits

A value judgment should be based on the best data available concerning the extent to which the program objectives are being reached. How many people are included in the fitness program? What kinds of body composition, CRF, and low back function changes have been made? Do the participants enjoy the activities? How many dropouts were there? Why? How many injuries? Why? What can be done to help more people make better fitness gains and decrease the number of dropouts and injuries? Are some staff members better than others in some of these areas? What can be done to help staff personnel maintain their strengths and improve in their weak areas?

In addition to this type of continuing evaluation of the program, it is helpful to have a formal evaluation of the program periodically (e.g., every 3-5 years). Mitchell and Blair (7) described the necessary steps and offered helpful suggestions for developing and conducting a program evaluation. They provided assistance in setting up the evaluation (questions to be asked, evaluation design) as well as collecting, analyzing, and reporting the information.

Evaluating the Cost-Effectiveness of Fitness Programs

Good fitness programs cost a substantial amount of money for personnel, facilities, equipment, and supplies, in addition to the cost of clothing, time, and travel for the participant. Gettman (3) summarized the economic benefits from fitness programs. Shephard (11) reviewed the potential benefits for the individual and for businesses that sponsor a fitness program for their employees. Program directors should ask the questions in the box titled Evaluating Cost-Effectiveness to determine if their program is cost-effective. Shephard summarized **cost-effectiveness** research evidence indicating that research on the economics of physical activity has found improved health and *lower* health care costs, absenteeism, and disability associated with exercise and fitness programs.

form
26.7

Sample Accident Injury Form

1. ______________________________ ______________________
Name of victim Date

2. Describe, in detail, the nature of the injury or health problem:

3. Describe, in detail, how the accident occurred:

4. List, in order, the things you or other staff members did in response to the incident:

5. Describe any problems encountered in dealing with the situation:

6. List the names of people who witnessed the accident and emergency procedures performed:

Turn in this form, within 24 hr of the accident, to ______________________________

Your suggestions concerning safety, emergency procedures, and/or this form are welcome. Please talk to ____.

From Edward T. Howley and B. Don Franks, 2003, *Health Fitness Instructor's Handbook,* 4th ed. (Champaign, IL: Human Kinetics).

Evaluating Cost-Effectiveness

Have the individuals in our programs achieved these benefits?

- Enhanced quality of life
- Better health
- Improved mood
- Increased range of experiences
- Improved personal appearance, self-image, and health
- Lower risk of major health problems
- Potential increase in the length of their life

Has the industry in which our participants work experienced these benefits?

- Improved corporate image, worker satisfaction, and productivity
- Decrease in absenteeism, employee turnover, injury rate, and medical costs

Evaluating Quality

The most important element of a program is setting up procedures to ensure a high standard of quality in all information, personal contact, and activities that are conducted in the name of the fitness program. One aspect of establishing high standards is to ensure the inclusiveness of the program. All people should feel welcome in the program regardless of sex, ethnic background, or social class. The administrator should ask these questions to determine if the program is achieving this atmosphere:

- Have I employed staff with varied backgrounds?
- Are the staff trained to be sensitive to people from different backgrounds?
- Are our programs scheduled at convenient times and places?
- Do we try to contact various groups within the community?
- Have we provided ways for people with low incomes to participate?
- Do we have a policy whereby inappropriate (e.g., sexist or racist) comments or actions by staff members or participants will not be tolerated?

8 In Review

Evaluation of the program is a continuing process to ensure that quality information and inclusive programs are being provided in a cost-effective manner.

Case Studies

You can check your answers by referring to appendix A.

26.1

The fitness director where you work asks you to evaluate four part-time fitness instructors. What steps would you take?

26.2

The fitness program board of directors asks for an evaluation of the fitness goals of the program. The program director asks you to be in charge of the evaluation. What would you do?

Source List

1. American College of Sports Medicine. (2000). *ACSM's guidelines for exercise testing and prescription* (6th ed.). Philadelphia: Lippincott Williams & Wilkins.
2. Ancharski, F. (1998). Financial considerations. In J.L. Roitman (Ed.), *ACSM's resource manual for guidelines for exercise testing and prescription* (3rd ed., pp. 602-609). Philadelphia: Lippincott Williams & Wilkins.
3. Gettman, L.R. (1999). Economic benefits of physical activity. In C.B. Corbin & R.P. Pangrazi (Eds.), *Toward a better understanding of physical fitness and activity* (pp. 145-149). Scottsdale, AZ: Holcomb Hathaway.
4. Herbert, D.L., & Herbert, W.G. (1998). Legal considerations. In J.L. Roitman (Ed.), *ACSM's resource manual for guidelines for exercise testing and prescription* (3rd ed., pp. 610-615). Philadelphia: Lippincott Williams & Wilkins.
5. Howley, E.T. (1988). The exercise testing laboratory. In S.N. Blair, P. Painter, R.R. Pate, L.K. Smith, & C.B. Taylor (Eds.), *Resource manual for guidelines for exercise testing and prescription* (2nd ed., pp. 406-413). Philadelphia: Lea & Febiger.
6. Minor, S. (1998). Health and fitness program development. In J.L. Roitman (Ed.), *ACSM's resource manual for guidelines for exercise testing and prescription* (3rd ed., pp. 587-594). Philadelphia: Lippincott Williams & Wilkins.
7. Mitchell, B.S., & Blair, S.N. (1988). Evaluation of preventive and rehabilitation exercise programs. In S.N. Blair, P. Painter, R.R. Pate, L.K. Smith, & C.B. Taylor (Eds.), *Resource manual for guidelines for exercise testing and prescription* (2nd ed., pp. 414-420). Philadelphia: Lea & Febiger.
8. Musser, J.W. (1988). Budget considerations. In S.N. Blair, P. Painter, R. Pate, L.K. Smith, & C.B. Taylor (Eds.), *Resource manual for guidelines for exercise testing and prescription* (2nd ed., pp. 390-394). Philadelphia: Lea & Febiger.
9. Patton, R.W., Corry, J.M., Gettman, L.R., & Graf, J. (1986). *Implementing health/fitness programs*. Champaign, IL: Human Kinetics.
10. Peterson, J.A., & Tharrett, S.J. (Eds.). (1998). *ACSM's health/fitness facility standards and guidelines*. Champaign, IL: Human Kinetics.
11. Shephard, R.J. (1990). Costs and benefits of an exercising versus a nonexercising society. In C. Bouchard, R.J. Shephard, T. Stephens, J.R. Sutton, & B.D. McPherson (Eds.), *Exercise, fitness, and health* (pp. 49-60). Champaign, IL: Human Kinetics.

part six

Scientific Foundations

Part VI provides the basic scientific foundation for understanding the structure and function of the human body. We review the bones, joints, and muscles of the body and how they are used biomechanically in common physical activities in **chapter 27**. In **chapter 28**, we cover the basic concepts of energy, muscle function, and the physiological response to acute and chronic physical activity. Differences due to gender, type of exercise, and temperature are described.

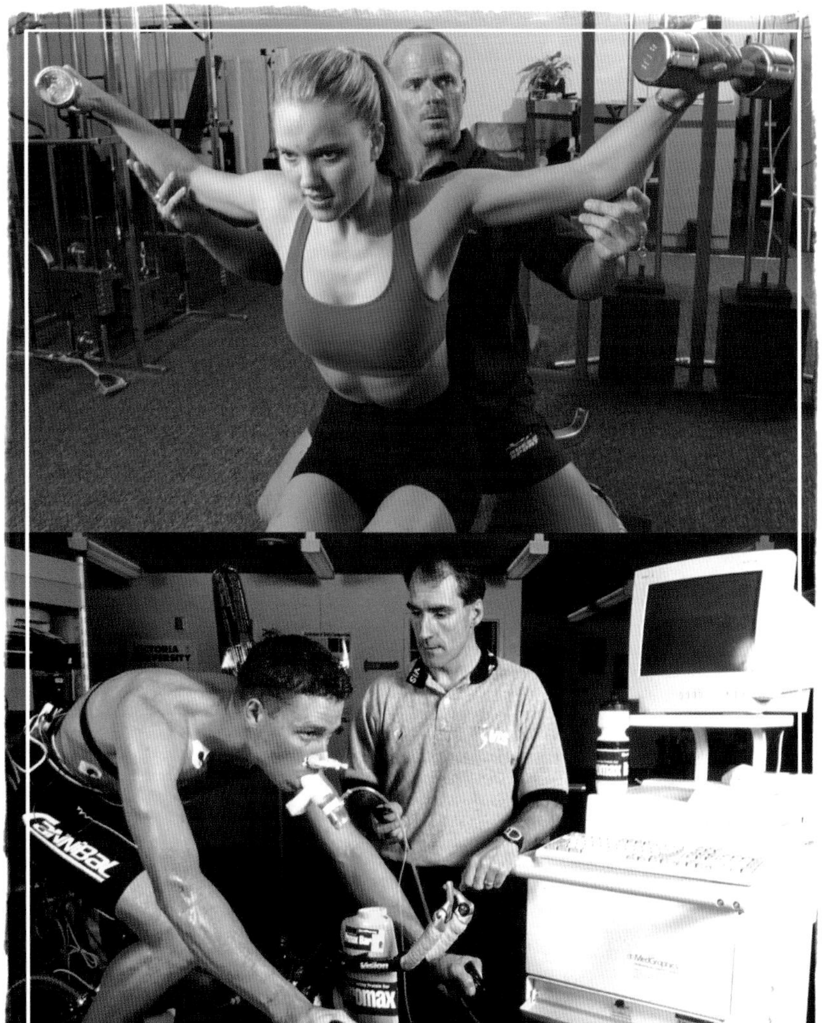

twenty-seven

Functional Anatomy and Biomechanics

Jean Lewis

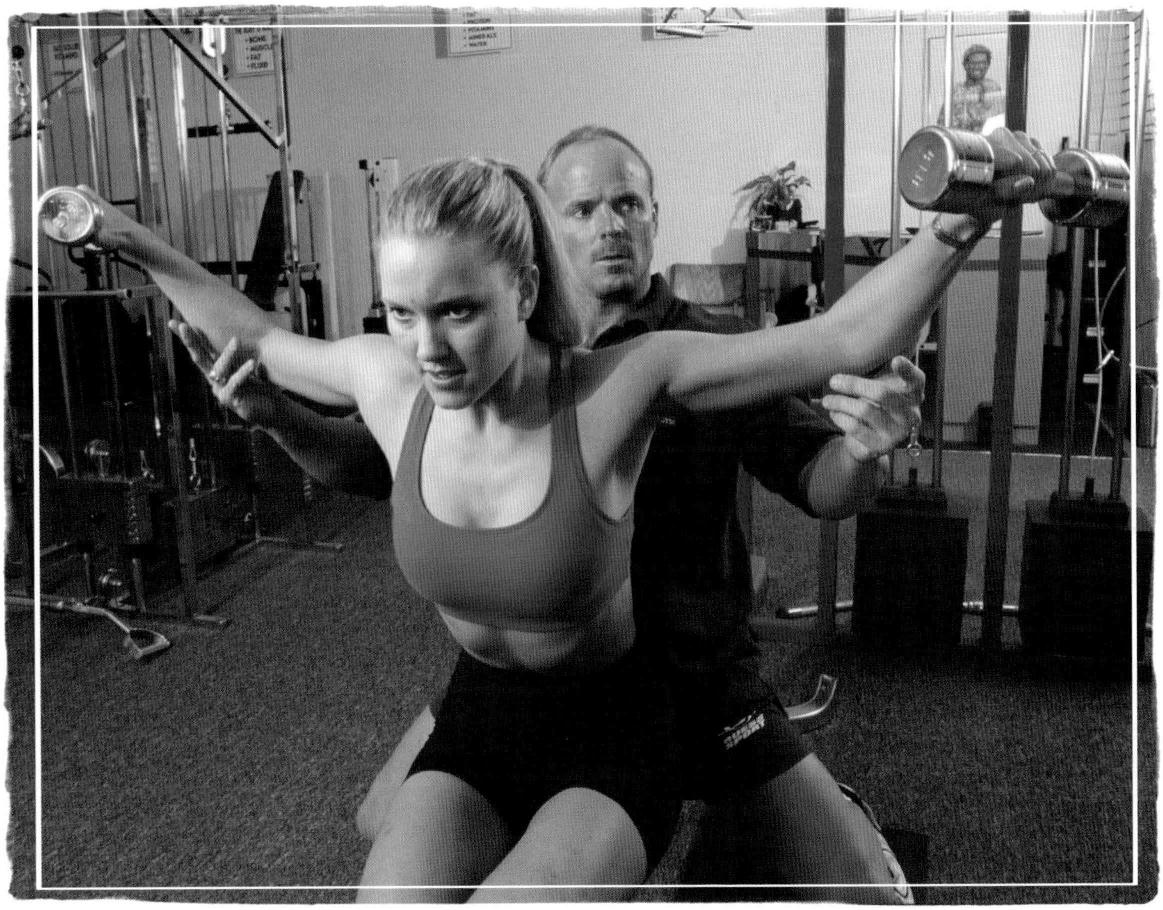

© Jason Wise/SportsChrome USA

Objectives

The reader will be able to do the following:

1. Describe the general structure of long bones.
2. Identify the major bones of the skeletal system and classify them by shape.
3. Describe the process of ossification of long bones.
4. Distinguish between synarthrodial, amphiarthrodial, and diarthrodial joints, both structurally and functionally, and identify the structures of a diarthrodial joint.
5. List the factors that determine range and direction of motion at the joints.
6. Name and demonstrate the movements possible at each joint.
7. Describe forces that can cause joint movement and that can resist movement caused by another force.
8. Describe the gross structure of a muscle.
9. Explain how muscle tension can be increased.
10. Describe the phases of a ballistic movement including the type of muscle action.
11. Explain the differences between concentric, eccentric, and isometric muscle actions.
12. Describe the roles of muscles.
13. List the major muscles in each muscle group, and identify the major actions and joints of involvement of the following muscles: trapezius, serratus anterior, deltoid, pectoralis major, latissimus dorsi, biceps brachii, brachialis, triceps brachii, flexor and extensor carpi radialis and ulnaris, rectus abdominis, external oblique, erector spinae, gluteus maximus, gluteus medius, iliopsoas, rectus femoris, the three vasti muscles, the three hamstring muscles, tibialis anterior, soleus, and gastrocnemius.
14. Cite specific errors that occur during exercise for the vertebral column, lumbosacral joints, and knee joint.
15. Analyze locomotion, throwing, cycling, jumping, and swimming for the movements and muscle involvement.
16. Describe good lifting techniques.
17. Describe the three factors that determine stability; identify the interrelationships among line of gravity, base of support, balance, and stability; and describe the practical applications of these interrelationships during physical activity.
18. Describe torque and its relationship to muscle actions.
19. Describe how an exerciser can change body segment positions to alter the resistive torque.
20. Explain how the mechanical principles of rotational inertia and angular momentum apply to movement.
21. Discuss the common errors seen in locomotion, throwing, and striking.

The HFI must have knowledge of the bones, joints, and muscles; must understand the involvement of muscle forces and other forces; and must be able to apply biomechanical principles to human movement. With this knowledge and understanding, the instructor will be better equipped to lead and direct physical activity safely for participants seeking the health-related effects of exercise. This knowledge will also help the instructor earn the respect of clients, who will view the instructor as a professional in the field, rather than a technician who may know what to do and how but not why. This chapter is but a summary; for detailed presentations of these topics, see the references (1-9).

Understanding Skeletal Anatomy

Most of the 200 distinct bones in the human skeleton are involved in producing movement. Their high mineral component gives them rigidity; the protein component makes them resistant to tension. The two types of bone tissue are (a) compact tissue, which is the dense, hard, outer layer of bone, and (b) spongy, or cancellous tissue, which has a latticelike structure to allow greater structural strength along the lines of stress at a reduced weight. Bones are often divided into four classifications according to their shapes: long, short, flat, and irregular.

Long Bones

The long bones, found in the limbs and digits, serve primarily as levers for movement. Each long bone consists of the **diaphysis**, or shaft, which is made up of thick, compact bone around the hollow medullary cavity; the expanded ends, or **epiphyses**, composed of spongy bone with a thin, outer layer of compact bone; the **articular cartilage**, a thin layer of hyaline cartilage covering the articulating surfaces (the surfaces of a bone that meet or come into contact with another bone to form a joint) that provides a friction-free surface and helps absorb shock; and the **periosteum**, a fibrous membrane covering the entire bone (except where the articular cartilage is present) that serves as an attachment site for many muscles (see figure 27.1).

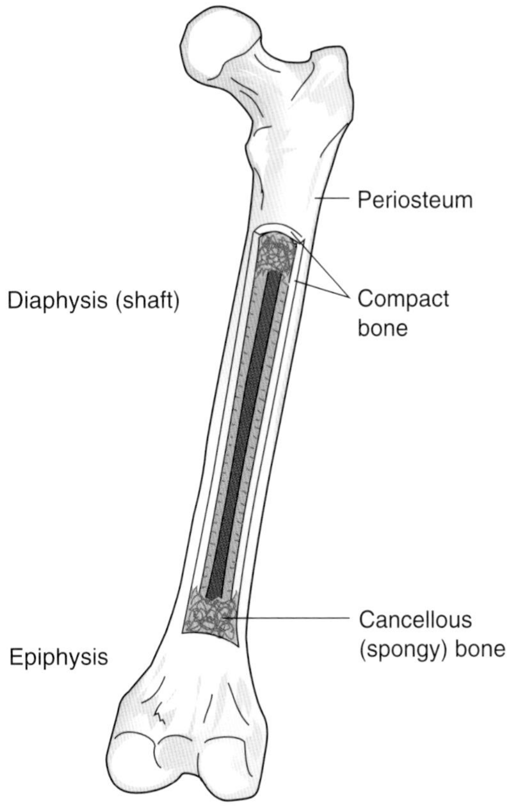

Figure 27.1 The femur, an example of a long bone.

1 In Review

The structures of a long bone include the diaphysis, or shaft; the epiphyses, or expanded ends; the periosteum, which covers the bone except at the articulating surfaces; and the articular cartilage that covers the articulating surfaces to provide a friction-free surface and help absorb shock.

Short, Flat, and Irregular Bones

In addition to long bones, the skeleton is made up of short bones, flat bones, and irregular-shaped bones (see figure 27.2).

The tarsals (ankle) and carpals (wrist) are the short bones. Their composition (spongy bone with a thin outside layer of compact bone) provides greater strength, but their cubic shape decreases their movement potential.

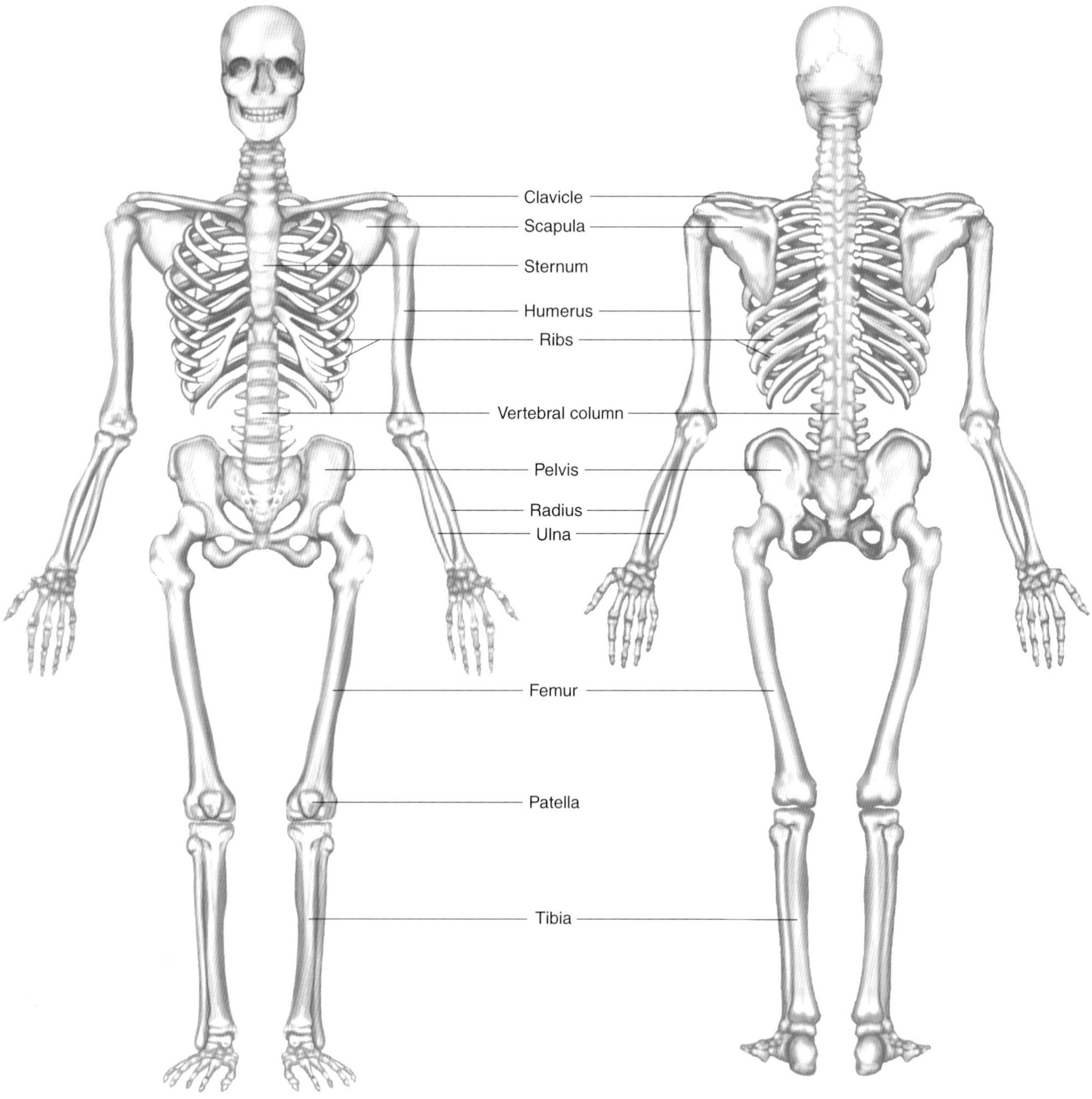

Figure 27.2 Front and back view of the human skeleton, with bones classified by shape.

The flat bones, such as the ribs, ilia, and scapulae, serve primarily as broad sites for muscle attachments and, in the case of the ribs and ilia, to enclose cavities and protect internal organs. These bones are also spongy and covered with a thin layer of compact bone.

The ischium, pubis, and vertebrae are irregular shaped bones that serve special purposes such as protecting internal parts and supporting the body in addition to being sites for muscle attachments.

2 In Review

Figure 27.2 shows the major skeletal bones, long bones, short bones, flat bones, and irregular bones classified by shape. Each particular type of bone has a specific structure and purpose.

Ossification of Bones

The skeleton begins as a cartilaginous structure, which is replaced gradually by bone (**ossification**). This process begins at the diaphysis of long bones (in centers of ossification) and spreads toward the epiphyses. The **epiphyseal plates** between the diaphyses and epiphyses are the growth areas where the cartilage is replaced by bone; bone growth in length and width continues until the epiphyseal plates are completely ossified. During growth, additional cartilage is laid down to be replaced eventually by bone. When no further cartilage is produced, and the cartilage present is replaced by bone, growth ceases. Other secondary centers of ossification develop in the epiphyses and in some bony protuberances, such as the tibial tuberosity and the articular condyles of the humerus. Short bones have one center of ossification. Dates of closure vary. Although bone fusion at some centers of ossification may occur by puberty or earlier, most of the long bones do not have complete ossification until the late teens. Premature closing, which results in a shorter bone length, can be caused by trauma, abnormal stresses, malnutrition, and drugs.

3 In Review

Ossification is the replacement of cartilage with bone. Generally, bone growth is completed by the late teens.

Structure and Function of the Joints

Joints, the places where bones meet or articulate, are often classified according to the amount of movement that can take place at those sites. The classifications are synarthrodial, amphiarthrodial, and diarthrodial joints. The **synarthrodial joints** are the immovable joints. The bones merge into each other and are bound together by fibrous tissue that is continuous with the periosteum. The sutures, or the lines of junction, of the cranial (skull) bones are prime examples of this type of joint. The **amphiarthrodial** (or **cartilaginous**) **joints** allow only slight movement in all directions. Usually a fibrocartilage disk separates the bones, and movement can occur only by deformation of the disk. Examples of these joints are the tibiofibular and sacroiliac joints and the joints between the bodies of the vertebrae of the spine. **Ligaments**, which are tough, fibrous bands of connective tissue, connect the bones to each other, not only in this type of joint but also in all joints.

Diarthrodial (or **synovial**) **joints** (see figure 27.3) are freely movable joints that allow a variety of movement direction and range; therefore, most of the joint movements during physical activity occur at diarthrodial joints. The diarthrodial joints are the most common and include most joints of the extremities. Strong and fairly inelastic ligaments, along with connective and muscle tissue that crosses the joint, are responsible for maintaining the stability of the joint. Diarthrodial joints have distinct physical characteristics that also differentiate them from the other types of joints. The articulating surfaces of the bones are covered by articular cartilage, a type of hyaline cartilage that reduces friction and acts somewhat as a shock absorber. Each joint is enclosed by an **articular capsule**, a ligamentous structure that may be fairly thin in spots or thick enough to be considered separate ligaments. The **synovial membrane** lines the inner surface of the capsule. It secretes synovial fluid into the **joint cavity**, the space enclosed by the articular capsule, to bathe (or lubricate) the joint to allow for ease of movement.

Normally, the joint cavity is small and therefore contains little synovial fluid, but an injury to the joint can increase secretion of synovial fluid and cause swelling. Some diarthrodial joints, such as the sternoclavicular, distal radioulnar, and knee joints, also have a partial or complete fibrocartilage disk between the bones to aid in the absorption of shock

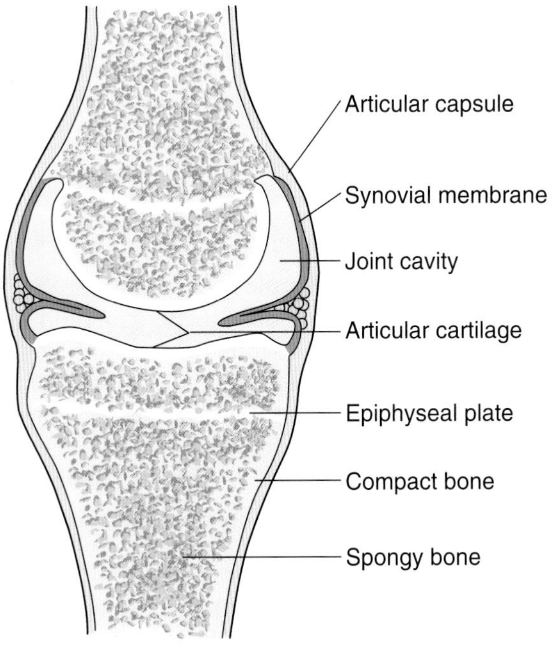

Figure 27.3 A diarthrodial or synovial joint.

and, in the case of the knee, to give greater stability to the joint. The partial, semilunar-shaped disks between the femur and tibia at the knee are called **menisci**.

To reduce frictional rubbing that occurs as the lengths of tendons change during muscle action, tendons often are surrounded by tendinous sheaths—cylindrical, tunnel-like sacs lined with synovial membrane. For example, the two proximal tendons of the biceps brachii muscle pass through these tunnels in the bicipital groove of the humerus. **Bursae**, or sacs of synovial fluid that lie between muscles, tendons, and bones, also reduce friction between the tissues and act as shock absorbers. Many bursae are found around the shoulder, elbow, hip, and knee. Bursitis, or the inflammation of a bursa, can be caused by repeated friction or mechanical irritation, or as a result of inflammatory or degenerative conditions of the tendons.

4 In Review

The types of joints are synarthrodial, which do not allow movement; amphiarthrodial, which allow only slight movement; and diarthrodial, or synovial, which are characterized functionally by their wide range of movement and structurally by the presence of articular cartilage, an articular capsule, synovial membrane, and synovial fluid within the joint cavity.

Factors That Determine Direction and Range of Motion

Most of the movement at a joint is rotary in nature: The bone moves around a fixed axis, the joint. The structures of the bones at and near their articulating ends largely determine both the direction and the range of movement. Ball-and-socket joints, which are found at the hip and shoulder, allow a wide range of movement in all directions; but a hinge joint, such as the elbow joint, restricts both direction and range of movement because bone impinges on bone. The length of the ligaments, and to a lesser extent their **elasticity**, or ability to lengthen (stretch) passively and return to their normal length, are also factors in range of movement. For example, the iliofemoral ligament at the anterior hip joint is a strong but short ligament that prohibits much hip hyperextension. Elasticity can be changed by appropriate exercise; the amount of elasticity is determined by the amount and type of physical activity in which an individual engages.

5 In Review

The potential range and direction of motion are related to the shape of the articulating ends of the bones, the length of ligaments, and the elasticity of connective tissue.

Specific Joint Movements

Specific terminology is used to describe the direction of movement at the different joints. The anatomical position (standing with arms at sides and turned so the palm of the hand faces forward) serves as a point of reference. Although different terminology may be used for specific joints, **flexion** in general is anterior or posterior movement from the anatomical position that brings two bones together, **extension** is the return from flexion, and **hyperextension** is the continuation of extension past the anatomical position. **Abduction** is the movement of a bone laterally from the anatomical position; **adduction** is the return back toward the anatomical position. **Rotation** occurs when the bone spins around its longitudinal axis so that its surface faces a different direction.

Shoulder Girdle

This joint complex includes the articulations between the sternum and clavicle and between the clavicle and scapula. Rotary joint movement occurs at those articulations, but the movement terms *elevation, depression, abduction, adduction,* and *upward* and *downward rotation* describe the resulting movements of the scapulae (see figure 27.4). Abduction, adduction, and scapular elevation and depression all can occur without shoulder joint movement but may enhance it. Upward and downward rotation can occur only when the humerus is moved upward, outward, and downward. If the scapulae cannot rotate upward, the arms cannot be elevated sideways above the horizon (beyond 90°).

Shoulder Joint

Because of its ball-and-socket structure, the shoulder joint can move in all directions—flexion, extension, hyperextension, abduction, adduction, lateral (outward, away from the midline) and medial (inward, toward the midline) rotation, and circumduction, which is the circular movement of the arm in a

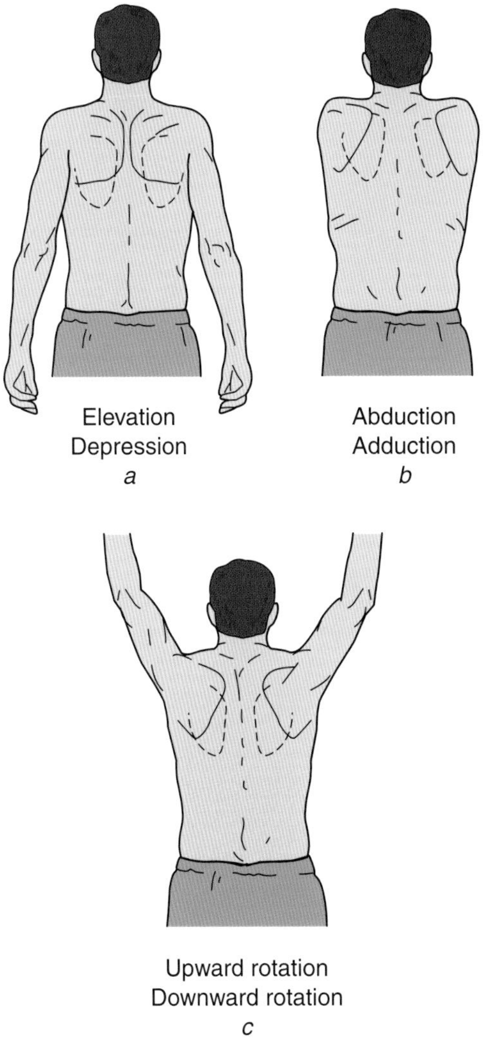

Figure 27.4 Movements of the scapulae.

wide arc. Horizontal extension and horizontal flexion are movements of the arm parallel to the ground (see figure 27.5).

Scapular movements can enhance shoulder joint movements. As the arm flexes or horizontally flexes, scapular abduction can move the hand out farther in front. Scapular adduction can allow the arm to move back more during hyperextension and horizontal extension. Elevation of the scapula can allow the hand to reach higher. Medial rotation may be accompanied by scapular abduction; lateral rotation may be accompanied by scapular adduction.

Elbow Joint

Sometimes referred to as the humeroulnar joint for the bones involved in elbow joint movement, the elbow joint allows only flexion and extension because of its bony arrangement (see figure 27.6). The ability of some individuals to hyperextend the elbow joint is attributable to the shape of the articulating surfaces.

Radioulnar Joints

Pronation and supination are the movements of the radius around the ulna in the lower arm (see figure 27.7). Although the wrist is not involved in these movements, the position of the radioulnar joints can be identified by the direction in which the palm of the hand is facing. When the arms are hanging down alongside the trunk, the palm faces forward in the supinated position and toward the back in the pronated position. In the supinated position, the radius and ulna are parallel to each other; in the pronated position, the radius lies across and on top of the ulna. Pronation combined with shoulder joint medial rotation, and supination combined with shoulder joint lateral rotation, move the hand around the midline even farther.

Wrist Joint

Movement at the wrist joint can occur in two planes of direction: flexion, extension, and hyperextension; and abduction (sometimes referred to as radial flexion) and adduction (ulnar flexion; see figure 27.8).

Metacarpophalangeal and Interphalangeal Joints

The second through the fifth metacarpophalangeal joints allow flexion and extension as well as abduction and adduction of the fingers. The metacarpophalangeal joint of the thumb allows only flexion and extension, but it is the only digit that also allows movement at the carpometacarpal joint (which gives the thumb its movement ability). All the interphalangeal joints of the fingers and toes only flex and extend.

Vertebral Column

Movements of the trunk—flexion, extension, hyperextension, lateral flexion, and rotation—occur at all the joints of the vertebral column (see figure 27.9).

Lumbosacral Joint: Pelvis Movement

The tilts of the pelvis (see figure 27.10) occur mainly at the joint formed by the fifth lumbar vertebra and the pelvis. The reference point for the direction of the tilts is the iliac crest. As the crest moves forward and down, the pelvis has a forward, or anterior,

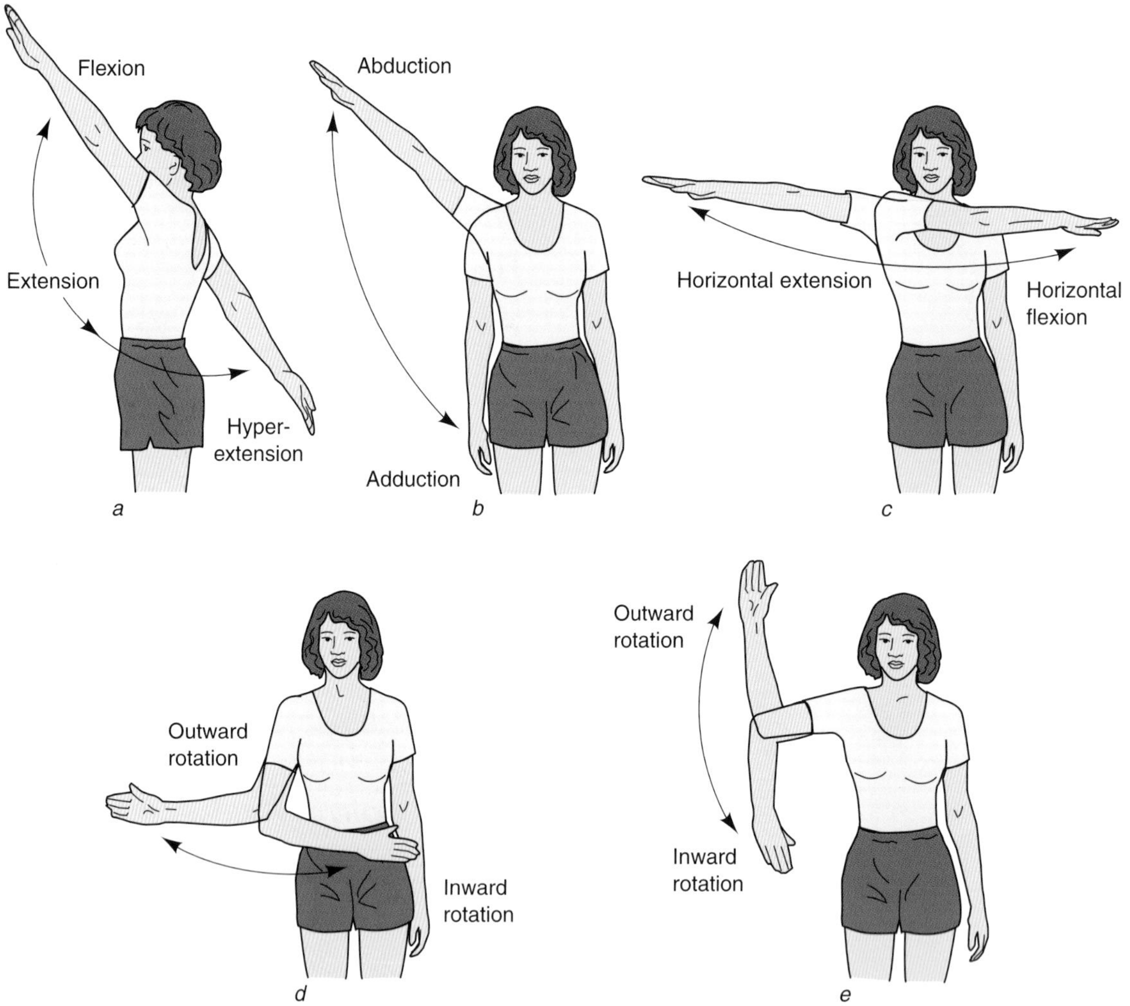

Figure 27.5 Movements of the shoulder joint.

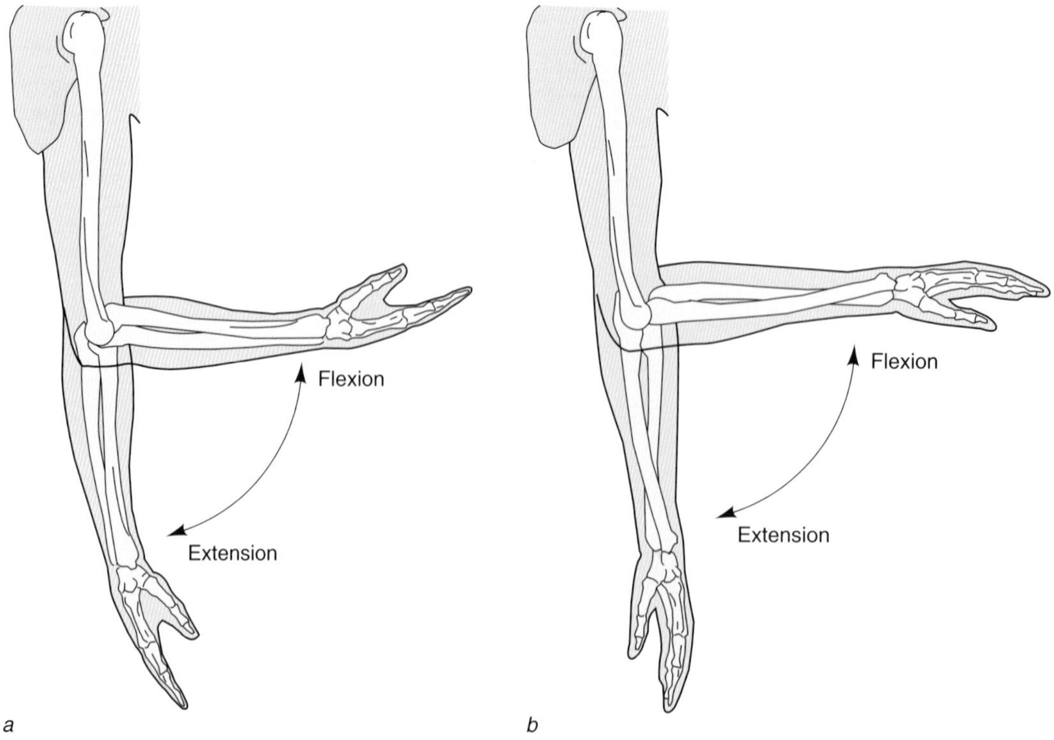

Figure 27.6 Movements of the elbow joint.

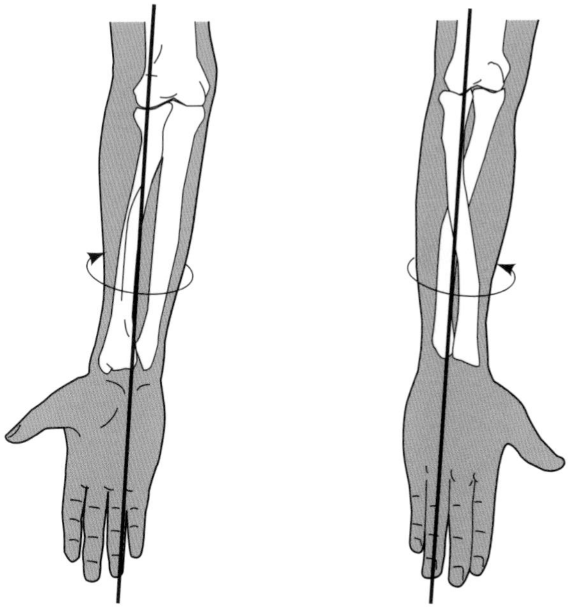

Figure 27.7 Movements of the radioulnar joints.

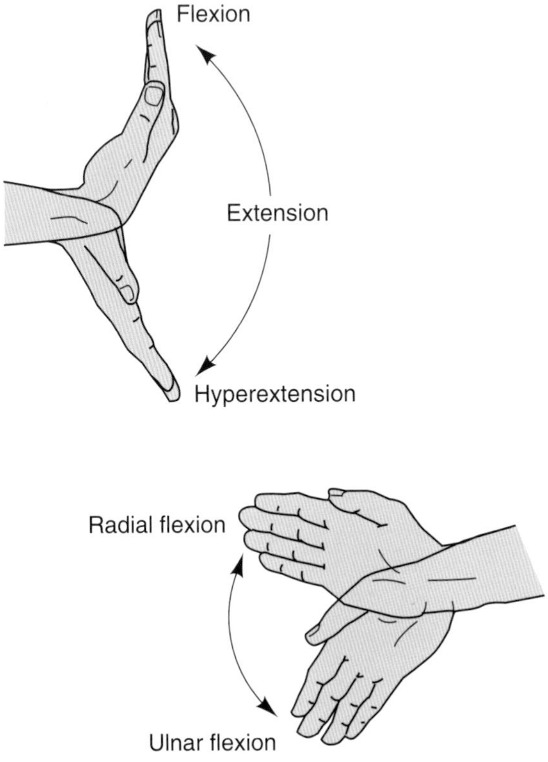

Figure 27.8 Movements of the wrist joint.

pelvic tilt; as the crest rotates toward the back, the pelvis has a backward, or posterior, tilt. The anterior pelvic tilt usually is accompanied by a hyperextension of the lumbar vertebrae, whereas a backward tilt usually results in a flattening out of the lumbar vertebrae.

Hip Joint

The hip joint structure is similar to the shoulder joint, a ball-and-socket arrangement, and the same movements are possible (see figure 27.11). Because of the deepness of the socket and the tightness of the ligaments at the hip joint, ROM at this joint, especially for hyperextension, is less than at the shoulder joint. True hip abduction is also limited to about 45° by bony impingement. The leg can be abducted higher only by rotating the hip laterally.

Knee Joint

Flexion and extension are the major movements at the knee. Although some hyperextension may be possible, it should be avoided (see figure 27.12). When the knee is in a flexed position, a limited amount of rotation, abduction, and adduction is possible.

Ankle Joint

Also called the talocrural joint, the ankle is limited to movement in one plane only. Plantar flexion (pointing the toes downward) is still sometimes referred to as extension; dorsiflexion (flexing the toes back) is also referred to as flexion (see figure 27.13).

Intertarsal Joints

The sideways movements of the foot occur between the different tarsal joints in the foot (see figure 27.14). Inversion can be considered a combination of pronation and adduction; eversion is a combination of supination and abduction.

6 In Review

The possible movements at each joint are summarized in this table.

Joint	Movements
Shoulder girdle	Elevation, depression; abduction, adduction; upward rotation, downward rotation
Shoulder joint	Flexion, extension, hyperextension; abduction, adduction; medial rotation, lateral rotation; horizontal flexion, horizontal extension
Elbow joint	Flexion, extension
Radioulnar joint	Pronation, supination
Wrist joint	Flexion, extension, hyperextension; radial flexion, ulnar flexion
Metatarsophalangeal joints	Flexion, extension, abduction,adduction
Vertebral column	Flexion, extension, hyperextension; lateral flexion; rotation
Lumbosacral joint	Forward pelvic tilt, backward pelvic tilt
Hip joint	Flexion, extension, hyperextension; abduction, adduction; medial rotation, lateral rotation
Knee joint	Flexion, extension
Ankle joint	Plantar flexion, dorsiflexion
Intertarsal joint	Eversion, inversion

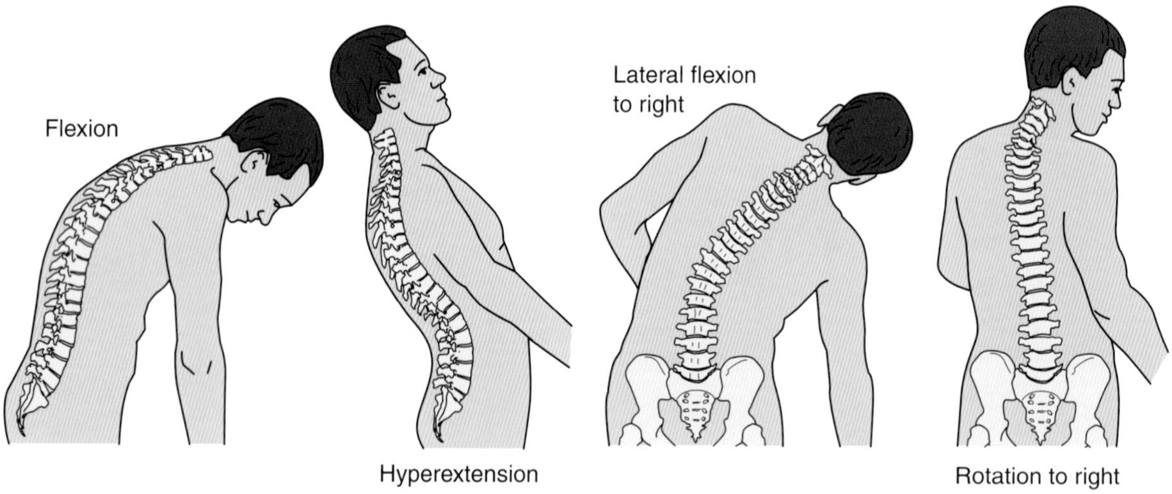

Figure 27.9 Movements of the vertebral column.

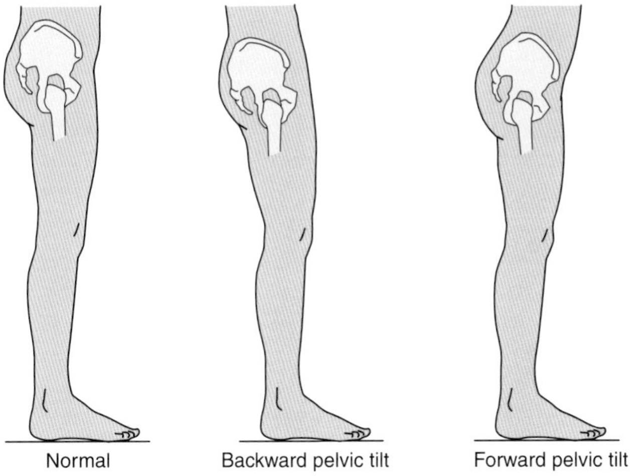

Figure 27.10 Movements of the lumbosacral joint.

Forces That Cause Movement

Joint movement is caused primarily by either a muscle-shortening action or gravitational pull, although other forces, such as another person pushing or pulling on a body part, may cause joint movement. Whether a muscle action will cause the movement depends on the force of that action and the amount of resistance from the other forces.

Forces That Resist or Prevent Movement Caused by Another Force

The same forces that can cause movement also resist or prevent movement. Joint movement caused by gravity can be resisted or decelerated by eccentric muscle action (which lengthens the muscle; see the

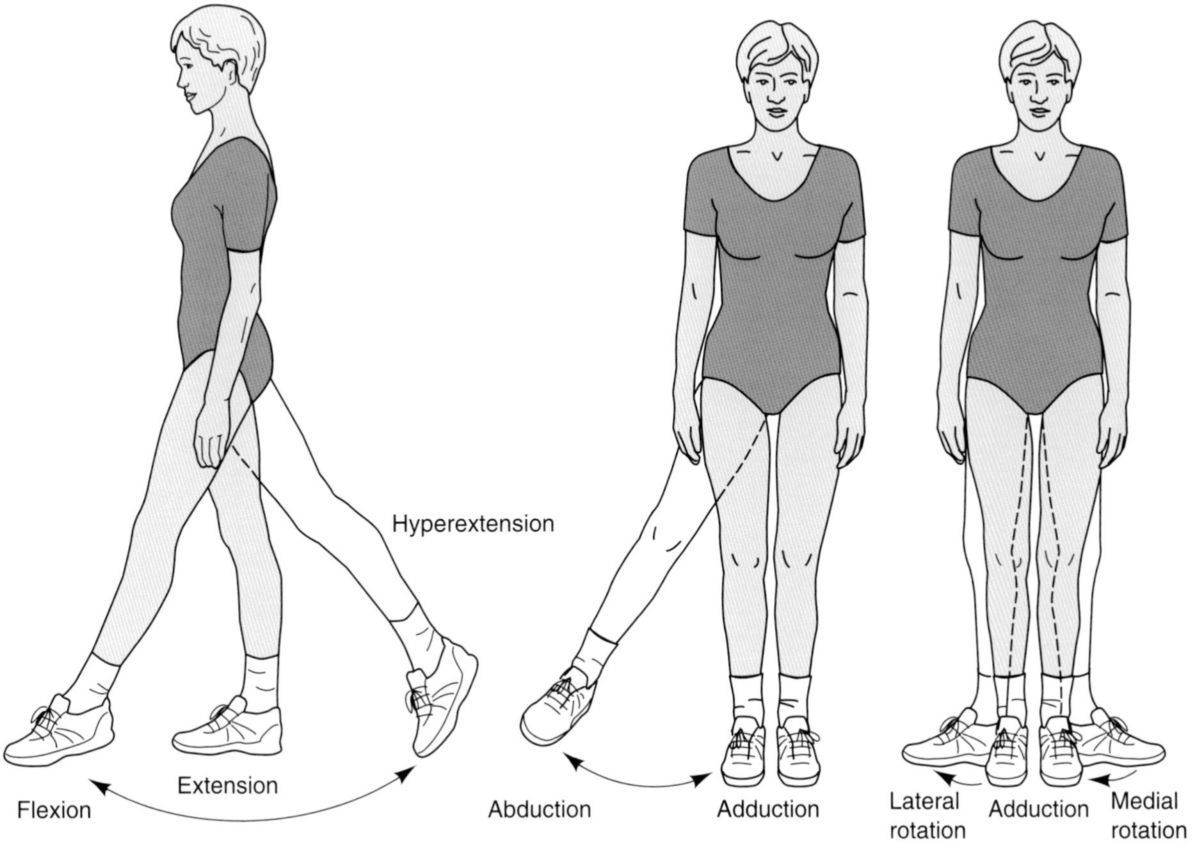

Figure 27.11 Movements of the hip joint.

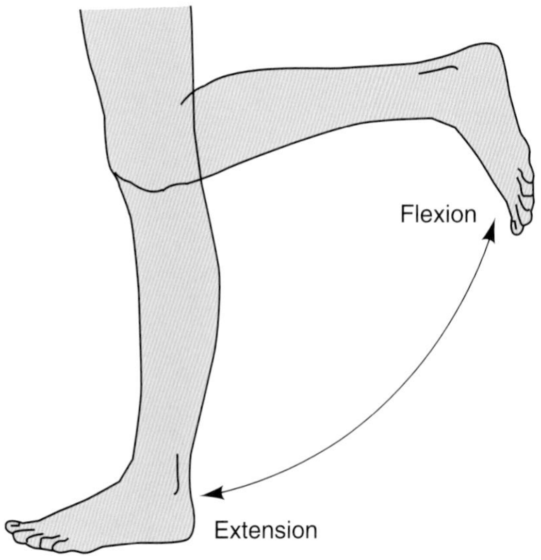

Figure 27.12 Movements of the knee joint.

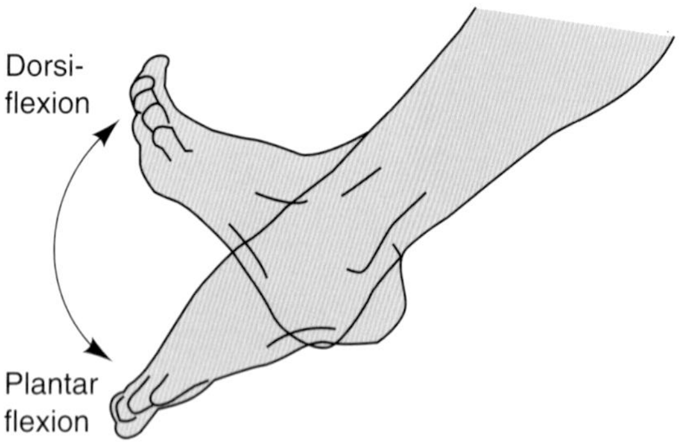

Figure 27.13 Movements of the ankle joint.

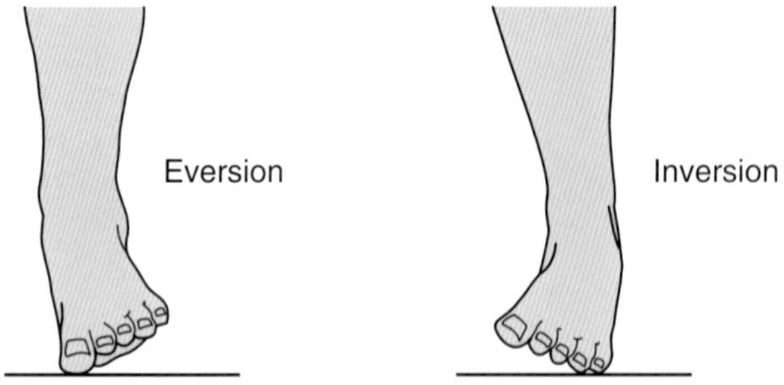

Figure 27.14 Movements of the intertarsal joints.

section on eccentric action later in the chapter). Gravity always resists movement occurring in the direction away from the earth. Other forces that can resist movement include internal tissue restriction by tight ligaments and tendons, exercise bands, hydraulic or air pressure devices on resistance training equipment, and the drag provided by air and water against bodies moving through them.

7 In Review

Forces that can both cause and resist joint movements include muscle action and gravity.

Voluntary (Skeletal) Muscle

A skeletal muscle that is involved in joint movements consists of thousands of muscle fibers (e.g., the brachioradialis has approximately 130,000 fibers; the gastrocnemius has more than 1 million) and connective tissue. Each fiber is enclosed by the connective tissue endomysium. The **fasciculi**, or bundles of fibers grouped together, are surrounded by the **perimysium**, and the entire muscle is enclosed by the **epimysium**. The **tendon** is the passive part of the muscle made up of the elastic connective tissues. Each muscle is attached either to the bone itself, to the periosteum of the bone, or to deep, thick fascia by tendons and the perimysium and epimysium connective tissues. The sizes and the shapes of the tendons vary and depend on their functions and the shape of the muscle itself. Some tendons (e.g., the hamstring muscle tendons found at the sides of the posterior knee and the Achilles tendon) are obvious and significant parts of the entire muscle length, but other muscles such as the supraspinatus and infraspinatus (muscles that abduct and rotate the arm) seem to lie directly on the bone with no observable tendon. Many of the distal attachments (attachments farthest away from the body part being moved) that are usually found on bones that show the largest movements have a more defined tendinous structure than the proximal attachments (attachments nearest to the body part being moved). Broad and flat tendons, such as the proximal tendinous sheath of the latissimus dorsi, are called **aponeuroses**. Refer to figure 27.15 for anterior and posterior views of surface muscles. Other muscles lie underneath the surface muscles.

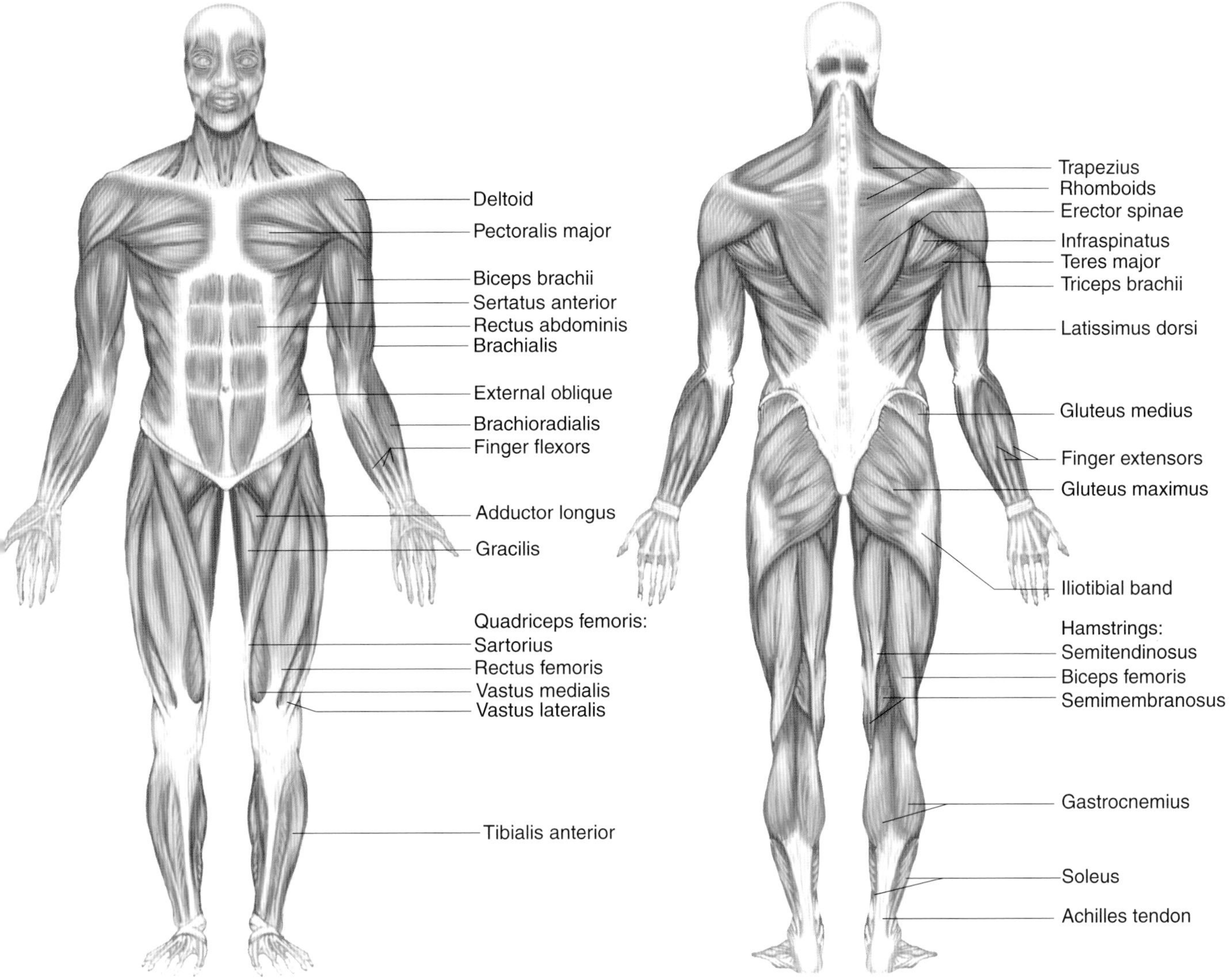

Figure 27.15 Front and back views of the surface muscles of the human body.

8 In Review

The structures associated with muscle include fasciculi, perimysium, epimysium, tendons, and aponeuroses.

Muscle Action

Each muscle fiber is innervated, or receives its stimulus, by a branch of a motor neuron. The functional organization, or **motor unit**, consists of a single motor neuron and its branches and all the muscle fibers innervated by that motor neuron. With a sufficiently strong stimulus, each muscle fiber within that motor unit responds maximally; muscular tension increases as a result of the stimulation of more motor units (**recruitment**) or an increased rate of stimulation (summation). A muscle that has as its primary purpose a strength or power movement (as does the gastrocnemius) rather than a delicate movement (as do any of the finger muscles) has a large number of muscle fibers and also has many muscle fibers per motor unit. When a muscle develops tension, it tends to shorten toward the middle, pulling on all of its bony attachments. Whether the bones of attachment move as a result of that muscle action depends on the amount of the force of the action and the resistance to that movement from other forces. Muscles act in three major ways: concentric actions, eccentric actions, and isometric actions.

9 **In Review**

The motor unit consists of a single motor neuron and its branches and all the muscle fibers innervated by that motor neuron. Muscular tension is increased by recruitment and summation.

Concentric Action

A **concentric action** occurs when a muscle acts forcibly enough to actually shorten. This shortening pulls the bones of attachment closer to each other, causing movement at the joint. Figure 27.16 illustrates elbow flexion against gravity as a result of a concentric action: The muscles responsible for the flexion are able to act with sufficient force to shorten, which pulls the lower arm toward the humerus. Although the pull is on all the bones of attachment, usually only the bone farthest from the trunk (e.g., a limb) will move in a concentric action. To stand up from a semisquat position, the body must initiate extension at the hip joints and knee joints, but gravity resists that extension. The muscles must develop sufficient force to overcome the gravitational force; if sufficient force is developed, the muscle will shorten in a concentric action, pulling on the bones to cause extension. Resistance training with free weights uses gravitational pull as the resistance; the use of pulleys changes the direction of the gravitational pull, offering resistance to movement in other directions. Water resists movement of submerged body parts in all directions.

To exercise muscles by using gravity as the resisting force, the movements must be done in the direction opposite the pull of gravity (i.e., away from the earth). Arm abduction from a standing position is a movement opposite the pull of gravity, so a concentric action is required by the muscles that will pull the humerus into the abducted position. Movements such as shoulder horizontal flexion and horizontal extension (see figure 27.5) executed from a standing position occur parallel to the ground and therefore are not resisted by gravity. Internal tissue friction is the only resistance, but concentric action by the muscles responsible for these movements is still necessary. During these movements, gravity is still trying to draw the arm toward the earth, but it is not interfering with the horizontal movement. To perform horizontal flexion and extension against the resistance of gravity, the performer must get into a position in which the movements are away from the pull of gravity. To horizontally extend the shoulder joints against gravity, the performer can be lying prone on a bench or floor or standing with the trunk flexed at the hip. Horizontal flexion against gravity can be done from a supine position on the floor.

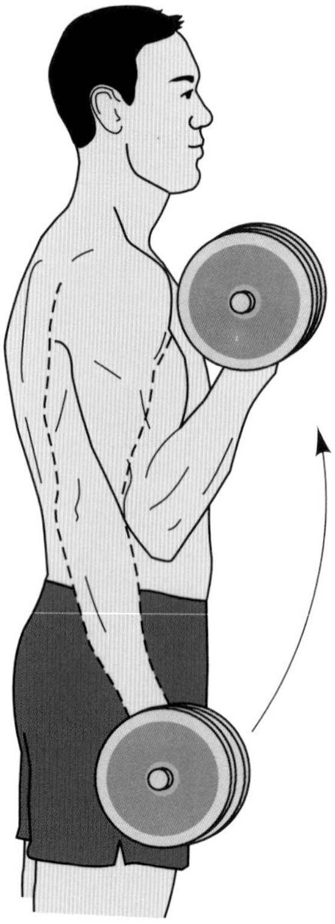

Figure 27.16 Concentric action by the elbow flexors.

A concentric action is also necessary for a rapid movement, regardless of the direction of another force. When an external force could cause the desired movement without any muscular action, but too slowly, concentric actions produce the desired speed. An example of this is seen in the arm movements during the second count of a jumping jack, when the arms adduct from their abducted position: Gravity would adduct the arms, but concentrically acting muscles cause the movement to occur much more quickly.

A muscle that is very effective in causing a certain joint movement is a prime mover, or **agonist**. Assistant movers are muscles that are not as effective for the same movement. For example, the peroneus longus and brevis are prime movers for eversion of the intertarsal joints, but they can offer only a little assistance in plantar flexion of the ankle joint. During a concentric action, muscles that act opposite to the muscles causing the concentric action, the **antagonist** muscles, are basically passive and lengthen as the agonists shorten. For example, for elbow flexion to occur against the pull of gravity, the muscles responsible for elbow flexion act concentrically; the antagonists, or the muscles responsible for elbow extension, relax and lengthen passively during the movement. In some fitness activities, such as aerobic dance, however, the antagonist muscles can respond in a manner to offer more resistance to the concentrically acting muscles. This resistance is done by having all the muscles activated (as in a bodybuilder's pose) during the movements.

Eccentric Action

An **eccentric action** occurs when a muscle generates tension that is not great enough to cause movement but instead acts as a brake to control the speed of movement caused by another force (see figure 27.17). The muscle exerts force, but its length increases. Arm abduction requires a concentric action of muscles; gravity will adduct the arm back down to the side. To adduct the arm more slowly than gravity, the same muscles that acted concentrically to abduct the arm now act eccentrically to control the speed of the lowering arm. Eccentric actions also may occur when a muscle's maximum effort still is not great enough to overcome the opposing force; movement will be caused by that force despite the maximally activated muscle, which is still lengthening. An example of this is if someone, with the elbow joint flexed to a 90° position, is handed a heavy weight. The exerciser tries to flex the elbow joint or even maintain the position but lacks the strength to do so. The elbow joint extends despite the efforts to flex it. Muscles antagonist to the eccentrically acting muscles passively shorten during the movement.

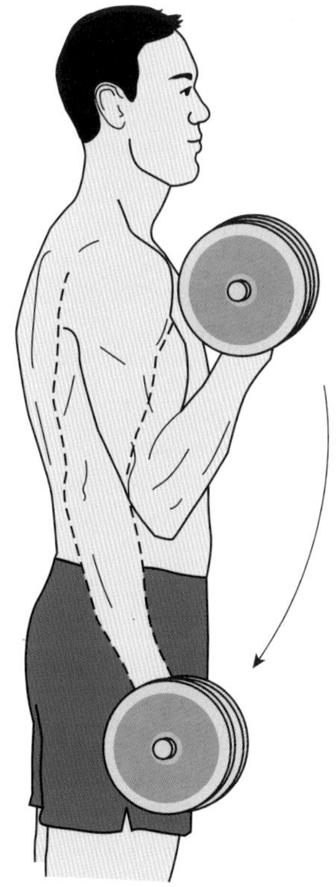

Figure 27.17 Eccentric action by the elbow flexors.

Ballistic Movements and Muscle Action

A **ballistic**, or fast, **movement** occurs when resistance is insignificant, as in throwing a ball, and requires a burst of concentric actions to initiate the movement. Once movement has begun, the muscles that caused the movement basically shut down; any further action slows the movement. Other muscles actively guide the movement in the appropriate direction. Eccentric actions of muscles that are antagonist, or opposite, to the muscles that initiated the movement decelerate and eventually stop the movement. For example, one of the most important movements in throwing is medial rotation of the shoulder joint. The muscles responsible for medial rotation act quickly in a concentric manner to begin the throwing motion. After the ball is released, the muscles responsible for lateral rotation act eccentrically to slow and eventually stop the movement; this is called the follow-through. The reverse is true for the windup, or preparation for the actual throw. All of this occurs in an exceedingly short period of time.

Jumping jacks require repeated ballistic movements in which opposing muscles come into play. The arm movements require concentric action by the agonist muscles to initiate the rapid movement. Once the movement is initiated, these muscles basically shut down. To stop the abduction movement and initiate the arm movement in the opposite direction, muscles antagonistic to those that acted concentrically to initiate the movement come into play. They act eccentrically to decelerate the movement and then act concentrically to initiate the next arm movement (adduction).

10 **In Review**

A ballistic movement is a rapid movement that begins with the agonist muscles acting concentrically to initiate movement; then "coasting," in which there is minimal muscle activity; and last, follow-through with an eccentric action of the antagonist muscles to decelerate the movement.

Isometric Action

During an **isometric**, or static, **action**, the muscle exerts a force that counteracts an opposing force. The muscle length does not change, so no movement occurs, and the joint position is maintained. The contractile part of the muscle shortens, but the elastic connective tissue lengthens proportionately; no overall change in the entire muscle length occurs. Holding the arm in an abducted position or maintaining a semisquat position requires an isometric action, producing just enough muscle force to counteract the pull of gravity and resulting in no movement. The effort involved in trying to move an immovable object (e.g., pushing against a wall) is another example of isometric actions; although the amount of muscular force can be maximal, no joint movement will occur (see figure 27.18).

Quad sets, a rehabilitation exercise in which the knee extensor muscles are activated with the knee already in the extended position, provide another example of a static action. A backward pelvic tilt desired during some exercises is maintained by isometric action of the abdominal muscles after they have acted concentrically to tilt the pelvis backward. During all resistance exercises that involve the arms or legs, the trunk muscles should be activated isometrically to stabilize the trunk and help prevent injury.

11 In Review

A concentric action, which shortens the muscle and therefore pulls the bones of attachment, is necessary if joint movement is to be in a direction opposite another force, such as gravity, and if joint movement is to be rapid, regardless of the direction of any other forces. An eccentric action, which lengthens the muscle, controls the velocity of movement caused by another force. An isometric action, which does not change the length of a muscle, prevents movement.

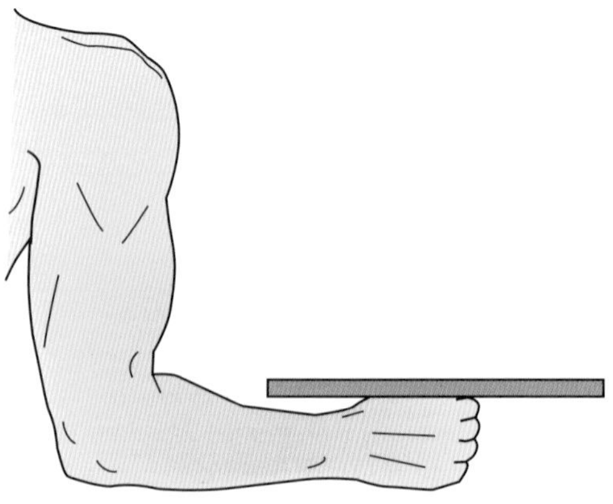

Figure 27.18 Isometric action by the elbow flexors.

Roles of Muscles

As previously mentioned in the discussion of muscular actions, muscles can act in several ways and have several functions. They can cause movement (concentric action), decelerate movement caused by another force (eccentric action), or prevent movement (isometric action). Muscles may also act isometrically to stabilize or prevent an undesirable body segment movement. For example, during a push-up exercise, gravity tends to cause hyperextension of the vertebral column and hip joint. Isometric action of the abdominal muscles prevents this sagging; activating the abdominal muscles stabilizes the trunk in its proper position.

Another function of the muscle is to counteract an undesirable action caused by the concentric action of another muscle. The concentric action of most muscles causes more than one movement at the same joint, or movement at more than one joint. If only one of those movements is intended, another muscle would act to prevent the undesirable movement. For example, concentric action of the upper trapezius fibers would cause elevation and some adduction of the scapula. If only adduction is desired, the lower trapezius fibers, which cause depression and adduction, neutralize the undesirable elevation to avoid unnecessary discomfort. In this example, the different fibers of the trapezius neutralize the unwanted action and help the desired action. The biceps brachii muscle causes elbow flexion and radioulnar supination; for only flexion to occur with biceps brachii action, the pronator teres counteracts the supination.

Muscles also guide movements initiated or caused by other muscles. During activities against a great resistance, such as lifting free weights, muscles help maintain balance or proper direction of the movement. After muscle force has initiated a ballistic movement, other muscles can help guide the movement in the proper direction.

12 In Review

The major roles of the muscles are to cause movement (concentric action) regardless of an opposing force, decelerate or control the speed of movement (eccentric action) caused by another force, and prevent movement (isometric action). Other muscle functions include counteracting an undesirable action caused by the concentric action of another muscle and guiding movements initiated or caused by another muscle.

Muscle Groups

A **muscle group** includes all of the muscles that cause the same movement at the same joint. The group is named for the joint where the movement takes place and the common movement that is caused by the concentric action of those muscles. The elbow flexors, for example, are a muscle group composed of the specific muscles responsible for flexion at the elbow joint when the muscles act concentrically. Table 27.1 lists the muscles that are prime (and assistant) movers of the muscle groups. Note that a movement being observed at a joint does not necessarily involve the muscle group for the movement that is occurring. The muscle group responsible for the opposite action may be acting eccentrically to control the movement. For example, the elbow flexor muscle group exerts force to flex the elbow joint during the elbow curl exercise. To return to the starting position, the pull of gravity extends the joint to the original position, but the elbow flexor muscle group is still exerting force to control the speed of that movement with eccentric actions. To maintain the elbow in a flexed position requires an isometric action by those same elbow flexors.

Specific muscles that cause more than one action at a joint or cause movement at more than one joint belong to more than one muscle group. For example, the flexor carpi ulnaris muscle belongs in both the wrist flexor and wrist adductor muscle groups. The biceps brachii is part of the elbow flexor and radioulnar supinator muscle groups.

13 In Review

A muscle group includes all the muscles that act concentrically to cause a specific movement at a specific joint. Table 27.1 lists the muscles in each muscle group, including the major actions that occur at each joint.

Tips for Exercising Muscle Groups and Some Common Exercise Mistakes

Many of the errors in exercise and movement result from a lack of knowledge rather than a lack of muscular strength or coordination. By applying basic knowledge, an exerciser can perform better and more safely. This section offers specific tips and things to be aware of for each major muscle group.

Shoulder Girdle and Shoulder Joint Complex

Movement can be enhanced and more muscles involved if a deliberate effort is made to incorporate shoulder girdle movements with shoulder joint movements. Optimal involvement of these muscles can be achieved in the following exercises and movements:

- *Forward reaching.* Flexion can be accompanied by scapular abduction if the exerciser reaches the fingertips as far forward as possible.
- *Push-up.* At the completion of a push-up, the scapulae can be abducted to raise the chest a little bit more off the floor.
- *Overhead reaching.* Normally, some scapular elevation is involved when the arm is overhead. A conscious effort to reach as high as possible will involve the scapulae elevators more; conversely, a deliberate attempt to keep the shoulders down for a "long neck" look requires concentric action by the scapulae depressors.
- *Sideward arm reaching.* During shoulder joint horizontal extension in movement or a specific exercise, the arm can be moved farther back with scapular adduction.

Elbow and Radioulnar Joints

Flexion against a resistance requires concentric action of the flexor muscles at the elbow joint. The position of the radioulnar joints, whether the arm is supinated or pronated, does not affect the involvement of the elbow joint muscles. The degree to which these muscles are strengthened, however, is affected by supination and pronation—a good point to remember when instructing participants on how to do curls. Normally, elbow flexion with the radioulnar joint in a pronated position (reverse curls) is a weaker movement because the biceps brachii muscle cannot act as strongly as when the radioulnar joints are in a supinated position. (The distal tendon of the biceps brachii muscle is wrapped around the radius somewhat in the pronated position, which diminishes its pulling force.) The brachialis muscle, though, is not affected by the radioulnar joint position because it is attached to the ulna, which is the nonmoving bone in radioulnar joint movements. Furthermore, the brachioradialis

Table 27.1 Muscles That Are Prime Movers (and Assistant Movers)

Joint	Prime movers (and assistant movers)
Shoulder girdle	Abductors—serratus anterior, pectoralis minor
	Adductors—middle fibers of trapezius, rhomboids (upper and lower fibers of trapezius)
	Upward rotators—upper and lower fibers of trapezius, serratus anterior
	Downward rotators—rhomboids, pectoralis minor
	Elevators—levator scapulae, upper fibers of trapezius, rhomboids
	Depressors—lower fibers of trapezius, pectoralis minor
Shoulder joint	Flexors—anterior deltoid, clavicular portion of pectoralis major (short head of biceps brachii)
	Extensors—sternal portion of pectoralis major, latissimus dorsi, teres major (posterior deltoid, long head of triceps brachii, infraspinatus/teres minor)
	Hyperextensors—latissimus dorsi, teres major (posterior deltoid, infraspinatus, teres minor)
	Abductors—middle deltoid, supraspinatus (anterior deltoid, long head of biceps brachii)
	Adductors—latissimus dorsi, teres major, sternal portion of pectoralis major (short head of biceps brachii, long head of triceps brachii)
	Lateral rotators—infraspinatus,* teres minor* (posterior deltoid)
	Medial rotators—pectoralis major, subscapularis,* latissimus dorsi, teres major (anterior deltoid, supraspinatus*)
	Horizontal flexors—both portions of pectoralis major, anterior deltoid
	Horizontal extensors—latissimus dorsi, teres major, infraspinatus, teres minor, posterior deltoid
Elbow joint	Flexors—brachialis, biceps brachii, brachioradialis (pronator teres, flexor carpi ulnaris and radialis)
	Extensors—triceps brachii (anconeus, extensor carpi ulnaris and radialis)
Radioulnar joint	Pronators—pronator quadratus, pronator teres, brachioradialis
	Supinators—supinator, biceps brachii, brachioradialis
Wrist joint	Flexors—flexor carpi ulnaris, flexor carpi radialis (flexor digitorum superficialis and profundus)
	Extensors and hyperextensors—extensor carpi ulnaris, extensor carpi radialis longus and brevis (extensor digitorum)
	Abductors (radial flexors)—flexor carpi radialis, extensor carpi radialis longus and brevis (extensor pollicis)
	Adductors (ulnar flexors)—flexor carpi ulnaris, extensor carpi ulnaris
Lumbosacral joint	Forward pelvic tilters—iliopsoas (rectus femoris)
	Backward pelvic tilters—rectus abdominis, internal oblique (external oblique, gluteus maximus)
Spinal column (thoracic and lumbar areas)	Flexors—rectus abdominis, external oblique, internal oblique
	Extensors and hyperextensors—erector spinae group
	Rotators—internal oblique, external oblique, erector spinae, rotatores, multifidus
	Lateral flexors—internal oblique, external oblique, quadratus lumborum, multifidus, rotatores (erector spinae group)
Hip joint	Flexors—iliopsoas, pectineus, rectus femoris (sartorius, tensor fascia latae, gracilis, adductor longus and brevis)
	Extensors and hyperextensors—gluteus maximus, biceps femoris, semitendinosus, semimembranosus
	Abductors—gluteus medius (tensors fascia latae, iliopsoas, sartorius)

(continued)

Table 27.1 *(continued)*

Joint	Prime movers (and assistant movers)
	Lateral rotators—gluteus maximus, the six deep lateral rotator muscles (iliopsoas, sartorius)
	Medial rotators—gluteus minimus, gluteus medius (tensor fascia latae, pectineus)
Knee joint	Flexors—biceps femoris, semimembranosus, semitendinosus (sartorius, gracilis, gastrocnemius, plantaris)
	Extensors—rectus femoris, vastus medialis, vastus lateralis, vastus intermedius
Ankle joint	Plantar flexors—gastrocnemius, soleus (peroneus longus, peroneus brevis, tibialis posterior, flexor digitorum, flexor hallucis longus)
	Dorsiflexors—tibialis anterior, extensor digitorum longus, peroneus tertius (extensor hallucis longus)
Intertarsal joint	Inverters—tibialis anterior, tibialis posterior (extensor and flexor hallucis longus, flexor digitorum longus)
	Everters—extensor digitorum longus, peroneus brevis, peroneus longus, peroneus tertius

*Rotator cuff muscles.

muscle can act with more force when the radioulnar joint is in a semipronated, semisupinated position. None of the elbow extensor muscles are affected by the radioulnar joint positions, but the radioulnar joint position will affect the amount of weight that may be pressed (moved) on the lat machine because of strength limitations of the wrist muscles. Triceps push-downs, when elbow extension occurs with the radioulnar joints in the pronated position, require the wrist flexors to stabilize the wrist joint; triceps pull-downs (supinated position) utilize the wrist extensors, which are usually much weaker than the flexors. If an exerciser wanted to concentrate more on building the elbow extensors, he or she should perform triceps push-downs.

Wrist Joint

The wrist muscles during wrist flexion and extension curl exercises are affected by the position of the radioulnar joints. Gravity acts as a resistance for wrist flexion when the radioulnar joints are in the supinated position and a resistance for extension when the radioulnar joints are in the pronated position. Remind exercise participants that the position of the radioulnar joints affects which wrist muscles are strengthened during these exercises.

Vertebral Column and Lumbosacral Joints

In general, neither neck hyperextension nor hyperflexion is desirable. The same pairs of muscles that act concentrically to cause flexion and extension can be strengthened or stretched, one side at a time, by cervical lateral flexion and rotation. The instructor should ask participants to tilt or turn the head from side to side rather than to bend the neck forward or back. Although hyperextension may not be contraindicated for the young, no benefits can be gained and it teaches bad habits.

Many exercises require appropriate positioning of the lumbosacral joint and lumbar vertebrae and actions by the abdominal muscles for either movement or stabilization. An abdominal curl-up or crunch exercise should begin with a backward pelvic tilt that is maintained throughout the curl-up and return movement. If there is any indication that a backward pelvic tilt cannot be maintained, or if the exerciser feels tightness or an ache in the lumbar area, the exercise should be stopped. If the problem is inadequate strength to maintain the backward tilt position, the exercise should be modified to one that requires less abdominal muscle strength, one that the exerciser has sufficient abdominal strength to do correctly.

A full curl-up, in which the exerciser comes up to a sitting position, requires hip flexion by the hip flexor muscles during the last stages of the exercise. Initially, the abdominal muscles act concentrically to tilt the pelvis backward and then to flex the vertebral column. Once flexion is achieved, these muscles act isometrically to keep the pelvis tilted backward and the trunk in a flexed position. There is a "sticking point" that can be felt by the exerciser during a full curl-up. This occurs when the trunk flexion is complete and the hip flexors begin to bring the trunk to an upright position. Doing partial curl-ups or crunches will help eliminate the role of the hip flexors and focus solely on strengthening the abdominals.

The exercise called leg lifts is considered to be an abdominal exercise, but it is often not taught correctly. From a supine position on the floor, the legs are lifted and held up by concentric and then isometric action of the hip flexors. Some of the hip flexor muscles also pull the lumbosacral joint into a forward-tilted position. It is the role of the abdominal muscles to prevent that forward tilt and to maintain a flattened lumbar spine and posterior pelvic tilt. The backward pelvic tilt should precede the hip flexion, and, as in the case of the curl-up exercise, if the proper tilt cannot be maintained, the exercise should not be done in that fashion.

There is also a tendency for the pelvis to tilt forward during overhead arm movements from a standing position. This can be prevented by keeping the arms in front of the ears and by flexing the knees slightly.

When weights are lifted from a supine position, as in the bench press, there is a tendency to hyperextend the lumbar spine and tilt the pelvis forward. Although this can allow the exerciser to lift a somewhat heavier weight, it does not increase the work of the arm and chest muscles, and it puts the lower back into a compromising position. Bench presses are best done with the hips and knees in a flexed position and feet on the bench or a bench extension. Upright presses are best done seated with the back supported.

Hip Joint

A common error during side-lying leg raises to exercise the hip abductor muscles is the attempt to move the foot as high as possible. Because the ROM for true abduction is limited (about 45°), the exerciser often rotates the top leg laterally, which turns the foot out and allows it to go higher. However, this rotation changes the muscle involvement more to the hip flexor muscles. To exercise the primary abductor muscles, the leg should not be rotated; the toes should face forward, not up. Turning the feet out comes from lateral rotation of the hips; there should be no attempt to rotate the knee or the ankle joints.

In backward leg movements to strengthen the gluteus muscles, hyperextension is limited primarily by the tightness of the hip ligaments. A leg can appear to be more hyperextended if it is accompanied by a forward pelvic tilt. The exerciser should be cautioned to keep the pelvis in its proper neutral position, even though some apparent hip hyperextension is lost.

A common exercise position is standing with feet shoulder-width apart. The exerciser should have the feet turned slightly outward (from hip lateral rotation). Too much rotation is potentially dangerous. During any squatting or standing movement, the knee should be directly over the foot (not in front of the foot) to prevent strain to the lateral and medial knee ligaments. Although the knee can be kept over the foot even in the toed-out position during a squat, some individuals tend to let the knees move toward the inside of the feet. It is easier to determine whether the knee position is correct when the feet are almost parallel to each other. During the squat, the exerciser should be able to see the big toe on each foot.

Knee Joint

Hyperflexion can strain and stretch knee ligaments and put pressure on the menisci; therefore, a full squat that creates an angle at the knee joint of less than 90°, especially with additional weights, should not be attempted, nor should sitting on the lower legs. During any lunging movements or forward-back stride positions in which the front knee is in a flexed position, the knee should be over or in back of the foot, not in front. Any knee position that puts a twisting pressure on the knee joint should also be avoided. The hurdler position, with one leg out to the back and side with a flexed knee, should be avoided; that leg should also be in front.

Ankle Joint

If the squat exercise is performed with the heels of the feet resting on a low block, the soleus muscles are exercised more than they would be if the feet were flat. This "heels up" position shortens the gastrocnemius muscles even more (they already are shortened by the flexed knee positions), limiting their ability to generate force. The soleus muscles, which do not cross the knees, aren't shortened to the extent that it affects the force generation. The gastrocnemius muscles are weaker in this position, so more of the work is done by the soleus muscles. To increase the force production of the gastrocnemius muscles, the squat could be done with the balls of the feet on the block. A mountain climber especially would benefit from this because it mimics the knee and ankle joint positions in climbing.

Intertarsal Joints

Walking on the insides or outsides of the foot should never be done. Not only does this stress the knees, it can cause ankle sprains. A better way of exercising the invertors and evertors is to walk back and forth, instead of up and down, across a ramp or hill.

14 In Review

During the following exercises involving the vertebral column and lumbosacral joints, participants should remember the following:

- Maintain backward pelvic tilt during the abdominal crunch/curl-up.
- Tilt the pelvis backward before hip flexion in the curl-up and leg lifts.
- Keep the pelvis tilted backward during overhead arm movements performed in a standing position.
- Keep the lumbar spine flat on bench during weightlifting in a supine position.

For exercise involving the knee, participants should remember the following:

- Keep the knee over the foot (not beyond) during lunging and squatting movements.
- Maintain foot/knee alignment.

Muscle Group Involvement in Selected Activities

Human movement is caused or controlled by muscle forces. The following sections briefly analyze the involvement of muscle groups in some common physical activities.

Walking, Jogging, and Running

Jogging can be looked at as a modification of walking, and running as a fast jog. The different phases and the muscle groups involved in walking, jogging, and running are similar, but more forceful muscle actions are needed to increase speed. The three basic phases are the push-off, the recovery of the push-off leg, and the landing.

The push-off is accomplished by the concentric action of the hip hyperextensors, the talocrural plantar flexors, and, to a lesser extent, the foot metatarsophalangeal flexors (see the back leg in figure 27.19). Because the knee of the back leg is almost in the extended position at push-off, little work is done by the knee extensors to help propel the body forward. The gluteus maximus may assume a greater role in hip hyperextension as speed increases. Medial rotation takes place at the hip joint, but because the foot is fixed on the ground, this movement is seen at the pelvis.

At the beginning of the recovery phase, the hip flexors act concentrically to begin the forward leg swing. This is basically a ballistic movement, so the momentum initiated by the hip flexors continues the motion. The knee flexors bend the knee at the beginning of hip flexion, the extensors initiate the straightening of the knee, and the flexors then work eccentrically to control the knee extension at the end of the recovery phase. The talocrural joint is dorsiflexed to clear the foot from the ground and prepare for the landing (see the recovery leg in figure 27.19). Running speed is a product of stride length and stride frequency. To increase both factors in running, the hip is flexed to a greater extent and with a much greater velocity (see figure 27.20, the recovery leg).

Just before landing, the hip extensors act eccentrically to decelerate the forward leg swing. On contact, the knee extensors act eccentrically to cushion the impact. The heel should touch the ground first during walking and jogging; as running speed increases, the ball of the foot or the entire foot may

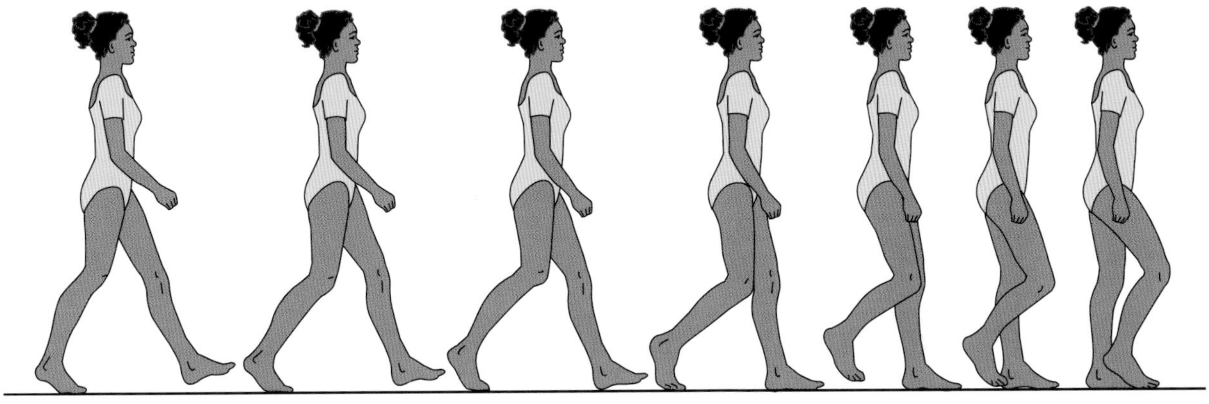

Figure 27.19 Walking movements.

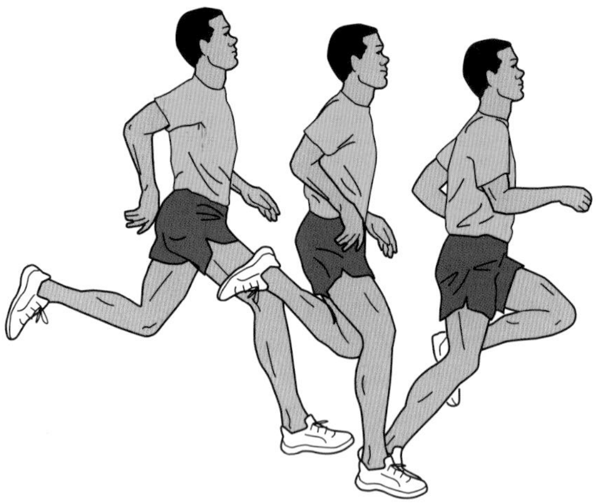

Figure 27.20 Running movements.

make contact. During the landing phase in walking and jogging, the talocrural dorsiflexors act eccentrically to control the speed of movement of the ball of the foot to the ground.

The arm swing requires shoulder flexion and extension to hyperextension. As speed increases, the swing becomes more vigorous, and there is more elbow flexion. For the greatest efficiency, the arms should move in an anterior/posterior direction. To increase the upper limb muscle involvement for exercise, a walker can exaggerate the flexion and hyperextension movements or can abduct and adduct or horizontally flex and extend the shoulder joint.

Walking or running up an incline elicits a greater force of action from the gluteus maximus muscle at the hip and from the knee extensors. The talocrural dorsiflexors are more active immediately before landing to position the talocrural joint to conform with the angle of the incline. Because the talocrural joint is in a more dorsiflexed position, the plantar flexors begin acting during push-off from a more stretched position. For these reasons, hill climbing requires greater flexibility in the plantar flexors, especially the soleus muscle, and greater strength in the dorsiflexors. There is also more eccentric action by the knee extensors during landing in downhill than in uphill running. As a result, these muscle groups are more apt to become fatigued and to be sore afterward.

Jogging in place requires the talocrural plantar flexors to propel the body upward; they work more than any of the other lower extremity muscle groups in this activity. The knee extensors are primarily active in eccentric action to cushion the landing. During walking and jogging, the heel is the first part of the foot to make contact with the surface, but during jogging in place, the ball of the foot touches first. The plantar flexors therefore are also active during the landing, acting eccentrically to control the speed and amount of dorsiflexion. It is better to have sufficient dorsiflexion so the heel touches the ground briefly rather than to always stay up on the toes, which can put quite a strain on the plantar flexors. Additional muscles can be involved in executing movements with the leg immediately after push-off and before the foot lands again: hip flexion with flexed or extended knee, hip hyperextension with flexed or extended knee, hip abduction/adduction, hip lateral rotation along with hip and knee flexion that brings the foot to the front of the trunk, and medial rotation with knee flexion that brings the foot behind and to the side of the trunk.

Cycling

The main force in cycling comes from the hip and knee extensor muscles during the downward push. With toe clips, the rider can use the hip and talocrural dorsiflexors to help return the pedal to the up position, but only if she or he makes a conscious effort to do so.

Jumping

The hip and knee extensors, followed by the talocrural plantar flexors, forcibly act to propel the body upward. The lean of the trunk primarily determines the angle of takeoff. The trunk extends, and the arms flex from a hyperextended position just before the leg action. If the reach height of the arms is important, as in a jump ball in basketball or a tennis smash, the scapulae elevate. During the landing, the hip and knee extensors and the talocrural plantar flexors act eccentrically.

Overarm Throwing

There are three phases in throwing: the windup, or preparation; the execution, or actual throw; and the follow-through, or recovery. Figure 27.21 illustrates the sequence of the actual throw.

In preparation for throwing, there is a weight shift to the back foot, a medial rotation of the back leg (because the leg is fixed to the ground, rotation is seen at the pelvis), trunk rotation and some lateral flexion and hyperextension, shoulder lateral rotation, some horizontal extension of the throwing arm accompanied by adduction of the scapula, flexion of the elbow, and hyperextension of the wrist. The movements of the throwing arm are all ballistic. The lateral rotation at the shoulder is remarkably fast and powerful. Toward the end of the windup, the medial rotators begin to act eccentrically to decelerate the rotation in preparation for the actual throw.

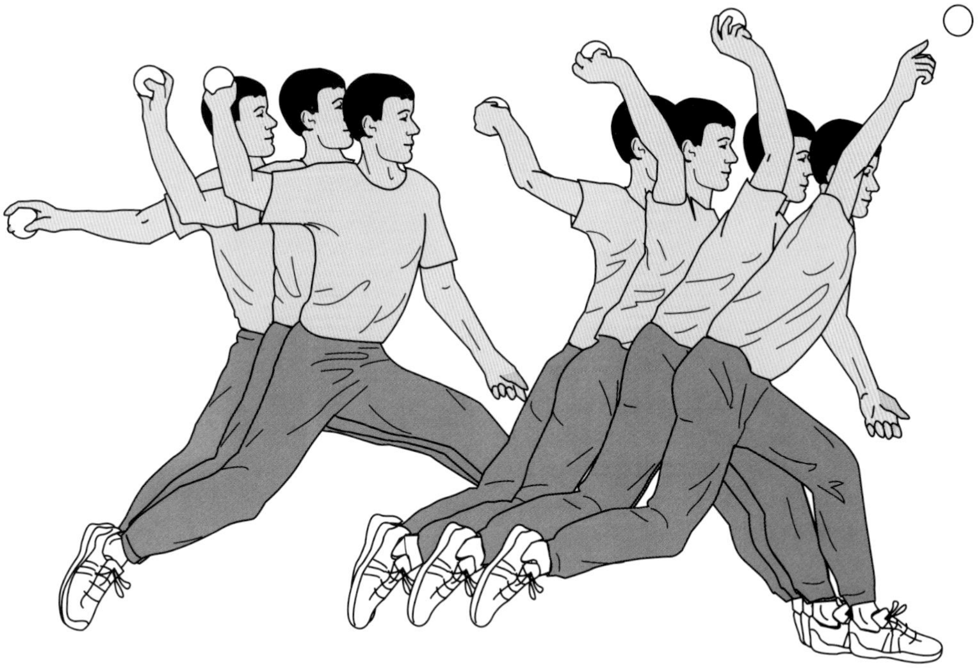

Figure 27.21 Overarm throwing movements.

The weight shift forward is the initial movement in the throwing pattern. This is accomplished by the hip abductors, hyperextensors, and lateral rotators; the talocrural plantar flexors; and the intertarsal everters of the back leg. The front hip rotates laterally. The trunk then flexes laterally in the direction opposite that of the windup and rotates, beginning at the lumbar area and continuing through the thoracic vertebrae, and then flexes. There is a forcible medial rotation of the shoulder, along with scapular abduction. Although there is some horizontal flexion, most of the force of the shoulder in an overhand throw comes from this medial rotation. The elbow extends, and the wrist moves toward flexion. Depending on the desired spin on the ball, the radioulnar pronators and the wrist abductors or adductors also may be involved.

Because the actions at the shoulder and elbow joints are vigorous ballistic movements, the shoulder lateral rotators and horizontal extensors act eccentrically to decelerate the movements; the elbow flexors act eccentrically to prevent elbow hyperextension.

Swimming and Exercise in Water

Swimming is a unique activity because the water medium offers resistance to movements of submerged body parts in all directions and at all speeds. Exercises or movements performed in water demand concentric actions. Gravity is less of a factor in water, so less stress is put on the weight-bearing joints.

Lifting and Carrying Objects

The weight to be lifted from the ground should be located close to the lifter's spread feet; the lifter squats, keeping the trunk as erect as possible. The actual lifting should be accomplished by the legs rather than spine or arm action. Proper lifting is begun by moving the trunk to a position as perpendicular to the floor as possible and then tilting the pelvis backward and keeping the abdominal muscles activated; the knee extensors along with the hip extensors then act concentrically. The lift should be slow, not jerky (see figure 27.22). Insufficient leg strength can result in an incorrect lifting technique. The weight should be carried close to the body, with the trunk assuming a position that allows the line of gravity to fall well within the area of the base. The trunk lateral flexors are more active when the weight is carried on one side; the extensors are more active when the weight is in front of the body; and the abdominals are more active when the weight is carried across the top of the back, as in backpacking.

15 In Review

The movements and muscle involvement for locomotion, throwing, cycling, jumping, and swimming are summarized here:

Major muscle group	Movement task
Hip extensor	Locomotion—push-off; cycling; jumping; swimming—front crawl, back crawl, sidestroke
Hip flexor	Locomotion—recovery; swimming—front crawl, back crawl, sidestroke
Hip abductors	Swimming—breaststroke; throwing
Hip adductors	Swimming—breaststroke
Hip lateral and medial rotators	Throwing
Knee extensor	Locomotion—landing; cycling; jumping
Knee flexor	Locomotion—recovery
Talocrural plantar flexor	Locomotion—push-off, landing; jumping
Talocrural dorsiflexor	Locomotion—recovery
Shoulder-joint flexor	Underhand throwing
Shoulder-joint extensors	Swimming—front crawl
Shoulder-joint medial and lateral rotators	Throwing
Anterior shoulder-joint muscles	Swimming—back crawl, sidestroke lead arm; throwing
Posterior shoulder-joint muscles	Swimming—sidestroke trailarm, breast stroke; throwing—windup
Shoulder girdle upward and downward rotator	Swimming—breast stroke, sidestroke lead arm, front crawl, back crawl
Shoulder-girdle abductor	Swimming—back crawl; throwing
Shoulder-girdle adductor	Swimming—front crawl, breast stroke; throwing—windup
Shoulder-girdle elevator	Swimming—front crawl, back crawl, sidestroke lead arm, breast stroke
Elbow flexor	Throwing
Elbow extensor	Throwing
Trunk flexor	Throwing
Trunk rotator	Throwing

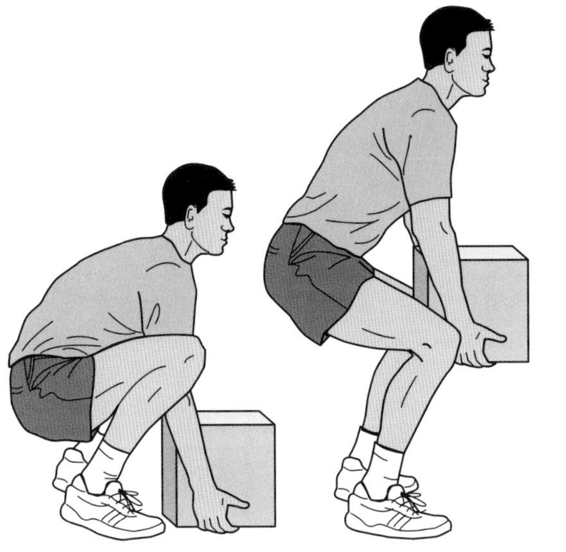

Figure 27.22 Lifting technique.

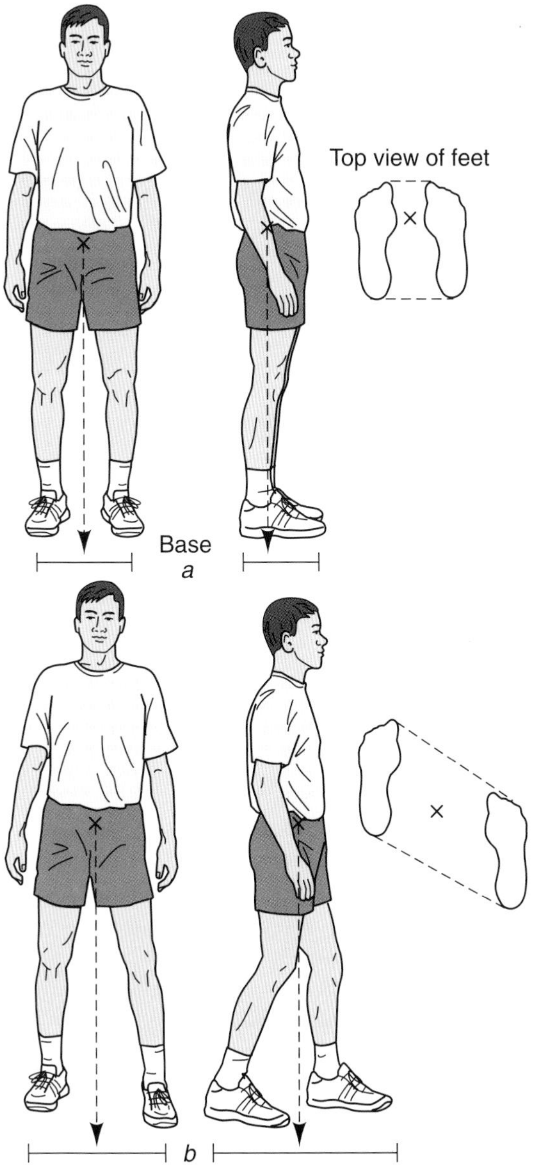

Figure 27.23 Bases of support.

16 In Review

The steps in proper lifting are to place the feet close to the object, move the vertebral column to an upright position perpendicular to the floor, tilt the pelvis backward, and slowly extend the hips and knees while activating the abdominals.

Basic Mechanical Concepts Related to Human Movement

Knowledge of the laws and principles of mechanics is also important to understanding human movement. Some of these basic but important concepts are described next.

Achieving Stability

For an individual to maintain balance, his or her line of gravity must fall within the area of the base of support. Figure 27.23a illustrates the area of the base of support in a standing position with feet together; figure 27.23b illustrates a position with feet apart and forward and back.

Stability, or the ease with which balance can be maintained, is proportional to the distance from the line of gravity to the outer limits of the base that is farthest from a potentially upsetting force. Figure 27.24 compares more stable positions with less stable positions. A wide base of support usually, but not necessarily, ensures greater stability. From a feet-apart position, if one leans so that the line of gravity falls directly over one foot and a pushing force is applied in the same direction of the lean, there is less stability than if the feet were together but with the line of gravity falling over the edge of the foot closer to the applied force.

The degree of stability is also indirectly proportional to the height of the center of gravity, which is approximately at the level of the naval, relative to the floor, in a standing position. The lower the center of gravity over the feet, the greater the force needed to upset the stability. The degree of stability is also directly proportional to the weight of the

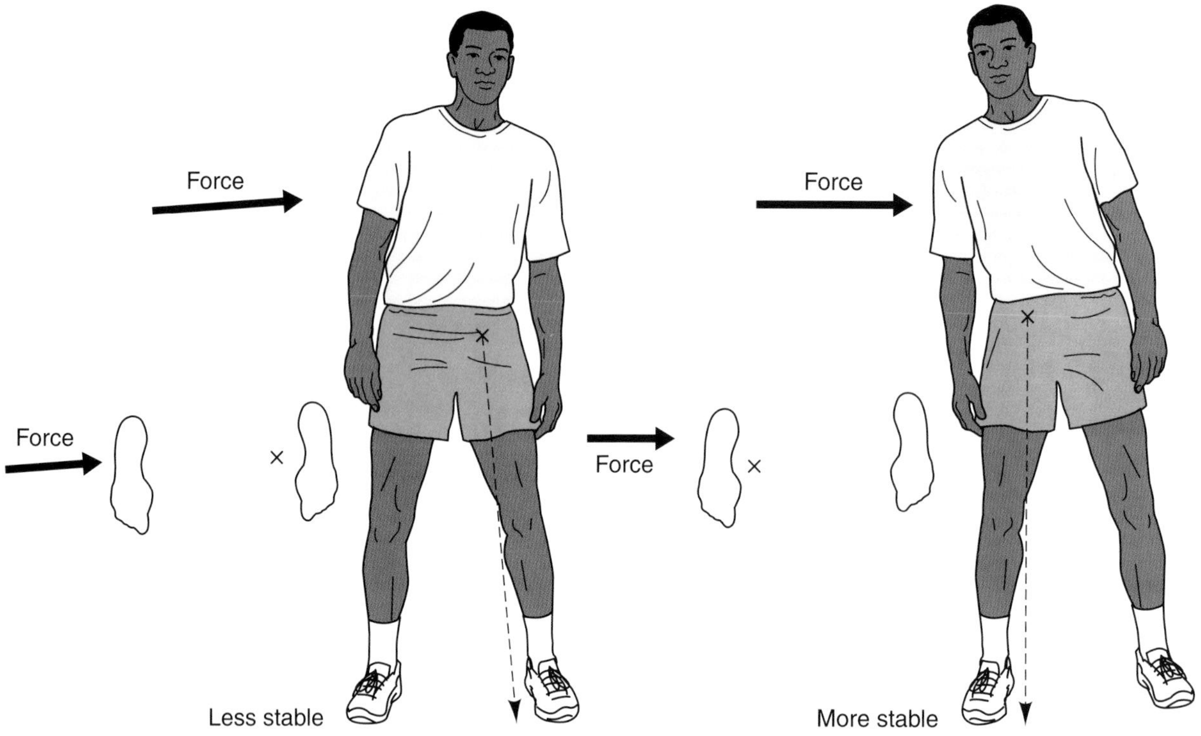

Figure 27.24 Relationship between line of gravity and outer limits of base of support.

body. With all other factors being equal, a heavy person is more stable than a lighter one.

Stability may be increased by moving the feet apart to widen the base of support and by flexing the knees and hips to lower the center of gravity. During standing exercises that require some degree of balance, stability can also be aided by having a nearby object such as a wall or chair to hold or push against if necessary. Many exercises can be executed from a sitting position, which increases the base and lowers the center of gravity. To help maintain stability against a potentially upsetting force, the weight should be shifted toward that force. When locomotion is going to occur, a position close to instability is attained by shifting the line of gravity closer to the outer limits of the base (which is the area of the push-off foot in walking, or the hands in a track start position) in the direction of the intended movement. During locomotion, as the line of gravity moves outside the limits of the base, a new base is established when the other foot lands, and stability is maintained. If something prevents the foot from establishing a new base, stability is lost. A basketball guard, in taking a charge from a forward, will fall down quicker and easier if the guard is in an unstable position—standing fairly erect with feet closer together and weight on heels—at the collision.

17 In Review

Stability in humans is directly proportional to the distance of the line of gravity from the limits of the base, indirectly proportional to the height of the center of gravity above the base, and directly proportional to the weight of the body. For stability in a standing position, the knees should be flexed to lower the center of gravity, the feet should be apart in the direction of an oncoming force to increase the distance of the line of gravity to the outer limits of the upsetting force, and the weight of the body (line of gravity) should be shifted toward the force.

Torque

A force is any push or pull that tends to cause movement. The effect produced when a force causes rotation is called **torque (T)**. It is the product of the magnitude of the force (F) and the **force arm (FA)**, which is the perpendicular distance from the axis to the direction of the application of that force. Algebraically, torque can be expressed as follows:

$$T = F \times FA$$

When two opposing forces act to produce rotation in opposite directions, one of the forces often is designated as the **resistance force (R)**; its force arm is called the **resistance arm (RA)**. When we consider the torque produced by sufficient muscle force to cause movement against gravity or some other external force, F and FA are designated for the muscle and R and RA for the gravitational or other opposing force.

Applying Torque to Muscle Action

Muscle action can be considered the force; the FA is the perpendicular distance from the joint (axis) to the direction of the force from its point of application (where the muscle attaches to the bone being moved). Figure 27.25 illustrates the direction of pull of the biceps brachii on the radius; the force arm is the perpendicular distance from the elbow joint to this line of force. If the muscle insertion were closer to the joint, the same force would produce less torque because of the shorter force arm; to produce the same torque, more muscle force must be produced.

Torque is also affected by joint position. Figure 27.26 again shows the direction of pull by the biceps brachii but with the elbow in a less flexed position. This results in a shorter force arm, so the same muscle force produces less torque at that joint angle.

Torque Resulting From Other Forces

The force from gravitational pull is treated as a resistance force. The resistance (R) produced by gravity pulling on a body part is the weight of the object; the resistance arm (RA) is the perpendicular distance from the axis of rotation to the point of the object that represents its center of gravity. The torque is the product of the resistive force and the resistance arm. Figure 27.27 illustrates the torque produced as a result of gravity acting on the arm. The torque that opposes limb movements can be increased by adding weight to increase both the magnitude of force and the length of the resistance arm or by adjusting the weight further from the axis. The resistance arm of a force applied by someone pushing or pulling on a limb is the perpendicular distance from the axis to the point of application of the push or pull.

For muscle action to move a bone, the muscle force must produce a torque greater than the opposing or resistance torque; the muscle action is concentric. A greater resistance torque results in movement, and the muscle acts eccentrically. Technically, it can be argued that the muscle force during an eccentric action should be considered the resistance, and the external force causing the movement should be considered the force. When the muscular torque equals the resistance torque, no movement occurs; the muscle is acting isometrically.

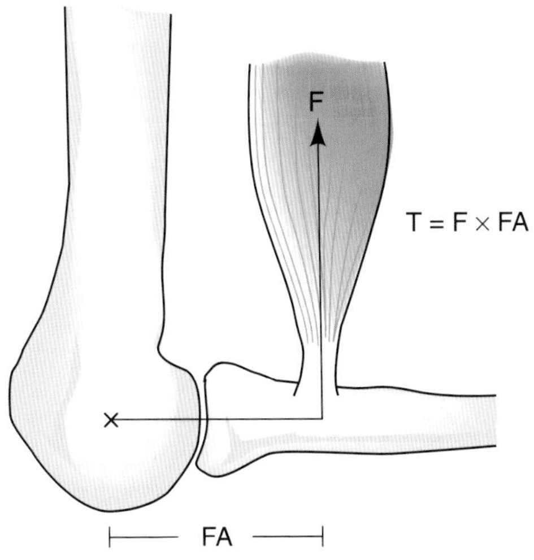

Figure 27.25 Force (F) and force arm (FA) of biceps brachii muscle.

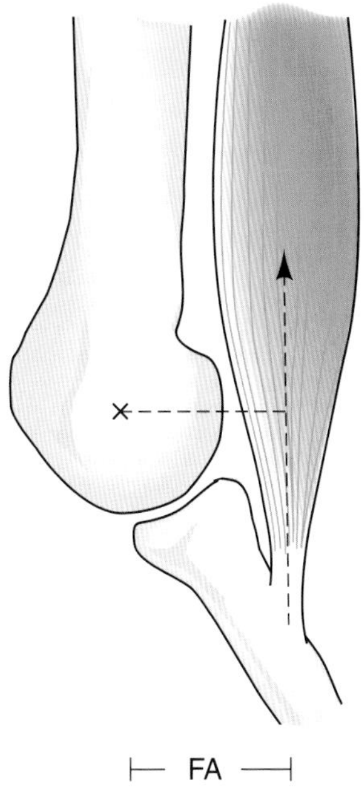

Figure 27.26 Effect of a less flexed position of the elbow joint on the force arm of the biceps brachii.

18 In Review

Torque can be expressed algebraically as T = F × FA, for the torque that produces the movement, or T = R × RA, for the torque that is opposing the movement. A concentric action produces a torque that is greater than the resistive torque. An eccentric action produces a torque that is less than the opposing torque. An isometric action produces a torque that is the same as the opposing torque.

Applying Torque to Exercising

Knowledge of torques can be used to modify exercises for different individuals. The amount of muscular action necessary during the exercise can be modified to fit an individual's needs by altering the amount of resistance or the resistance arm, or both, to change the resistive torque. For example, resistive torque can be increased with the use of external weights, which therefore would require stronger muscle actions. The resistance torque also can be changed by altering the position of the body parts. Figure 27.28 shows an exerciser making modifications to reduce the necessary muscle force by not using the weight, to reduce both the resistance and the resistance arm, and by flexing the elbow to reduce the length of the resistance arm.

The arm position during a curl-up exercise determines the length of the resistance arm and therefore the amount of resistance torque against which the abdominal muscles have to work. Arms may be held at the sides of the body to bring the upper body mass closer to the axis of rotation to reduce the necessary muscle force; arms can be put overhead with hands on the scapulae or straight out to increase the resistive torque, therefore increasing the required muscle force. Modifications to lessen the resistance torque do not necessarily make the exercise "easy" for all individuals. If an exerciser with a lower strength level finds the resistive torque too great to overcome for a sufficient number of repetitions, the limb positions can be altered to reduce the torque against which the muscles have to work; however, this individual is still working as hard, relative to his or her maximal ability, as a stronger individual who did not have to reduce the resistive torque.

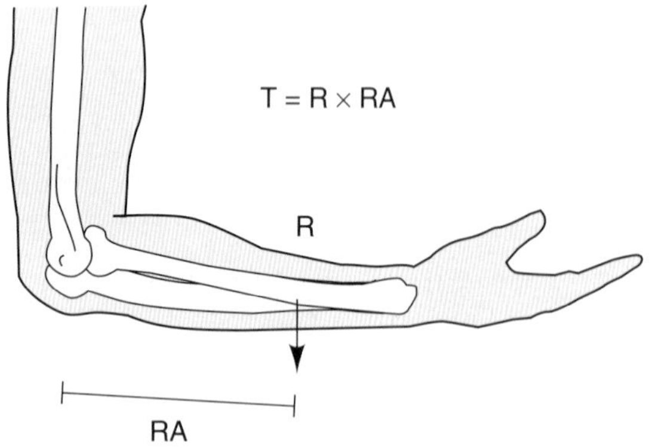

Figure 27.27 Resistance (R) and resistance arm (RA) of lower arm.

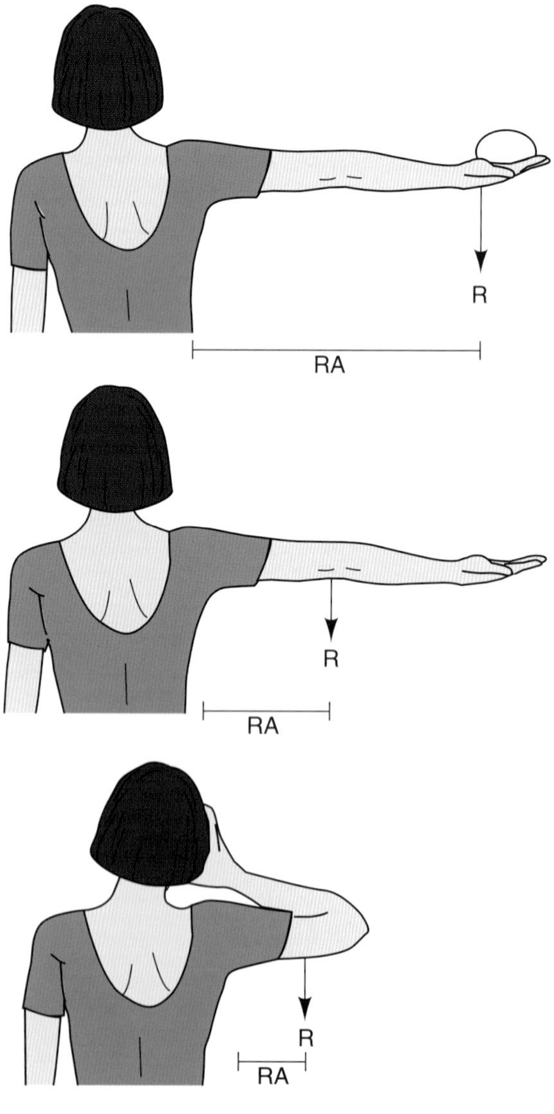

Figure 27.28 Modifications of resistive torque.

19 **In Review**

The torque that resists limb movements can be altered by increasing or decreasing the amount of the resistive force and changing the position of the resistive force relative to the joint to change the resistance arm.

Rotational Inertia

Rotational inertia (also referred to as the moment of inertia), or the reluctance of a body segment or segments to rotate around an axis or a joint, is dependent on the body's mass and the distribution of that mass around the joint. A leg, for example, has more rotational inertia than an arm, not only because of its heavier mass but also because its mass is concentrated a greater distance away from its axis. A softball bat held by its fat end has less rotational inertia than a bat grasped in the usual manner.

The rotational inertia of body segments before or during movement depends on the mass of the segments, which cannot be changed, and the distribution of the mass around the joints, which can be manipulated to alter the rotational inertia. For example, an arm with elbow, wrist, and fingers extended has a greater rotational inertia than an arm with elbow, wrist, and fingers flexed; a leg with extended knee and ankle has more inertia than if the knee were flexed and the ankle dorsiflexed. The amount of muscular force necessary to cause rapid limb movement is proportional to the rotational inertia of the limb to be moved. During jogging, in which speed of running is not a factor, the knee of the recovery leg is flexed to reduce the leg's rotational inertia around the hip joint. Less muscular force is needed to swing the recovery leg forward, which reduces the possibility of local fatigue of the hip flexor muscles. In sprinting, the quicker the recovery leg is brought forward, the faster the running speed. Powerful actions of the hip flexors, along with a greater knee flexion, result in the recovery leg coming through sooner with increased overall speed. Another example of rapid movement to which this principle can be applied is jumping jacks. Keeping the elbow flexed reduces the rotational inertia. This either reduces the amount of muscle force by the shoulder abductor and adductor muscle groups to maintain a certain cadence or, if maximum muscle force is still applied, it results in faster movements.

Angular Momentum

Angular momentum, or the quantity of angular motion, is expressed as the product of the rotational inertia, which is determined by both the mass of the moving part and the distribution of the mass around the joints and the angular velocity. A moving body part possesses angular momentum; the faster it is moving and the greater its rotational inertia, the greater the angular momentum. The amount of force necessary to change angular momentum is proportional to the amount of the momentum.

Applying Angular Momentum to Exercising

The concept of angular momentum can be applied to ballistic limb movements during exercise. A fast-moving body segment is decelerated by eccentric muscle actions; the faster the movement, the greater the mass, or the greater the desired deceleration, the greater the muscle force that must be applied. Care must be taken when rapid ballistic limb movements are performed, especially with added weights. A large amount of momentum may be generated, and considerable muscle strength may be required to decelerate and eventually stop the movement.

Transfer of Angular Momentum

Transfer of angular momentum from one body segment to another can be achieved by stabilizing the initial moving body part at a joint, which will result in angular movement of another body part. For example, when an athlete is performing a curl-up exercise for the trunk flexors, flinging the arms forward from an overhead position or the elbows from alongside the head transfers their momentum to the trunk. This decreases the amount of muscular action needed by the trunk flexors and makes the exercise seem easier, but the abdominal flexors do not work as hard. A jump with a turn in the air can be better achieved if the arms are swung forcibly across the body in the intended direction of the spin just before takeoff.

20 **In Review**

Rotational inertia during fast limb movements can be decreased by moving the mass of the limb closer to the axis or joints. The amount of angular momentum depends on the rotational inertia and angular velocity of a moving body segment. The amount of eccentric force necessary to decelerate the angular velocity of a body segment is proportional to the amount of the angular momentum of the body segment. Angular momentum can be transferred from one body segment to another by stabilizing the initial moving body part at a joint.

Common Mechanical Errors During Locomotion, Throwing, and Striking

Success in activities depends in part on the proper execution of movements. Some of the more common errors that violate the laws of mechanics to some degree are discussed in the next sections.

Errors in Locomotion

Some beginning joggers have a tendency to run "stiff legged," or with insufficient knee flexion of the recovery leg. This results in a greater rotational inertia of the leg; the hip flexor muscles must exert more force than if the knee were more flexed to bring the mass of the leg closer to the hip axis.

Another potential problem is direction of the arm and leg movements. All movements should be executed in the anterior and posterior directions. Swinging the hands across the trunk rotates the upper trunk; in reaction, the lower trunk rotates in the opposite direction. The recovery leg may also tend to rotate medially at the hip; this swings the recovery foot to the outside. The touchdown foot should land in a forward-backward direction and not pointed to the outside. Sometimes runners are not aware of this tendency, and the HFI should instruct them to "toe in" somewhat when landing, which will result in the correct foot alignment.

Some joggers and runners propel themselves too high off the ground during the airborne phase; this results in a shorter stride length. Although the length of time the body is airborne may be the same as when running with less lift, less horizontal distance is covered.

Overstriding, in which the line of gravity from the runner's center of gravity falls in front of the touchdown foot, can decrease running speed. No propulsion force against the ground for forward movement can take place until the line of gravity is over and ahead of the foot. Under-striding, in which the line of gravity falls well in back of the foot at touchdown, shortens the period of time during which the propulsion muscles can work.

Errors in Throwing and Striking

A ball is thrown for accuracy, speed, or distance, which depends in part on the speed of the ball when it leaves the hand. The speed of the ball in the hand just before release is the speed of the ball immediately after it leaves the hand. The more joints that can be involved in the throwing motions, the greater the speed of the ball when it is released. Proper throwing and striking techniques are the same for females and males. Most throwing problems that result in low velocity, such as pushing the ball rather than throwing it, stem from a lack of sufficient trunk rotation or from poor timing of this rotation with the shoulder joint movements. The thrower should rotate the trunk and hips during the windup so that the pelvis is sideways to the intended direction of the throw and the shoulders are rotated even more to the back. As the hips and then the different sections of the spinal column rotate back to begin the execution of the throw, the arm lags behind. This sets up for a whiplike action of the arm and allows an adequate length of time for the important medial rotation. Without this trunk rotation, the resulting inadequate arm rotation produces a pushing motion during the throw. The vertebral column also has to rotate in a wavelike fashion, with the thoracic vertebrae being the last to rotate.

The same sequence of motion applies to striking events, such as tennis and badminton stroking and softball batting. A common fault in learning how to serve a tennis ball or smash a birdie is insufficient trunk rotation. It is easier to hit an object without trunk rotation, but the impact of the racket on the projectile will not be as great. In batting, a common error is the lack of fluid timing between the different body segment movements. The hip, trunk, and arm movements follow one another so the bat is moving with great velocity on contact with the ball. Beginners often stop one motion before beginning the next.

21 In Review

Common mechanical errors in locomotion include running "stiff legged," "toeing out," swinging the arms across the trunk, overstriding, understriding, and lifting too high off the ground. The most common mechanical errors in throwing and striking are insufficient trunk rotation and poor timing among the trunk, hip, and arm movements.

Case Studies

You can check your answers by referring to appendix A.

27.1

You are supervising the resistance training area when you hear a lot of clanging noise coming from the seated leg press area. You discover that the exerciser at that machine is not controlling the descent of the weights. You suggest that he slowly return the weights rather than just letting them drop. He asks you for the reason for the suggestion—he doesn't see any benefit in a controlled return other than reduced noise. What do you tell him?

27.2

Alice wants to know why she can move a heavier weight when she does wrist curls with her palms up than with her palms down, and why she can do more pull-ups with her palms facing her than with her palms away. How would you explain both to her?

27.3

José complains that his lower back aches somewhat when he reaches overhead while standing in place during the cool-down portion of an aerobics class. What would you suggest he do during this movement to prevent the aching?

Source List

1. Gowitzke, B.A., & Milner, M. (1988). *Scientific bases of human movement* (3rd ed.). Baltimore: Williams & Wilkins.
2. Gray, H. (1994). *Anatomy of the human body*. Philadelphia: Lea & Febiger.
3. Hall, S.J. (1995). *Basic biomechanics* (2nd ed.). St. Louis: Mosby.
4. Hamill, J., & Knutzen, K. (1995). *Biomechanical basis of human movement*. Baltimore: Williams & Wilkins.
5. Hay, J.G., & Reid, J.G. (1988). *The anatomical and mechanical bases of human motion*. Englewood Cliffs, NJ: Prentice Hall.
6. Kreighbaum, E., & Barthels, K.M. (1996). *Biomechanics* (4th ed.). Minneapolis: Burgess.
7. Luttgens, K. Deutsch, H., & Hamilton, N. (1992). *Kinesiology* (8th ed.). Madison, WI: Brown & Benchmark.
8. Rasch, P.J. (1989). *Kinesiology and applied anatomy* (7th ed.). Philadelphia: Lea & Febiger.
9. Thompson, C.W. (1994). *Manual of structural kinesiology*. St. Louis: Mosby.

twenty-eight

Exercise Physiology

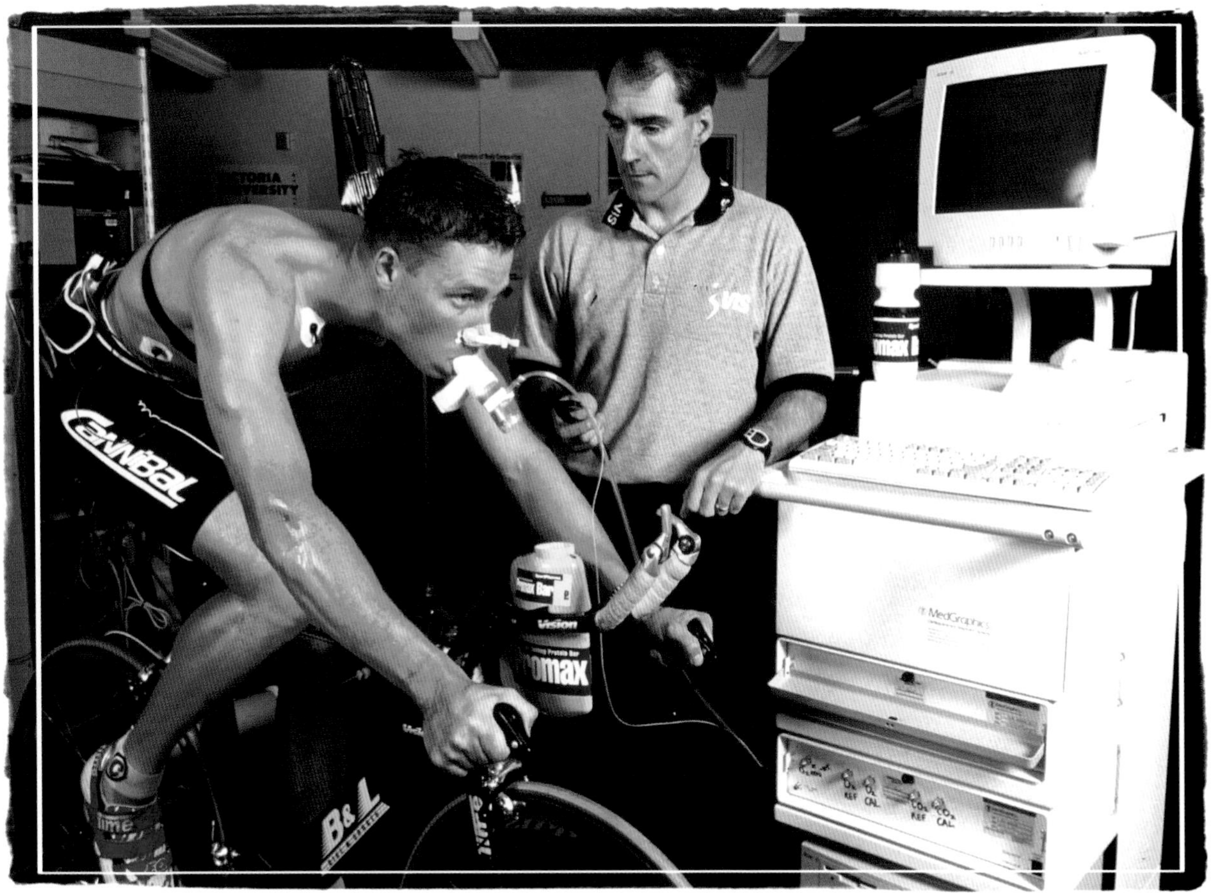

© Sport the Library/Tom Putt

Objectives

The reader will be able to do the following:

1. Indicate the methods by which muscle produces energy aerobically and anaerobically and evaluate the importance of each type of energy production in fitness and sport activities.
2. Describe the structure of skeletal muscle and the sliding-filament theory of muscle contraction.
3. Describe the power, speed, endurance, and metabolism of the different types of muscle fibers.
4. Describe tension development in terms of twitch, summation, and tetanus, and describe the role of recruitment of muscle fiber types in exercise of increasing intensities.
5. Describe the various fuels for muscle work and the effect of exercise intensity and duration on the respiratory exchange ratio.
6. Describe the means by which ATP is supplied to the muscle during the transition from rest to steady-state work and the effects of training on those responses.
7. Describe the effect of types of exercise tests, training, heredity, sex, age, altitude, carbon monoxide, and cardiovascular and pulmonary diseases on $\dot{V}O_2$max.
8. Describe how the ventilatory threshold and the lactate threshold indicate fitness as well as predict performance in endurance events.
9. Explain the changes in HR, stroke volume, cardiac output, and oxygen extraction during a GXT and the effect of training on those responses. Link the variation in $\dot{V}O_2$max in the population to differences in maximal cardiac output and oxygen extraction.
10. Describe the changes in SBP and the double product during a GXT and how they differ for arm and leg work.
11. Summarize the effects of endurance training on muscle, metabolic and cardiovascular responses to submaximal work, and $\dot{V}O_2$max. Describe the effect of reduced training or cessation of training on $\dot{V}O_2$max and the degree to which endurance training effects are specific to the muscles involved in the training.
12. Describe how men and women differ in their cardiovascular responses to graded exercise.
13. Contrast the cardiovascular responses measured during dynamic exercise with those measured during isometric exercise or heavy resistance training exercises.
14. Contrast the importance of the different mechanisms for heat loss during heavy exercise and during submaximal exercise in a hot environment. Describe the effect of training in a hot and humid environment on heat tolerance.

HFIs and PFTs need to know the basic aspects of exercise physiology to prescribe appropriate activities, deal with weight loss concerns, and explain to participants what happens as a result of training or when exercise is done in a hot and humid environment. This chapter can't possibly cover the extensive detail found in an exercise physiology text; instead we summarize major topics and, where possible, apply the discussion to exercise testing and exercise prescription. We refer the interested reader to the exercise physiology texts listed in the references (2, 8, 22, 41, 46, 49, 52, 64).

Relationship of Energy and Work

Energy is what makes a body go. Several kinds of energy exist in biological systems: electrical energy in nerves and muscles; chemical energy in the synthesis of molecules; mechanical energy in the contraction of a muscle to move an object; and thermal energy, derived from all of these processes, that helps to maintain body temperature. The ultimate source of the energy for biological systems is the sun. The radiant energy from the sun is captured by plants and used to convert simple atoms and molecules into carbohydrates, fats, and proteins. The sun's energy is trapped within the chemical bonds of these food molecules.

For the cells to use this energy, the foodstuffs must be broken down in a manner that conserves most of the energy contained in the bonds of the carbohydrates, fats, and proteins. In addition, the final product must be in a form that can be used by the cell—adenosine triphosphate, or ATP. Cells use ATP as the primary energy source for biological work, whether electrical, mechanical, or chemical. ATP is a molecule that has three phosphates linked together by high-energy bonds. When the bond between the phosphates is broken, energy is released and may be used by the cell. At this point the ATP has been reduced to a lower energy state: adenosine diphosphate (ADP) and inorganic phosphate (P_i).

When a muscle is doing work, ATP is constantly being broken down to ADP and P_i. The ATP must be replaced as fast as it is used if the muscle is to continue to generate force. The muscle cell has a great capacity to replace ATP under a wide variety of circumstances, from a short, quick dash to a marathon. Edington and Edgerton (18) devised a logical approach to the topic of supplying energy for muscle contraction. They divided the energy sources into immediate, short-term, and long-term sources of ATP (energy).

Immediate Sources of Energy

The very limited amount of ATP stored in a muscle might meet the energy demands of a maximal effort lasting about 1 s. **Creatine phosphate (CP)**, another high-energy phosphate molecule stored in the muscle, is the most important immediate source of energy. CP can donate its phosphate molecule (and the energy therein) to ADP to make ATP, allowing the muscle to continue to develop force.

$$\text{CP} + \text{ADP} \rightarrow \text{ATP} + \text{C}$$

This reaction takes place as fast as the muscle forms ADP. Unfortunately, the CP store in muscle lasts only 3 to 5 s when the muscle is working maximally. This process does not require oxygen and is one of the **anaerobic** (without oxygen) mechanisms for producing ATP. CP would be the primary source of ATP during a shot put, a vertical jump, or the first seconds of a sprint.

Short-Term Sources of Energy

As the muscle store of CP decreases, the muscle fibers break down glucose (a simple sugar) to produce ATP at a very high rate. The glucose is obtained from blood or the muscle glycogen store. The multienzyme pathway involved in glucose metabolism is called **glycolysis**, and it does not require oxygen to function (like the breakdown of CP, it too is an anaerobic process).

$$\text{Glucose} \rightarrow 2 \text{ pyruvic acid} + 2 \text{ ATP}$$

In glycolysis, glucose is broken down to two pyruvic acid molecules; in the process, ADP is converted to ATP and the muscle can maintain a high rate of work. But this can only continue for a limited period of time. When glycolysis is operating at a high speed, pyruvic acid is converted to lactic acid to keep the process going. This results in the accumulation of lactic acid (lactate) in the muscle and the blood. This accumulation of lactic acid in the muscle slows the rate at which glycogen can be broken down and actually may interfere with the mechanism involved in muscle contraction. Supplying ATP via glycolysis has its obvious shortcomings, but it does allow a person to run at high rates of speed for short distances. This short-term source of energy is of primary importance in events involving maximal work of about 2 min.

Long-Term Sources of Energy

The long-term source of energy involves the production of ATP from a variety of fuels, but this method requires the utilization of oxygen (it is **aerobic**). The primary fuels include muscle glycogen, blood glucose, plasma free fatty acids, and intramuscular fats. Glucose is broken down in glycolysis (as described previously), but in this case the pyruvic acid is taken into the **mitochondria** of the cell, where it is converted to a 2-carbon fragment (acetyl CoA) and enters the Krebs cycle. Fats are taken into the mitochondria where they are broken down to the same 2-carbon fragment, which enters the Krebs cycle. The energy originally contained in the glucose and fats is extracted from the acetyl CoA and is used to generate ATP in the electron transport chain in a process called oxidative phosphorylation, in which oxygen must be used.

$$\text{Carbohydrates and fat} + O_2 \rightarrow \text{ATP}$$

ATP production via aerobic mechanisms is slower than from the immediate and short-term sources of energy, and during submaximal work it may be 2 or 3 min before the ATP needs of the cell are met completely by this aerobic process. One reason for this lag is the time it takes for the heart to increase the delivery of oxygen-enriched blood to the muscles at the rate needed to meet the ATP demands of the muscle. The aerobic production of ATP is the primary means of supplying energy to the muscle in maximal work lasting more than 2 min and for all types of submaximal work.

Interaction of Exercise Intensity, Duration, and Energy Production

The proportion of energy coming from the anaerobic sources (immediate and short-term energy) is very much influenced by the intensity and duration of the activity. Figure 28.1 shows that during an all-out activity lasting less than 1 min (e.g., a 400-m dash), the muscles obtain most of the ATP from anaerobic sources. In a 2-min maximal effort, approximately 50% of the energy comes from anaerobic sources and 50% comes from aerobic sources; in a 10-min maximal effort, the anaerobic component drops to 15%. Thus, the anaerobic component is considerably less than 15% in a typical submaximal training session.

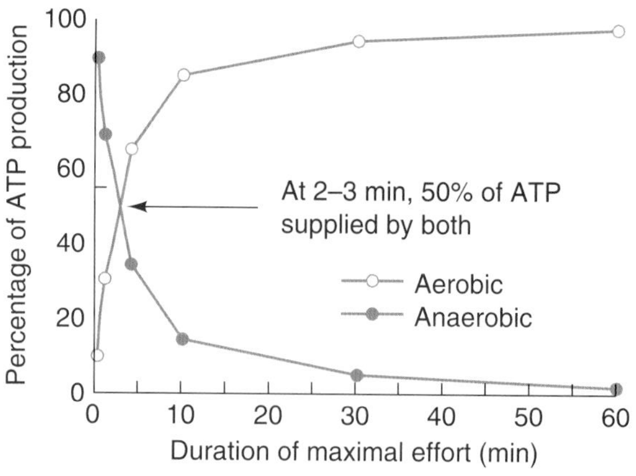

Figure 28.1 Percentage of contribution to total energy supply during maximal work of various durations (49). ATP = adenosine triphosphate.

1 In Review

ATP is supplied at a high rate by the anaerobic processes: creatine phosphate breakdown and glycolysis. Anaerobic energy production is important in short explosive events (e.g., shot put) and in athletic competitions requiring maximal effort for less than 2 min. ATP is supplied during prolonged exercise by the aerobic metabolism of carbohydrates and fats in the mitochondria of the muscle. This is the primary means of supplying energy to the muscle in maximal work lasting more than 2 min and in all submaximal work.

Understanding Muscle Structure and Function

Exercise means movement, and movement requires muscle action. To discuss human physiology related to exercise and endurance training, we must start with skeletal muscle, the tissue that converts the chemical energy of ATP to mechanical work. How does a muscle do this? We begin with a presentation of the structure of skeletal muscle.

Figure 28.2 shows the structure of skeletal muscle, from the intact muscle to the smallest functional unit. A **muscle fiber** is a cylindrical cell that has repeating light and dark bands, giving it the name *striated muscle*. The striations are attributable to a more basic structural component called the **myofibril**, which runs the length of the muscle. Each

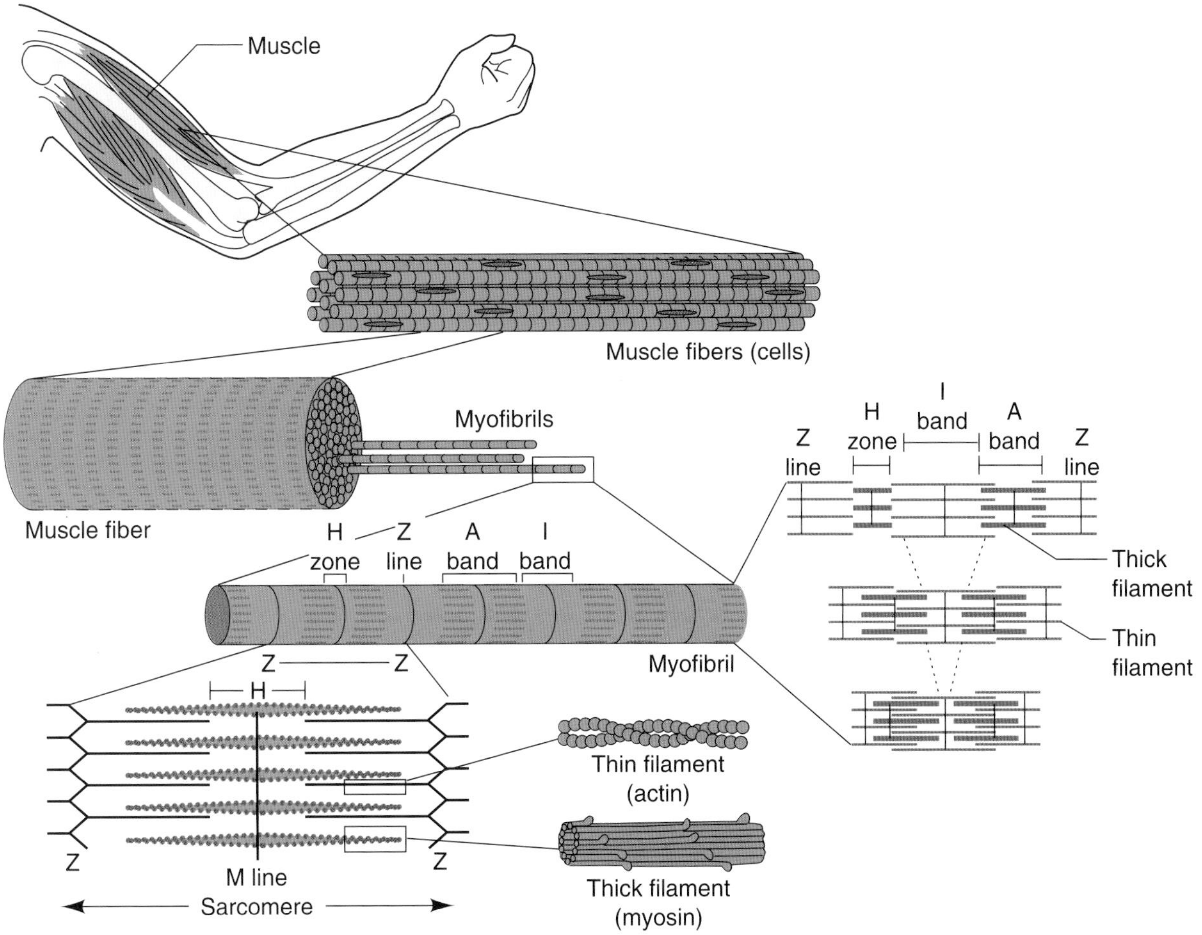

Figure 28.2 Levels of fibrillar organization within a skeletal muscle, and changes in filament alignment and banding pattern in a myofibril during shortening.

Reprinted, by permission of McGraw-Hill, from Vander, Sherman, and Luciano, 1980, *Human physiology* (3rd ed.).

myofibril is composed of a long series of **sarcomeres**, the fundamental unit of muscle contraction. Figure 28.2 shows that the sarcomere is composed of the thick filament **myosin** and the thin filament **actin** and is bounded by connective tissue called the **Z line** (63).

An enlargement of two sarcomeres in Figure 28.2 shows the **A band**, **I band**, and **H zone** and the changes that take place when the sarcomere goes from the resting state to the contracted state. The I band is composed of actin and is bisected by the Z line, and the A band is composed of myosin and actin. According to the **sliding-filament theory** of muscle contraction, the thin actin filaments slide over the thick myosin filaments, pulling the Z lines toward the center of the sarcomere. In this way the entire muscle shortens, but the contractile proteins do not change size. How does the muscle release the energy in ATP to make this happen?

If ATP is the energy supply, then an ATPase (an enzyme) must exist in muscle to split ATP and release the potential energy contained within its structure. The ATPase is found in an extension of the thick myosin filament, the **cross-bridge**, which also possesses the ability to bind to actin. Figure 28.3 shows the interaction of ATP, the cross-bridge, and actin that leads to the shortening of the sarcomere (63).

Because all of the components needed for muscle contraction are present (ATP, actin, myosin), why aren't the cross-bridges always moving and the muscle always in the state of contraction? At rest, two proteins that are associated with actin block the interaction of myosin with actin: **troponin**, which has the capacity to bind calcium, and **tropomyosin**. Figure 28.4 shows that when a muscle is depolarized (excited) by a motor nerve, the action potential spreads over the surface of the muscle fiber and

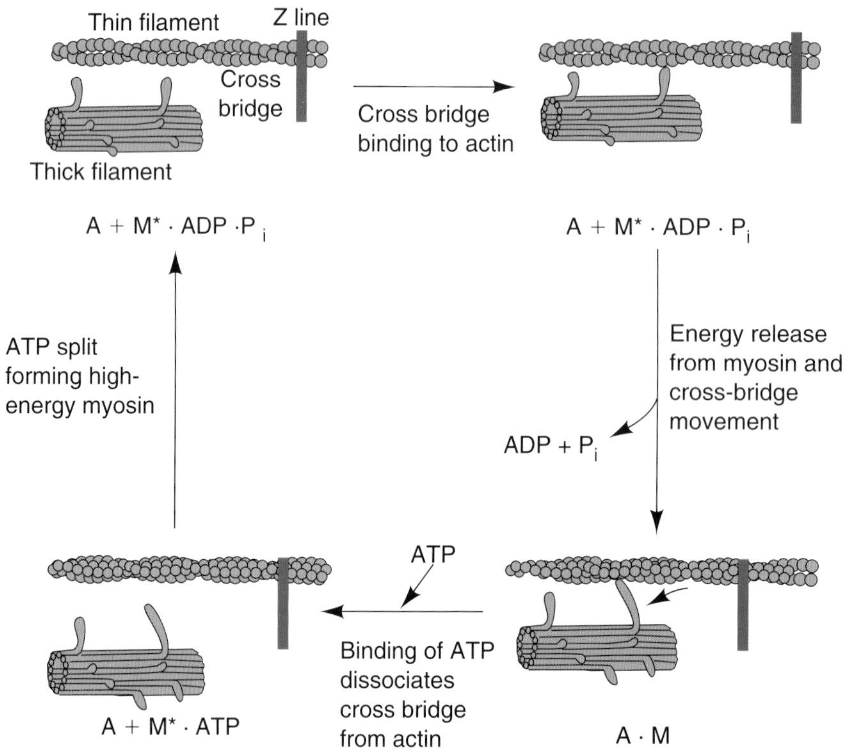

Figure 28.3 Chemical and mechanical changes during the four stages of a single cross-bridge cycle. Start reading the figure at the lower left. A = actin; M* = energized form of myosin; ATP = adenosine triphosphate; ADP = adenosine diphosphate; P_i = inorganic phosphate.

Reprinted, by permission of McGraw-Hill, from Vander, Sherman, and Luciano, 1985, *Human physiology* (4th ed.).

enters the fiber through special channels called **transverse tubules** (shown as item 1 in the figure). Once inside the muscle fiber, this wave of depolarization spreads over the **sarcoplasmic reticulum (SR)**, a membrane that surrounds the myofibril, and calcium is released from the SR into the sarcoplasm (item 2 in the figure). When the calcium binds with troponin, the tropomyosin aligns the binding site on actin so the myosin cross-bridge can interact with it (item 3 in the figure). The binding of the cross-bridge to actin results in the release of energy, the cross-bridge moves, and the sarcomere shortens (item 4 in figure). This sequence is repeated as long as there is calcium present and the muscle has ATP to replace what is used. Muscle relaxation is achieved when the calcium is pumped back into the sarcoplasmic reticulum and troponin and tropomyosin can again block the interaction of actin and myosin (items 5 and 6 in the figure) (63). The muscle needs ATP for cross-bridge movement, to pump the calcium back to the SR, and to maintain the resting membrane potential that allows the muscle to be depolarized.

2 In Review

Muscle contraction occurs when ATP is split to form a high-energy myosin-ATP cross-bridge; the myosin-ATP cross-bridge binds to actin and energy is released; the cross-bridge moves and pulls actin toward the center of the sarcomere; finally, ATP binds to and releases the cross-bridge from actin to start the process over again. Calcium release from the sarcoplasmic reticulum blocks inhibitory proteins (troponin and tropomyosin) and allows the cross-bridge to bind to actin to initiate movement of the cross-bridge. Relaxation occurs when calcium is pumped back into the sarcoplasmic reticulum and ATP binds to the cross-bridge.

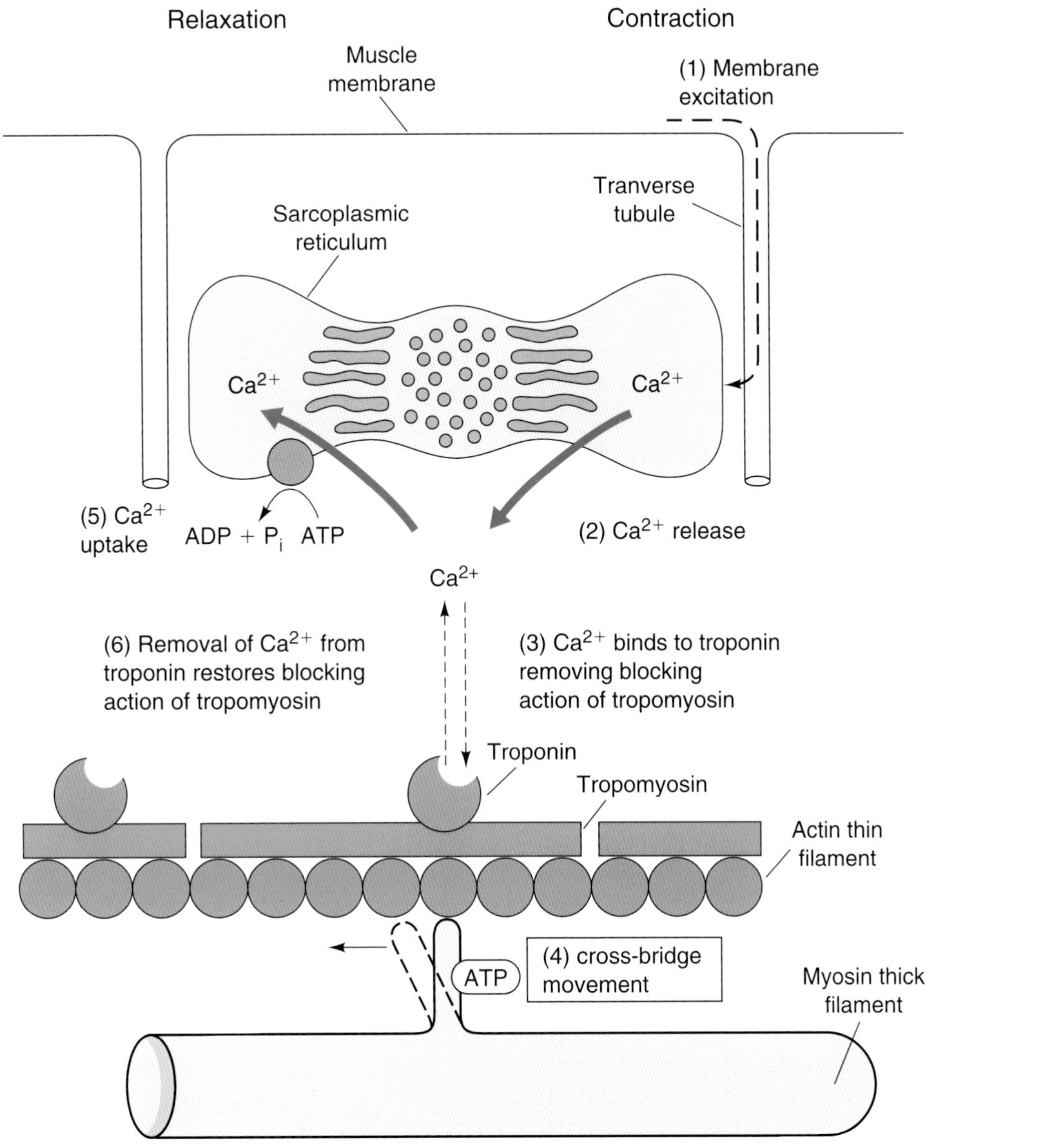

Figure 28.4 Role of calcium in muscle excitation-contraction coupling. ADP = adenosine diphosphate; P_i = inorganic phosphate; ATP = adenosine triphosphate.

Reprinted, by permission of McGraw-Hill, from Vander, Sherman, and Luciano, 1985, *Human physiology* (4th ed.).

Muscle Fiber Types and Performance

Muscle fibers vary in their abilities to produce ATP by the different aerobic and anaerobic mechanisms described earlier in the chapter. Some muscle fibers contract quickly and have an innate capacity to produce great amounts of force, but they fatigue quickly. These muscle fibers produce most of their ATP by creatine phosphate breakdown and glycolysis, and they are termed **fast glycolytic**, or **type IIb**, fibers. Other muscle fibers contract slowly and produce only small amounts of force, but they have great resistance to fatigue. These fibers produce most of their ATP aerobically in the mitochondria and are called **slow oxidative**, or **type I**, fibers. They have many mitochondria and a relatively large number of capillaries helping to deliver oxygen to the mitochondria. Last, there is a fiber with a combination of type I and type IIb characteristics. It is a fast-contracting muscle fiber that not only produces a great force when stimulated but also is resistant to fatigue because of its large number of mitochondria and capillaries. These fibers are called **fast oxidative glycolytic**, or **type IIa**, fibers.

3 In Review

Muscle fibers differ in speed of contraction, force, and resistance to fatigue. Type I fibers are slow, have low force, and are fatigue resistant. Type IIa fibers are fast, have high force, and are fatigue resistant. Type IIb fibers are fast twitch, have high force, and have a low resistance to fatigue.

Muscle Fiber Types: Genetics, Sex, and Training

In the average male and female, about 52% of the muscle fibers are type I, with the fast-twitch fibers divided into approximately 33% type IIa and approximately 13% type IIb (57, 58). There is great variation, however, in the distribution of fiber types in the overall population. On the basis of studies comparing identical to fraternal twins, the distribution of fast and slow fibers seems to be genetically fixed. In addition, fast-twitch fibers cannot be converted to slow-twitch fibers, and vice versa, with endurance training programs (3). In contrast, the capacity of the muscle fiber to produce ATP aerobically (its oxidative capacity) seems to be easily altered by endurance training. In fact, in some elite endurance athletes type IIb fibers can't be found; they have been converted to the oxidative version, type IIa (57). The increase in mitochondria and capillaries in endurance-trained muscles allows an individual to meet ATP demands via the aerobic processes, with less glycogen depletion and lactate formation (30).

Tension (Force) Development in the Muscle

The tension, or force, generated by a muscle depends on more than the fiber type. When a single threshold-level stimulus excites a muscle fiber, a single, low-tension twitch results, a brief contraction followed by relaxation. If the frequency of stimulation is increased, the muscle fiber can't relax between stimuli, and the tension of one contraction is added to the previous one. This is called **summation**. A further increase in the frequency of stimulation results in the contractions fusing together into a smooth, sustained, high-tension contraction called **tetanus**. The typical means by which muscle fibers develop tension is through tetanic contractions. The force of contraction is dependent on more than just the frequency of stimulation; it depends also on the degree to which the muscle fibers contract simultaneously (synchronous firing) and the number of muscle fibers recruited. This latter factor is the most important.

Figure 28.5 shows the order of recruitment of the different muscle fiber types as the intensity of exercise increases. The order is from the most to the least oxidative, from the slowest fiber to the fastest (type I → type IIa → type IIb) (55). Consequently, at higher work rates when the type IIb fibers are being recruited, there is a greater chance of producing lactic acid. Although chronic light exercise (less than 40% $\dot{V}O_2$max) recruits and causes a training effect in only the type I fibers, exercise beyond 70% $\dot{V}O_2$max involves all fiber types. This has important implications in the specificity of training and the potential for transferring training effects from one activity to another. Obviously, if you don't use a muscle fiber, it can't become "trained."

4 In Review

Muscle tension depends on the frequency of stimulation leading to a tetanus contraction, the synchronous firing of muscle fibers, and the recruitment of muscle fibers. The order of recruitment of muscle fibers is from the most to the least oxidative. Light-to-moderate exercise uses type I muscle fibers, whereas moderate-to-vigorous exercise requires the recruitment of type IIa fibers. Both favor the aerobic metabolism of carbohydrates and fats. Heavy exercise requires the involvement of type IIb fibers that favor anaerobic glycolysis, which increases the likelihood of lactate production.

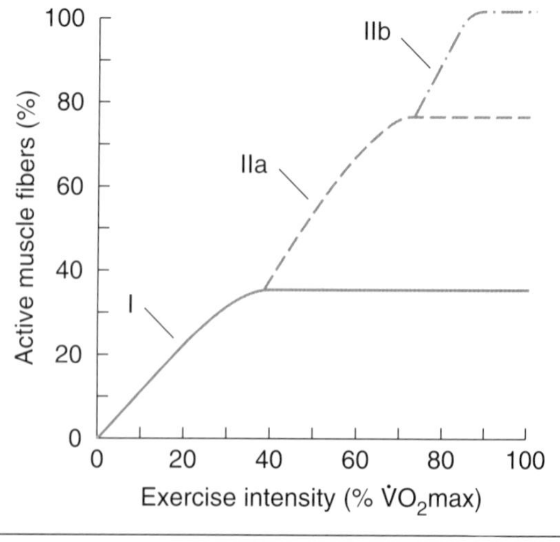

Figure 28.5 Order of muscle fiber type recruitment in exercise of increasing intensity.

From Sale, 1987, Influence of exercise and training on motor unit activation. In *Exercise and sport sciences reviews*, vol. 15, edited by Pandolf. Adapted by permission of Macmillan Publishing Company.

Metabolic, Cardiovascular, and Respiratory Responses to Exercise

A primary task of the HFI or PFT is to recommend physical activities that increase or maintain cardiorespiratory function. Activities that demand the production of energy (ATP) by aerobic mechanisms automatically cause the circulatory and respiratory systems to deliver oxygen to the muscle to meet the demand. The selected aerobic activities must be strenuous enough to challenge the cardiorespiratory systems to cause them to improve. This crucial link between aerobic activities and cardiorespiratory function provides the basis for much of exercise programming. The following sections summarize selected metabolic, cardiovascular, and respiratory responses to submaximal work and to a GXT taken to maximum. We begin with a discussion of how oxygen uptake is measured.

Measuring Oxygen Uptake

How does oxygen get to the mitochondria? Oxygen enters the lungs when a person inhales; it then diffuses from the alveoli of the lungs into the blood. Oxygen is bound to hemoglobin in the red blood cells, and the heart delivers the oxygen-enriched blood to the muscles. Oxygen then diffuses into the muscle cells to the mitochondria, where it is used (consumed) in the production of ATP. How is oxygen consumption measured during exercise?

Oxygen consumption ($\dot{V}O_2$) is measured by subtracting the volume of oxygen exhaled from the volume of oxygen inhaled.

$$\dot{V}O_2 = \text{volume } O_2 \text{ inhaled} - \text{volume } O_2 \text{ exhaled}$$

In the classic approach to measuring $\dot{V}O_2$, the subject breathes through a two-way valve that allows room air (containing 20.93% O_2 and 0.03% CO_2) to be inhaled into the lungs while directing exhaled air to a meteorological balloon, or Douglas bag (see figure 28.6). A volume meter measures the liters of air inhaled per minute, which is called the **pulmonary ventilation**. The exhaled air contained in the meteorological balloon is analyzed for its oxygen and carbon dioxide content, and the oxygen consumption (uptake) is calculated by simply multiplying the volume of air breathed by the percentage of oxygen extracted. Oxygen extraction is the percentage of oxygen extracted from the inhaled air, the difference between the 20.93% O_2 in room air and the percentage of O_2 in the meteorological balloon.

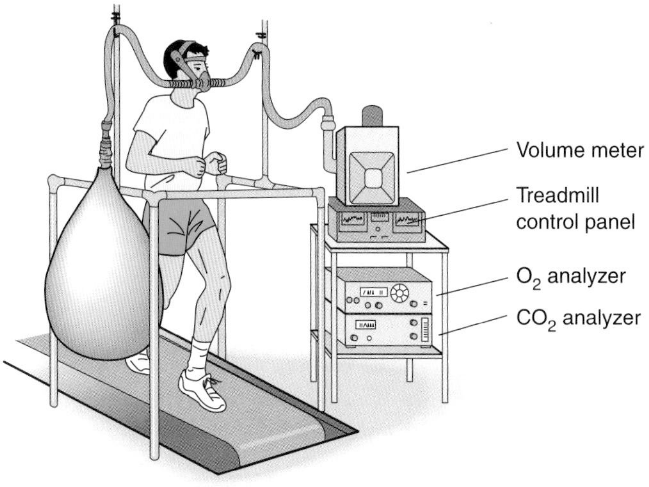

Figure 28.6 Conventional equipment involved in the measurement of oxygen uptake.

The following is a simplified presentation of the general steps used to calculate $\dot{V}O_2$; a more detailed presentation is found in Appendix B.

$$\dot{V}O_2 = \text{pulmonary ventilation } (L \cdot min^{-1}) \cdot O_2 \text{ extraction}$$

If ventilation = 60 $L \cdot min^{-1}$, and exhaled O_2 = 16.93%, then

$$\dot{V}O_2 = 60\ L \cdot min^{-1} \cdot (20.93\%\ O_2 - 16.93\%\ O_2)$$

$$\dot{V}O_2 = 60\ L \cdot min^{-1} \cdot 4.00\%\ O_2 = 2.4\ L \cdot min^{-1}$$

CO_2 is produced in the mitochondria and diffuses out of the muscle into the venous blood, where it is carried back to the lungs. There it diffuses into the alveoli and, in this example, is exhaled into the meteorological balloon. CO_2 production ($\dot{V}CO_2$) can be calculated as described for the $\dot{V}O_2$.

If ventilation = 60 $L \cdot min^{-1}$, and exhaled CO_2 = 3.03%, then

$$\dot{V}CO_2 = 60\ L \cdot min^{-1} \cdot (3.03\%\ CO_2 - 0.03\%\ CO_2)$$

$$\dot{V}CO_2 = 60\ L \cdot min^{-1} \cdot 3.00\%\ CO_2 = 1.8\ L \cdot min^{-1}$$

The ratio of CO_2 production ($\dot{V}CO_2$) to oxygen consumption ($\dot{V}O_2$) at the cell is called the **respiratory quotient (RQ)**. Because $\dot{V}CO_2$ and $\dot{V}O_2$ are measured at the mouth rather than at the tissue, this ratio is called the **respiratory exchange ratio (R)**. R is an important measure in that it can tell us what type of fuel is being used during exercise (see the next section).

$$R = \dot{V}CO_2 \div \dot{V}O_2$$

Using the values already calculated,

$$R = 1.8\ L \cdot min^{-1} \div 2.4\ L \cdot min^{-1} = 0.75$$

Fuel Utilization During Exercise

In general, protein contributes less than 5% to total energy production during exercise, and for the purpose of our discussion it will be ignored (49). This leaves carbohydrate (muscle glycogen and blood glucose, which is derived from liver glycogen) and fat (adipose tissue and intramuscular fat) as the primary fuels for exercise. The ability of the respiratory exchange ratio to provide good information about the metabolism of fats and carbohydrates during exercise is attributable to the following observations about the metabolism of fats and glucose.

When R = 1.0, 100% of the energy is derived from carbohydrates, 0% from fat; when R = 0.7, it is the reverse. When R = 0.85, approximately 50% of the energy is derived from carbohydrates and 50% from fat (see the box below). For the measurement to be correct, the subject must be in a steady state. If lactic acid is increasing in the blood, the plasma bicarbonate HCO_3^- buffer store will react with the acid (H^+) and produce CO_2, which is exhaled as we are stimulated to hyperventilate:

$$H^+ + HCO_3^- \rightarrow H_2CO_3 \rightarrow H_2O + CO_2$$

This CO_2 is not the result of the aerobic metabolism of carbohydrate and fat, and when the CO_2 is exhaled it will result in an overestimation of the true value of R. During strenuous work, lactic acid is produced in great amounts, and the R can exceed 1.0.

Effect of Exercise Intensity on Fuel Utilization

Figure 28.7 shows the changes in R during progressive work up to $\dot{V}O_2max$. In the progressive test, R increases at about 40 to 50% $\dot{V}O_2max$, indicating that type IIa fibers are being recruited and carbohydrates (CHO) are becoming a more important fuel source. This has an adaptive advantage—the muscle obtains about 6% more energy from each liter of O_2 when carbohydrates are used (5 kcal · L^{-1}) compared with when fat is used (4.7 kcal · L^{-1}).

The carbohydrate fuels for muscular exercise include muscle glycogen and blood glucose. Muscle glycogen is the primary carbohydrate fuel for heavy exercise lasting less than 2 hr, and inadequate muscle glycogen results in premature fatigue (11). As muscle glycogen is used during prolonged heavy exercise, blood glucose becomes more important in supplying the carbohydrate fuel. Towards the end of heavy

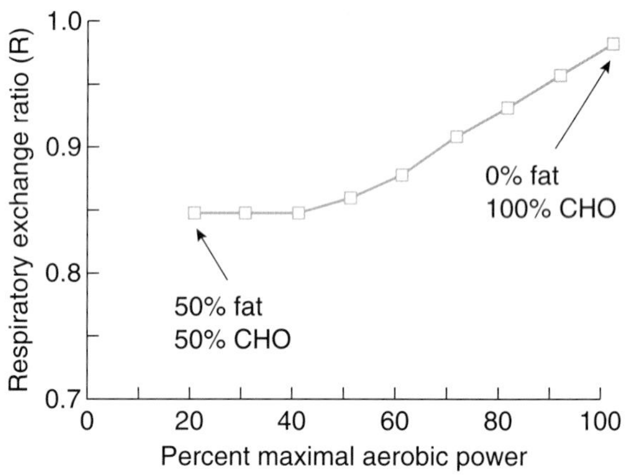

Figure 28.7 Changes in the respiratory exchange ratio with increasing exercise intensity (2).

Respiratory Quotients for Carbohydrate and Fat

For glucose

$$C_6H_{12}O_6 + 6\ O_2 \rightarrow 6\ CO_2 + 6\ H_2O + \text{energy}$$

$$R = \frac{6\ CO_2}{6\ O_2} = 1.0$$

For palmitate (a fatty acid)

$$C_{16}H_{32}O_2 + 23\ O_2 \rightarrow 16\ CO_2 + 16\ H_2O + \text{energy}$$

$$R = \frac{16\ CO_2}{23\ O_2} = 0.7$$

exercise lasting 3 hr or more, blood glucose provides almost all the carbohydrate used by the muscles. Therefore, heavy exercise is limited by the availability of carbohydrate fuels, which must be either stored in abundance prior to exercise (muscle glycogen) or replaced through ingestion of carbohydrates during exercise (blood glucose) (10).

Effect of Exercise Duration on Fuel Utilization

Figure 28.8 shows the change in R during a 90-min test at 60 to 70% of the subject's $\dot{V}O_2$max (50). R decreases over time, indicating a greater reliance on fat as a fuel. The fats are derived from both intramuscular fat stores and adipose tissue, which releases free fatty acids into the blood to be carried to the muscle. This increased use of fat spares the remaining carbohydrate stores and extends the time to exhaustion.

Effect of Diet and Training on Fuel Utilization

The type of fuel used during exercise depends on diet. It has been demonstrated clearly that a high-carbohydrate diet increases the muscle glycogen content and extends the time to exhaustion, compared with an average diet (33). Furthermore, the capacity of the muscle to increase its glycogen store is increased if a person performs strenuous exercise before eating the high-carbohydrate diet (33, 61). Finally, during prolonged heavy exercise, carbohydrate drinks help to maintain the blood glucose concentration and extend the time to fatigue (10).

Endurance training increases the number of mitochondria in the muscles involved in the training program. This increases the capacity of the muscle to use fat as a fuel and the ability to process the available carbohydrate aerobically. This spares the carbohydrate store and reduces lactate production, both of which favorably influence performance (30).

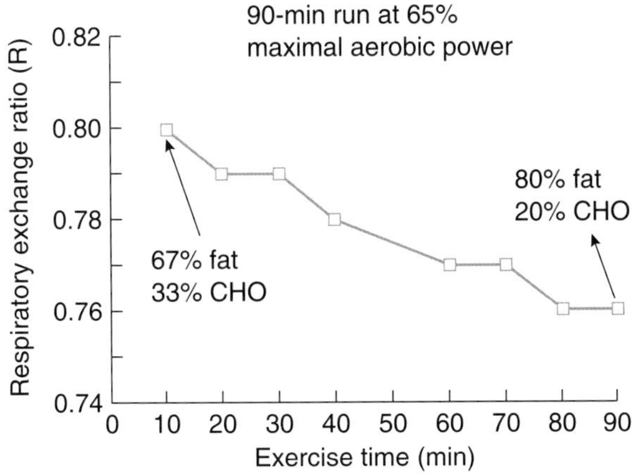

Figure 28.8 Changes in the respiratory exchange ratio during prolonged steady-state exercise (50). CHO = carbohydrate.

5 In Review

The respiratory exchange ratio (R) can be used as an index of fuel use during steady-state exercise. When R = 1.0, 100% of the energy is derived from carbohydrate; when R = 0.7, 100% of the energy is derived from fat. When lactic acid increases in the blood during heavy exercise, the acid is buffered by plasma bicarbonate. This causes CO_2 to be produced and invalidates the use of R as an indicator of fuel use during exercise. As exercise intensity increases, the R increases, indicating that carbohydrates become more important in generating ATP. During prolonged moderately strenuous exercise, the R decreases over time, indicating that fat is being used more and carbohydrates are being spared.

Transition From Rest to Steady-State Work

Some readers might mistakenly assume from the discussion of the immediate, short-, and long-term sources of energy that these various sources of ATP are used in distinct activities and do not work together to allow a person to make the transition from rest to exercise. When an individual steps onto a treadmill belt moving at a velocity of 200 m · min^{-1} (7.5 miles · hr^{-1}), the ATP requirement increases from the low level needed to stand alongside the treadmill to the new level of ATP required by the muscles to run at 200 m · min^{-1}. This change in the ATP supply to the muscle must take place in the first step onto the treadmill. If the person fails to do so, he or she will drift off the back of the treadmill. What energy sources supply ATP during the first minutes of work?

Oxygen Uptake

The cardiovascular and respiratory systems cannot instantaneously increase the delivery of oxygen to the muscles to completely meet the ATP demands by aerobic processes. In the interval between the time a person steps onto the treadmill and the time his or her cardiovascular and respiratory systems deliver the correct amount of oxygen, the immediate and short-term sources of energy supply the needed ATP. The volume of oxygen "missing" in the first few minutes of work is the **oxygen deficit** (figure 28.9). Creatine phosphate supplies some of the needed ATP, and the anaerobic breakdown of glycogen to lactic acid provides the rest until the oxidative mechanisms meet the ATP requirement. When the oxygen uptake levels off during submaximal work, the oxygen uptake value is said to represent the **steady-state oxygen requirement** for the activity. At this point, the ATP need of the cell is being met by the production of ATP with oxygen in the mitochondria of the muscle on a "pay as you go" basis.

When the individual stops running and steps off the treadmill, the ATP need of the muscles that were involved in the activity drops suddenly back toward the resting value. The oxygen uptake decreases quickly at first and then more gradually approaches the resting value. This elevated oxygen uptake in recovery from exercise is called the oxygen repayment, **oxygen debt**, or excess postexercise oxygen consumption (figure 28.9). In part, the elevated oxygen uptake is being used to make additional ATP to bring the CP store of the muscle back to normal (remember that it was depleted somewhat at the onset of work). Some of the "extra" oxygen taken in during recovery from exercise is used to pay the ATP requirement for the higher HR and breathing during recovery (compared with rest). A small part of the oxygen repayment is used by the liver to convert a portion of the lactic acid produced at the onset of work into glucose (49).

If an individual reaches the steady-state oxygen requirement earlier during the first minutes of work, she or he incurs a smaller oxygen deficit. This results in less CP depletion and the production of less lactic acid. Endurance training speeds up the kinetics of oxygen transport; that is, it decreases the time needed to reach a steady state of oxygen uptake. People in poor condition, as well as people with cardiovascular or pulmonary disease, take longer to reach the steady-state oxygen requirement. As a result, they incur a larger oxygen deficit and must produce more ATP by the immediate and short-term sources of energy at the onset of work or during the transition from one intensity to the next in a GXT (26, 47).

Heart Rate and Pulmonary Ventilation

The link between the cardiorespiratory responses to work and the time it takes to reach the steady-state oxygen requirement should be no surprise. Figure 28.10 shows the typical HR and pulmonary ventilation responses to a submaximal run test. The shape of the curve in each case resembles the curve for oxygen uptake described earlier.

In addition, the muscle has something to do with the lag in the oxygen-uptake response at the onset of work. An untrained muscle has relatively few mitochondria available to produce ATP aerobically and also has relatively few capillaries per muscle fiber to bring the oxygen-enriched arterial blood to those mitochondria. Following an endurance training program, both of these factors increase, so the muscle can produce more ATP aerobically at the onset of work. The result is a reduction in lactic acid production at the onset of work and a lowering of the blood lactic acid concentration for a fixed submaximal work rate following an endurance training program (26, 30, 47).

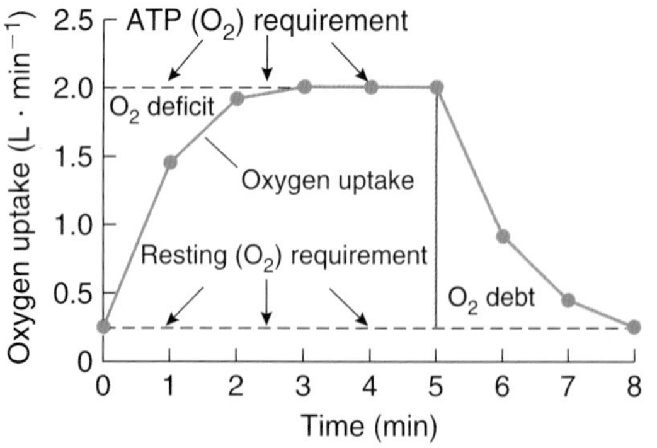

Figure 28.9 Oxygen deficit and oxygen debt (repayment) during a 5-min run on a treadmill. ATP = adenosine triphosphate.

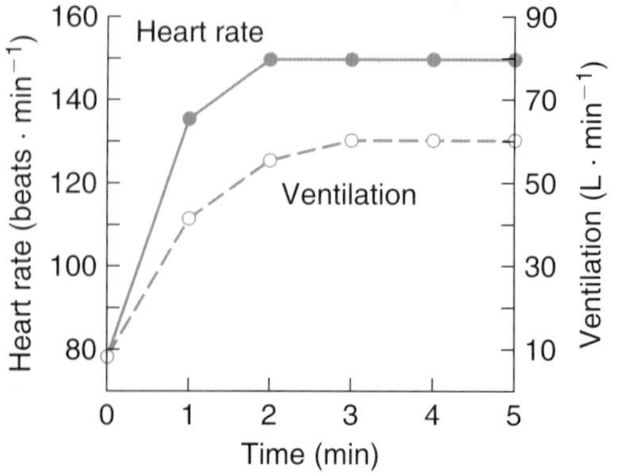

Figure 28.10 Heart-rate and pulmonary ventilation responses during a 5-min run on a treadmill.

6 In Review

At the onset of submaximal exercise, the $\dot{V}O_2$ does not increase immediately (oxygen deficit), and some of the ATP must be supplied anaerobically by CP and glycolysis. At the end of exercise, the $\dot{V}O_2$ remains elevated for some time to (a) replenish CP stores, (b) support the energy cost of the elevated HR and breathing, and (c) synthesize glucose from lactic acid. With training, the oxygen deficit is reduced because of a more rapid increase in $\dot{V}O_2$ at the onset of work, allowing the steady-state oxygen requirement to be reached more quickly.

Graded Exercise Test

A clear link exists between oxygen consumption and cardiorespiratory fitness, because oxygen delivery to tissue is dependent on lung and heart function. One of the most common tests used to evaluate cardiorespiratory function is a GXT, in which the individual exercises at progressively increasing work rates until maximum work tolerance is reached. During the test the individual may be monitored for cardiovascular variables (ECG, HR, BP), respiratory variables (pulmonary ventilation, respiratory frequency), and metabolic variables (oxygen uptake, blood lactic acid level). The manner in which an individual responds to the GXT gives important information about cardiorespiratory function and the capacity for prolonged work.

Oxygen Uptake and Maximal Aerobic Power

Oxygen uptake, measured as described earlier, is expressed per kilogram of body weight to facilitate comparisons between people and for the same person over time. The $\dot{V}O_2$ value in liters per minute is simply multiplied by 1000 to convert the $\dot{V}O_2$ to ml $\cdot$ min^{-1}; that value is divided by the subject's body weight in kilograms to yield a value expressed in milliliters per kilogram per minute.

$$\dot{V}O_2 = 2.4\ L \cdot min^{-1} \cdot 1000\ ml \cdot L^{-1}$$
$$\dot{V}O_2 = 2400\ ml \cdot min^{-1}$$

For a 60-kg subject,

$$\dot{V}O_2 = 2400\ ml \cdot min^{-1} \div 60\ kg = 40\ ml \cdot kg^{-1} \cdot min^{-1}$$

Figure 28.11 shows a GXT conducted on a treadmill in which the speed is constant (3 miles $\cdot$ hr^{-1}) and the grade changes 3% every 3 min. With each stage of a GXT, the oxygen uptake increases to meet the ATP demand of the work rate. Also, the individual incurs a small oxygen deficit at each stage as the cardiovascular system tries to adjust to the new demand placed on it by the increased work rate.

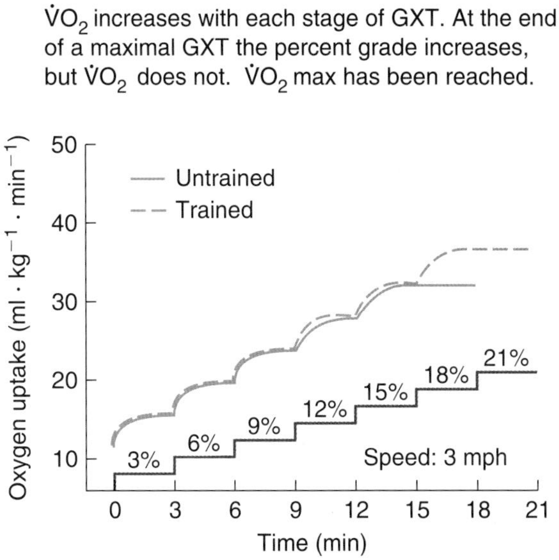

Figure 28.11 Oxygen uptake responses to a graded exercise test (GXT) (38).

It has been shown that apparently healthy individuals reach the steady-state oxygen requirement by 1.5 min or so of each stage of the test up to moderately heavy work (44, 45). People who have low cardiorespiratory fitness or cardiovascular and pulmonary diseases may not be able to reach the expected values in the same amount of time and might incur larger oxygen deficits with each stage of the test. The oxygen uptake measured at various stages of the test on these latter individuals is lower than expected because they could not reach the expected steady-state demands of the test at each stage.

Toward the end of a GXT, a point is reached at which the work rate changes (i.e., the grade on the treadmill is increased) but the oxygen uptake does not. In effect, the limits of the cardiovascular system to transport oxygen to the muscle have been reached. This point is called **maximal aerobic power**, or **maximal oxygen uptake ($\dot{V}O_2$max).** A complete leveling off in the oxygen consumption is not seen in all cases because it requires the individual to work one stage past the actual point at which $\dot{V}O_2$max is reached. This requires the subject to be highly motivated. In some GXT protocols, the "plateau" in oxygen uptake is judged against the criterion of less than 2.1 ml · kg^{-1} · min^{-1} increase in $\dot{V}O_2$ from one stage to the next (62). Other criteria for having achieved $\dot{V}O_2$max include an R greater than 1.15 (34) and a blood lactate concentration greater than 8 mmol · L^{-1}, about 8 times the resting value (1). These and other criteria have been used alone and in combination to increase the likelihood that the individual has really achieved $\dot{V}O_2$max (32). Participation in a 10- to 20-week endurance training program increases $\dot{V}O_2$max. If this trained person were to retake the GXT, he or she would reach the steady state sooner at light to moderate work rates and then would go one or more stages further into the test, at which time the greater $\dot{V}O_2$max is measured.

Maximal aerobic power is the greatest rate at which the body (primarily muscle) can produce ATP aerobically. It is also the upper limit at which the cardiovascular system can deliver oxygen-enriched blood to the muscles. Thus, maximal aerobic power is not only a good index of cardiorespiratory fitness; it is also a good predictor of performance capability in aerobic events such as distance running, cycling, cross-country skiing, and swimming (4, 5). In the apparently healthy person, maximal aerobic power is usually understood as the quantitative limit at which the cardiovascular system can deliver oxygen to tissues. This usual interpretation must be tempered by the mode of exercise (test type) used to impose the work rate on the individual subject.

Test Type

For the average person, the highest value for maximal aerobic power is measured when the subject completes a GXT involving uphill running. A GXT conducted at a walking speed usually results in a $\dot{V}O_2$max value 4 to 6% below the graded running value, and a test on a cycle ergometer may yield a value 10 to 12% lower than the graded running value (20, 42, 43). Last, if a subject works to exhaustion using an arm ergometer, then the highest oxygen uptake value is less than 70% of that measured with the legs (23). Knowledge of these variations in maximal aerobic power is helpful in making recommendations about the intensity of different exercises needed to achieve THR. At any given submaximal work rate, most physiological responses (HR, BP, and blood lactic acid) are higher for arm work than for leg work (23, 60). Maximal aerobic power is influenced by more than the type of test used in its measurement. Other factors include endurance training, heredity, sex, age, altitude, pollution, and cardiovascular and pulmonary disease.

Training and Heredity

Typically, endurance training programs increase $\dot{V}O_2$max by 5 to 25%, with the magnitude of the change depending primarily on the initial level of fitness. A person with a low $\dot{V}O_2$max makes the largest percentage change as a result of a training program. Eventually, a point is reached where further training does not increase $\dot{V}O_2$max. It has been demonstrated that approximately 40% of the extremely high values of maximal aerobic power found in elite cross-country skiers and distance runners are related to a genetic predisposition for having a superior cardiovascular system (6). Because typical endurance training programs may increase $\dot{V}O_2$max by only 20% or so, it is unrealistic to expect a person with a $\dot{V}O_2$max of 40 ml · kg^{-1} · min^{-1} to increase the value to 80 ml · kg^{-1} · min^{-1}, a value measured in some elite cross-country skiers and distance runners (56). On the other hand, those who do severe interval training can achieve gains of 44% in $\dot{V}O_2$max (25).

Sex and Age

Women have $\dot{V}O_2$max values about 15% lower than men's; that difference exists across ages 20 to 60 years. The primary reasons for the sex difference relate to differences in percentage of body fat and hemoglobin levels (see later discussion). The 15% difference between men and women is an average difference, and a considerable overlap in $\dot{V}O_2$max values exists in these populations (2). The aging effect indicates a gradual but systematic 1%-per-year reduction in $\dot{V}O_2$max in most people. The $\dot{V}O_2$max of a given individual is influenced by the level of physical activity and percentage of body fat. Those who remain active and maintain body weight (which is not the usual case) have higher $\dot{V}O_2$max values across the age span. In fact, the impact of an endurance-training program implemented in middle-aged individuals gives the appearance of reversing the aging effect because $\dot{V}O_2$max is elevated to a new level consistent with a younger, sedentary individual (35-37).

Altitude and Pollution

$\dot{V}O_2$max decreases with increasing altitude. At 7400 ft (2300 m), $\dot{V}O_2$max is only 88% of the sea-level value. This decrease in $\dot{V}O_2$max is attributable primarily to the reduction in arterial oxygen content that occurs as the oxygen pressure decreases with increasing altitude. With the lower arterial oxygen content at high altitudes, the heart must pump more blood per minute to meet the oxygen needs of any task. As a result, the HR response is higher at submaximal intensities when performed at higher altitudes (31).

Carbon monoxide, produced from the burning of fossil fuel as well as from cigarette smoke, binds readily to hemoglobin and can decrease oxygen transport to muscles. The critical concentration of carbon monoxide in blood needed to decrease $\dot{V}O_2max$ is about 4%. After that, there is approximately a 1% decrease in $\dot{V}O_2max$ for every 1% increase in the carbon monoxide concentration in the blood (51).

Cardiovascular and Pulmonary Diseases

Cardiovascular and pulmonary diseases decrease $\dot{V}O_2max$ by diminishing the delivery of oxygen from the air to the blood and reducing the capacity of the heart to deliver blood to the muscles. Patients with cardiovascular disease have some of the lowest $\dot{V}O_2max$ (functional capacity) values, but they also experience the largest percentage changes in $\dot{V}O_2max$ in endurance training programs. Table 28.1 shows common values for $\dot{V}O_2max$ in a variety of populations (2, 22, 64).

Table 28.1 Maximal Aerobic Power Measured in Healthy and Diseased Populations

Population	$\dot{V}O_2max$ (ml · kg^{-1} · min^{-1}) Men	Women
Cross-country skiing	82	68
Distance runners	79	68
College students	45	38
Middle-aged adults	35	30
Postmyocardial infarction patients	22	18
Severe pulmonary diseased patients	13	13

Data compiled from Åstrand and Rodahl, 1986; Fox, Bowers, and Foss, 1993; Wilmore and Costill, 1999; the Fort Sanders Cardiac Rehabilitation Program; and J.T. Daniels (personal communication).

7 In Review

Maximal oxygen uptake, $\dot{V}O_2max$, is the greatest rate at which O_2 can be delivered to working muscles during dynamic exercise. $\dot{V}O_2max$ is influenced by heredity and training, decreases about 1% per year as we age, and is about 15% lower in women compared with men of the same age. $\dot{V}O_2max$ is lower at high altitude, and carbon monoxide decreases $\dot{V}O_2max$ because of its ability to bind to hemoglobin and limit oxygen transport. Cardiovascular and pulmonary diseases negatively affect $\dot{V}O_2max$; however, large improvements can be attained through endurance training for individuals with cardiovascular disease.

Blood Lactic Acid and Pulmonary Ventilation

Lactic acid produced by a muscle is released into the blood. Figure 28.12 shows that during a GXT, blood lactate concentration changes little or not at all at the lower work rates; the lactate is metabolized as fast as it is produced (7). As the GXT increases in intensity, a point is reached at which the blood lactate concentration suddenly increases. The work rate at which the lactate concentration suddenly increases is called the **lactate threshold**. It is also called the anaerobic threshold, but because several conditions other than an oxygen lack (hypoxia) at the muscle cell can result in lactate production and release into the blood, lactate threshold is the preferred term. An endurance training program increases the number of mitochondria in the trained muscles, facilitating the aerobic metabolism of carbohydrates and the use of more fat as fuel. As a result, when the subject takes the GXT again, less lactate is produced and the lactate threshold occurs at a later stage of the test. The lactate threshold is a good indicator of endurance performance and has been used to predict performance in endurance races (4, 5).

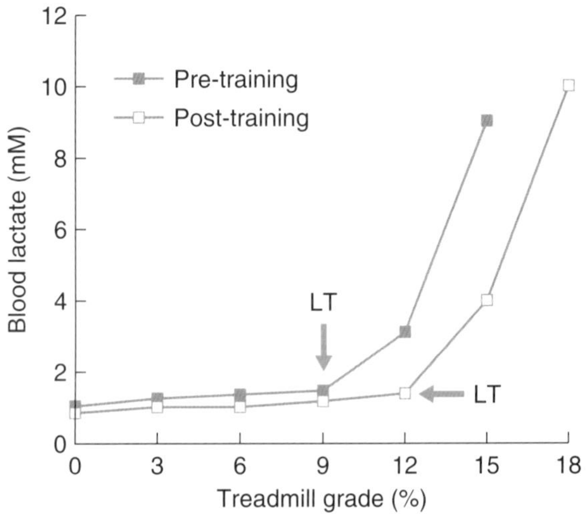

Figure 28.12 Training causes the lactate threshold (LT) to occur at a higher exercise intensity (19).

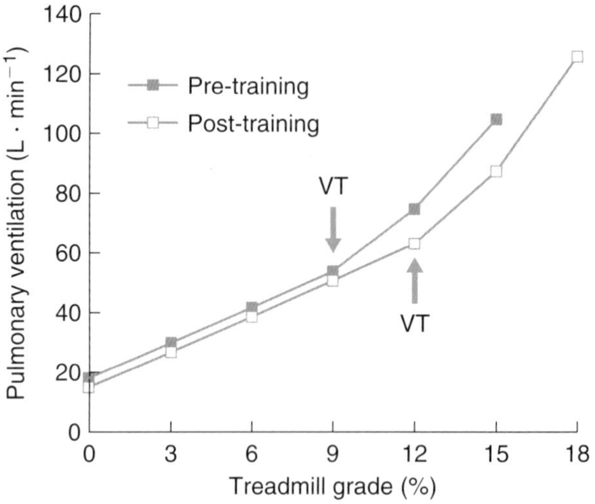

Figure 28.13 The ventilatory threshold (VT) occurs later in the GXT following training.

Pulmonary ventilation is the volume of air inhaled or exhaled per minute and is calculated by multiplying the frequency (f) of breathing by the tidal volume (TV), the volume of air moved in one breath. For example,

$$\text{Ventilation } (L \cdot min^{-1}) = TV\ (L \cdot breath^{-1}) \cdot f\ (breaths \cdot min^{-1})$$

$$30\ (L \cdot min^{-1}) = 1.5\ L \cdot breath^{-1} \cdot 20\ breaths \cdot min^{-1}$$

Pulmonary ventilation increases linearly with work rate until 50 to 80% of $\dot{V}O_2$max, at which point a relative **hyperventilation** results (see figure 28.13). The inflection point in the pulmonary ventilation response is called the **ventilatory threshold.** The ventilatory threshold has been used as a noninvasive indicator of the lactate threshold and as a predictor of performance (17, 48). The increase in pulmonary ventilation is mediated by changes in the frequency of breathing (from about 10-12 breaths $\cdot$ min^{-1} at rest to 40-50 breaths $\cdot$ min^{-1} during maximal work) and the tidal volume (from 0.5 L $\cdot$ breath^{-1} at rest to 2-3 L $\cdot$ breath^{-1} in maximal work). Endurance training programs result in a lower pulmonary ventilation during submaximal work; the ventilatory threshold occurs later into the GXT. The maximal value for pulmonary ventilation tends to change in the direction of $\dot{V}O_2$max.

8 In Review

The points at which the blood lactic acid concentration and the pulmonary ventilation increase suddenly during a GXT are called the lactate and ventilatory thresholds, respectively. The lactate and ventilatory thresholds are good predictors of performance in endurance events (e.g., 10K runs, marathons).

Heart Rate

Once the HR reaches about 110 beats $\cdot$ min^{-1}, it increases linearly with work rate during a GXT until near-maximal efforts. Figure 28.14 shows the influence of a training program on the subject's HR response at the same work rates. The lower HR at submaximal work rates is a beneficial effect because it decreases the oxygen needed by the heart muscle. Maximal HR shows no change or is slightly reduced as a result of an endurance training program.

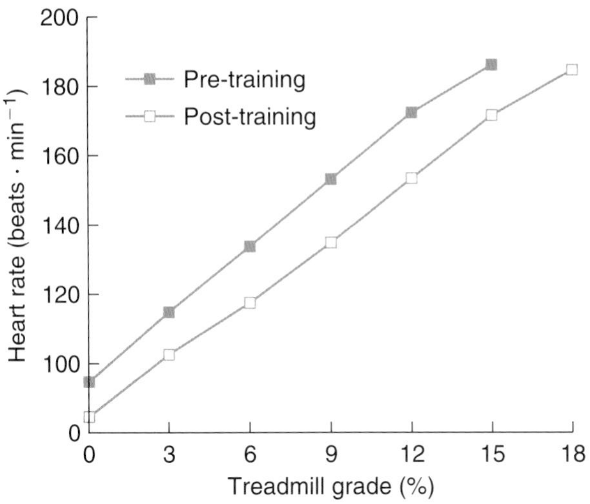

Figure 28.14 Training causes a reduction in the heart rate response to submaximal exercise (19).

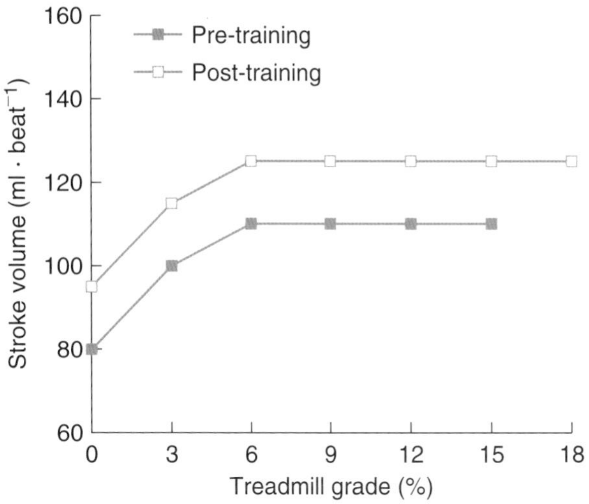

Figure 28.15 Stroke volume increases with training due to increases in the volume of the ventricle (19).

Stroke Volume

The volume of blood pumped by the heart per beat (ml · beat^{-1}) is called the stroke volume (SV). For individuals doing work in the upright position (cycling, walking), SV increases in the early stages of the GXT until about 40% $\dot{V}O_2$max is reached and then levels off (see figure 28.15) (2). Consequently, HR is the sole factor responsible for the increased flow of blood from the heart to the working muscles for work rates greater than 40% $\dot{V}O_2$max. This is what makes the HR a good indicator of the metabolic rate during exercise; it is linearly related to exercise intensity from light to heavy exercise. One of the primary effects of an endurance training program is an increase in SV at rest and during work; this is caused, in part, by an increase in the volume of the ventricle (19). This increases the **end-diastolic volume**, the volume of blood in the heart just before contraction. So even if the same fraction of blood in the ventricle is pumped per beat (**ejection fraction**) following endurance training, the heart pumps more blood per minute at the same HR.

Cardiac Output

Cardiac output is the volume of blood pumped by the heart per minute and is calculated by multiplying the HR (beats · min^{-1}) by the SV (ml · beat^{-1}).

Cardiac output (Q) = HR · SV
= 60 beats · min^{-1} · 80 ml · beat^{-1}
= 4800 ml · min^{-1} or 4.8 L · min^{-1}

Cardiac output increases linearly with work rate. Generally, the cardiac output response to light and moderate work is not affected by an endurance training program. What is changed is the manner in which the cardiac output is achieved, with a lower HR and a higher SV.

The maximal cardiac output (highest value reached in a GXT) is the most important cardiovascular variable determining maximal aerobic power because the oxygen-enriched blood (carrying about 0.2 L of O_2 per liter of blood) must be delivered to the muscle for the mitochondria to use. If a person's maximal cardiac output is 10 L · min^{-1}, only 2 L of O_2 would leave the heart for the tissues per minute (i.e., 0.2 L of O_2 per liter of blood times a cardiac output of 10 L · min^{-1} = 2 L of O_2 · min^{-1}). A person with a maximal cardiac output of 30 L · min^{-1} would deliver 6 L of O_2 per minute to the tissues. One of the effects of an endurance training program is to increase the maximal cardiac output and thus the delivery of oxygen to the muscles (see figure 28.16). This increase in maximal cardiac output is matched by an increase in the capillary number in the muscle to allow the blood to move slowly enough through the muscle to maintain the time needed for oxygen to diffuse from the blood to the mitochondria (57). The increase in maximal cardiac output accounts for 50% of the increase in maximal oxygen uptake that occurs in previously sedentary individuals who engage in endurance training (54).

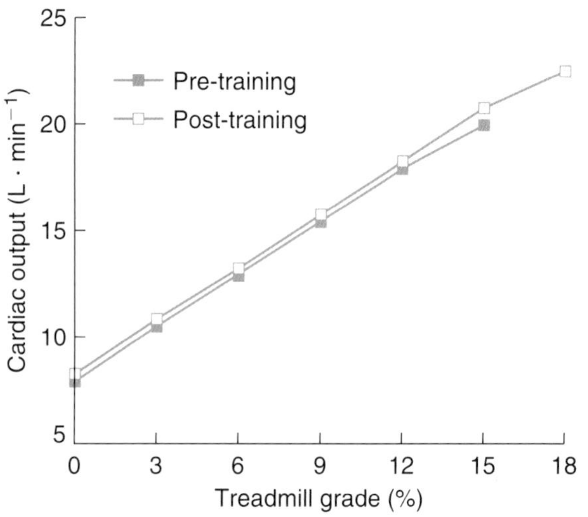

Figure 28.16 Maximal cardiac output is increased following training (19).

In the normal population, SV is the major variable influencing maximal cardiac output. Differences in maximal cardiac output and maximal aerobic power that exist between females and males, between trained and untrained individuals, and between the world-class endurance athlete and the average person can be explained to a large degree on the basis of differences in maximal stroke volume. This is shown in table 28.2, where $\dot{V}O_2$max varies by a factor of 3 among three distinct groups, whereas maximal HR is almost the same for all three groups. Clearly, maximal SV is the primary factor related to the differences that exist among individuals in $\dot{V}O_2$max.

Oxygen Extraction

Two factors determine the oxygen uptake at any time: the volume of blood delivered to the tissues per minute (cardiac output) and the volume of oxygen extracted from each liter of blood. Oxygen extraction is calculated by subtracting the oxygen content of mixed venous blood (as it returns to the heart) from the oxygen content of the arterial blood. This is called the arteriovenous oxygen difference, or the (a-$\bar{v}$)O_2 difference.

$$\dot{V}O_2 = \text{cardiac output} \cdot (\text{a-}\bar{v})O_2 \text{ difference}$$

$$\text{At rest, cardiac output} = 5 \text{ L} \cdot \text{min}^{-1}$$

$$\text{arterial oxygen content} = 200 \text{ ml of } O_2$$

$$\text{per liter of blood (ml} \cdot \text{L}^{-1})$$

$$\text{mixed venous oxygen content} = 150 \text{ ml of } O_2 \cdot \text{L}^{-1}$$

$$\dot{V}O_2 = 5 \text{ L} \cdot \text{min}^{-1} \cdot (200 - 150 \text{ ml of } O_2 \cdot \text{L}^{-1})$$
$$\dot{V}O_2 = 5 \text{ L} \cdot \text{min}^{-1} \cdot 50 \text{ ml of } O_2 \cdot \text{L}^{-1}$$
$$\dot{V}O_2 = 250 \text{ ml} \cdot \text{min}^{-1}$$

The (a-$\bar{v}$)O_2 difference is a measure of the ability of the muscle to extract oxygen, and it increases with exercise intensity. The ability of a tissue to extract oxygen is a function of the capillary-to-muscle-fiber ratio and the number of mitochondria in the muscle fiber. Endurance training programs increase all of these factors (see figure 28.17), thus increasing the maximal capacity to extract oxygen in the last stage of the GXT (57). This increase in the (a-$\bar{v}$)O_2 difference accounts for about 50% of the increase in $\dot{V}O_2$max that occurs with endurance training programs in previously sedentary individuals (54).

Table 28.2 Maximal Values of $\dot{V}O_2$max, Heart Rate, Stroke Volume, and Arteriovenous (a-$\bar{v}$) Oxygen Difference in Three Groups With Very Low, Normal, and High Maximal $\dot{V}O_2$max

Group	$\dot{V}O_2$max (L · min⁻¹)	=	Heart rate (beats · min⁻¹)	×	Stroke volume (ml · beat⁻¹)	×	(a-$\bar{v}$) Oxygen difference (ml · L⁻¹)
Mitral stenosis	1.60	=	190	×	50	×	170
Sedentary	3.20	=	200	×	100	×	160
Athlete	5.20	=	190	×	160	×	170

From L. Rowell, "Circulation," *Medicine and Science in Sports,* 1 pp. 15–22, 1969, © by the American College of Sports Medicine.

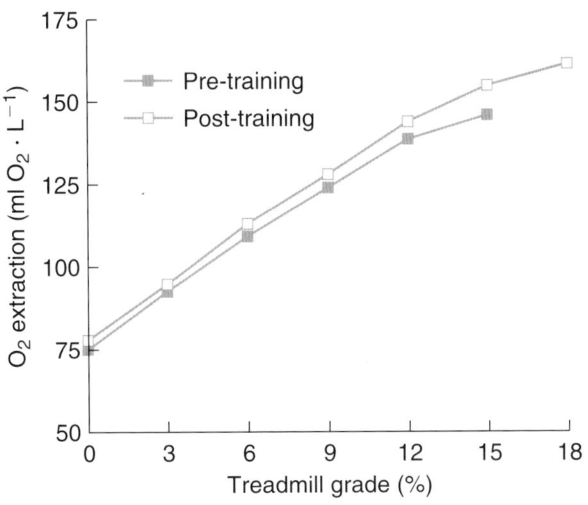

Figure 28.17 Maximal O_2 extraction is increased following training due to increase in capillary and mitochondrial density in the trained muscles (19).

9 In Review

During acute exercise, HR increases linearly with work rate once an HR of 110 beats · min^{-1} has been achieved. During exercise in the upright position, SV increases until an intensity of about 40% $\dot{V}O_2max$ is reached. Cardiac output (HR × SV) increases linearly with work rate. Following an endurance training program, HR is lower and SV is higher at rest and during submaximal work; in addition, maximal cardiac output is increased, because of an increase in maximal SV, with no change or a slight decrease in maximal HR. Variations in $\dot{V}O_2max$ across the population are attributed primarily to differences in maximal SV. Fifty percent of the increase in $\dot{V}O_2max$ attributable to endurance training is a result of an increase in maximal SV; the other 50% is attributable to an increase in oxygen extraction.

Blood Pressure

BP is dependent on the balance between cardiac output and the resistance the blood vessels offer to blood flow (total peripheral resistance). The resistance to blood flow is altered by the constriction or dilation of blood vessels called **arterioles,** located between the artery and the capillary.

BP = cardiac output × total peripheral resistance

BP is sensed by **baroreceptors** in the arch of the aorta and in the carotid arteries. If there is a change in BP, signals from the baroreceptors go to the cardiovascular control center in the brain, which in turn alters cardiac output or the diameter of arterioles. For example, when a person who has been lying supine suddenly stands, blood pools in the lower extremities, SV decreases, and, with it, BP. If BP is not restored, blood flow to the brain will be reduced and the person might faint. The baroreceptors monitor this decrease in BP, and the cardiovascular control center simultaneously increases the HR and reduces the diameter of the arterioles (to increase total peripheral resistance) to try to return BP to normal values. During exercise, the arterioles dilate in the active muscle to increase blood flow and meet metabolic demands. This dilation is matched with a constriction of arterioles in the liver, kidneys, and gastrointestinal tract and an increase in HR and SV, as already mentioned. These coordinated changes maintain BP and direct most of the cardiac output to the working muscles.

BP is monitored at each stage of a GXT. Figure 28.18 shows that **systolic blood pressure (SBP)** increases with each stage until maximum work tolerance is reached. At that point, SBP might decrease. A fall in SBP with an increase in work rate is used as one of the indicators of maximal cardiovascular function and can aid in determining the end point for an exercise test. **Diastolic blood pressure (DBP)** tends to remain the same or decrease during a GXT. An increase in DBP toward the end of the test

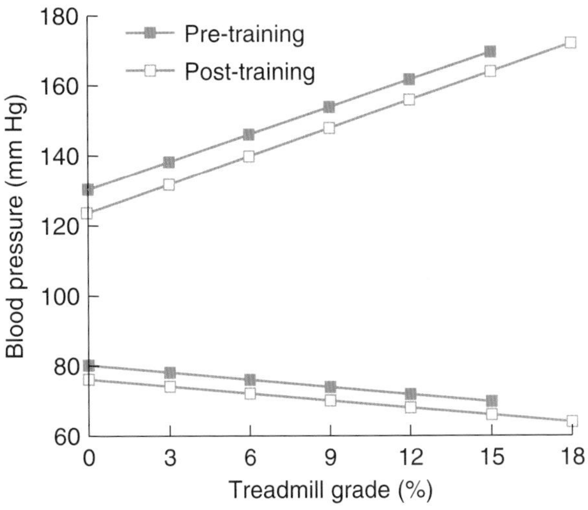

Figure 28.18 Systolic BP increases until maximum work tolerance is reached. Diastolic BP remains steady or decreases.

is another indicator that the limits of an individual's functional capacity have been reached. Endurance training programs reduce the BP responses at fixed submaximal work rates.

Two factors that determine the oxygen demand (work) of the heart during aerobic exercise are the HR and the SBP. The product of these two variables is called the **rate-pressure product**, or the **double product**, and is proportional to the myocardial oxygen demand (i.e., the volume of oxygen needed by the heart muscle per minute to function properly). Factors that decrease the HR and BP responses to work increase the chance that the coronary blood supply to the heart muscle will adequately meet the oxygen needs of the heart. Endurance training decreases the HR and BP responses to fixed submaximal work tasks and is seen as protective against any diminished blood supply (ischemia) to the myocardium. Drugs are also used to reduce HR and BP responses to try to reduce the work of the heart (see chapter 24).

When a person does the same rate of work with the arms as with the legs, the HR and BP responses are considerably higher during the arm work. This is shown in figure 28.19, in which the rate-pressure product is plotted for various levels of arm and leg work. Given that the load on the heart and the potential for fatigue are greater for arm work, an HFI should choose activities that use the large-muscle groups of the legs; this would result in lower HR and BP responses and reduced perception of fatigue (23, 60).

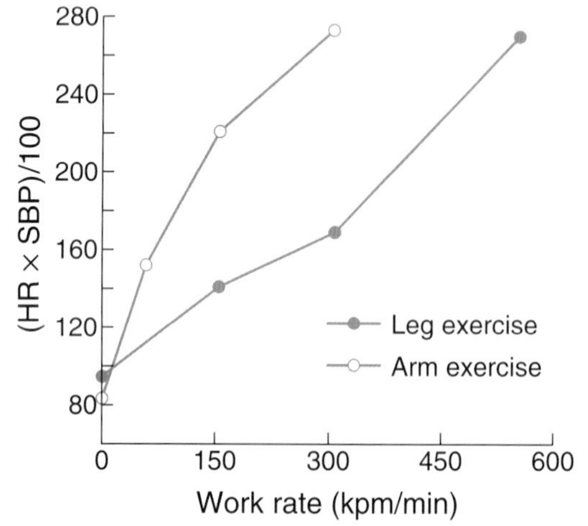

Figure 28.19 Rate-pressure product at rest and during arm and leg exercise.

Adapted from Schwade, Blomqvist, and Shapiro 1977.

10 In Review

SBP increases with each stage of a GXT, whereas DBP remains the same or decreases. The work of the heart is proportional to the product of the HR and the SBP. Training lowers both, making it easier for the coronary arteries to meet the oxygen demand of the heart. HR and BP are higher during arm work compared with leg work at the same work rate.

Effects of Endurance Training and Detraining on Physiological Responses to Exercise

Many observations have been made about the effects of endurance training on various physiological responses to exercise. In this section we show how some of the effects of endurance training are interrelated.

- *Endurance training increases the number of mitochondria and capillaries in muscle, causing all active fibers to become more oxidative.* This effect is manifested by the increase in the type IIa fibers and a decrease in type IIb fibers. These changes increase the endurance capacity of the muscle by allowing fat to be used for a greater percentage of energy production, sparing the muscle glycogen store and reducing lactate production. The lactate threshold is shifted to the right, and performance times in endurance events improve.
- *Endurance training decreases the time it takes to achieve a steady state in submaximal exercise.* This reduces the oxygen deficit and reduces reliance on CP and anaerobic glycolysis for energy.
- *Endurance training increases the volume of the ventricle.* This accommodates an increase in the end-diastolic volume, such that more blood is pumped out per beat. The increased SV is accompanied by a decrease in HR during submaximal work, so the cardiac output remains the same. The oxygen needs of the tissues are met with less work by the heart.
- *Maximal aerobic power increases with endurance training, the increase being inversely related to the initial $\dot{V}O_2max$.* In formerly sedentary individuals, about 50% of the increase in $\dot{V}O_2$max is attributable to an increase in maximal cardiac output, a change brought about by an increase in maximal SV, given that

maximal HR either remains the same or is decreased slightly. The other 50% of the increase in $\dot{V}O_2max$ is attributable to an increase in oxygen extraction at the muscle, shown by an increase in the $(a-\bar{v})O_2$ difference. This occurs as a result of increases in the number of capillaries and mitochondria in the trained muscles.

Transfer of Training

The training effects that have been discussed are observed only when trained muscles are used in the exercise test. Although this may appear obvious for the decrease in blood lactate that is attributable, in part, to the increase in the mitochondria of the trained muscles, it is also linked to the changes that occur in the HR response to submaximal work following the training program. Figure 28.20 shows the results of repeated submaximal exercise tests conducted on individuals who trained only one leg on a cycle ergometer for 13 days. The HR response to a fixed submaximal work rate using the trained leg decreased as expected. At the end of the 13 days of training, the untrained leg was subjected to the same exercise test. The HR responded as if a training effect had not occurred. This indicates that part of the reason the HR response to submaximal exercise decreases as a result of the training program is because of signals coming back from the trained muscles to the cardiovascular control center. This results in less sympathetic nervous system stimulation of the heart (9, 54). This has important implications for evaluating the effects of a training program. The expected training responses (lower lactate production, lower HR, more fat use) are linked to doing an exercise test that uses the same muscle groups that were involved in the training. The probability of some carryover of the training effect to another activity depends on the degree to which the new activity uses the muscles that are already trained.

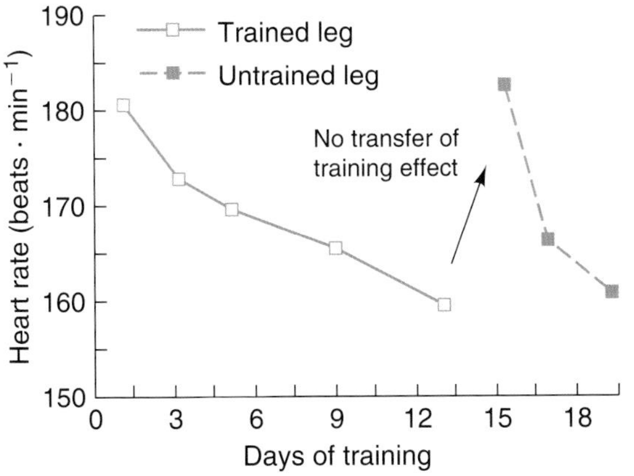

Figure 28.20 Lack of transfer of training effect (9).

Detraining

How fast is a training effect lost? A number of investigations have explored this question by having subjects either reduce or completely cease training. Maximal oxygen uptake usually is used as the principal measure to evaluate changes attributable to detraining, but an individual's response to a submaximal work rate also has been used to track these changes over time.

Cessation of Training

The following study used subjects who had trained for 10 ± 3 years and agreed to cease training for 84 days (15). They were tested on days 12, 21, 56, and 84 of the detraining period. Figure 28.21 shows that $\dot{V}O_2max$ decreased 7% within the first 12 days of detraining. [Remember that $\dot{V}O_2max$ = cardiac output · $(a-\bar{v})O_2$ difference.] The decrease in $\dot{V}O_2max$ was attributable entirely to a decrease in maximal cardiac output because the maximal oxygen extraction [$(a-\bar{v})O_2$ difference] was unchanged. In turn, the decrease in maximal cardiac output was attributable entirely to a decrease in maximal SV because maximal HR actually increased during the period of no training. A subsequent study showed that the reduced SV was caused by a reduction in plasma volume that occurred in the first 12 days of no training (13). In contrast, the decrease in $\dot{V}O_2max$ that occurred between days 21 and 84 was attributable to a decrease in the maximal oxygen extraction [$(a-\bar{v})O_2$ difference] because maximal cardiac output was unchanged (see figure 28.21). This decrease in oxygen extraction appeared to result from a reduction in the number of mitochondria in the muscle, given that the number of capillaries surrounding each muscle fiber was unchanged (12).

The same subjects also completed a standard (fixed work rate) submaximal exercise test during the 84 days of no training (14). Figure 28.22 shows that HR and blood lactic acid responses to this work test increased throughout the period of detraining. The higher responses are related to the fact that the same work rate required a greater percentage of $\dot{V}O_2max$ because the latter variable decreased throughout the period of detraining. The magnitude of change in HR and blood lactic acid responses to this submaximal work bout, however, makes them very sensitive indicators of the training state of an individual.

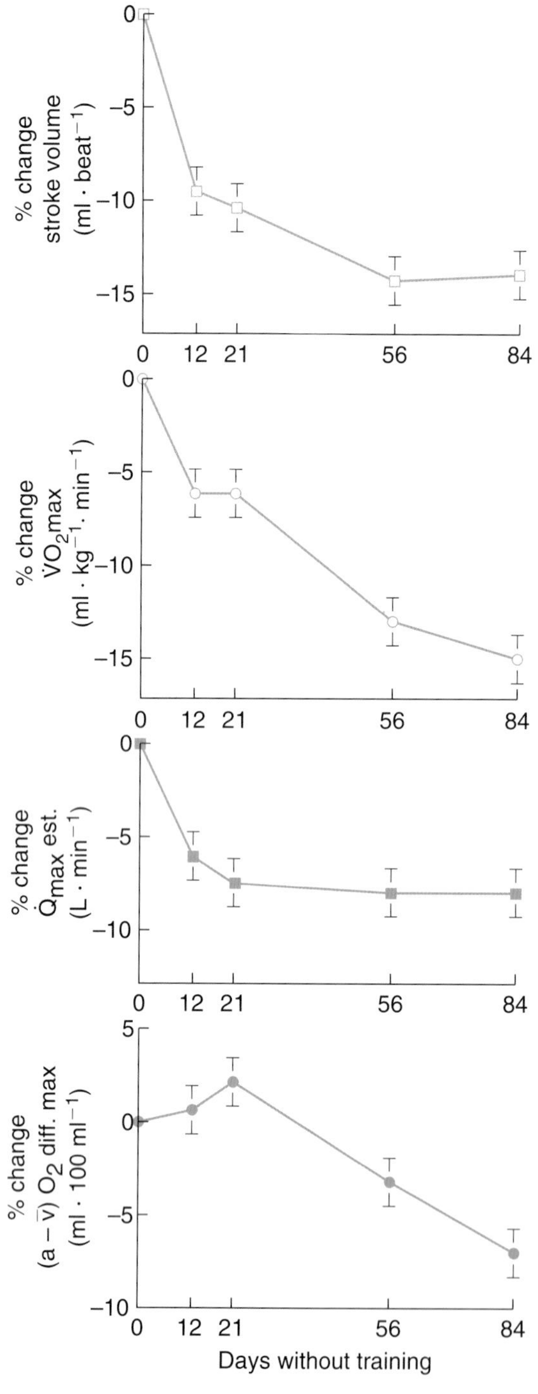

Figure 28.21 Effects of detraining on percentage changes in stroke volume during exercise, maximal oxygen uptake ($\dot{V}O_2max$), maximal cardiac output ($\dot{Q}_{2max}$ est.), and maximal arteriovenous oxygen difference [(a-v̄) O_2 diff. max].

Adapted from Coyle 1984.

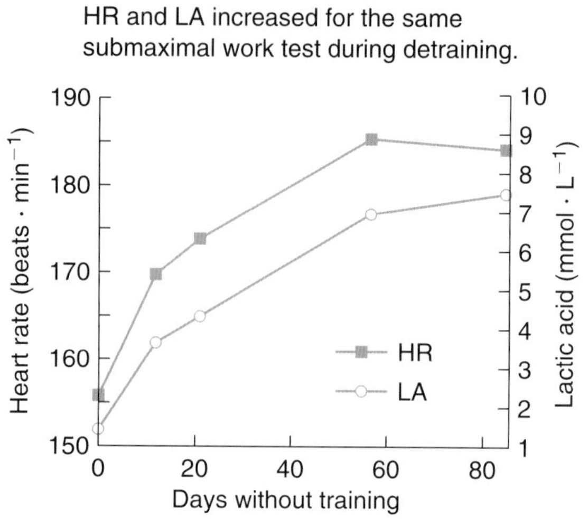

Figure 28.22 Changes in the heart rate and blood lactic acid concentration responses to a standard exercise test taken during 84 days of detraining (14).

Reduced Training

To evaluate the effect of a reduction in training, Hickson and colleagues (27-29) first trained subjects for 10 weeks to increase $\dot{V}O_2$max. The training program was conducted 40 min per day, 6 days per week. Three days involved running at near maximum intensity for 40 min; the other 3 days required six 5-min bouts at near-maximum intensity on a cycle ergometer, with a 2-min rest between work bouts. Subjects expended about 600 kcal per day of exercise, or 3600 kcal per week. At the end of this 10-week training program, the subjects were divided into groups that trained at either a one-third or a two-thirds reduction in the previous frequency (4 and 2 days per week, respectively), duration (26 and 13 min per day, respectively), or intensity (a one-third or two-thirds reduction in work done or distance run per 40-min session). Data collected on the maximal treadmill tests showed that the reduction in duration from 40 to 26 or 13 min, or a reduction in frequency from 6 to 4 or 2 days per week, did not affect $\dot{V}O_2$max. In contrast, $\dot{V}O_2$max clearly was decreased when the intensity of training was reduced by either one third or two thirds. What is interesting is that the subjects were able to maintain $\dot{V}O_2$max when the total exercise done per week was reduced from 3600 to 1200 kcal in the two-thirds reduced frequency and duration group, but they were not able to maintain $\dot{V}O_2$max when the intensity was reduced, even though the subjects were still expending about 1200 kcal per week. This points to the importance of the exercise intensity in maintaining $\dot{V}O_2$max and confirms that it takes less exercise to maintain than to achieve a specific level of $\dot{V}O_2$max.

11 In Review

Endurance training increases the ability of a muscle to use fat as a fuel and spare carbohydrate, decreases the time it takes to achieve a steady state during submaximal work, increases the size of the ventricle, and increases $\dot{V}O_2$max by increasing SV and oxygen extraction. Endurance training effects (lower HR, lower blood lactate) do not "transfer" when untrained muscles are used to perform the work. Maximal oxygen uptake decreases with cessation of training. The initial decrease is caused by a decrease in SV and, later, a reduction in oxygen extraction. Maximal oxygen uptake can be maintained by doing intense exercise, even when exercise duration and frequency are reduced.

Cardiovascular Responses to Exercise for Females and Males

Generally, little difference exists between prepubescent boys and girls in $\dot{V}O_2$max or in their cardiovascular responses to submaximal exercise. During puberty, differences between girls and boys appear and are related to the female's higher percentage of body fat, lower hemoglobin, and smaller heart size relative to body weight (2). These latter factors also affect a woman's cardiovascular responses to submaximal work. For example, if an 80-kg male were walking on a 10% grade on a treadmill at 3 miles · hr^{-1}, his $\dot{V}O_2$ would be 2.07 L · min^{-1} or 25.9 ml · kg^{-1} · min^{-1}.

The HR might be 140 beats · min^{-1} for this person. If he had to carry a backpack weighing 15 kg, the $\dot{V}O_2$ expressed per kilogram would not change (25.9 ml · kg^{-1} · min^{-1}), but the total oxygen requirement would increase 389 ml · min^{-1} (i.e., 15 kg · 25.9 ml · kg^{-1} · min^{-1}) to carry the 15-kg load. His HR obviously would be higher with this load than without, even though the $\dot{V}O_2$ expressed per kilogram of body weight is the same. Likewise, performance in the 12-min run test to evaluate maximal aerobic power was decreased by 89 m when body weight was experimentally increased to simulate a 5% gain in body fat (16). When a woman walks on a treadmill at a given grade and speed, her HR is higher than a comparable male's HR because of the additional fat weight she carries. The lower hemoglobin and smaller relative heart size also cause the HR to be higher at the same oxygen uptake expressed per unit of body weight.

The differences between males and females in the cardiovascular response to submaximal work become more exaggerated when work is done on a cycle ergometer where a given work rate demands a similar $\dot{V}O_2$ in liters per min, independent of sex or training. As previously mentioned, the average woman has less hemoglobin and a smaller heart volume than the average male. To deliver the same volume of oxygen to the muscles, the woman must have a higher HR to compensate for the smaller SV and must have a slightly higher cardiac output to compensate for the lower hemoglobin concentration (2). These differences between women and men in the cardiovascular responses to cycle ergometry are shown in figure 28.23.

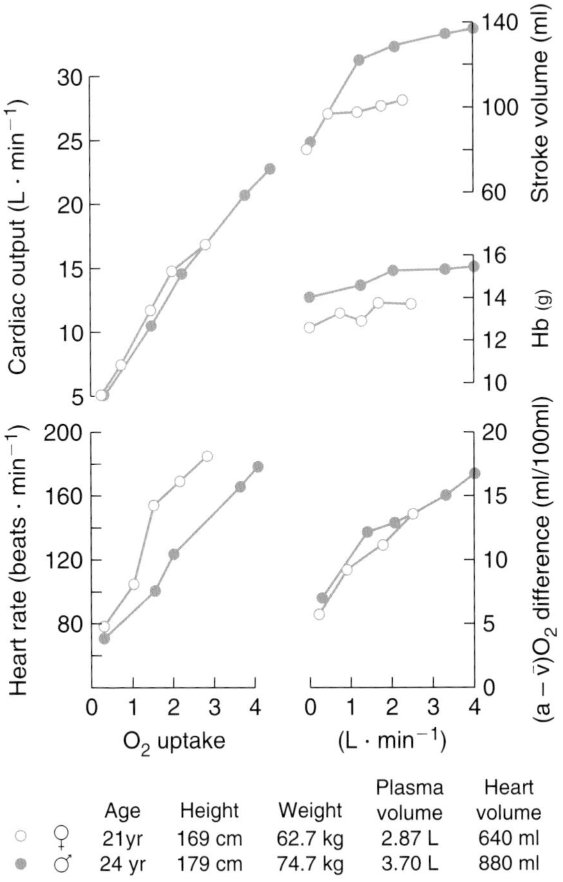

Figure 28.23 The cardiovascular responses of well-trained men and women to cycle ergometry exercise.

Adapted, by permission of McGraw-Hill, from Åstrand and Rodahl, 1986, *Textbook of work physiology* (3rd ed.).

12 In Review

At the same work rate, or $\dot{V}O_2$, women respond with a higher HR to compensate for a lower SV. The cardiac output is slightly higher to compensate for the lower hemoglobin level (and oxygen content) of the arterial blood.

Cardiovascular Responses to Isometric Exercise and Weightlifting

Most endurance exercise programs use dynamic activities involving large-muscle masses to place loads on the cardiorespiratory system. The previous summary of the physiological responses to a GXT indicates the rather proportional nature of the cardiovascular load to the exercise intensity. But this is not necessarily the case for activities that fall into the strength training category, in which a person can have a disproportionately high cardiovascular load relative to the exercise intensity. In the previous discussion of cardiovascular responses to a GXT, a progressive increase in the HR and SBP responses was observed with each stage of the test. Figure 28.24 shows the HR and BP responses to an isometric exercise test (sustained handgrip) at only 30% maximal voluntary contraction strength and to a treadmill test at two exercise intensities. The most impressive change during the sustained handgrip is in BP; the SBP and DBP increase over time, and the magnitude of the SBP exceeds 220 mm Hg. This kind of exercise places an additional load on the heart and is not recommended in strength training programs for older adults or people with heart disease (39).

Dynamic, heavy-resistance exercises can also cause extreme BP responses. Figure 28.25 shows the peak BP response achieved during exercises done at 95 to 100% of the maximum weight that could be lifted one time (1RM). Note that both DBP and SBP are elevated, with average values exceeding 300/200 mm Hg for the two-leg leg press done to fatigue. The elevation in pressure was believed to be caused by the compression of the arteries by the muscles, a reflex response attributable to the "static" component associated with near-maximal dynamic lifts, and the Valsalva maneuver, which, independently, can elevate BP (40). Another study reported peak values of about 190/140 mm Hg for exercises of 50%, 70%, and 80% of 1RM done to fatigue in novice and untrained lifters. Bodybuilders responded with lower pressures, indicating a cardiovascular adaptation to weight training (21).

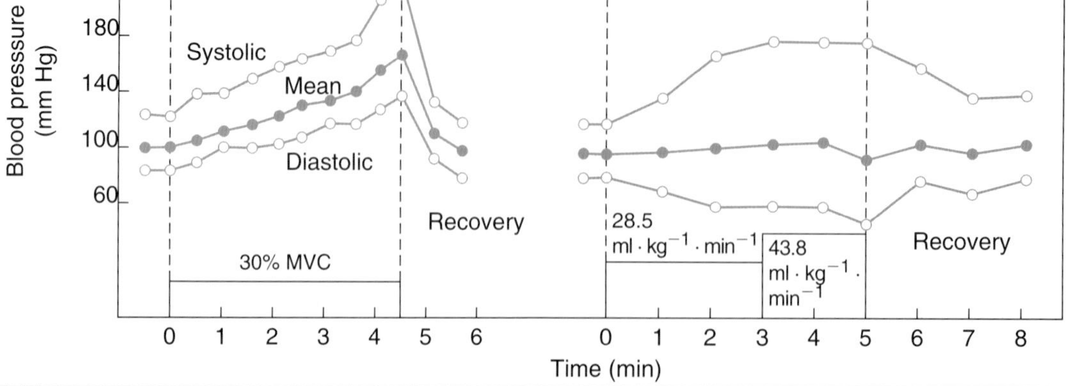

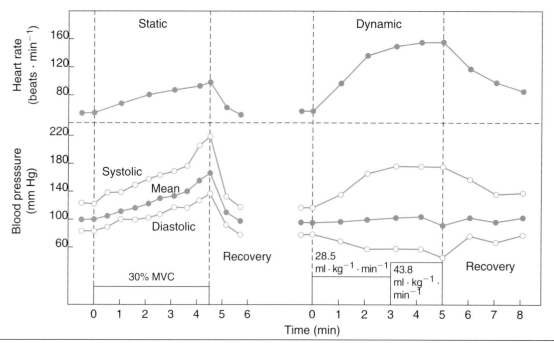

Figure 28.24 Comparison of the heart rate and blood pressure responses to a fatiguing, sustained hand-grip contraction at 30% of maximal voluntary contraction strength (30% MVC) and an exhausting treadmill test.

Adapted from Lind and McNichol 1967.

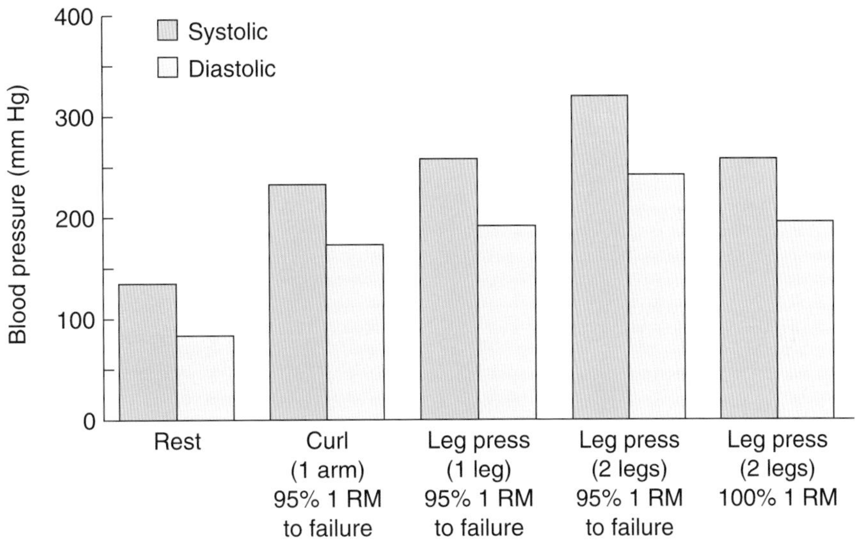

Figure 28.25 Blood pressure responses during weightlifting (RM = repetition maximum) (40).

13 In Review

Isometric exercise and heavy-resistance training exercises cause very high BP responses compared with those measured during dynamic endurance exercise. Both SBP and DBP are increased with isometric and dynamic resistance-training exercises.

Regulating Body Temperature

Under resting conditions, the body's core temperature is 37° C, and there is a balance between heat production and heat loss. Heat production mechanisms include the basal metabolic rate, shivering, work, and exercise. When exercise is done, the mechanical efficiency is about 20% or less, which means that 80% or more of the energy production ($\dot{V}O_2$) is converted to heat. For example, if you are working on a cycle ergometer at a rate requiring a $\dot{V}O_2$ of 2.0 L · min^{-1}, your energy production is about 10 kcal · min^{-1}. At 20% efficiency, 2 kcal · min^{-1} is used to do work, and 8 kcal · min^{-1} is converted to heat. If most of this added heat is not lost, core temperature might rise quickly to dangerous levels. How does the body lose excess heat?

Heat-Loss Mechanisms

Heat is lost from the body by four processes. In **radiation**, heat is transferred from the surface of one object to the surface of another, with no physical contact between the objects. Heat loss depends on the temperature gradient, that is, the temperature difference between the surfaces of the objects. When a person is seated at rest in a comfortable environment (21-22° C), about 60% of body heat is lost through radiation to cooler objects. **Conduction** is the transfer of heat from one object to another by direct contact, and, like radiation, conduction depends on a temperature gradient. When we sit on cold marble benches, we lose heat from our bodies by conduction. **Convection** is a special case of conduction in which heat is transferred to air (or water) molecules, which become lighter and rise away from the body to be replaced by cold air (or water). Heat loss can be increased by increasing the movement of the air (or water) over the surface of the body. For example, a fan enhances heat loss by placing more cold air molecules into contact with the skin. It should be clear that all of these heat-loss mechanisms can be heat-gain mechanisms as well. We gain heat from the sun by radiation across 93 million miles of space, and we gain heat by conduction when we sit on hot sand at the beach because the sand temperature is greater than skin temperature. Similarly, if a fan were to place more hot air (warmer than skin temperature) into contact with the skin, we would gain, not lose, heat. Heat gained from the environment is added to that generated by exercise and puts an additional strain on heat-loss mechanisms.

The last heat-loss mechanism is the evaporation of sweat. **Sweating** is the process of producing a watery solution over the surface of the body. **Evaporation** is a process in which liquid water is converted to a gas. This conversion requires about 580 kcal of heat per liter of sweat evaporated. The heat for this comes from the body and, thus, the body is cooled. At rest, about 25% of heat loss is caused by evaporation, but during exercise it becomes the primary mechanism for heat loss.

Evaporation depends on the **water vapor pressure gradient** between the skin and the air and is not directly dependent on temperature. The water vapor pressure of the air is dependent on the **relative humidity** and the **saturation pressure** at that air temperature. For example, the relative humidity can be 90% in winter, but because the saturation pressure of cold air is low, on such a day the water vapor pressure of the air is also low, and you can see water vapor rising from your body following exercise. In warm temperatures, however, the relative humidity is a good indicator of the water vapor pressure of the air. If the water vapor pressure of the air is too high, sweat will not evaporate, and sweat that does not evaporate does not cool the body (49).

Body Temperature Response to Exercise

Figure 28.26 shows that during exercise in a comfortable environment, the core temperature increases to a level proportional to the relative intensity (% $\dot{V}O_2max$) of the exercise and then levels off (59). The gain in body heat that occurs early in exercise triggers the heat-loss mechanisms discussed in the preceding section. After 10 to 20 min, heat loss equals heat production, and the core temperature remains steady (24). What are the most important heat-loss mechanisms during exercise?

Heat Loss During Exercise

Exercise intensity and environmental temperature influence the heat-loss mechanism that is primarily responsible for maintaining a steady core temperature during exercise. When a person participates in a series of progressively more difficult exercise tests in an environment that allows heat loss by all the mechanisms just mentioned, the contribution that convection and radiation make to overall heat loss is modest. Because the temperature gradient between the skin and the room is not altered much during exercise, the rate of heat loss is relatively constant. To compensate for this, evaporation picks up when heat loss by convection and radiation levels off, and it is responsible for most of the heat loss in heavy exercise (figure 28.27).

When a person performs steady-state exercise in a warm environment compared with a cool one, the role that evaporation plays becomes even more important. Figure 28.28 shows that as environmental temperature increases, the gradient for heat loss by convection and radiation decreases, and, with it, the rate of heat loss by these processes also decreases. As a result, evaporation must compensate to maintain core temperature.

An important insight to be gained from this discussion is that in strenuous exercise or hot environments, evaporation is the most important process for losing heat and maintaining body temperature in the safe range. It should be no surprise, then, that factors which affect sweat production (such as dehydration) or interfere with the evaporation of sweat (such as impermeable clothing) are causes for concern. Chapter 10 provides the specifics on how to deal with heat and humidity when prescribing exercise, and chapter 25 provides important information on preventing and treating heat-related disorders.

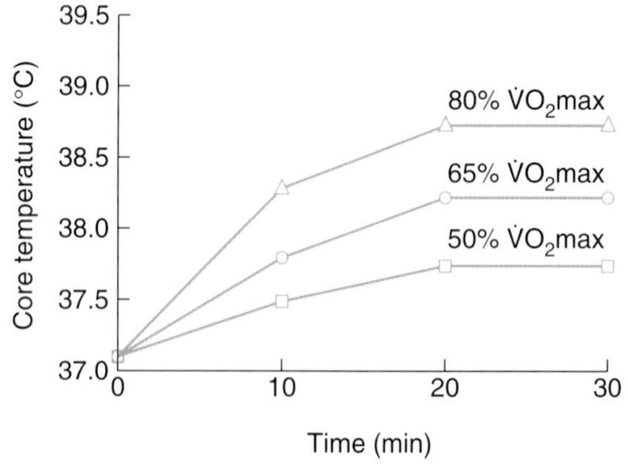

Figure 28.26 Core temperature increases over time to a level proportional to the relative work rate (59).

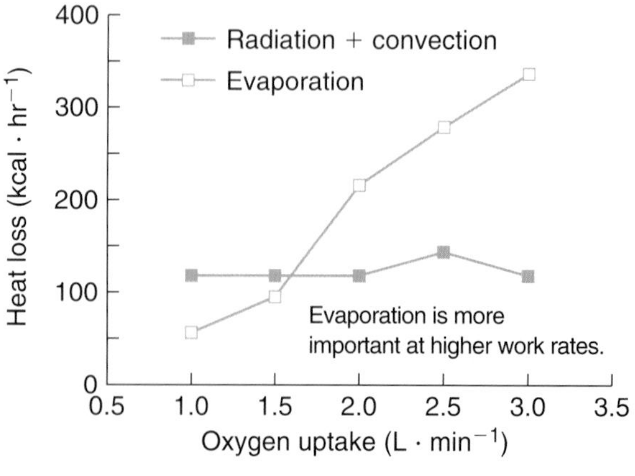

Figure 28.27 Importance of evaporation as a heat loss mechanism as exercise intensity increases (2).

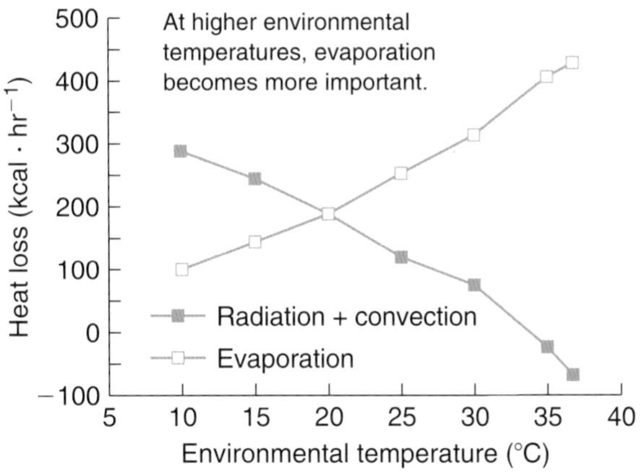

Figure 28.28 Importance of evaporation as a heat loss mechanism during exercise as environmental temperature increases (2).

Training in a hot and humid environment for as little as 7 to 12 days results in specific adaptations that improve heat tolerance and, as a result, the trained individual's body temperature is lower during submaximal exercise (24). Adaptations that improve heat tolerance include the following:

- An increase in plasma volume
- An earlier onset of sweating
- A higher sweat rate
- A reduction in salt loss in sweat
- Reduced blood flow to the skin

14 In Review

Heat can be lost from the body by radiation and convection when a temperature gradient exists from the skin to the environment; however, evaporation is the primary mechanism of heat loss during high-intensity exercise or during exercise in a hot environment. Body temperature increases during submaximal exercise and achieves a new level proportional to the exercise intensity. Acclimatization to heat can be achieved in 7 to 12 days of training in a hot and humid environment and improves one's ability to exercise safely.

Case Studies

You can check your answers by referring to appendix A.

28.1

A female competitive distance runner took a GXT on a motor-driven treadmill in which the speed of the run increased 0.5 miles · hr^{-1} each minute, with the test starting at 5 miles · hr^{-1}. Blood samples for lactic acid determination were obtained each minute, and the lactate threshold was found to occur at the 8 mph stage of the test. Unfortunately, no one at the testing center knew what this meant relative to performance, and she has come to you for help. What would you tell her?

28.2

A client with whom you have been working retakes a maximal GXT following 10 weeks of endurance training and finds his HR lower at each stage of the test. He is bothered by this because he thought his heart would be stronger and beat more times per minute. How would you help him understand what happened?

28.3

A female client is bothered by the fact that elite women runners who train as hard as elite male runners don't achieve the same performance times in distance races. She wants to know why and has come to you for the answer. How would you respond?

Source List

1. Åstrand, P-O. (1952). *Experimental studies of physical working capacity in relation to sex and age*. Copenhagen: Ejnar Munksgaard.
2. Åstrand, P-O., & Rodahl, K. (1986). *Textbook of work physiology* (3rd ed.). New York: McGraw-Hill.
3. Bassett, D.R., Jr. (1994). Skeletal muscle characteristics: Relationships to cardiovascular risk factors. *Medicine and Science in Sports and Exercise, 26,* 957-966.
4. Bassett, D.R., & Howley, E.T. (1997). Maximal oxygen uptake: Classical versus contemporary viewpoints. *Medicine and Science in Sports and Exercise, 29,* 591-603.
5. Bassett, D.R., & Howley, E.T. (2000). Limiting factors for maximal oxygen uptake and determinants of endurance performance. *Medicine and Science in Sports and Exercise, 32,* 70-84.
6. Bouchard, C., Lesage, R., Lortie, G., Simoneau, J., Hamel, P., Boulay, M., Perusse, L., Theriault, G., & Leblank, C. (1986). Aerobic performance in brothers, dizygotic and monozygotic twins. *Medicine and Science in Sports and Exercise, 18,* 639-646.
7. Brooks, G.A. (1985). Anaerobic threshold: Review of the concept, and directions for future research. *Medicine and Science in Sports and Exercise, 17,* 22-31.
8. Brooks, G.A., Fahey, T.D., & White, T.P. (2000). *Exercise physiology: Human bioenergetics and its application* (3rd ed.). Mountain View, CA: Mayfield.
9. Claytor, R.P. (1985). *Selected cardiovascular, sympathoadrenal, and metabolic responses to one-leg exercise training*. Unpublished doctoral dissertation, University of Tennessee, Knoxville.
10. Coggan, A.R., & Coyle, E.F. (1991). Carbohydrate ingestion during prolonged exercise: Effects on metabolism and performance. *Exercise and Sport Sciences Reviews, 19,* 1-40.
11. Costill, D.L. (1988). Carbohydrates for exercise: Dietary demands of optimal performance. *International Journal of Sports Medicine, 9,* 1-18.
12. Coyle, E.F. (1988). Detraining and retention of training-induced adaptations. In S.N. Blair, P. Painter, R.R. Pate, L.K. Smith, & C.B. Taylor (Eds.), *Resource manual for guidelines for exercise testing and prescription* (pp. 83-89). Philadelphia: Lea & Febiger.
13. Coyle, E.F., Hemmert, M.K., & Coggan, A.R. (1986). Effects of detraining on cardiovascular responses to exercise: Role of blood volume. *Journal of Applied Physiology, 60,* 95-99.
14. Coyle, E.F., Martin, W.H., III, Bloomfield, S.A., Lowry, O.H., & Holloszy, J.O. (1985). Effects of detraining on responses to submaximal exercise. *Journal of Applied Physiology, 59,* 853-859.
15. Coyle, E.F., Martin, W.H., III, Sinacore, D.R., Joyner, M.J., Hagberg, J.M., & Holloszy, J.O. (1984). Time course of loss of adaptation after stopping prolonged intense endurance training. *Journal of Applied Physiology, 57,* 1857-1864.
16. Cureton, K.J., Sparling, P.B., Evans, B.W., Johnson, S.M., Kong, U.D., & Purvis, J.W. (1978). Effect of experimental alterations in excess weight on aerobic capacity and distance-running performance. *Medicine and Science in Sports, 10,* 194-199.
17. Davis, J.H. (1985). Anaerobic threshold: Review of the concept and directions for future research. *Medicine and Science in Sports and Exercise, 17,* 6-18.
18. Edington, D.W., & Edgerton, V.R. (1976). *The biology of physical activity*. Boston: Houghton Mifflin.
19. Ekblom, B., Åstrand, P-O., Saltin, B., Stenberg, J., & Wallstrom, B. (1968). Effect of training on circulatory response to exercise. *Journal of Applied Physiology, 24,* 518-528.
20. Faulkner, J.A., Roberts, D.E., Elk, R.L., & Conway, J. (1971). Cardiovascular responses to submaximum and maximum effort cycling and running. *Journal of Applied Physiology, 30,* 457-461.
21. Fleck, S.J., & Dean, L.S. (1987). Resistance-training experience and the pressor response during resistance exercise. *Journal of Applied Physiology, 63,* 116-120.
22. Fox, E.L., Bowers, R.W., & Foss, M.L. (1993). *The physiological basis for exercise and sport* (5th ed.). Madison, WI: Brown & Benchmark.
23. Franklin, B.A. (1985). Exercise testing, training, and arm ergometry. *Sports Medicine, 2,* 100-119.
24. Gisolfi, C., & Wenger, C.B. (1984). Temperature regulation during exercise: Old concepts, new ideas. *Exercise and Sport Sciences Reviews, 12,* 339-372.
25. Hickson, R.C., Bomze, H.A., & Holloszy, J.O. (1977). Linear increase in aerobic power induced by a strenuous program of endurance exercise. *Journal of Applied Physiology: Respiratory, Environmental and Exercise Physiology, 42,* 372-376.
26. Hickson, R.C., Bomze, H.A., & Holloszy, J.O. (1978). Faster adjustment of O_2 uptake to the energy requirement of exercise in the trained state. *Journal of Applied Physiology: Respiratory, Environmental and Exercise Physiology, 44,* 877-881.
27. Hickson, R.C., Foster, C., Pollock, M.L., Galassi, T.M., & Rich, S. (1985). Reduced training intensities and loss of aerobic power, endurance, and cardiac growth. *Journal of Applied Physiology, 58,* 492-499.
28. Hickson, R.C., Kanakis, C., Jr., Davis, J.R., Moore, A.M., & Rich, S. (1982). Reduced training duration effects on aerobic power, endurance, and cardiac growth. *Journal of Applied Physiology, 53,* 225-229.
29. Hickson, R.C., & Rosenkoetter, M.A. (1981). Reduced training frequencies and maintenance of increased aerobic power. *Medicine and Science in Sports and Exercise, 13,* 13-16.
30. Holloszy, J.O., & Coyle, E.F. (1984). Adaptations of skeletal muscle to endurance exercise and their metabolic consequences. *Journal of Applied Physiology: Respiratory, Environmental and Exercise Physiology, 56,* 831-838.
31. Howley, E.T. (1980). Effect of altitude on physical performance. In G.A. Stull & T.K. Cureton (Eds.), *Encyclopedia of physical education, fitness, and sports: Training, environment, nutrition, and fitness* (pp. 177-187). Salt Lake City: Brighton.
32. Howley, E.T., Bassett, D.R., Jr., & Welch, H.G. (1995). Criteria for maximal oxygen uptake—Review and commentary. *Medicine and Science in Sports and Exercise, 24,* 1055-1058.
33. Hultman, E. (1967). Physiological role of muscle glycogen in man, with special reference to exercise. *Circulation Research, 20-21*(Suppl. 1), 99-114.
34. Issekutz, B., Birkhead, N.C., & Rodahl, K. (1962). The use of respiratory quotients in assessment of aerobic power capacity. *Journal of Applied Physiology, 17,* 47-50.
35. Kasch, F.W., Boyer, J.L., Van Camp, S.P., Verity, L.S., & Wallace, J.P. (1990). The effects of physical activity and inactivity on aerobic power in older men (a longitudinal study). *The Physician and Sportsmedicine, 18*(4), 73-83.
36. Kasch, F.W., Wallace, J.P., & Van Camp, S.P. (1985). Effects of 18 years of endurance exercise on the physical work capacity of older men. *Journal of Cardiopulmonary Rehabilitation, 5,* 308-312.
37. Kasch, F.W., Wallace, J.P., Van Camp, S.P., & Verity, L.S. (1988). A longitudinal study of cardiovascular stability in active men aged 45 to 65 yrs. *The Physician and Sportsmedicine, 16*(1), 117-126.

38. Katch, F.I., & McArdle, W.D. (1977). *Nutrition and weight control*. Boston: Houghton Mifflin.
39. Lind, A.R., & McNicol, G.W. (1967). Muscular factors which determine the cardiovascular responses to sustained and rhythmic exercise. *Canadian Medical Association Journal, 96,* 706-713.
40. MacDougall, J.D., Tuxen, D., Sale, D.G., Moroz, J.R., & Sutton, J.R. (1985). Arterial blood-pressure response to heavy resistance exercise. *Journal of Applied Physiology, 58,* 785-790.
41. McArdle, W.D., Katch, F.I., & Katch, V.L. (1996). *Exercise physiology, energy, nutrition, and human performance* (4th ed.). Baltimore: Williams & Wilkins.
42. McArdle, W.D., Katch, F.I., & Pechar, G.S. (1973). Comparison of continuous and discontinuous treadmill and bicycle tests for max VO_2. *Medicine and Science in Sports, 5*(3), 156-160.
43. McArdle, W.D., & Magel, J.R. (1970). Physical work capacity and maximum oxygen uptake in treadmill and bicycle exercise. *Medicine and Science in Sports, 2*(3), 118-123.
44. Montoye, H.J., Ayen, T., Nagle, F., & Howley, E.T. (1986). The oxygen requirement for horizontal and grade walking on a motor-driven treadmill. *Medicine and Science in Sports and Exercise, 17,* 640-645.
45. Nagle, F.J., Balke, B., Baptista, G., Alleyia, J., & Howley, E. (1971). Compatibility of progressive treadmill, bicycle, and step tests based on oxygen-uptake responses. *Medicine and Science in Sports, 3,* 149-154.
46. Plowman, S.A., & Smith, D.L. (1997). *Exercise physiology for fitness and performance*. Needham Heights, MA: Allyn & Bacon.
47. Powers, S.K., Dodd, S., & Beadle, R.E. (1985). Oxygen-uptake kinetics in trained athletes differing in VO_2max. *European Journal of Applied Physiology, 54,* 306-308.
48. Powers, S., Dodd, S., Deason, R., Byrd, R., & McKnight, T. (1983). Ventilatory threshold, running economy, and distance-running performance of trained athletes. *Research Quarterly for Exercise and Sport, 54,* 179-182.
49. Powers, S.K., & Howley, E.T. (2001). *Exercise physiology* (4th ed.). New York: McGraw-Hill.
50. Powers, S., Riley, W., & Howley, E. (1980). A comparison of fat metabolism in trained men and women during prolonged aerobic work. *Research Quarterly for Exercise and Sport, 52,* 427-431.
51. Raven, P.B., Drinkwater, B.L., Ruhling, R.O., Bolduan, N., Taguchi, S., Gliner, J., & Horvath, S.M. (1974). Effect of carbon monoxide and peroxyacetyl nitrate on man's maximal aerobic capacity. *Journal of Applied Physiology, 36,* 288-293.
52. Robergs, R.A., & Roberts, S.O. (1997). *Exercise physiology*. St. Louis: Mosby-Year Book.
53. Rowell, L.B. (1969). Circulation. *Medicine and Science in Sports, 1,* 15-22.
54. Rowell, L.B. (1986). *Human circulation-regulation during physical stress*. New York: Oxford University Press.
55. Sale, D.G. (1987). Influence of exercise and training on motor unit activation. *Exercise and Sport Sciences Reviews, 15,* 95-151.
56. Saltin, B. (1969). Physiological effects of physical conditioning. *Medicine and Science in Sports, 1,* 50-56.
57. Saltin, B., & Gollnick, P.D. (1983). Skeletal muscle adaptability: Significance for metabolism and performance. In L.D. Peachey, R.H. Adrian, & S.R. Geiger (Eds.), *Handbook of physiology* (pp. 555-631). Baltimore: Williams & Wilkins.
58. Saltin, B., Henriksson, J., Nygaard, E., Anderson, P., & Jansson, E. (1977). Fiber types and metabolic potentials of skeletal muscles in sedentary man and endurance runners. *Annals of the New York Academy of Science, 301,* 3-29.
59. Saltin, B., & Hermansen, L. (1966). Esophageal, rectal, and muscle temperature during exercise. *Journal of Applied Physiology, 21,* 1757-1762.
60. Schwade, J., Blomqvist, C.G., & Shapiro, W. (1977). A comparison of the response to arm and leg work in patients with ischemic heart disease. *American Heart Journal, 94,* 203-208.
61. Sherman, W.M. (1983). Carbohydrates, muscle glycogen, and muscle glycogen supercompensation. In M.H. Williams (Ed.), *Ergogenic aids in sports* (pp. 3-26). Champaign, IL: Human Kinetics.
62. Taylor, H.L., Buskirk, E.R., & Henschel, A. (1955). Maximal oxygen intake as an objective measure of cardiorespiratory performance. *Journal of Applied Physiology, 8,* 73-80.
63. Vander, A.J., Sherman, J.H., & Luciano, D.S. (1985). *Human physiology* (4th ed.). New York: McGraw-Hill.
64. Wilmore, J.H., & Costill, D.L. (1999). *Physiology of sport and exercise* (2nd ed.). Champaign, IL: Human Kinetics.

Case Study Answers

1.1

You might respond by admitting that there are risks related to exercise, with 7 deaths per year for every 100 000 exercisers. However, more people die while sleeping, or after eating and yet few people advocate the cessation of those activities. In addition, the risks of deterioration of the cardiovascular system through sedentary living causes a much higher risk of major health problems than being active. Finally, risks can be minimized by starting very slowly and gradually increasing the amount and intensity of work done during exercise.

1.2

You might begin by stating that the CDC recommendations were aimed at individuals who are currently sedentary and not individuals who are habitually active and involved in strenuous exercise. In addition, you might indicate that participation in more strenuous exercise is associated with other health-related benefits (increases in cardiorespiratory fitness [$\dot{V}O_2$]) that cannot be realized with moderate exercise.

2.1

You would help Fred to see that his goals are primarily health-related goals at this time. After engaging in moderate-intensity exercise, he may want to add fitness goals to his list. Susan, on the other hand, has already reached her health and fitness goals—she now has performance goals. You would help her analyze the various underlying factors and skills needed to compete in soccer, and suggest some training to help her improve in these areas.

3.1

Encourage the woman to begin moderate-intensity exercise, using the walking program in chapter 14. Recommend that she get a health screening, including body composition, blood pressure, and blood profile. If the breathlessness continues or gets worse with regular exercise, she should see her personal physician. After she reaches the final stage of the walking program, recommend that she have physical fitness testing to determine appropriate vigorous-intensity exercise.

3.2

It appears that his elevated heart rate and blood pressure may be an anxious response to a new environment. Talk with him about the kinds of activities he enjoys. Explain the procedures of the GXT, indicating again that he can stop whenever he wants to and that the fitness center has never had problems on the test. Have him walk around the center to look at the various fitness stations. When he returns, have him sit, and show him how to relax when he exhales. Retake his HR and BP. If they are lower, then continue with the GXT, giving him extra attention (e.g., frequently asking how he is doing during the test). If HR and BP remain high, ask him to come back for a second visit at a time that is convenient for him when the center will not be busy. Give him a relaxation program to try at home.

3.3

a. John's major risk factors include age, hypertension, cigarette smoking, physical inactivity, and total/HDL ratio > 5. Secondary risk factors include percent body fat, stress, and gender (male).

b. Nonpharmacological intervention programs might include smoking cessation classes, stress management classes, dietary counseling, and initiation of moderate physical activity.

4.1

$$3.5\ \text{mi} \cdot \text{hr}^{-1} \cdot 26.8\ \text{m} \cdot \text{min}^{-1} = 93.8\ \text{m} \cdot \text{min}^{-1}$$

$$93.8\ \text{m} \cdot \text{min}^{-1}\left(\frac{0.1\ \text{ml} \cdot \text{kg}^{-1} \cdot \text{min}^{-1}}{\text{m} \cdot \text{min}^{-1}}\right) +$$

$$3.5\ \text{ml} \cdot \text{kg}^{-1} \cdot \text{min}^{-1} = 12.9\ \text{ml} \cdot \text{kg}^{-1} \cdot \text{min}^{-1}$$

$$12.9\ \text{ml} \cdot \text{kg}^{-1} \cdot \text{min}^{-1} \cdot 75\ \text{kg} =$$

$$968\ \text{ml} \cdot \text{min}^{-1}\ \text{or}\ .97\ \text{L} \cdot \text{min}^{-1}$$

$$.97\ \text{L} \cdot \text{min}^{-1} \cdot 5\ \text{kcal} \cdot \text{L}^{-1} = 4.85\ \text{kcal} \cdot \text{min}^{-1}$$

$$4.85\ \text{kcal} \cdot \text{min}^{-1} \cdot 30\ \text{min} = 146\ \text{kcal}$$

$$100\ \text{W} \cdot \frac{6.1\ \text{kpm} \cdot \text{min}^{-1}}{\text{W}} = 610\ \text{kpm} \cdot \text{min}^{-1}$$

$$(610\ \text{kpm} \cdot \text{min}^{-1} \cdot 2\ \text{ml} \cdot \text{kpm}^{-1}) +$$

$$(60\ \text{kg} \cdot 3.5\ \text{ml} \cdot \text{kg}^{-1} \cdot \text{min}^{-1}) = 1430\ \text{ml} \cdot \text{min}^{-1}$$

$$\text{or } 1.43\ \text{L} \cdot \text{min}^{-1}$$

$$3\ \text{mi} \cdot 1610\ \text{m} \cdot \text{mi}^{-1} = 4830\ \text{m} \div 24\ \text{min} = 201\ \text{m} \cdot \text{min}^{-1}$$

$$201\ \text{m} \cdot \text{min}^{-1}\left(\frac{0.2\ \text{ml} \cdot \text{kg}^{-1} \cdot \text{min}^{-1}}{\text{m} \cdot \text{min}^{-1}}\right) +$$

$$3.5\ \text{ml} \cdot \text{kg}^{-1} \cdot \text{min}^{-1} = 43.7\ \text{ml} \cdot \text{kg}^{-1} \cdot \text{min}^{-1}$$

$$43.7\ \text{ml} \cdot \text{kg}^{-1} \cdot \text{min}^{-1} \cdot 70\ \text{kg} =$$

$$3059\ \text{ml} \cdot \text{min}^{-1} \text{ or } 3.06\ \text{L} \cdot \text{min}^{-1}$$

$$3.06\ \text{L} \cdot \text{min}^{-1} \cdot 5\ \text{kcal} \cdot \text{L}^{-1} =$$

$$15.3\ \text{kcal} \cdot \text{min}^{-1} \cdot 24\ \text{min} = 367\ \text{kcal}$$

$$12\ \text{METs} = 12\ \text{kcal} \cdot \text{kg}^{-1} \cdot \text{hr}^{-1} \cdot 70\% = 8.4\ \text{kcal} \cdot \text{kg}^{-1} \cdot \text{hr}^{-1}$$

$$8.4\ \text{kcal} \cdot \text{kg}^{-1} \cdot \text{hr}^{-1} \cdot 85\ \text{kg} = 714\ \text{kcal} / \text{hr} \cdot 0.5\ \text{hr} = 357\ \text{kcal}$$

4.5

You might indicate the cost of jogging 1 m/min (0.2 ml · kg^{-1} · min^{-1}) is about twice that for walking (0.1 ml · kg^{-1} · min^{-1}) due to the extra energy needed to propel the body off the ground and absorb the force of impact on each step. You might provide a summary table he can use describing the caloric cost of walking and running 1 mi.

5.1

The requirement that sedentary middle-age participants take a maximal, unmonitored test at the beginning of their fitness program is inappropriate. You might suggest, in place of the 1.5-mi run, the use of the 1-mi-walk test, which should be used after the participants have demonstrated that they can comfortably walk 1 mi.

5.2

His estimated $\dot{V}O_2max$ = 37.8 ml · kg^{-1} · min^{-1}. His level of cardiorespiratory fitness is adequate for most activities and just short of being "good" for his age group.

5.3

The heart rate response of 100 beats · min^{-1} at the work rate of 300 kpm · min^{-1} should have been ignored. The heart rate values should have been extrapolated to 170 beats · min^{-1}, and the vertical line dropped from that point would indicate a work rate of about 1050 kpm · min^{-1}, equal to a $\dot{V}O_2$ of 2.4 L · min^{-1}. This equals 8.4 METs (2400 ml · min^{-1} ÷ 81.7 kg = 29.4 ml · kg^{-1} · min^{-1} ÷ 3.5 ml · kg^{-1}·min^{-1} = 8.4 METs).

5.4

The graph should have ignored the heart rate value of 96 beats · min^{-1}. The line was extrapolated to 190 beats · min^{-1} and the vertical line dropped from that point indicated a value of about 16.75% grade, which is equal to a $\dot{V}O_2$ of about 35.6 ml · kg · min^{-1} (see chapter 7). This is 10.2 METs, or 1.94 L · min^{-1}.

5.5

The reference point for the scale is the "zero" established when the free-swinging pendulum stops, with the cycle on a flat surface. All scale values are relative to this zero, and if the zero is off, all scale readings will be off. If the pendulum is not at zero when no weight is attached, the entire scale is off by the amount the zero value is off. For example, if the scale reads .25 kg when no weight is attached each value is shifted .25 kg upward when known weights are attached.

6.1

a. BMI

71 inches × 2.54 cm/inch = 180.3 cm = 1.803 m

230 pounds / 2.2 lbs/kg = 104.5 kg

$104.5\ \text{kg} / (1.803\ \text{m})^2 = 32.1\ \text{kg/m}^2$

This value places Mr. Jackson in the obese range.

WHR

43 in / 36 in = 1.19

This value places Mr. Jackson at increased risk for cardiovascular disease.

%BF

The correct formula to use can be found in chapter 6:

$$D_b = 1.10938 - 0.0008267\ (\text{sum of skinfolds}) + 0.0000016\ (\text{sum of skinfolds})^2 - 0.0002574\ (\text{age})$$

Using 92 as the sum of Mr. Jackson's skinfolds and an age of 48 years, you will calculate a body density of 1.0345 kg/L.

Using the Siri equation (%BF = 495 / D_b − 450), you will calculate a body fat percentage of 28.5%.

b. Target body weight

Fat mass = 230 × .285 = 65.55 lbs

Fat-free mass = 230 – 65.55 = 164.45 lbs

Target body weight = Fat mass
= 230 × .285 = 65.55 lbs

Fat-free mass = 230 – 65.55 = 164.45 lbs

Using the equation above, you will calculate a target body weight for this *initial* goal of 216 pounds.

7.1

This athlete weighs 86.4 kg. The ACSM, ADA, and Dietitians of Canada position statement (3) suggests that such an athlete may benefit from ingesting 1.2 to 1.4 g of protein per kg body weight. This athlete is consuming approximately 525 kcal of protein each day (3500 kcal × 0.15 = 525 kcal). This is roughly equal to 131 g of protein (525 kcal / 4 kcal/g = 131.25 g). This is approximately 1.5 g/kg (131.25 g / 86.4 kg = 1.52 g/kg). Additional protein intake appears unwarranted.

9.1

Sacral angle should be at least 80º (a book or a board on edge placed against the sacrum would be snug if it were 90º). Next examine the curvature of the spine; it should be smooth with no evident flatness or hypermobility in any one particular area. Arm-leg length discrepancy might also be a factor (e.g., long arms in relation to legs).

9.2

Most false positives in the administration of the Thomas test result when the individual being tested brings his/her thigh too close to the chest. This can result in excessive posterior rotation of the pelvis which, in turn, can make it appear that the hip flexors are tight.

10.1

If a person has a normal response to a GXT, HR and systolic blood pressure increase with each stage of the test, whereas the diastolic pressure remains the same or decreases slightly. In addition, the ECG response shows no significant S-T segment depression or elevation, and no significant arrhythmias occur. In these cases it can be assumed that the last load achieved on the test represents the true functional capacity (max METs). The GXT presented in Case Study 10.1 is representative of such a test.

Paul has normal resting BP and a negative family history for CHD. Risk factors include a relatively high percentage of body fat (indicating obesity), sedentary lifestyle, and a poor blood lipid profile. Based on these findings, THR range of 158 to 177 beats · min^{-1} was calculated (60%-80% $\dot{V}O_2max$ as measured during the maximal GXT); this HR range corresponds to work rates equal to 6.3 to 8.4 METs. Initially, he will work at or below the lower end of the calculated THR range, with the emphasis on the duration of activity. As he becomes more active he will be able to work within the THR range, depending, of course, on his interests. He was referred for nutritional counseling to improve his blood lipid profile. Paul has an estimated HRmax of 174 beats · min^{-1}; his measured HR was 24 beats · min^{-1} higher. Given the inherent biological variation in the estimated HRmax, use the measured values when they are available.

10.2

Mary's maximal aerobic power was estimated to be about 1.65 L · min^{-1} by extrapolating the HR/work rate relationship to the predicted maximal heart rate (see chapter 5). This is equivalent to a $\dot{V}O_2max$ of 27 ml · kg^{-1} · min^{-1}, or 7.7 METs.

Her blood chemistry values and BP are normal. Her family history is negative for CHD. Her HR response to the test is normal and indicates poor cardiorespiratory fitness. The low maximal aerobic power is related to the sedentary lifestyle, the cigarette smoking (carbon monoxide), and the 30% body fatness. She was encouraged to participate in a smoking-cessation program and was given the names of two local professional groups.

The recommended exercise program emphasized the low end of the THR zone (70% HRmax: 127 beats · min^{-1}) with long duration. She preferred a walking program to begin with because of the freedom it gave her schedule. She was given the walking program in chapter 14 and was asked to record her HR response to each of the exercise sessions.

A body fatness goal of 22% resulted in a target body weight of 121 lb (55 kg). She did not feel the need for dietary counseling at this time, but she agreed to record her food intake for 10 days to determine the patterns of eating behavior that would be beneficial to change (see chapters 7 and 11). She made an appointment for a meeting with the HFI in 2 weeks to discuss the progress with her program.

11.1

Resting Metabolic Rate (see box on page 193)

$$65 \text{ in} \times 2.54 \text{ cm/in} = 165.1 \text{cm}$$

$$160 \text{ lb} / 2.2 \text{ lb/kg} = 72.7 \text{ kg}$$

$$655 + (1.8 \times 165.1) + (9.6 \times 72.7) - (4.7 \times 52) = \text{RMR } 1406 \text{ kcal}$$

Daily Caloric Needed (see box on page 194)

$$1406 \text{ kcal} \times 1.3 = 1828 \text{ kcal}$$

12.1

Beginners can make relatively large gains in strength by following any reasonable strength training program. Over time, however, it becomes more challenging to continually make strength gains, because as training proceeds, individuals approach their genetic potential. This member appears to have become "stale" because he has performed the same workout for 6 months. Changing the intensity, volume, and choice of exercise can help to keep the exercise stimulus effective. Although there are many different ways to alter this individual's workout plan, following a nonlinear periodized workout routine is an effective training method and easy for fitness members to follow. Thus, advising this member to vary his choice of exercises throughout the week and/or use moderate (8-10RM), heavy (4-6RM), and light loads (13-15RM) on alternate days would promote additional gains and prevent boredom. This can help to maximize gains and prevent the staleness that sometimes occurs after the initial adaptation period.

12.2

Despite preconceived concerns regarding the safety and appropriateness of strength training for children and seniors, conclusive research findings indicate that strength training can be safe, effective, and highly beneficial for people of all ages provided that appropriate training guidelines are followed. Although some children and seniors have been injured while strength training, a majority of injuries reported in the literature appear to be the result of improper exercise technique and/or inadequate supervision. Thus, your recommendations for program development regarding strength training for children and seniors should include the use of qualified instructors who understand the uniqueness of special populations and who would supervise program activities to ensure safe strength training procedures. Participants should be screened to identify any medical condition that may limit safe participation in the program activities. The training environment should be free of any potential hazards (e.g., free weights on the floor, broken or malfunctioning equipment), and the room should be adequately ventilated. Beginners should start with a light weight on all exercises, and the program should focus on learning proper exercise technique and having fun. Strength training 2 or 3 times a week on nonconsecutive days is recommended. If free weights are used, spotters should be nearby in case of a failed repetition. In addition to undertaking strength-building activities, children and seniors should be encouraged to participate in other physical activities that enhance aerobic fitness, flexibility, agility, and balance.

13.1

Although it is possible that this exercise might be appropriate for some individuals with well-developed abdominal musculature, it is not an appropriate exercise to give the masses since the quality of the movement is so critical. The individual with extremely well-developed abdominal muscles may be able to perform this exercise and keep his or her low back in contact with the exercise surface throughout its execution; however, the individual with weaker abdominals and/or tight hip flexors will invariably anteriorly tilt the pelvis, and the resulting lumbar lordosis places the lumbar vertebra in a potentially compromising position. Undoubtedly the physical therapists that use this activity use it only as a test on a one-to-one basis; this enables them to immediately stop the activity if they believe it is compromising to any individual.

13.2

It is good that the exercise leader emphasizes the importance of not doing ballistic stretches even from the sitting position; however, there are other factors that he/she should also consider. This maneuver is a fair exercise for use in attempting to improve hamstring extensibility. However, if the individual has extremely tight hamstrings (i.e., if the sacrum should be less than 80 to 90º with the exercise surface in the sit-and-reach), the forward stretching from this position could potentially stretch the tissues of the low back instead of the hamstrings. Therefore, for the individual with fairly tight hamstrings the sit-and- reach exercise may be contraindicated; the standing toe touch could be worse because of the effect of gravity on the moment arm of force.

13.3

Although isometric exercises have become less popular as a strength development activity in most applications (joint injury would be an exception), they can be used most appropriately for strengthening trunk musculature, assuming the exerciser does not have high blood pressure. The oblique curl could be particularly advantageous since the internal and external oblique muscles would have an important role in stabilization of the spine. This factor may decrease the likelihood of having low-back problems; for the individual who is symptomatic, the development of these muscles in this way may enable the individual to better maintain his/her neutral spine and avoid postures which exacerbate his/her condition.

14.1

Topics to address include

- attention to signs and symptoms that indicate problems and directions to act on them with a visit to their physician,
- proper shoes,
- clothing appropriate for the season, site (e.g., safety, surface, lighting),
- buddy system, where possible, to encourage participation, and
- alternate place in poor weather (shopping mall).

14.2

Before beginning an aerobic dance class, the participant should be able to walk 4 miles at a brisk pace with comfort. The appropriate transition from a walking program would be into a low-intensity, low-impact aerobics class. The participant should stay at the low end of the THR zone during this transition period and increase the intensity of the class only after these low-intensity, low-impact sessions can be comfortably completed.

15.1

Refer the parent to the recommendations for children, indicating that the emphasis should be on proper form, supervision, and endurance at this age. After puberty, he can include resistance training with fewer reps.

15.2

Acknowledge that reading and math are very important. The school needs to provide a good foundation in these areas, but it cannot possibly do it all—some will need to be done at home and in the community. The inclusion of physical activity (through physical education and recess) is essential for the health of the children (refer to table 15.4). Basic health is a prerequisite for other learning. In the same way, the school cannot provide all the physical activity recommended, but can provide a foundation that can be supplemented in the home and community.

16.1

You should begin by finding out when he had his last physical and what his physician told him relative to his arthritis. A submaximal cycle ergometer test should be carried out to obtain some base-line measures (heart rate, RPE) to use as reference points for subsequent follow-ups. Establish a target heart rate zone for him (50-70% of HRR), and verify that this elicits an RPE of about 10 to13. Have him begin his exercise program at 50% HRR, doing work/relief intervals (5-min on, 1 minute off) to determine if he can do a series of these with little or no joint discomfort. The goal is for 30 min of continuous activity as long as the discomfort is little or nothing. Increase the work interval to 10 min in the second week. If joint discomfort is a problem, stay with intervals within his tolerance. Intensity can be increased after he has achieved 30 min of total exercise time. Introduce him to a variety of weight-supported exercise modes (cycle, rower, water aerobics) that he should be able to use with less joint discomfort than he experienced with jogging. Workouts should be done 3 to 4 times per week and include regular warm-up and flexibility activities.

17.1

Since John is a 46-year old male with typical effort-induced angina and elevated total cholesterol/HDL ratio over 5.0 (signifying increased risk), he has a high likelihood of CHD. A reasonable step to take next would be to refer him for a graded exercise test (GXT) in the presence of a physician, to see if signs and/or symptoms of CHD occur. If they do, a more definitive diagnostic test such as coronary angiography might be recommended.

17.2

Jane's GXT results indicated that her maximal aerobic capacity was 7 METs; therefore, prescribing exercise at about 60% of this value, or around 4 METs, would be appropriate. Appropriate exercises would be treadmill walking, stationary cycling, and arm cranking. Realize that her maximal heart rate is low due to the fact that she is taking a beta-blocker. Thus, exercise could be prescribed on the basis of RPE (e.g., a target rating of "somewhat hard" on Borg's RPE scale). Light resistance exercises using dumbbells and elastic bands, as tolerated, would also be acceptable. The resistance should be selected so as to allow her to perform 12 to 15 repetitions with good form.

18.1

a. Because Marsha is hypertensive, has Class II obesity, is inactive, has a strong family history of cardiovascular disease and diabetes, and has not undergone a medical examination in several years, medical clearance prior to beginning an exercise program is recommended. The medical examination should be used to reveal if there are any underlying medical conditions that would make it unsafe for Marsha to engage in moderate to vigorous exercise.

b. In addition to height and weight, measurement of waist and hip circumference should be performed. In addition to BMI calculations, an estimate of body fat percentage could be useful, but only if methods are chosen that are both reliable and accurate for obese individuals (see chapter 6). Skinfold measurements are often not possible with obese clients. Bioelectrical impedance analysis could be used if obesity-specific equations are chosen. Air displacement plethysmography is also a good choice if available. Standard flexibility and strength tests should be performed. Cardiovascular fitness could be assessed with either a submaximal cycle ergometer or treadmill protocol.

c. The program design should incorporate Marsha's goals and exercise interests. Assuming that she is willing to invest in coming to your facility 3 times per week for one hour and then exercising on her own on other days, the following program would target a weight loss goal of 1 pound per week.

    - Exercise 6 days per week with approximately 300 kcal expended per session. Three days per week attend classes designed to address cardiorespiratory, strength, and flexibility needs. Three days per week walk approximately one hour (may be divided into two, 30-min sessions). This increase in activity will increase her caloric expenditure by approximately 1800 kcal per week.
    - Reduce caloric consumption to 250 kcal below estimated caloric need. Using formulas in chapter 11, Marsha's calculated daily caloric need is approximately 2175 kcal / d. Targeting her daily caloric intake to approximately 1925 kcal / d will result in a caloric deficit of 1750 kcal per week.

19.1

Dave displays many of the symptoms of overweight, inactive Americans including elevated plasma glucose, blood pressure, and LDL-C. As might be expected, his HDL-C and aerobic fitness are lower than recommended. His high BMI (38.7 kg / m^2) and low level of physical activity are the issues which Dave's physician wants to be addressed with his exercise program. His estimated daily caloric need is around 3000 kcal / day (see chapter 11). To lose approximately 1.5 pounds per week, he will need to establish a caloric deficit of around 5250 kcals. This will be accomplished through dietary restriction and increasing physical activity. This will lead to a weight reduction of approximately 18 pounds in 3 months.

Dietary plan—Limit total intake to 2250 to 2500 kcal / day. He will be particularly encouraged to reduce saturated fats and trans fatty acids. He will probably need educational materials on making healthy food choices.

Exercise plan—Begin aerobic and resistance training program. Dave will attend the exercise facility 3 days per week. On these days he will use a variety of aerobic exercise equipment to complete a total of 30 to 40 minutes (increase as tolerated and time available up to 60 min) of aerobic activity. Low-to-moderate intensity should be used. He will also use resistance training equipment to complete at least 1 set of 10 to 15 repetitions on 8 to 10 exercises (e.g., bench press, leg press, shoulder press, lat pulldowns). On at least 2 other days per week, he will be encouraged to walk briskly 2 to 3 miles. He may divide this distance into 2 sessions if desired. (Note: Because of Dave's low level of fitness and previous inactivity, he will probably need a few weeks of progression to meet these goals.)

20.1

It would be important to find out if she has worked with her physician and is currently not experiencing problems with her current medication. In addition, ask if she carries a bronchodilator with her to class, and determine that she knows how to use it at the onset of wheezing. Lastly, pay special attention to her during the early phases of the class.

20.2

The patient likely has emphysema and possibly bronchitis, two forms of chronic obstructive pulmonary disease (COPD) that commonly result from cigarette smoking. This is shown by his reduced ability to exhale air quickly ($FEV_{1.0}$). The logical course of treatment is a smoking cessation program, followed by a pulmonary rehabilitation program to help him regain his ability to exercise so that he can carry out functional activities of daily living (ADLs).

20.3

The patient has a limited ability to exercise, but intermittent treadmill walking on the level, cycle ergometry, and rowing would be suitable. Arm exercises with very light weights and stretch cord protocols for upper body conditioning are also appropriate. During physical training his oxygen saturation, ECG, and symptoms of dyspnea should be closely monitored. Supplemental oxygen will help to increase his oxygen saturation, maintaining it above 90%.

21.1

A resistance training program as well as impact-oriented aerobic activity is appropriate. A good start for this woman would be brisk walking (2+ miles) on most days of the week combined with resistance training focused on the large muscle groups of the chest, arms, legs, and back. Good resistance exercises include leg press (maybe squats if adequately taught and supervised), back extension, bench press, and military press. After an initial progression period, her goal should be 3 sets at around 70% of 1RM on three nonconsecutive days each week.

22.1

Dana is in the preparation stage and has low exercise self-efficacy. She has had a bad experience with exercise in the past, so you want to educate her about what to expect at the beginning of an exercise program and make sure the prescription is appropriate for her fitness level. Use the fitness evaluation to give her a realistic idea of her current fitness level and how much progress she can expect based on a sensible prescription. In setting goals with her, find out what *she* wants to achieve and activities she might enjoy. Brainstorm about barriers to exercise and how to counter them. Identify supports and ways she could reward herself during the program. Target her low exercise self-efficacy with a beginners' exercise class where she would have social support. Make sure she gets individual attention and encouragement, especially during the first few weeks. A behavioral contract with Mike doing something she wants him to do when she meets short-term goals could provide incentives and support she will need to keep her program going.

22.2

Jack is in the action stage and is especially susceptible to relapse. You could make a point of walking with Jack the next time he comes in to provide support and education about relapse prevention. Extra work at the end of the term is a high risk situation for him; he is discouraged and at risk of relapse. Talk with him about setting short-term goals that can be readjusting during exams. Help him to make the goals realistic and reachable. He might want to take "walk breaks" for 10 to 15 min during the days he can't get to the facility. Point out that these breaks will help him stay on track and give him a way to manage stress at work. Praise him for how far he has come and for continuing even though he is very busy. Help him see that the high risk situation is time limited, and brainstorm about ways he can reward himself for the walking he can do. Recruit veteran walkers to provide support and encouragement.

23.1

You might guess that Linda's days are full of interaction with people—children, employees, employers, and the public. The walking and jogging programs provided her with some time to be alone with her own thoughts without dealing with other people. You might start the conversation by telling Linda that you have missed her the past couple of weeks. Ask her what she liked about the first few months of the fitness program, what her fitness goals are, and what could be done to help her. If your guess about her wanting to be alone is correct, then emphasize that continuing in the running program is a good option for her exercise. You might suggest that she try cycling or swimming laps just for variety for some of her workouts. It is important for her to realize that it's okay for her to choose to have her individual exercise schedule and to tailor her program to her own interests.

24.1

a. HR = 1500 / 12 = 125 beats · min^{-1}
   P-R interval duration = 0.12 s
   QRS complex duration = 0.08 s
   Q-T interval duartion = 0.32 s
b. Sinus tachycardia—Fast heart rate over 100 beats · min^{-1}.
c. Common causes of sinus tachycardia are anziety, nervousness, caffeine, or low fitness level.

24.2

a. Atrial fibrillation—Jagged baseline with irregularly spaced PVCs.
b. Ventricular rate = 6 cardiac cycles in a 6-s strip × 10 = 60 beats · min^{-1}.

24.3

a. Trigeminy—Every third heart beat is a PVC.
b. You should gradually decrease treadmill speed and grade, and notify the physician.

24.4

Because the person was on Inderal (a nonselective β-blocker) at the time of his exercise test, his heart rate would have been suppressed. Now that he is no longer taking the medication, his previously calculated target HR will be too low. The exercise intensity should be adjusted upward.

24.5

Isordil contains nitroglycerin and is used to reduce the chance of having an angina attack. The drug relaxes vascular smooth muscle and might cause pooling of blood in the extremities. This pooling could cause a decrease in blood pressure and result in symptoms of dizziness.

25.1

a. Suspect insulin shock.
b. Ask the following questions: What happened? Are you a diabetic? Have you taken your insulin today? Have you eaten?
c. Check her Medic Alert tag. If insulin shock is still suspected, administer sugar (orange juice, candy, sugar granules). If she is unconscious or her recovery is slow (greater than 1-2 min), refer to a physician.

25.2

a. Suspect heat stroke.
b. Implement EMS—call 911. This is a medical emergency. Cool quickly, starting at the head and work down. Expose as much skin surface as possible. Monitor vital signs. Treat cramps by stretching and applying ice, direct pressure, and gentle massage. Treat for shock. Wrap in cold wet sheets for transport.
c. Emergency plans and materials should include
    - access to cooling agents, such as water, ice, ice towels, cool environment;
    - access to phone, with knowledge of EMS
    - knowledge of roles in emergency: person in charge, who assists person in charge, person responsible for making emergency phone call, who is to meet and direct the emergency vehicle to the injured; and
    - knowledge of rules to move person if necessary

26.1

You might use the following steps in your evaluation:

a. What are the expectations (based on written job descriptions and conversations with both the fitness director and the instructors)?
b. How can each expectation be evaluated?
c. Set up a procedure (including communication with both the fitness director and instructors) to evaluate each component of the job.
d. Share your evaluation with the Instructors, giving them a chance to add comments, before submitting it to the fitness director.

26.2

You might include the following in your evaluation:

a. Clearly describe of the fitness goals (long-range plan, official mission statements, statement from the program director).
b. Identify aspects of the program that relate to each goal (e.g., exercise to music and improvement in cardiorespiratory fitness).
c. Set up specific tests to determine each of the fitness goals, measuring before and after various experiences.
d. Set up systematic ways to determine individual satisfaction, enjoyment, and injuries associated with various aspects of the program.
e. Analyze the positive (and negative) changes that have occurred.
f. Recommend ways to improve future fitness goals.

27.1

Explain to the exerciser that the hip and knee extensor muscles that are used to push against the weights are also working to control the descent. The press requires concentric contraction; the return requires eccentric contraction. Both kinds of contractions lead to increases in strength.

27.2

When she's doing the wrist curls with her palms down (radioulnar pronated position), the wrist extensors are the contracting muscles; in the palms up position (supinated position), the wrist flexors are the working muscles. The wrist flexors are usually stronger than the wrist extensors.

The explanation is different for the pull-ups. The elbow flexor muscles are working regardless of the radioulnar joint position. However, when the palms are facing away (pronation), the distal tendon of the biceps brachii muscle is wrapped around the radius bone and therefore this muscle cannot exert as much force as when the palms are facing toward the body (supinated position).

27.3

He should make a conscious effort to maintain a backward pelvic tilt. He should also keep his arms in front of his head instead of by his ears and his knees slightly flexed to help him maintain the backward tilt.

28.1

The lactate threshold is the point during a graded exercise test when the blood lactic acid concentration suddenly increases. The lactate threshold has been used as an indicator of performance, in that the speed at which it occurs is closely related to the speed that can be maintained in distance runs (10K or marathon). As she improves her training, the lactate threshold occurs later into the GXT, indicating that she can maintain a faster pace in distance runs.

28.2

You need to confirm your client's feeling that the heart is stronger after training and, as a result, can pump more blood out per beat (increased stroke volume). As a result, the heart does not have to beat as many times to deliver the same amount of oxygen to the tissues. This is a more efficient way for the heart to pump blood, and in fact, the heart does not have to work as hard.

28.3

You might begin with a brief statement indicating that running speed in distance races is related to the amount of oxygen the runner can deliver to the muscles. The more oxygen that can be delivered, the faster the running speed. The elite female distance runner differs from the elite male distance runner in three ways that have a bearing on this issue: Heart size is smaller and she cannot pump as much oxygen-rich blood to the muscle per minute; the oxygen content of her blood is lower due to the lower hemoglobin concentration; and she is also carrying relatively more body fat that would have a negative impact on sustained running speed, even at the same level of fitness.

Calculation of Oxygen Uptake and Carbon Dioxide Production

Calculation of Oxygen Consumption ($\dot{V}O_2$)

The air we breathe is composed of 20.93% oxygen (O_2), 0.03% carbon dioxide (CO_2), and the balance, 79.04%, nitrogen (N_2). When we exhale, the fraction of the air represented by O_2 is decreased and the fraction represented by CO_2 is increased. To calculate the volume of O_2 used by the body ($\dot{V}O_2$), we simply subtract the number of liters of O_2 exhaled from the number of liters of O_2 inhaled. Equation 1 summarizes these words.

(1) Oxygen consumption =

[Volume of O_2 inhaled] –

[Volume of O_2 exhaled]

Now, using VO_2 to mean volume of *oxygen* used, V_I to mean volume of *air* inhaled, V_E to mean volume of *air* exhaled, F_{IO_2} to mean fraction of oxygen in inhaled air, and F_{EO_2} to mean fraction of oxygen in exhaled air, equation 1 can be written:

$$(2)\ VO_2 = [V_I \cdot F_{IO_2}] - [V_E \cdot F_{EO_2}]$$

You know that F_{IO_2} = 0.2093 and F_{EO_2} will be determined on an oxygen analyzer. Consequently, you are left with only two unknowns, the volume of air (liters) inhaled (V_I) and the volume of air (liters) exhaled (V_E). It appears that you must measure both volumes, but fortunately, this is not necessary. It was determined years ago that N_2 is neither used nor produced by the body. Consequently, the number of liters of N_2 inhaled must equal the number of liters of N_2 exhaled. Equation 3 states this equality using the symbols mentioned earlier.

$$(3)\ V_I \cdot F_{IN_2} = V_E \cdot F_{EN_2}$$

This is a very important relationship because it permits you to calculate V_E when V_I is known or vice versa. Using equation 3 here are two formulas, one to give V_E when V_I is known, and one to give V_I when V_E is known.

$$V_I = \frac{V_E \cdot F_{EN_2}}{F_{IN_2}} \qquad V_E = \frac{V_I \cdot F_{IN_2}}{F_{EN_2}}$$

Now that you know how to do this, there is only one other piece to the puzzle needed to permit you to calculate $\dot{V}O_2$. The value for F_{IN_2} is constant (0.7904) so we must determine F_{EN_2}. When the expired gas sample is analyzed you will obtain a value for F_{EO_2} and F_{ECO_2}, but not F_{EN_2}. However, since all the gas fractions must add up to 1.0000, you can calculate F_{EN_2}. (In the same way, we calculated F_{IN_2}: 1.0000 – .0003 (CO_2) – .2093 (O_2) = .7904.)

Problem: Calculate F_{EN_2} when F_{EO_2} = .1600 and F_{ECO_2} = .0450

Answer: F_{EN_2} = 1.0000 – .1600 – .0450 = .7950

The following problem shows how these equations are used. Given that V_I equals 100 L, F_{EO_2} = .1600, and F_{ECO_2} = .0450, calculate V_E.

$$V_E \cdot F_{EN_2} = V_I \cdot F_{IN_2}, \text{so } V_E = \frac{V_I \cdot F_{IN_2}}{F_{EN_2}}$$

$$F_{IN_2} = .7904 \text{ and}$$

$$F_{EN_2} = 1.0000 - .1600 - .0450 = .7950$$

$$V_E = 100 \text{ L} \cdot \frac{.7904}{.7950} = 99.4 \text{ L}$$

At this point, the equation for VO_2 can be rewritten, using V_I, V_E, F_{IO_2}, and F_{EO_2}.

$$VO_2 = V_I \cdot F_{IO_2} - V_E \cdot F_{EO_2}$$

Assuming that you measure only V_I this formula is rewritten:

$$VO_2 = V_I \cdot F_{IO_2} - \frac{V_I \cdot F_{IN_2}}{F_{EN_2}} \cdot F_{EO_2}$$

V_I can be factored out of this equation, so:

$$VO_2 = V_I \left[F_{IO_2} - \frac{F_{IN_2}}{F_{EN_2}} \cdot F_{EO_2} \right]$$

We will repeat the last two steps assuming that V_E is the volume that is measured and then factor out V_E.

$$VO_2 = \frac{V_E \cdot F_{EN_2}}{F_{IN_2}} \cdot F_{IO_2} - V_E \cdot F_{EO_2}$$

$$= V_E \left[\frac{F_{EN_2}}{F_{IN_2}} \cdot F_{IO_2} - F_{EO_2} \right]$$

At this point you know how to calculate VO_2. If you ever get stuck, always go back to the formula:

$VO_2 = V_I \cdot F_{IO_2} - V_E \cdot F_{EO_2}$ and simply substitute for V_E or V_I, depending on what was measured.

Some comments:

1. You must always match the volume measurement with the F_{EO_2} and F_{ECO_2} values measured in that expired volume. If you measure V_I for 2 min, you must have a single 2-min bag of expired gas to get F_{EO_2} and F_{ECO_2} values. If you measure a 30-s volume your expired bag must be collected over those 30 s.
2. VO_2 and VCO_2 are usually expressed in liters/min: the *rate* at which O_2 is used or CO_2 is produced per minute. To signify this *rate*, we write $\dot{V}O_2$ (read Vee dot). You would convert 30-s or 2-min volumes to 1-min values before making calculations of $\dot{V}O_2$.

Sample problem:

$\dot{V}_I = 100$ L/min, $F_{EO_2} = .1600$, $F_{ECO_2} = .0450$

Calculate $\dot{V}O_2$:

$$\dot{V}O_2 = \dot{V}_I \cdot F_{IO_2} - \dot{V}_E \cdot F_{EO_2}$$

$$\dot{V}_E = \frac{\dot{V}_I \cdot F_{IN_2}}{F_{EN_2}}$$

$$\dot{V}O_2 = \dot{V}_I \cdot F_{IO_2} - \frac{\dot{V}_I \cdot F_{IN_2}}{F_{EN_2}} \cdot F_{EO_2}$$

$$= \dot{V}_I \left[F_{IO_2} - \frac{F_{IN_2}}{F_{EN_2}} \cdot F_{EO_2} \right]$$

$$F_{EN_2} = 1.0000 - .1600 - .0450 = .7950$$

$$\dot{V}O_2 = 100 \text{ L/min} \left[.2093 - \frac{.7904}{.7950} \cdot .1600 \right]$$

$$= 5.02 \text{ L/min}$$

The volume (let's assume that $\dot{V}_E$ was measured) used in the above equations was measured at room temperature (23 °C) and at the barometric pressure of that moment (740 mmHg). The environmental conditions under which the volume was measured are called ambient conditions. If this volume of gas were transported to 10 000 feet above sea level, where the barometric pressure is lower, the volume would increase because of the reduced pressure. The volume of a gas varies inversely with pressure (at a constant temperature). Another factor influencing the volume of a gas is the temperature. If that volume, measured at 23 °C, were placed in a refrigerator at 0 °C, the volume of gas would decrease. The volume of gas varies directly with the temperature (at constant pressure).

Since the volume ($\dot{V}_E$) is influenced by both pressure and temperature, the value measured as O_2 used ($\dot{V}O_2$) might reflect changes in pressure or temperature, rather than a change in workload, training, and so on. Consequently, it would be convenient to express $\dot{V}_E$ in such a way as to make measurements comparable when they are obtained under different environmental conditions. This is done by standardizing the temperature, barometric pressure, and water vapor pressure at which the volume is expressed. By convention, volumes are expressed at Standard Temperature and Pressure, Dry (STPD): 273 °K (equals 0 °C), 760 mmHg pressure (sea level), and with no water vapor pressure. When $\dot{V}O_2$ is expressed STPD, you can calculate the number of molecules of oxygen actually used by the body because *at STPD one mole of oxygen equals 22.4 L.*

Let's make the correction to STPD one step at a time. Let's assume that a volume ($\dot{V}_E$) was measured at 740 mmHg, 23 °C and equaled 100 L/min. This *expired* volume is *always* saturated with water vapor.

To correct for temperature you use 273 °K as the standard (0 °C).

$$\text{Volume} \times \frac{273\ °\text{K}}{273\ °\text{K} + x\ °\text{C}} = \frac{273\ °\text{K}}{273 + 23}$$

$$100\ \text{L/min} \times \frac{273\ °\text{K}}{296\ °\text{K}} = 92.23\ \text{L/min}$$

When we make corrections for pressure we must remove the effect of water vapor pressure because the gas volume is adjusted on the basis of the standard pressure (760 mmHg), which is a dry pressure.

To correct the volume to the standard 760 mmHg pressure (dry) use:

$$\text{Volume} \times \frac{\text{barometric pressure} - \text{water vapor pressure}}{760\ \text{mmHg (dry)}}$$

Water vapor pressure is dependent on two things: the temperature and the relative humidity. In expired gas the gas volume is saturated (100% relative humidity). Consequently, you can obtain a value for water vapor pressure directly from the table below.

Going back to our pressure correction:

$$92.23\ \text{L/min} \times \frac{740 - 21.1}{760} = 87.24\ \text{L/min (STPD)}$$

To combine the temperature and pressure correction:

Temperature (°C)	Saturation water vapor pressure (mmHg)
18	15.5
19	16.5
20	17.5
21	18.7
22	19.8
23	21.1
24	22.4
25	23.8
26	25.2
27	26.7

$$100\ \text{L/min} \times \frac{273\ °\text{K}}{273\ °\text{K} + 23} \times \frac{740 - 21.1}{760} = 87.24\ \text{L/min (STPD)}$$

A special note must be made here. If you are using an inspired (inhaled) volume ($\dot{V}_I$), you are rarely dealing with a gas saturated with water vapor. Consequently, when you correct for pressure you must find what the water vapor is in the inspired air. You do this by finding the relative humidity of the air. You then multiply this value by the water vapor pressure value for saturated air at whatever the temperature is. To clarify, if your volume in the above example was $\dot{V}_I$ and had a relative humidity of 50%, the pressure correction would have been:

$$\text{Volume} \times \frac{740 - (.50 \times 21.1\ \text{mmHg})}{760\ \text{mmHg}}$$

While this may seem like a minor point, it is critical to the accurate measurement of $\dot{V}O_2$ that the proper water vapor correction be used. When you do calculations for $\dot{V}O_2$ you usually find the STPD factor first since you will be multiplying this factor by each volume measured.

Problem: Given $\dot{V}_I = 100$ L/min, $F_{EO_2} = .1700$, $F_{ECO_2} = .0385$. The temperature = 20 °C, barometric pressure = 740 mmHg, and the relative humidity = 30%.

Answer:

$$\text{STPD factor} = \frac{740\ \text{mmHg} - (.30)17.5\ \text{mmHg}}{760} \times \frac{273\ °\text{K}}{273\ °\text{K} + 20\ °\text{C}} = .900$$

$$100\ \text{L/min} \times .900 = 90\ \text{L/min STPD}$$

$$\dot{V}O_2 = \dot{V}_{I_{STPD}} \left[F_{IO_2} - \frac{F_{IN_2}}{F_{EN_2}} \cdot F_{EO_2} \right]$$

$$\dot{V}O_2 = 90\ \text{L/min} \left[.2093 - \frac{.7904}{.7915} \cdot .1700 \right]$$

$$\dot{V}O_2 = 3.56\ \text{L/min}$$

Carbon Dioxide Production ($\dot{V}CO_2$)

When O_2 is used, CO_2 is produced. The ratio of CO_2 production ($\dot{V}CO_2$) to O_2 consumption ($\dot{V}O_2$) is an important measurement in metabolism. This ratio ($\dot{V}CO_2 \div \dot{V}O_2$) is called the respiratory exchange ratio and is abbreviated as "R."

How do we measure $\dot{V}CO_2$? We start at the same step as for $\dot{V}O_2$:

$$\dot{V}CO_2 = \text{liters of } CO_2 \text{ expired} - \text{liters of } CO_2 \text{ inspired}$$

$$= \dot{V}_E \cdot F_{ECO_2} - \dot{V}_I \cdot F_{ICO_2}$$

The steps to follow are the same as for measuring $\dot{V}O_2$. Always use an STPD volume in your calculations. The following is the equation to use when $\dot{V}_I$ is measured:

$$\dot{V}CO_2 = \dot{V}_{I_{STPD}} \left[\frac{F_{IN_2}}{F_{EN_2}} \cdot F_{ECO_2} - F_{ICO_2} \right]$$

The following steps summarize the calculations for $\dot{V}CO_2$ and R for the previous problem.

$$\dot{V}CO_2 = 90 \text{ L / min} \left[\frac{.7904}{.7915} \cdot .0385 - .0003 \right]$$

$$= 3.43 \text{ L / min}$$

$$R = \dot{V}CO_2 \div \dot{V}O_2 = 3.43 \text{ L / min} \div 3.56 \text{ L / min}$$

$$R = .96$$

Energy Costs of Various Physical Activities

METS	SPECIFIC ACTIVITY	EXAMPLES
8.5	bicycling,	bicycling, BMX or mountain
4.0	bicycling,	bicycling, <10 mph, leisure, to work or for pleasure (Taylor Code 115)
8.0	bicycling,	bicycling, general
6.0	bicycling,	bicycling, 10-11.9 mph, leisure, slow, light effort
8.0	bicycling,	bicycling, 12-13.9 mph, leisure, moderate effort
10.0	bicycling,	bicycling, 14-15.9 mph, racing or leisure, fast, vigorous effort
12.0	bicycling,	bicycling, 16-19 mph, racing/not drafting or > 19 mph drafting, very fast, racing general
16.0	bicycling,	bicycling, >20 mph, racing, not drafting
5.0	bicycling,	unicycling
7.0	conditioning exercise,	bicycling, stationary, general
3.0	conditioning exercise,	bicycling, stationary, 50 watts, very light effort
5.5	conditioning exercise,	bicycling, stationary, 100 watts, light effort
7.0	conditioning exercise,	bicycling, stationary, 150 watts, moderate effort
10.5	conditioning exercise,	bicycling, stationary, 200 watts, vigorous effort
12.5	conditioning exercise,	bicycling, stationary, 250 watts, very vigorous effort
8.0	conditioning exercise,	calisthenics (e.g. pushups, sit ups, pull ups, jumping jacks), heavy, vigorous effort
3.5	conditioning exercise,	calisthenics, home exercise, light or moderate effort, general (example: back exercises), going up & down from floor (Taylor Code 150)
8.0	conditioning exercise,	circuit training, including some aerobic movement with minimal rest, general
6.0	conditioning exercise,	weight lifting (free weight, Nautilus or universal-type), power lifting or body building, vigorous effort (Taylor Code 210)
5.5	conditioning exercise,	health club exercise, general (Taylor Code 160)
9.0	conditioning exercise,	stair-treadmill ergometer, general
7.0	conditioning exercise,	rowing, stationary ergometer, general
3.5	conditioning exercise,	rowing, stationary, 50 watts, light effort
7.0	conditioning exercise,	rowing, stationary, 100 watts, moderate effort
8.5	conditioning exercise,	rowing, stationary, 150 watts, vigorous effort
12.0	conditioning exercise,	rowing, stationary, 200 watts, very vigorous effort
7.0	conditioning exercise,	ski machine, general
6.0	conditioning exercise,	Slimnastics, Jazzercise
2.5	conditioning exercise,	stretching, hatha yoga

(continued)

METS	SPECIFIC ACTIVITY	EXAMPLES
2.5	conditioning exercise,	mild stretching
6.0	conditioning exercise,	teaching aerobic exercise class
4.0	conditioning exercise,	water aerobics, water calisthenics
3.0	conditioning exercise,	weight lifting (free, Nautilus or universal-type), light or moderate effort, light workout, general
1.0	conditioning exercise,	whirlpool, sitting
4.8	dancing,	ballet or modern, twist, jazz, tap, jitterbug
6.5	dancing,	aerobic, general
8.5	dancing,	aerobic, step, with 6-8 inch step
10.0	dancing,	aerobic, step, with 10-12 inch step
5.0	dancing,	aerobic, low impact
7.0	dancing,	aerobic, high impact
4.5	dancing,	general, Greek, Middle Eastern, hula, flamenco, belly, swing
5.5	dancing,	ballroom, fast (Taylor Code 125)
4.5	dancing,	ballroom, fast (disco, folk, square), line dancing, Irish step dancing, polka, contra, country
3.0	dancing,	ballroom, slow (e.g. waltz, foxtrot, slow dancing), samba, tango, 19th C, mambo, chacha
5.5	dancing,	Anishinaabe Jingle Dancing or other traditional American Indian dancing
3.0	fishing and hunting,	fishing, general
4.0	fishing and hunting,	digging worms, with shovel
4.0	fishing and hunting,	fishing from river bank and walking
2.5	fishing and hunting,	fishing from boat, sitting
3.5	fishing and hunting,	fishing from river bank, standing (Taylor Code 660)
6.0	fishing and hunting,	fishing in stream, in waders (Taylor Code 670)
2.0	fishing and hunting,	fishing, ice, sitting
2.5	fishing and hunting,	hunting, bow and arrow or crossbow
6.0	fishing and hunting,	hunting, deer, elk, large game (Taylor Code 170)
2.5	fishing and hunting,	hunting, duck, wading
5.0	fishing and hunting,	hunting, general
6.0	fishing and hunting,	hunting, pheasants or grouse (Taylor Code 680)
5.0	fishing and hunting,	hunting, rabbit, squirrel, prairie chick, raccoon, small game (Taylor Code 690)
2.5	fishing and hunting,	pistol shooting or trap shooting, standing
3.3	home activities,	carpet sweeping, sweeping floors
3.0	home activities,	cleaning, heavy or major (e.g. wash car, wash windows, clean garage), vigorous effort
3.5	home activities,	mopping
2.5	home activities,	multiple household tasks all at once, light effort
3.5	home activities,	multiple household tasks all at once, moderate effort
4.0	home activities,	multiple household tasks all at once, vigorous effort
3.0	home activities,	cleaning, house or cabin, general
2.5	home activities,	cleaning, light (dusting, straightening up, changing linen, carrying out trash)
2.3	home activities,	wash dishes–standing or in general (not broken into stand/walk components)

(continued)

METS	SPECIFIC ACTIVITY	EXAMPLES
2.5	home activities,	wash dishes; clearing dishes from table–walking
3.5	home activities,	vacuuming
6.0	home activities,	butchering animals
2.0	home activities,	cooking or food preparation–standing or sitting or in general (not broken into stand/walk components), manual appliances
2.5	home activities,	serving food, setting table–implied walking or standing
2.5	home activities,	cooking or food preparation–walking
2.5	home activities,	feeding animals
2.5	home activities,	putting away groceries (e.g. carrying groceries, shopping without a grocery cart), carrying packages
7.5	home activities,	carrying groceries upstairs
3.0	home activities,	cooking Indian bread on an outside stove
2.3	home activities,	food shopping with or without a grocery cart, standing or walking
2.3	home activities,	non-food shopping, standing or walking
2.3	home activities,	ironing
1.5	home activities,	sitting–knitting, sewing, light wrapping (presents)
2.0	home activities,	implied standing–laundry, fold or hang clothes, put clothes in washer or dryer, packing suitcase
2.3	home activities,	implied walking–putting away clothes, gathering clothes to pack, putting away laundry
2.0	home activities,	making bed
5.0	home activities,	maple syruping/sugar bushing (including carrying buckets, carrying wood)
6.0	home activities,	moving furniture, household items, carrying boxes
3.8	home activities,	scrubbing floors, on hands and knees, scrubbing bathroom, bathtub
4.0	home activities,	sweeping garage, sidewalk or outside of house
3.5	home activities,	standing–packing/unpacking boxes, occasional lifting of household items light–moderate effort
3.0	home activities,	implied walking–putting away household items–moderate effort
2.5	home activities,	watering plants
2.5	home activities,	building a fire inside
9.0	home activities,	moving household items upstairs, carrying boxes or furniture
2.0	home activities,	standing–light (pump gas, change light bulb, etc.)
3.0	home activities,	walking–light, non-cleaning (readying to leave, shut/lock doors, close windows, etc.)
2.5	home activities,	sitting–playing with child(ren)–light, only active periods
2.8	home activities,	standing–playing with child(ren)–light, only active periods
4.0	home activities,	walk/run–playing with child(ren)–moderate, only active periods
5.0	home activities,	walk/run–playing with child(ren)–vigorous, only active periods
3.0	home activities,	carrying small children
2.5	home activities,	child care: sitting/kneeling–dressing, bathing, grooming, feeding, occasional lifting of child–light effort, general
3.0	home activities,	child care: standing–dressing, bathing, grooming, feeding, occasional lifting of child–light effort
4.0	home activities,	elder care, disabled adult, only active periods
1.5	home activities,	reclining with baby
2.5	home activities,	sit, playing with animals, light, only active periods

(continued)

METS	SPECIFIC ACTIVITY	EXAMPLES
2.8	home activities,	stand, playing with animals, light, only active periods
2.8	home activities,	walk/run, playing with animals, light, only active periods
4.0	home activities,	walk/run, playing with animals, moderate, only active periods
5.0	home activities,	walk/run, playing with animals, vigorous, only active periods
3.5	home activities,	standing–bathing dog
3.0	home repair,	airplane repair
4.0	home repair,	automobile body work
3.0	home repair,	automobile repair
3.0	home repair,	carpentry, general, workshop (Taylor Code 620)
6.0	home repair,	carpentry, outside house, installing rain gutters, building a fence, (Taylor Code 640)
4.5	home repair,	carpentry, finishing or refinishing cabinets or furniture
7.5	home repair,	carpentry, sawing hardwood
5.0	home repair,	caulking, chinking log cabin
4.5	home repair,	caulking, except log cabin
5.0	home repair,	cleaning gutters
5.0	home repair,	excavating garage
5.0	home repair,	hanging storm windows
4.5	home repair,	laying or removing carpet
4.5	home repair,	laying tile or linoleum, repairing appliances
5.0	home repair,	painting, outside home (Taylor Code 650)
3.0	home repair,	painting, papering, plastering, scraping, inside house, hanging sheet rock, remodeling
4.5	home repair,	painting, (Taylor Code 630)
3.0	home repair,	put on and removal of tarp–sailboat
6.0	home repair,	roofing
4.5	home repair,	sanding floors with a power sander
4.5	home repair,	scraping and painting sailboat or powerboat
5.0	home repair,	spreading dirt with a shovel
4.5	home repair,	washing and waxing hull of sailboat, car, powerboat, airplane
4.5	home repair,	washing fence, painting fence
3.0	home repair,	wiring, plumbing
1.0	inactivity,	lying quietly and watching television
1.0	quiet inactivity,	lying quietly, doing nothing, lying in bed awake, listening to music (not talking or reading)
1.0	quiet inactivity,	sitting quietly and watching television
1.0	quiet inactivity,	sitting quietly, sitting smoking, listening to music (not talking or reading), watching a movie in a theater
0.9	quiet inactivity,	sleeping
1.2	quiet inactivity,	standing quietly (standing in a line)
1.0	quiet inactivity,	reclining–writing
1.0	light inactivity,	reclining–talking or talking on phone
1.0	light inactivity,	reclining–reading
1.0	light inactivity,	meditating
5.0	light lawn and garden,	carrying, loading or stacking wood, loading/unloading or carrying lumber
6.0	lawn and garden,	chopping wood, splitting logs

(continued)

METS	SPECIFIC ACTIVITY	EXAMPLES
5.0	lawn and garden,	clearing land, hauling branches, wheelbarrow chores
5.0	lawn and garden,	digging sandbox
5.0	lawn and garden,	digging, spading, filling garden, composting, (Taylor Code 590)
6.0	lawn and garden,	gardening with heavy power tools, tilling a garden, chain saw
5.0	lawn and garden,	laying crushed rock
5.0	lawn and garden,	laying sod
5.5	lawn and garden,	mowing lawn, general
2.5	lawn and garden,	mowing lawn, riding mower (Taylor Code 550)
6.0	lawn and garden,	mowing lawn, walk, hand mower (Taylor Code 570)
5.5	lawn and garden,	mowing lawn, walk, power mower
4.5	lawn and garden,	mowing lawn, power mower (Taylor Code 590)
4.5	lawn and garden,	operating snow blower, walking
4.5	lawn and garden,	planting seedlings, shrubs
4.5	lawn and garden,	planting trees
4.3	lawn and garden,	raking lawn
4.0	lawn and garden,	raking lawn (Taylor Code 600)
4.0	lawn and garden,	raking roof with snow rake
3.0	lawn and garden,	riding snow blower
4.0	lawn and garden,	sacking grass, leaves
6.0	lawn and garden,	shoveling snow, by hand (Taylor Code 610)
4.5	lawn and garden,	trimming shrubs or trees, manual cutter
3.5	lawn and garden,	trimming shrubs or trees, power cutter, using leaf blower, edger
2.5	lawn and garden,	walking, applying fertilizer or seeding a lawn
1.5	lawn and garden,	watering lawn or garden, standing or walking
4.5	lawn and garden,	weeding, cultivating garden (Taylor Code 580)
4.0	lawn and garden,	gardening, general
3.0	lawn and garden,	picking fruit off trees, picking fruits/vegetables, moderate effort
3.0	lawn and garden,	implied walking/standing–picking up yard, light, picking flowers or vegetables
3.0	lawn and garden,	walking, gathering gardening tools
1.5	miscellaneous,	sitting–card playing, playing board games
2.3	miscellaneous,	standing–drawing (writing), casino gambling, duplicating machine
1.3	miscellaneous,	sitting–reading, book, newspaper, etc.
1.8	miscellaneous,	sitting–writing, desk work, typing
1.8	miscellaneous,	standing–talking or talking on the phone
1.5	miscellaneous,	sitting–talking or talking on the phone
1.8	miscellaneous,	sitting–studying, general, including reading and/or writing
1.8	miscellaneous,	sitting–in class, general, including note-taking or class discussion
1.8	miscellaneous,	standing–reading
2.0	miscellaneous,	standing–miscellaneous
1.5	miscellaneous,	sitting–arts and crafts, light effort
2.0	miscellaneous,	sitting–arts and crafts, moderate effort
1.8	miscellaneous,	standing–arts and crafts, light effort
3.0	miscellaneous,	standing–arts and crafts, moderate effort
3.5	miscellaneous,	standing–arts and crafts, vigorous effort
1.5	miscellaneous,	retreat/family reunion activities involving sitting, relaxing, talking, eating

(continued)

METS	SPECIFIC ACTIVITY	EXAMPLES
2.0	miscellaneous,	touring/traveling/vacation involving walking and riding
2.5	miscellaneous,	camping involving standing, walking, sitting, light-to-moderate effort
1.5	miscellaneous,	sitting at a sporting event, spectator
1.8	music playing,	accordion
2.0	music playing,	cello
2.5	music playing,	conducting
4.0	music playing,	drums
2.0	music playing,	flute (sitting)
2.0	music playing,	horn
2.5	music playing,	piano or organ
3.5	music playing,	trombone
2.5	music playing,	trumpet
2.5	music playing,	violin
2.0	music playing,	woodwind
2.0	music playing,	guitar, classical, folk (sitting)
3.0	music playing,	guitar, rock and roll band (standing)
4.0	music playing,	marching band, playing an instrument, baton twirling (walking)
3.5	music playing,	marching band, drum major (walking)
4.0	occupation,	bakery, general, moderate effort
2.5	occupation,	bakery, light effort
2.3	occupation,	bookbinding
6.0	occupation,	building road (including hauling debris, driving heavy machinery)
2.0	occupation,	building road, directing traffic (standing)
3.5	occupation,	carpentry, general
8.0	occupation,	carrying heavy loads, such as bricks
8.0	occupation,	carrying moderate loads up stairs, moving boxes (16-40 lbs)
2.5	occupation,	chambermaid, making bed (nursing)
6.5	occupation,	coal mining, drilling coal, rock
6.5	occupation,	coal mining, erecting supports
6.0	occupation,	coal mining, general
7.0	occupation,	coal mining, shoveling coal
5.5	occupation,	construction, outside, remodeling
3.0	occupation,	custodial work–buffing the floor with electric buffer
2.5	occupation,	custodial work–cleaning sink and toilet, light effort
2.5	occupation,	custodial work–dusting, light effort
4.0	occupation,	custodial work–feathering arena floor, moderate effort
3.5	occupation,	custodial work–general cleaning, moderate effort
3.5	occupation,	custodial work–mopping, moderate effort
3.0	occupation,	custodial work–take out trash, moderate effort
2.5	occupation,	custodial work–vacuuming, light effort
3.0	occupation,	custodial work–vacuuming, moderate effort
3.5	occupation,	electrical work, plumbing
8.0	occupation,	farming, baling hay, cleaning barn, poultry work, vigorous effort
3.5	occupation,	farming, chasing cattle, non-strenuous (walking), moderate effort
4.0	occupation,	farming, chasing cattle or other livestock on horseback, moderate effort

(continued)

METS	SPECIFIC ACTIVITY	EXAMPLES
2.0	occupation,	farming, chasing cattle or other livestock, driving, light effort
2.5	occupation,	farming, driving harvester, cutting hay, irrigation work
2.5	occupation,	farming, driving tractor
4.0	occupation,	farming, feeding small animals
4.5	occupation,	farming, feeding cattle, horses
4.5	occupation,	farming, hauling water for animals, general hauling water
6.0	occupation,	farming, taking care of animals (grooming, brushing, shearing sheep, assisting with birthing, medical care, branding)
8.0	occupation,	farming, forking straw bales, cleaning corral or barn, vigorous effort
3.0	occupation,	farming, milking by hand, moderate effort
1.5	occupation,	farming, milking by machine, light effort
5.5	occupation,	farming, shoveling grain, moderate effort
12.0	occupation,	fire fighter, general
11.0	occupation,	fire fighter, climbing ladder with full gear
8.0	occupation,	fire fighter, hauling hoses on ground
17.0	occupation,	forestry, ax chopping, fast
5.0	occupation,	forestry, ax chopping, slow
7.0	occupation,	forestry, barking trees
11.0	occupation,	forestry, carrying logs
8.0	occupation,	forestry, felling trees
8.0	occupation,	forestry, general
5.0	occupation,	forestry, hoeing
6.0	occupation,	forestry, planting by hand
7.0	occupation,	forestry, sawing by hand
4.5	occupation,	forestry, sawing, power
9.0	occupation,	forestry, trimming trees
4.0	occupation,	forestry, weeding
4.5	occupation,	furriery
6.0	occupation,	horse grooming
8.0	occupation,	horse racing, galloping
6.5	occupation,	horse racing, trotting
2.6	occupation,	horse racing, walking
3.5	occupation,	locksmith
2.5	occupation,	machine tooling, machining, working sheet metal
3.0	occupation,	machine tooling, operating lathe
5.0	occupation,	machine tooling, operating punch press
4.0	occupation,	machine tooling, tapping and drilling
3.0	occupation,	machine tooling, welding
7.0	occupation,	masonry, concrete
4.0	occupation,	masseur, masseuse (standing)
7.5	occupation,	moving, pushing heavy objects, 75 lbs or more (desks, moving van work)
12.0	occupation,	skindiving or SCUBA diving as a frogman (Navy Seal)
2.5	occupation,	operating heavy duty equipment/automated, not driving
4.5	occupation,	orange grove work
2.3	occupation,	printing (standing)

(continued)

METS	SPECIFIC ACTIVITY	EXAMPLES
2.5	occupation,	police, directing traffic (standing)
2.0	occupation,	police, driving a squad car (sitting)
1.3	occupation,	police, riding in a squad car (sitting)
4.0	occupation,	police, making an arrest (standing)
2.5	occupation,	shoe repair, general
8.5	occupation,	shoveling, digging ditches
9.0	occupation,	shoveling, heavy (more than 16 lbs/min)
6.0	occupation,	shoveling, light (less than 10 lbs/min)
7.0	occupation,	shoveling, moderate (10 to 15 lbs/min)
1.5	occupation,	sitting–light office work, general (chemistry lab work, light use of hand tools, watch repair or micro-assembly, light assembly/repair), sitting, reading, driving at work
1.5	occupation,	sitting–meetings, general, and/or with talking involved, eating at a business meeting
2.5	occupation,	sitting; moderate (heavy levers, riding mower/forklift, crane operation), teaching stretching or yoga
2.3	occupation,	standing; light (bartending, store clerk, assembling, filing, duplicating, putting up a Christmas tree), standing and talking at work, changing clothes when teaching physical education
3.0	occupation,	standing; light/moderate (assemble/repair heavy parts, welding, stocking, auto repair, pack boxes for moving, etc.), patient care (as in nursing)
4.0	occupation,	lifting items continuously, 10-20 lbs, with limited walking or resting
3.5	occupation,	standing; moderate (assembling at fast rate, intermittent, lifting 50 lbs, hitch/twisting ropes)
4.0	occupation,	standing; moderate/heavy (lifting more than 50 lbs, masonry, painting, paper hanging)
5.0	occupation,	steel mill, fettling
5.5	occupation,	steel mill, forging
8.0	occupation,	steel mill, hand rolling
8.0	occupation,	steel mill, merchant mill rolling
11.0	occupation,	steel mill, removing slag
7.5	occupation,	steel mill, tending furnace
5.5	occupation,	steel mill, tipping molds
8.0	occupation,	steel mill, working in general
2.5	occupation,	tailoring, cutting
2.5	occupation,	tailoring, general
2.0	occupation,	tailoring, hand sewing
2.5	occupation,	tailoring, machine sewing
4.0	occupation,	tailoring, pressing
3.5	occupation,	tailoring, weaving
6.5	occupation,	truck driving, loading and unloading truck (standing)
1.5	occupation,	typing, electric, manual or computer
6.0	occupation,	using heavy power tools such as pneumatic tools (jackhammers, drills, etc.)
8.0	occupation,	using heavy tools (not power) such as shovel, pick, tunnel bar, spade
2.0	occupation,	walking on job, less than 2.0 mph (in office or lab area), very slow

(continued)

METS	SPECIFIC ACTIVITY	EXAMPLES
3.3	occupation,	walking on job, 3.0 mph, in office, moderate speed, not carrying anything
3.8	occupation,	walking on job, 3.5 mph, in office, brisk speed, not carrying anything
3.0	occupation,	walking, 2.5 mph, slowly and carrying light objects less than 25 lbs
3.0	occupation,	walking, gathering things at work, ready to leave
4.0	occupation,	walking, 3.0 mph, moderately and carrying light objects less than 25 lbs
4.0	occupation,	walking, pushing a wheelchair
4.5	occupation,	walking, 3.5 mph, briskly and carrying objects less than 25 lbs
5.0	occupation,	walking or walk downstairs or standing, carrying objects about 25 to 49 lbs
6.5	occupation,	walking or walk downstairs or standing, carrying objects about 50 to 74 lbs
7.5	occupation,	walking or walk downstairs or standing, carrying objects about 75 to 99 lbs
8.5	occupation,	walking or walk downstairs or standing, carrying objects about 100 lbs or more
3.0	occupation,	working in scene shop, theater actor, backstage employee
4.0	occupation,	teach physical education, exercise, sports classes (non-sport play)
6.5	occupation,	teach physical education, exercise, sports classes (participate in the class)
6.0	running,	jog/walk combination (jogging component of less than 10 min) (Taylor Code 180)
7.0	running,	jogging, general
8.0	running,	jogging, in place
4.5	running,	jogging on a mini-tramp
8.0	running,	running, 5 mph (12 min/mile)
9.0	running,	running, 5.2 mph (11.5 min/mile)
10.0	running,	running, 6 mph (10 min/mile)
11.0	running,	running, 6.7 mph (9 min/mile)
11.5	running,	running, 7 mph (8.5 min/mile)
12.5	running,	running, 7.5 mph (8 min/mile)
13.5	running,	running, 8 mph (7.5 min/mile)
14.0	running,	running, 8.6 mph (7 min/mile)
15.0	running,	running, 9 mph (6.5 min/mile)
16.0	running,	running, 10 mph (6 min/mile)
18.0	running,	running, 10.9 mph (5.5 min/mile)
9.0	running,	running, cross country
8.0	running,	running (Taylor Code 200)
15.0	running,	running, stairs, up
10.0	running,	running, on a track, team practice
8.0	running,	running, training, pushing a wheelchair
2.0	self care,	standing–getting ready for bed, in general
1.0	self care,	sitting on toilet
1.5	self care,	bathing (sitting)
2.0	self care,	dressing, undressing (standing or sitting)
1.5	self care,	eating (sitting)
2.0	self care,	talking and eating or eating only (standing)

(continued)

METS	SPECIFIC ACTIVITY	EXAMPLES
1.0	self care,	taking medication, sitting or standing
2.0	self care,	grooming (washing, shaving, brushing teeth, urinating, washing hands, putting on make-up), sitting or standing
2.5	self care,	hairstyling
1.0	self care,	having hair or nails done by someone else, sitting
2.0	self care,	showering, toweling off (standing)
1.5	sexual activity,	active, vigorous effort
1.3	sexual activity,	general, moderate effort
1.0	sexual activity,	passive, light effort, kissing, hugging
3.5	sports,	archery (non-hunting)
7.0	sports,	badminton, competitive (Taylor Code 450)
4.5	sports,	badminton, social singles and doubles, general
8.0	sports,	basketball, game (Taylor Code 490)
6.0	sports,	basketball, non-game, general (Taylor Code 480)
7.0	sports,	basketball, officiating (Taylor Code 500)
4.5	sports,	basketball, shooting baskets
6.5	sports,	basketball, wheelchair
2.5	sports,	billiards
3.0	sports,	bowling (Taylor Code 390)
12.0	sports,	boxing, in ring, general
6.0	sports,	boxing, punching bag
9.0	sports,	boxing, sparring
7.0	sports,	broomball
5.0	sports,	children's games (hopscotch, 4-square, dodge ball, playground apparatus, t-ball, tetherball, marbles, jacks, acrace games)
4.0	sports,	coaching: football, soccer, basketball, baseball, swimming, etc.
5.0	sports,	cricket (batting, bowling)
2.5	sports,	croquet
4.0	sports,	curling
2.5	sports,	darts, wall or lawn
6.0	sports,	drag racing, pushing or driving a car
6.0	sports,	fencing
9.0	sports,	football, competitive
8.0	sports,	football, touch, flag, general (Taylor Code 510)
2.5	sports,	football or baseball, playing catch
3.0	sports,	Frisbee playing, general
8.0	sports,	Frisbee, ultimate
4.5	sports,	golf, general
4.5	sports,	golf, walking and carrying clubs
3.0	sports,	golf, miniature, driving range
4.3	sports,	golf, walking and pulling clubs
3.5	sports,	golf, using power cart (Taylor Code 070)
4.0	sports,	gymnastics, general
4.0	sports,	hacky sack
12.0	sports,	handball, general (Taylor Code 520)
8.0	sports,	handball, team

(continued)

METS	SPECIFIC ACTIVITY	EXAMPLES
3.5	sports,	hang gliding
8.0	sports,	hockey, field
8.0	sports,	hockey, ice
4.0	sports,	horseback riding, general
3.5	sports,	horseback riding, saddling horse, grooming horse
6.5	sports,	horseback riding, trotting
2.5	sports,	horseback riding, walking
3.0	sports,	horseshoe pitching, quoits
12.0	sports,	jai alai
10.0	sports,	judo, jujitsu, karate, kick boxing, tae kwan do
4.0	sports,	juggling
7.0	sports,	kickball
8.0	sports,	lacrosse
4.0	sports,	motor-cross
9.0	sports,	orienteering
10.0	sports,	paddleball, competitive
6.0	sports,	paddleball, casual, general (Taylor Code 460)
8.0	sports,	polo
10.0	sports,	racquetball, competitive
7.0	sports,	racquetball, casual, general (Taylor Code 470)
11.0	sports,	rock climbing, ascending rock
8.0	sports,	rock climbing, rappelling
12.0	sports,	rope jumping, fast
10.0	sports,	rope jumping, moderate, general
8.0	sports,	rope jumping, slow
10.0	sports,	rugby
3.0	sports,	shuffleboard, lawn bowling
5.0	sports,	skateboarding
7.0	sports,	skating, roller (Taylor Code 360)
12.5	sports,	roller blading (in-line skating)
3.5	sports,	sky diving
10.0	sports,	soccer, competitive
7.0	sports,	soccer, casual, general (Taylor Code 540)
5.0	sports,	softball or baseball, fast or slow pitch, general (Taylor Code 440)
4.0	sports,	softball, officiating
6.0	sports,	softball, pitching
12.0	sports,	squash (Taylor Code 530)
4.0	sports,	table tennis, ping pong (Taylor Code 410)
4.0	sports,	tai chi
7.0	sports,	tennis, general
6.0	sports,	tennis, doubles (Taylor Code 430)
5.0	sports,	tennis, doubles
8.0	sports,	tennis, singles (Taylor Code 420)
3.5	sports,	trampoline
4.0	sports,	volleyball (Taylor Code 400)
8.0	sports,	volleyball, competitive, in gymnasium

(continued)

METS	SPECIFIC ACTIVITY	EXAMPLES
3.0	sports,	volleyball, non-competitive, 6-9 member team, general
8.0	sports,	volleyball, beach
6.0	sports,	wrestling (one match = 5 min)
7.0	sports,	wallyball, general
4.0	sports,	track and field (shot, discus, hammer throw)
6.0	sports,	track and field (high jump, long jump, triple jump, javelin, pole vault)
10.0	sports,	track and field (steeplechase, hurdles)
2.0	transportation,	automobile or light truck (not a semi) driving
1.0	transportation,	riding in a car or truck
1.0	transportation,	riding in a bus
2.0	transportation,	flying airplane
2.5	transportation,	motor scooter, motorcycle
6.0	transportation,	pushing plane in and out of hangar
3.0	transportation,	driving heavy truck, tractor, bus
7.0	walking,	backpacking (Taylor Code 050)
3.5	walking,	carrying infant or 15 lb load (e.g. suitcase), level ground or down stairs
9.0	walking,	carrying load upstairs, general
5.0	walking,	carrying 1 to 15 lb load, upstairs
6.0	walking,	carrying 16 to 24 lb load, upstairs
8.0	walking,	carrying 25 to 49 lb load, upstairs
10.0	walking,	carrying 50 to 74 lb load, upstairs
12.0	walking,	carrying 74+ lb load, upstairs
3.0	walking,	loading unloading a car
7.0	walking,	climbing hills with 0 to 9 lb load
7.5	walking,	climbing hills with 10 to 20 lb load
8.0	walking,	climbing hills with 21 to 42 lb load
9.0	walking,	climbing hills with 42+ lb load
3.0	walking,	downstairs
6.0	walking,	hiking, cross country (Taylor Code 040)
2.5	walking,	bird watching
6.5	walking,	marching, rapidly, military
2.5	walking,	pushing or pulling stroller with child or walking with children
4.0	walking,	pushing a wheelchair, non-occupational setting
6.5	walking,	race walking
8.0	walking,	rock or mountain climbing (Taylor Code 060)
8.0	walking,	up stairs, using or climbing up ladder (Taylor Code 030)
5.0	walking,	using crutches
2.0	walking,	walking, household
2.0	walking,	walking, less than 2.0 mph, level ground, strolling, very slow
2.5	walking,	walking, 2.0 mph, level, slow pace, firm surface
3.5	walking,	walking for pleasure (Taylor Code 010)
2.5	walking,	walking from house to car or bus, from car or bus to go places, from car or bus to and from the worksite
2.5	walking,	walking to neighbor's house or family's house for social reasons
3.0	walking,	walking the dog

(continued)

METS	SPECIFIC ACTIVITY	EXAMPLES
3.0	walking,	walking, 2.5 mph, firm surface
2.8	walking,	walking, 2.5 mph, downhill
3.3	walking,	walking, 3.0 mph, level, moderate pace, firm surface
3.8	walking,	walking, 3.5 mph, level, brisk, firm surface, walking for exercise
6.0	walking,	walking, 3.5 mph, uphill
5.0	walking,	walking, 4.0 mph, level, firm surface, very brisk pace
6.3	walking,	walking, 4.5 mph, level, firm surface, very, very brisk
8.0	walking,	walking, 5.0 mph
3.5	walking,	walking, for pleasure, work break
5.0	walking,	walking, grass track
4.0	walking,	walking, to work or class (Taylor Code 015)
2.5	walking,	walking to and from an outhouse
2.5	water activities,	boating, power
4.0	water activities,	canoeing, on camping trip (Taylor Code 270)
3.3	water activities,	canoeing, harvesting wild rice, knocking rice off the stalks
7.0	water activities,	canoeing, portaging
3.0	water activities,	canoeing, rowing, 2.0-3.9 mph, light effort
7.0	water activities,	canoeing, rowing, 4.0-5.9 mph, moderate effort
12.0	water activities,	canoeing, rowing, >6 mph, vigorous effort
3.5	water activities,	canoeing, rowing, for pleasure, general (Taylor Code 250)
12.0	water activities,	canoeing, rowing, in competition, or crew or sculling (Taylor Code 260)
3.0	water activities,	diving, springboard or platform
5.0	water activities,	kayaking
4.0	water activities,	paddle boat
3.0	water activities,	sailing, boat and board sailing, windsurfing, ice sailing, general (Taylor Code 235)
5.0	water activities,	sailing, in competition
3.0	water activities,	sailing, Sunfish/Laser/Hobby Cat, Keel boats, ocean sailing, yachting
6.0	water activities,	skiing, water (Taylor Code 220)
7.0	water activities,	skimobiling
16.0	water activities,	skindiving, fast
12.5	water activities,	skindiving, moderate
7.0	water activities,	skindiving, scuba diving, general (Taylor Code 310)
5.0	water activities,	snorkeling (Taylor Code 320)
3.0	water activities,	surfing, body or board
10.0	water activities,	swimming laps, freestyle, fast, vigorous effort
7.0	water activities,	swimming laps, freestyle, slow, moderate or light effort
7.0	water activities,	swimming, backstroke, general
10.0	water activities,	swimming, breaststroke, general
11.0	water activities,	swimming, butterfly, general
11.0	water activities,	swimming, crawl, fast (75 yards/min), vigorous effort
8.0	water activities,	swimming, crawl, slow (50 yards/min), moderate or light effort
6.0	water activities,	swimming, lake, ocean, river (Taylor Codes 280, 295)
6.0	water activities,	swimming, leisurely, not lap swimming, general
8.0	water activities,	swimming, sidestroke, general
8.0	water activities,	swimming, synchronized

(continued)

METS	SPECIFIC ACTIVITY	EXAMPLES
10.0	water activities,	swimming, treading water, fast vigorous effort
4.0	water activities,	swimming, treading water, moderate effort, general
4.0	water activities,	water aerobics, water calisthenics
10.0	water activities,	water polo
3.0	water activities,	water volleyball
8.0	water activities,	water jogging
5.0	water activities,	whitewater rafting, kayaking, or canoeing
6.0	winter activities,	moving ice house (set up/drill holes, etc.)
5.5	winter activities,	skating, ice, 9 mph or less
7.0	winter activities,	skating, ice, general (Taylor Code 360)
9.0	winter activities,	skating, ice, rapidly, more than 9 mph
15.0	winter activities,	skating, speed, competitive
7.0	winter activities,	ski jumping (climb up carrying skis)
7.0	winter activities,	skiing, general
7.0	winter activities,	skiing, cross country, 2.5 mph, slow or light effort, ski walking
8.0	winter activities,	skiing, cross country, 4.0-4.9 mph, moderate speed and effort, general
9.0	winter activities,	skiing, cross country, 5.0-7.9 mph, brisk speed, vigorous effort
14.0	winter activities,	skiing, cross country, >8.0 mph, racing
16.5	winter activities,	skiing, cross country, hard snow, uphill, maximum, snow mountaineering
5.0	winter activities,	skiing, downhill, light effort
6.0	winter activities,	skiing, downhill, moderate effort, general
8.0	winter activities,	skiing, downhill, vigorous effort, racing
7.0	winter activities,	sledding, tobogganing, bobsledding, luge (Taylor Code 370)
8.0	winter activities,	snow shoeing
3.5	winter activities,	snowmobiling
1.0	religious activities,	sitting in church, in service, attending a ceremony, sitting quietly
2.5	religious activities,	sitting, playing an instrument at church
1.5	religious activities,	sitting in church, talking or singing, attending a ceremony, sitting, active participation
1.3	religious activities,	sitting, reading religious materials at home
1.2	religious activities,	standing in church (quietly), attending a ceremony, standing quietly
2.0	religious activities,	standing, singing in church, attending a ceremony, standing, active participation
1.0	religious activities,	kneeling in church/at home (praying)
1.8	religious activities,	standing, talking in church
2.0	religious activities,	walking in church
2.0	religious activities,	walking, less than 2.0 mph–very slow
3.3	religious activities,	walking, 3.0 mph, moderate speed, not carrying anything
3.8	religious activities,	walking, 3.5 mph, brisk speed, not carrying anything
2.0	religious activities,	walk/stand combination for religious purposes, usher
5.0	religious activities,	praise with dance or run, spiritual dancing in church
2.5	religious activities,	serving food at church
2.0	religious activities,	preparing food at church
2.3	religious activities,	washing dishes/cleaning kitchen at church

(continued)

METS	SPECIFIC ACTIVITY	EXAMPLES
1.5	religious activities,	eating at church
2.0	religious activities,	eating/talking at church or standing eating, American Indian Feast days
3.0	religious activities,	cleaning church
5.0	religious activities,	general yard work at church
2.5	religious activities,	standing–moderate (lifting 50 lbs., assembling at fast rate)
4.0	religious activities,	standing–moderate/heavy work
1.5	religious activities,	typing, electric, manual, or computer
1.5	volunteer activities,	sitting–meeting, general, and/or with talking involved
1.5	volunteer activities,	sitting–light office work, in general
2.5	volunteer activities,	sitting–moderate work
2.3	volunteer activities,	standing–light work (filing, talking, assembling)
2.5	volunteer activities,	sitting, child care, only active periods
3.0	volunteer activities,	standing, child care, only active periods
4.0	volunteer activities,	walk/run play with children, moderate, only active periods
5.0	volunteer activities,	walk/run play with children, vigorous, only active periods
3.0	volunteer activities,	standing–light/moderate work (pack boxes, assemble/repair, set up chairs/furniture)
3.5	volunteer activities,	standing–moderate (lifting 50 lbs., assembling at fast rate)
4.0	volunteer activities,	standing–moderate/heavy work
1.5	volunteer activities,	typing, electric, manual, or computer
2.0	volunteer activities,	walking, less than 2.0 mph, very slow
3.3	volunteer activities,	walking, 3.0 mph, moderate speed, not carrying anything
3.8	volunteer activities,	walking, 3.5 mph, brisk speed, not carrying anything
3.0	volunteer activities,	walking, 2.5 mph slowly and carrying objects less than 25 lbs
4.0	volunteer activities,	walking, 3.0 mph moderately and carrying objects less than 25 lbs, pushing something
4.5	volunteer activities,	walking, 3.5 mph, briskly and carrying objects less than 25 lbs
3.0	volunteer activities,	walk/stand combination, for volunteer purposes

From Ainsworth, B.E., Haskell, W.L., Whitt, M.C., Irwin, M.L., Swartz, A.M., Strath, S.J., O'Brien, W.L., Bassett, D.R., Jr., Schmitz, K.H., Emplaincourt, P.O., Jacobs, D.R., Jr., and Leon, A.S., Jacobs, D.R., Jr., (2000). Compendium of physical activities: An update of activity codes and MET intensities. *Medicine and Science in Sports and Exercise,* **32**(9):S498-S516. Additional values from Montoye, H.J., Kemper, H.C.G., Saris, W.H.M., and Washburn, R.A. (1996). *Measuring physical activity and energy expenditure.* Champaign, IL: Human Kinetics.

appendix D

Medications and Their Effects

Generic and Brand Names of Common Drugs by Class

Generic name	Brand name*
Beta blockers	
Acebutolol	Sectral
Atenolol	Tenormin
Betaxolal	Kerlone
Bisoprolol	Zebeta
Carteolol	Cartrol
Esmolol	Brevibloc
Metoprolol	Lopressor, Toprol
Nadolol	Corgard
Penbutolol	Levatol
Pindolol	Visken
Propranolol	Inderal
Sotalol	Betapace
Timolol	Blocadren
Beta blockers in combinations with	
Diuretics	Inderide, Lopressor Hydrochlorothiazide (HCTZ), Tenoretic, Timolide, Ziac, Corzide
Alpha- and beta-adrenergic blocking agents	
Carvedilol	Coreg
Labetalol	Trandate, Normodyne
Alpha$_1$-adrenergic blocking agents	
Doxazosin	Cardura
Prazosin	Minipress
Terazosin	Hytrin
Antiadrenergic agents without selective receptor blockade	
Clonidine	Catapres
Guanabenz	Wyntensin
Guanadrel	Hylorel
Guanethidine	Ismelin
Guanfacine	Tenex
Methyldopa	Aldomet
Reserpine	Serapasil
Nitrates and nitroglycerin	
Amyl nitrite	Amyl nitrite
Isosorbide mononitrate	Ismo, Monoket, Imdur

(continued)

Generic and Brand Names of Common Drugs by Class

Generic name	Brand name*
Isosorbide dinitrate	Isordil, Sorbitrate, Dilatrate
Nitroglycerin, sublingual	Nitrostat
Nitroglycerin, translingual	Nitrolingual
Nitroglycerin, transmucosal	Nitrogard
Nitroglycerin, sustained release	Nitrong, Nitrocine, Nitroglyn, Nitro-Bid
Nitroglycerin, transdermal	Minitran, Nitro-Dur, Transderm-Nitro, Deponit, Nitrodisc, Nitro-Derm
Nitroglycerin, topical	Nitro-Bid, Nitrol
Calcium channel blockers	
Amlodipine	Norvasc
Bepridil	Vascor
Diltiazem	Cardizem, Dilacor, Tiazac
Felodipine	Plendil
Isradipine	DynaCirc
Nicardipine	Cardene
Nifedipine	Adalat, Procardia
Nimodipine	Nimotop
Nisoldipine	Sular
Verapamil	Calan, Isoptin, Covera, Verelan
Cardiac Glycosides	
Digitoxin	Crystodigin
Digoxin	Lanoxin
Peripheral vasodilators (nonadrenergic)	
Hydralazine	Apresoline
Minoxidil	Loniten
Isoxsuprine	Vasodilan
Papaverine	Pavabid
Angiotensin-converting enzyme (ACE) inhibitors	
Benazepril	Lotensin
Captopril	Capoten
Enalapril	Vasotec
Fosinopril	Monopril
Lisinopril	Zestril, Prinivil
Moexipril	Univasc
Perindopril erbumine	Aceon
Quinapril	Accupril
Ramipril	Altace
Trandolapril	Mavik
ACE inhibitors + diuretics	
Captopril and HCTZ	Capozide
Enalapril maleate and HCTZ	Vaseretic
Lisinopril and HCTZ	Prinzide, Zestoric
Moexipril and HCTZ	Uniretic

(continued)

Generic and Brand Names of Common Drugs by Class

Generic name	Brand name*
Angiotensin II receptor antagonists	
Irbesartan	Avapro
Losartan	Cozaar
Valsartan	Diovan
Diuretics	
Thiazides	
Hydrochlorothiazide (HCTZ)	Esidrix
"Loop"	
Bumetanide	Bumex
Ethacrynic acid	Edecrin
Furosemide	Lasix
Potassium-sparing	
Amiloride	Midamor
Spironolactone	Aldactone
Triamterene	Dyrenium
Combinations	
Triamterene and HCTZ	Dyazide, Maxzide
Amiloride and HCTZ	Moduretic
Others	
Metolazone	Zaroxolyn
Antiarrhythmic agents	
Class I	
IA	
Disopyramide	Norpace
Moricizine	Ethmozine
Procainamide	Pronestyl, Procan SR
Quinidine	Quinora, Quinidex, Quinaglute, Quinalan, Cardioquin
IB	
Lidocaine	Xylocaine, Xylocard
Mexiletine	Mexitil
Phenytoin	Dilantin
Tocainide	Tonocard
IC	
Flecainide	Tambocor
Propafenone	Rythmol
Class II	
Beta-Blockers	
Class III	
Amiodarone	Cordarone
Bretylium	Bretylol
Sotalol	Betapace
Class IV	
Calcium channel blockers	

(continued)

Generic and Brand Names of Common Drugs by Class

Generic name	Brand name*
Antihyperlipidemic agents	
Atorvastatin	Lipitor
Cerivastatin	Baycol
Cholestyramine	Questran, Cholybar, Prevalite
Clofibrate	Atromid
Colestipol	Colestid
Fluvastatin	Lescol
Gemfibrozil	Lopid
Lovastatin	Mevacor
Nicotinic acid (niacin)	Nicobid, Nicolar, Slo-Niacin, Niaspan
Pravastatin	Pravachol
Simvastatin	Zocor
Sympathomimetic agents	
Albuterol	Proventil, Ventolin
Ephedrine	Primatene
Epinephrine	Adrenalin
Isoetharine	Bronkosol
Metaproterenol	Alupent
Terbutaline	Brethine
Others	
Clopidogrel	Plavix
Dipyridamole	Persantine
Pentoxifylline	Trental
Warfarin	Coumadin

*Represent selected brands; these are not necessarily all-inclusive.

Effects of Medications on Heart Rate, Blood Pressure, the Electrocardiogram (ECG), and Exercise Capacity

Medications	Heart rate	Blood pressure	ECG	Exercise capacity
I. Beta blockers (including carvedilol, labetalol)	↓* (R and E)	↓ (R and E)	↓ HR* (R) ↓ ischemia‡ (E)	↑ in patients with angina; ↓ or ↔ in patients without angina
II. Nitrates	↑ (R) ↑ or ↔ (E)	↓ (R) ↓ or ↔ (E)	↑ HR (R) ↑ or ↔ HR (E) ↓ ischemia‡ (E)	↑ in patients with angina; ↔ in patients without angina; ↑ or ↔ in patients with congestive heart failure (CHF)

(continued)

Medications	Heart rate	Blood pressure	ECG	Exercise capacity
III. Calcium channel blockers				
Amlodipine Felodipine Isradipine Nicardipine Nifedipine Nimodipine Nisoldipine	↑ or ↔ (R and E)	↓ (R and E)	↑ or ↔ HR (R and E) ↓ ischemia[‡] (E)	↑ in patients with angina; ↔ in patients without angina
Bepridil Diltiazem Verapamil	↓ (R and E)		↓ HR (R and E) ↓ ischemia[‡] (E)	
IV. Digitalis	↓ in patients with atrial fibrillation and possibly CHF Not significantly altered in patients with sinus rhythm	↔ (R and E)	May produce nonspecific ST-T wave changes (R) May produce ST segment depression (E)	Improved only in patients with atrial fibrillation or in patients with CHF
V. Diuretics	↔ (R and E)	↔ or ↓ (R and E)	↔ or PVCs (R) May cause PVCs and "false positive" test results if hypokalemia occurs May cause PVCs if hypomagnesemia occurs (E)	↔, except possibly in patients with CHF
VI. Vasodilators, nonadrenergic	↑ or ↔ (R and E)	↓ (R and E)	↑ or ↔ HR (R and E)	↔, except ↑ or ↔ in patients with CHF
ACE inhibitors	↔ (R and E)	↓ (R and E)	↔ (R and E)	↔, except ↑ or ↔ in patients with CHF
Alpha-adrenergic blockers	↔ (R and E)	↓ (R and E)	↔ (R and E)	↔
Antiadrenergic agents without selective blockade	↓ or ↔ (R and E)	↓ (R and E)	↓ or ↔ HR (R and E)	↔

(continued)

Medications	Heart rate	Blood pressure	ECG	Exercise capacity
VII. Antiarrhythmic agents		All antiarrhythmic agents may cause new or worsened arrhythmias (proarrhythmic effect)		
Class I				
Quinidine Disopyramide	↑ or ↔ (R and E)	↓ or ↔ (R) ↔ (E)	↑ or ↔ HR (R) May prolong QRS and QT intervals (R) Quinidine may result in "false negative" test results (E)	↔
Procainamide	↔ (R and E)	↔ (R and E)	May prolong QRS and QT intervals (R) May result in "false positive" test results (E)	↔
Phenytoin Tocainide Mexiletine	↔ (R and E)	↔ (R and E)	↔ (R and E)	↔
Flecainide Moricizine	↔ (R and E)	↔ (R and E)	May prolong QRS and QT intervals (R) ↔ (E)	↔
Propafenone	↓ (R) ↓ or ↔ (E)	↔ (R and E)	↓ HR (R) ↓ or ↔ HR (E)	↔
Class II				
Beta blockers (see I.)				
Class III				
Amiodarone	↓ (R and E)	↔ (R and E)	↓ HR (R) ↔ (E)	↔
Class IV				
Calcium channel blockers (see III.)				
VIII. Bronchodilators	↔ (R and E)	↔ (R and E)	↔ (R and E)	Bronchodilators ↑ exercise capacity in patients limited by bronchospasm
Anticholinergic agents Methylxanthines	↑ or ↔ (R and E)	↔	↑ or ↔ HR May produce PVCs (R and E)	
Sympathomimetic agents	↑ or ↔ (R and E)	↑, ↔, or ↓ (R and E)	↑ or ↔ HR (R and E)	↔
Cromolyn sodium	↔ (R and E)	↔ (R and E)	↔ (R and E)	↔
Corticosteroids	↔ (R and E)	↔ (R and E)	↔ (R and E)	↔

(continued)

Medications	Heart rate	Blood pressure	ECG	Exercise capacity
IX. Hyperlipidemic agents	Clofibrate may provoke arrhythmias, angina in patients with prior myocardial infarction Nicotinic acid may ↓ BP All other hyperlipidemic agents have no effect on HR, BP, and ECG			↔
X. Psychotropic medications				
Minor tranquilizers	May ↓ HR and BP by controlling anxiety.		No other effects.	
Antidepressants	↑ or ↔ (R and E)	↓ or ↔ (R and E)	Variable (R) May result in "false positive" test results (E)	
Major tranquilizers	↑ or ↔ (R and E)	↓ or ↔ (R and E)	Variable (R) May result in "false positive" or "false negative" test results (E)	
Lithium	↔ (R and E)	↔ (R and E)	May result in T wave changes and arrhythmias (R and E)	
XI. Nicotine	↑ or ↔ (R and E)	↑ (R and E)	↑ or ↔ HR May provoke ischemia, arrhythmias (R and E)	↔, except ↓ or ↔ in patients with angina
XII. Antihistamines	↔ (R and E)	↔ (R and E)	↔ (R and E)	↔
XIII. Cold medications with sympathomimetic agents		Effects similar to those described in sympathomimetic agents although magnitude of effects is usually smaller		↔
XIV. Thyroid medications Only levothyroxine	↑ (R and E)	↑ (R and E)	↑ HR. May provoke arrhythmias ↑ ischemia (R and E)	↔, unless angina worsened
XV. Alcohol	↔ (R and E)	Chronic use may have role in ↑ BP (R and E)	May provoke arrhythmias (R and E)	↔
XVI. Hypoglycemic agents Insulin and oral agents	↔ (R and E)	↔ (R and E)	↔ (R and E)	↔

Medications	Heart rate	Blood pressure	ECG	Exercise capacity
XVII. Dipyridamole	↔ (R and E)	↔ (R and E)	↔ (R and E)	↔
XVIII. Anticoagulants	↔ (R and E)	↔ (R and E)	↔ (R and E)	↔
XIX. Anti-gout medications	↔ (R and E)	↔ (R and E)	↔ (R and E)	↔
XX. Antiplatelet medications	↔ (R and E)	↔ (R and E)	↔ (R and E)	↔
XXI. Pentoxifylline	↔ (R and E)	↔ (R and E)	↔ (R and E)	↑ or ↔ in patients limited by intermittent claudication
XXII. Caffeine	Variable effects depending upon previous use Variable effects on exercise capacity May provoke arrhythmias			
XXIII. Anorexiants/ diet pills	↑ or ↔ (R and E)	↑ or ↔ (R and E)	↑ or ↔ HR (R and E)	

Key: ↑ = increase; ↔ = no effect; ↓ = decrease; R = rest; E = exercise; HR = heart rate; PVCs = premature ventricular contractions.

*Beta-blockers with ISA lower resting HR only slightly.

‡May prevent or delay myocardial ischemia (see text).

Evaluation of Fitness

This appendix provides a generic base for the specific areas of fitness evaluation covered in part II, making you better able to explain what fitness test scores really mean. In part II, we take a closer look at evaluation of energy cost, cardiorespiratory fitness, body composition and nutrition, muscular strength and endurance, and flexibility and low back function.

The first step toward relevant fitness testing is to choose your fitness tests wisely. You must consider the following factors in your test selection:

- **Reliability:** Can I get consistent results with this test?
- **Objectivity:** Would different test administrators get the same results on this test?
- **Validity:** Does the test measure the characteristic I'm interested in evaluating?

Although a test can be reliable and objective and still not be valid, tests that are unreliable or lack objectivity cannot be valid. Once the consistency of the test is ensured, there are ways to determine whether the test measures what it is supposed to measure. For example, do experts agree that a test is valid? Does the test compare favorably with an established test (a "standard") in the same area?

The fitness tests recommended in this book have been shown to be reliable and objective when carefully administered by trained professionals. There also is evidence that the tests are valid (experts recommend them or the tests compare with valid tests).

Fitness leaders can do several things to obtain more accurate results (i.e., less error) from testing:

- Properly prepare the person being tested.
- Organize the testing session.
- Attend to details.

Fitness testing has many uses in a fitness setting, from prescribing exercise to refining programs. Health fitness professionals must know how to interpret test scores and provide feedback to all program participants.

You can help participants evaluate their fitness test scores by doing the following (3, 4):

- Emphasize health status rather than comparison with others.
- Emphasize change rather than current status.
- Provide specific recommendations based on the test data and your understanding of the individual.

One common approach is to compare the fitness participant with people of the same gender and similar age (i.e., use percentiles). Much of the individual comparison with others is based on heredity and early experience. There are limits to how much change can be made even with a great deal of effort. It is unfortunate that many people in fitness programs try to use the *performance* model of being number one. The emphasis should not be on who can run the fastest or who has the lowest cholesterol, but rather on helping all people understand and try to obtain and maintain healthy levels of cardiorespiratory fitness, body composition, and low back function.

It should be noted that the sixth edition of the *ACSM Guidelines* (1) uses percentiles for fitness test evaluation. We understand that there is more research needed before the health criteria can be finalized; however, we think that attempting to set health criteria is a better approach, even with its limitations, than relying on percentiles. For example, a person could be significantly fatter now than in 1980 and be at the same percentile because the population has become fatter. In addition, a person could gain fat as he got older and stay at the same percentile, but that would not be healthy.

We have set fitness standards based on what is needed for good health. Although performance will decrease with age, the minimal fitness standards are the same for adults of all ages. It should be noted that more research is needed so that we can refine these standards; as we find out more about the relationship between test scores and positive health, some of these standards may need to be modified.

Fitness Test Standards for Ages 6 through 70

Test item	6-9	10-12	13-15	16-30	31-50	51-70
Mi run (min)						
Males						
Good	14	12	11	10	10	10
Borderline	16	14	13	12	12	12
Needs work	≥18	≥16	≥15	≥14	≥14	≥14
Females						
Good	14	12	13	12	12	12
Borderline	16	14	15	14	14	14
Needs work	≥18	≥16	≥17	≥16	≥16	≥16
Percent body fat (%)						
Males						
Good	7-18	7-18	7-18	7-18	7-18	7-18
Borderline	22	22	22	22	22	22
Needs work	<5	<5	<5	<5	<5	<5
	>25	>25	>25	>25	>25	>25
Females						
Good	7-18	7-18	16-25	16-25	16-25	16-25
Borderline	22	22	27	27	27	27
Needs work	<5	<5	<14	<14	<14	<14
	>25	>25	>30	>30	>30	>30
Curl-ups (#)						
Good	≥20	≥25	≥30	≥35	≥35	≥35
Borderline	12	15	22	25	25	25
Needs work	≤5	≤10	≤13	≤15	≤15	≤15
Sit-and-reach (in.)[a]						
Good	12	12	12	12	12	12
Borderline	8	8	8	8	8	8
Needs work	≤6	≤6	≤6	≤6	≤6	≤6
Modified pull-ups (#)						
Good	≥10	≥12	≥15	≥15	≥15	≥15
Borderline	6	8	10	10	10	10
Needs work	≤2	≤4	≤5	≤5	≤5	≤5

Note. [a]The feet touch the base of the box at 9 in. A score of 9 indicates the person can touch her feet.

Individuals over 70 years of age should be encouraged to do the walk test (see chapter 5) and strive to monitor the other fitness components.

Adapted from Corbin & Lindsey 2002,Cooper Institute for Aerobics Research 1992, President's Council on Physical Fitness and Sports 2001, and Franks 1989 (pp. 42-47).

The most important question for a fitness participant is not what her health status is at this moment in life, but rather what it will be 6 months, 2 years, or 20 years from now. In this way, the person is encouraged to deal with her status compared to health standards so that she can set reasonable, desirable, and achievable goals for the next testing period.

Test results can also help individuals meet specific goals. It may be that the health standards are not appropriate or reasonable for an individual. For example, the mile-run standards cannot be used for people who are swimming for their fitness workouts or for people who use wheelchairs. However, individual goals for covering a certain distance in the water or in a wheelchair can be established. Or the fitness leader may want to set intermediary goals for a person who is very unfit. For example, it would be discouraging to discuss mile-run standards for a person who can only walk a quarter of a mile without stopping. The initial goal for that person may be to work up to being able to walk a mile without stopping. As indicated in chapter 22, it is important to set goals and subgoals to help people begin and continue healthy behaviors.

Fitness and lifestyle behaviors (such as getting adequate exercise, nutrition, and rest; avoiding substance abuse; coping with stress) and fitness test scores are interrelated. The fitness leader should emphasize fitness *behaviors*. It is more important for people to begin and continue regular physical activity than to reach a certain level on a graded exercise test. Likewise, it is more important for people to develop healthy eating habits than to have a certain percentage of body fat. By emphasizing healthy behaviors, HFIs can recognize people for their efforts; and in the long run this will be the best way to improve their fitness test scores. An overemphasis on test scores can discourage some participants. Two good examples that recognize physical activity behavior are the Canadian *Active Living Challenge* (2) and the President's Council on Physical Fitness and Sports' *Presidential Sports Award* program (7). Both programs provide awards for people who do various physical activities for a certain number of hours, thus rewarding the behavior rather than some fitness test result.

Many individuals have one or more disabilities ranging from mild to severe limitations regarding physical activity and assessment. It is beyond the scope of this book to recommend specific activities and tests to deal with each possible condition (8). The HFI can, however, apply the following general principles:

- Almost all individuals with disabilities can benefit from regular physical activity.
- Most of these individuals can participate in a variety of activities with simple adaptations.
- Individuals with disabilities can gain motivation from periodic assessment.
- The same types of fitness tests can be used with simple adaptations.
- Adaptations in activity and assessment are often simply commonsense adjustments made by the HFI and the participant.
- Experts in adapted physical education and special education can provide additional assistance.

Analysis of test scores from different fitness classes can assist the HFI in deciding what revisions need to be made in the overall fitness program. How many people drop out of various classes? What kinds of aerobic, body fatness, and low back function changes are being made? How many injuries are related to the various classes? The answers to such questions help you to evaluate, revise, and improve your fitness programs. You might consider your programs to be improving steadily rather than having reached *perfection*. This improvement can result from program evaluation.

Another use of test scores is to help educate the public and to get positive attention for your program. What percentage of the participants stay with the program long enough to make important fitness gains? What is the total amount of fat lost by participants in 1 year? How many miles have the participants run during the year? Careful testing, record keeping, and analysis can provide helpful information about your program to the public.

Source List

1. American College of Sports Medicine. (2000). *ACSM's guidelines for exercise testing and prescription* (6th ed.). Philadelphia: Lippincott Williams & Wilkins.
2. Canadian Association for Health, Physical Education, Recreation and Dance. (1994). *The Canadian active living challenge*. Gloucester, Ontario: Author.
3. Cooper Institute for Aerobics Research. (1992). *Prudential FITNESSGRAM test administration manual*. Dallas: Author.
4. Corbin, C.B., & Lindsey, R. (2002). *Fitness for life* (4th ed updated). Champaign, IL: Human Kinetics.
5. Franks, B.D. (1989). *YMCA youth fitness test*. Champaign, IL: Human Kinetics.
6. President's Council on Physical Fitness and Sports. (2001). *President's challenge physical activity and fitness award program*. Washington, DC: Author.
7. President's Council on Physical Fitness and Sports. (1996). *Presidential sports award*. Washington, DC: Author.
8. Seaman, J.A. (1999). Physical activity and fitness for persons with disabilities. *PCPFS Research Digest, 3*(5).

β-adrenergic blocking medications (β-blockers)—Drugs that block receptors that respond to catecholamines (epinephrine and norepinephrine); slow HR.

β-adrenergic receptors—Receptors in the heart and lungs that respond to catecholamines (epinephrine and norepinephrine).

A band—Portion of the sarcomere composed of myosin and actin; the length of the A band remains constant during muscle shortening.

abduction—Movement of a bone laterally away from the anatomical position.

actin—The thin contractile filament of the sarcomere to which myosin binds to release the energy in the activated cross-bridges, leading to sarcomere shortening.

adduction—The return back to the anatomical position from the abducted position.

Adequate Intake (AI)—The amount of a nutrient considered adequate although insufficient data exist to establish an RDA.

adipose tissue—Tissue composed of fat cells.

adolescents—11 to 21 years of age, also called youth.

aerobic—Processes in which energy (ATP) is supplied when oxygen is utilized while a person is working.

agility—Ability to start, stop, and move the body quickly in different directions.

agonist—A muscle that is very effective in causing a certain joint movement. Also called the prime mover.

air displacement plethysmography—Method of body composition assessment that estimates body density from body volume and body weight.

airway obstruction—Blockage of the airway that can be caused by a foreign object. Swelling is secondary to direct trauma or allergic reaction.

alcohol—Ethanol; a depressant that may affect the response to an exercise tolerance test.

amenorrhea—A cessation of menses.

amino acids—Nitrogen-containing building blocks for proteins that can be used for energy.

amphiarthrodial joint—A type of joint that allows only slight movement in all directions. Also called the cartilaginous joint.

anaerobic—Energy (ATP) supplied without oxygen. Creatine phosphate and glycolysis supply ATP without the use of oxygen.

android-type obesity—Obesity in which there is a disproportionate amount of fat in the trunk and abdomen.

aneurysm—A spindle-shaped or saclike bulging of the wall of a blood-filled vein, artery, or ventricle.

angina pectoris—Severe cardiac pain that may radiate to the jaw, arms, or legs. Angina is caused by myocardial ischemia, which can be induced by exercise in susceptible individuals.

angular momentum—The quantity of rotation. Angular momentum is the product of the rotational inertia and the angular velocity.

anorexia nervosa—An eating disorder in which a preoccupation with body weight leads to self-starvation.

antagonist—A muscle that causes movement at a joint in a direction opposite to that of the joint's agonist (prime mover).

antiarrhythmics—Drugs that reduce the number of arrhythmias.

anticoagulant—A drug that delays blood clotting.

antihistamines—Drugs that relieve allergy symptoms, thus making it easier to breathe.

antihypertensives—Drugs that lower blood pressure.

antioxidant vitamins—Substances that attach to free radicals and diminish their effects. Antioxidants are touted to be effective in decreasing the risk of cardiovascular disease and cancer.

aortic valve—Heart valve located between the aorta and the left ventricle.

apnea—Temporary cessation of breathing; often caused by an excess amount of oxygen or too little carbon dioxide in the brain.

aponeuroses—Broad, flat, tendinous sheaths attaching muscles to each other.

arterioles—Blood vessels between the artery and the capillary; involved in the regulation of blood flow and blood pressure.

arteriosclerosis—An arterial disease characterized by the hardening and thickening of vessel walls.

arthritis—Inflammation of a joint.

articular capsule—A ligamentous structure that encloses a diarthrodial joint.

articular cartilage—Cartilage which covers bone surfaces that articulate (meet or come into contact) with other bone surfaces.

atherosclerosis—A form of arteriosclerosis in which fatty substances are deposited in the inner walls of the arteries.

atrial fibrillation—The atrial rate is 400 to 700, whereas the ventricle's rate is 60 to 160 beats · min^{-1}; P waves cannot be seen on the ECG.

atrial flutter—The atrial rate is 200 to 350, whereas the ventricle's rate is 60 to 160 beats · min^{-1}; ECG shows a sawtooth pattern between QRS complexes.

atrioventricular (AV) node—The origin of the bundle of His in the right atrium of the heart. Normal electrical activity of the heart passes through the AV node before depolarization of the ventricles.

atrophy—A reduction in muscle fiber size.

avascular—Without a blood supply.

balance—Ability to maintain a certain posture or to move without falling.

ballistic movement—A rapid movement with three phases: an initial concentric muscle action by agonists to begin movement, a coasting phase, and a deceleration by the eccentric action of the antagonist muscles.

baroreceptors—Receptors that monitor arterial BP.

behavioral contracts—Behavioral contracts are written, signed, public agreements to engage in specific goal-directed activities. Contracts include a designated time frame and clear consequences of meeting and not meeting the agreed upon objectives.

bench stepping—Can be used for both submaximal and maximal testing to evaluate cardiorespiratory function. The height of the bench and the number of steps per minute determine the intensity of the effort. Also a very popular conditioning exercise.

beta-carotene—A precursor of vitamin A and an important antioxidant.

binge eating disorder—An eating disorder characterized by consuming large amounts of food in a short period of time.

bioelectrical impedance analysis (BIA)—Method of body composition assessment based on the electrical conductivity of various tissues in the body.

black-globe temperature—A measure of radiant heat energy; measurement taken in the sunlight to evaluate the potential to gain or lose heat by radiation.

body composition—Description of the tissues that make up the body. It typically refers to the relative percentages of fat and nonfat tissues in the body.

body fat distribution (fat patterning)—Pattern of fat accumulation that often is inherited.

body mass index (BMI)—Measure of the relationship between height and weight; calculated by dividing the weight in kilograms by height in meters squared.

bodybuilding—A competitive sport in which the primary goal is to enhance muscular size, symmetry, and definition.

bone mineral density—Amount of bone mineral per unit area.Typically measured with DXA and used for clinical diagnosis of osteoporosis.

bradycardia—Slow HR, below 60 beats · min^{-1} at rest. Bradycardia is healthy if it is the result of physical conditioning.

bronchodilators—Drugs that dilate the bronchioles, providing relief from an asthma attack.

budget—A financial plan including estimated income and expenditure.

bulimia nervosa—An eating disorder characterized by consuming large amounts of food followed by periods of food purging.

bundle branch—Bundle of nerve fibers between both ventricles of the heart; conducts impulses.

bundle of His—Conduction pathway that connects the AV node with bundle branches in the ventricles.

bursae—Fibrous sacs lined with synovial membrane that contain a small quantity of synovial fluid. Bursae are found between tendon and bone, between skin and bone, and between muscle and muscle. Their function is to facilitate movement without friction between these surfaces.

calcium channel blockers—A class of medications that act by blocking the entry of calcium into the cell; used to treat angina, arrhythmias, and hypertension.

caloric equivalent of oxygen—Approximately 5 kcal of energy is produced per liter of oxygen consumed (5 kcal · L^{-1}).

carbohydrate loading—Practice of increasing carbohydrate intake and decreasing activity in the days preceding competition.

carbohydrate—An essential nutrient composed of carbon, hydrogen, and oxygen that is an essential energy source for the body.

carbon monoxide—A pollutant derived from the incomplete combustion of fossil fuels; binds to hemoglobin to reduce oxygen transport and thus reduce maximal aerobic power.

cardiopulmonary resuscitation (CPR)—Established procedures to restore breathing and blood circulation.

cardiorespiratory function—The ability of the circulatory and respiratory systems to supply fuel during sustained physical activity.

cholesterol—A fatty substance in which carbon, hydrogen, and oxygen atoms are arranged in rings, which may be deposited in the arterial walls, contributing to atherosclerosis.

chronic obstructive pulmonary diseases—A number of diseases that cause unremitting obstruction of air in the airways of the lung.

claudication—Interference with the blood supply to the legs, often resulting in limping.

closed-circuit spirometry—The subject breathes 100% oxygen from a spirometer while carbon dioxide is absorbed; the decrease in the volume of oxygen in the spirometer is proportional to the oxygen consumption.

communication—Interaction, often verbal, to share information and emotions.

compartment syndrome—Increased pressure within a muscular compartment that compromises blood flow and nerve supply.

concentric—A type of muscle action that occurs when the muscle shortens.

concentric action—A shortening of the muscle; causes movement at the joint.

conduction—Heat exchange mechanism in which heat is lost from warmer to cooler objects in direct contact with each other.

convection—Special case of conduction related to heat loss. Heat is transferred to air or water in direct contact with the skin; warm air or water is less dense and rises, carrying heat away from the body.

coordination—Ability to do a task integrating movements of the body and different parts of the body.

coronary arteries—Blood vessels that supply the heart muscle.

coronary artery bypass graft—Procedure in which arteries or veins are sutured above and below a blocked coronary artery to restore adequate blood flow to that portion of the myocardium.

coronary artery thrombosis—Occlusion of a coronary artery by a blood clot.

coronary heart disease (CHD)—Atherosclerosis of the coronary arteries. Also called coronary artery disease (CAD).

cost-effectiveness—Assessment of the cost versus the benefits of a program.

creatine phosphate (CP)—A high-energy phosphate compound that represents the primary immediate anaerobic source of ATP at the onset of exercise. Important in all-out activities lasting a few seconds.

creeping obesity—Slow accumulation of adipose tissue with age.

criterion method—Method used as the "gold standard" or the method against which other methods are compared.

cross-bridge—Part of myosin filament that binds to actin, releasing energy that results in shortening of the sarcomere.

cycle ergometer—A one-wheeled stationary cycle with adjustable resistance used as a work task for exercise testing or conditioning.

daily caloric need—Number of calories needed to maintain current body weight. It is composed of RMR, calories for activity, and the thermic effect of food.

decongestants—Drugs that reduces nasal and bronchial congestion and dry out the airways.

diabetes mellitus—Group of metabolic diseases characterized by high blood glucose concentrations.

diaphysis—The shaft of a long bone.

diarthrodial joint—A type of freely moving joint characterized by its synovial membrane and capsular ligament. Also called synovial joint.

diastolic blood pressure (DBP)—The pressure exerted by the blood on the vessel walls during the resting portion of the cardiac cycle, measured in millimeters of mercury by a sphygmomanometer.

dietary fiber—Substances found in plants that cannot be broken down by the human digestive system.

Dietary Reference Intake (DRI)—Set of values to be used in evaluation of dietary intake.

digitalis—A drug that augments the contraction of the heart muscle and slows the rate of conduction of cardiac impulses through the AV node.

direct calorimetry—A method of measuring the metabolic rate using a closed chamber in which a subject's heat loss is picked up by water flowing through the wall of a chamber; the gain in temperature of the water plus that lost in evaporation determines the metabolic rate.

disc—Located between vertebrae; acts as a shock absorber and frequently involved in low back pain.

disordered eating—Unhealthy eating pattern that can in some cases be a precursor to eating disorders.

diuretics—Drugs that increase urine production, thereby ridding the body of excess fluid.

dose—The quantity (intensity, frequency, and duration) of exercise needed to bring about a response (e.g., lower resting blood pressure).

dry-bulb temperature—The temperature of the air measured in the shade by an ordinary thermometer.

duration—The length of time for a fitness workout. Guidelines often include 20 to 60 min of aerobic work at THR; however, more importantly, the total work accomplished (e.g., distance covered) should be emphasized.

dyspnea—Difficult or labored breathing beyond what is expected for the intensity of work. The exercise test or activity should be stopped.

eating disorders—Clinical eating patterns that result in severe negative health consequences.

eccentric—A type of muscle action that occurs when the muscle lengthens.

eccentric action—Lengthening of the muscle during its action; controls speed of movement caused by another force.

ectopic focus—An irritated portion of the myocardium or electrical conducting system; gives rise to "extra beats" that do not originate from the sino-atrial (SA) node.

effect—The desired response resulting from exercise training (e.g., lower resting blood pressure).

ejection fraction—The fraction of the end diastolic volume ejected per beat (stroke volume divided by end-diastolic volume).

elasticity—Ability of ligaments and tendons to lengthen passively and return to their resting length.

electrocardiogram (ECG)—Graphic recording of the electrical activity of the heart, obtained with the electrocardiograph.

electrolytes—Particles that in solution convey an electrical charge. Most electrolyte drinks are diluted solutions of glucose, salt, and other minerals, with artificial flavoring. Other than sodium, the minerals provided by an electrolyte solution do not provide much benefit.

embolism—Sudden obstruction of a blood vessel by a solid body such as a clot carried in the bloodstream.

emergency medical system (EMS)—A system designed to handle medical emergencies; 911 or other community emergency number.

emergency procedures—Plan of action to follow in emergency situations.

empathy—Identification with the thoughts or feelings of another person, and the effective communication that the other person's feelings are understood.

end-diastolic volume—The volume of blood in the heart just prior to ventricular contraction; a measure of the stretch of the ventricle.

end-ROM—Point at which further movement stress may stretch ligaments or other soft tissue structures such as discs.

epimysium—The connective-tissue sheath surrounding a muscle.

epiphyseal plates—The sites of ossification in long bones.

epiphyses—The ends of long bones.

ergogenic aids—Substances taken in hopes of improving athletic performance.

essential amino acids—The eight amino acids that the body cannot synthesize and therefore must be ingested.

essential fat—The minimum amount of body fat needed for good health.

evaluation—The determination or judgment of the value or worth of something or someone. In a fitness setting, an evaluation determines the health or fitness status of an individual based on his or her characteristics, signs, symptoms, behaviors, and test results.

evaporation—Conversion from the liquid to the gaseous state by means of heat, as in evaporation of sweat; results in the loss of 580 kcal per liter of sweat evaporated.

Exercise Specialist®—A person certified by the ACSM to work in exercise rehabilitation settings with high-risk or diseased (e.g., cardiac and diabetic) populations.

exercise—Structured program of physical activity aimed at achieving some fitness goal.

extension—Increasing the angle at a joint, such as straightening the elbow.

facet joint—Junction of the superior and inferior articular processes of the vertebrae.

fasciculi—Bundles of muscle fibers surrounded by perimysium.

fat-free mass—Weight of the nonfat tissues of the body.

fats—Non-water-soluble substances composed of hydrogen, oxygen, and carbon that serve a variety of functions in the body including energy production.

female athlete triad—A condition sometimes observed in female athletes that is characterized by disordered eating patterns, amenorrhea, and osteoporosis.

first-degree AV block—The delayed transmission of impulses from atria to ventricles (in excess of 0.20 s).

flexibility—The ability to move a joint through the full range of motion without discomfort or pain.

flexion—Anterior or posterior movement that brings two bones together.

force arm (FA)—Perpendicular distance from the axis of rotation to the direction of the application of that force causing movement.

force—Any push or pull that causes movement.

forced expiratory volume in 1 s (FEV_1)—A person who can expel less than 75% of his or her VC in 1 s should be referred to a physician.

forced expiratory volume—The amount of air that can be exhaled forcibly in the first second of expiration.

free radicals—Molecules or fragments of molecules formed during metabolic processes that are highly reactive and can damage cellular components.

functional capacity—Maximal oxygen uptake, expressed in milliliters of oxygen per kilogram of body weight per minute, or in METs.

functional curve—Spinal curve (e.g., lordotic curve) that can be removed by assuming a different posture.

glucose—A simple sugar that is a vital energy source in the human body.

glycemic index—A rating system used to indicate how rapidly a food causes blood glucose to rise.

glycogen—The storage form of carbohydrates in the human body.

glycolysis—The metabolic pathway producing ATP from the anaerobic breakdown of glucose. This short-term source of ATP is important in all-out activities lasting less than 2 min.

goal setting—Goals are desired tasks we want to accomplish in a specific amount of time. Goals provide direction and foster persistence in the search for task strategies. Effective goal setting includes establishing objectives that can be measured, concretely defined, and practically achieved.

good nutrition—A diet in which foods are eaten in the proper quantities and with the needed distribution of nutrients to maintain good health in the present and in the future.

graded exercise test (GXT)—A multistage test that determines a person's physiological responses to different intensities of exercise and/or the person's maximal aerobic power.

gynoid-type obesity—Obesity in which there is a disproportionate amount of fat in the hips and thighs.

H zone—The middle area of the sarcomere that contains only myosin.

Health/Fitness Instructor[SM]—A person who is certified by the ACSM as qualified in exercise testing, prescription, and leadership in preventive programs.

health—Being alive with no major health problem. Also called *apparently healthy*.

heart rate (HR)—The number of beats of the heart per minute.

Heimlich maneuver—Procedure used to dislodge material caught in the respiratory passage that is blocking the airway.

hemorrhage—The escape of a large amount of blood from a vessel.

hepatitis B (HBV)—A type of hepatitis (viral infection of the liver) that is transmitted by sexual or blood-to-blood contact.

high-density lipoprotein cholesterol (HDL-C)—This form of cholesterol protects against the development of CHD, in that it helps transport cholesterol to the liver, where it is eliminated. Thus, low levels of HDL-C are related to a high risk of CHD.

high-risk situation—An event, thought, or interaction that challenges an individual's perceived ability to maintain a desired behavioral change.

human immunodeficiency virus (HIV)—A virus that destroys the body's ability to fight infection; this virus causes AIDS.

hydrostatic weighing—Method of body composition assessment based on Archimedes' principle that often is used as the criterion method. Also called underwater weighing.

hyperextension—A continuation of extension past the anatomical position.

hyperglycemia—Blood glucose concentrations above normal (fasting plasma glucose ≥110 mg/dl).

hypertension—High blood pressure. Normally systolic blood pressure exceeds 140 mmHg or diastolic pressure exceeds 90 mmHg in someone who has hypertension.

hyperthermia—An elevation of the core temperature; if unchecked can lead to heat exhaustion or heat stroke and death.

hypertrophy—An enlargement in muscle fiber size.

hyperventilation—A level of ventilation beyond that needed to maintain the arterial carbon dioxide level; can be initiated by a sudden increase in the hydrogen ion concentration attributable to lactic acid production during a progressive exercise test.

hypotension—Low blood pressure.

hypothermia—Below-normal body temperature.

hypoxemia—Abnormally low oxygen content in the arterial blood, but not total anoxia.

I band—An area of the sarcomere that is bisected by the Z line and is composed of actin; the I band decreases during muscle shortening as the actin slides over the myosin.

impaired glucose tolerance—A condition in which the body does not normally process glucose. Often an intermediate step before development of type 2 diabetes.

indirect calorimetry—The estimation of energy production on the basis of oxygen consumption.

inflammation—A reaction to injury; signs include heat, redness, pain, and swelling.

informed consent—A procedure used to obtain a person's voluntary permission to participate in a program. Informed consent requires a description of the procedures to be used as well as the potential benefits and risks and written consent of the participant.

insulin resistance—A condition in which the body's insulin receptors no longer respond normally to insulin.

intercalated disks—Special junctions between adjacent cardiac muscle cells that allow electrical impulses to pass from cell to cell into both ventricles (see bundle of His).

intracoronary stent—A device placed within the lumen of the artery, to maintain it in an open position.

iron-deficiency anemia—A condition characterized by a decreased amount of hemoglobin in red blood cells and a resultant decrease in the ability to transport oxygen by the blood.

isometric action—A muscle action in which the muscle length is unchanged; the muscle exerts a force that counteracts an opposing force. Also called a static action.

isometric—A type of muscle action in which the muscle length remains constant and no movement occurs.

J point—On an ECG, the point at which the S wave ends and the S-T segment begins.

joint cavity—The space between bones enclosed by the synovial membrane and articular cartilage.

kyphotic—Describes the condition of kyphosis, a convex curvature of the spine (e.g., the thoracic curve).

lactate threshold—The point during a GXT at which the blood lactate concentration suddenly increases; a good indicator of the highest sustainable work rate. Also called the anaerobic threshold.

leadership—The ability to influence and motivate people in a group to make decisions and to act on the basis of those decisions.

lean body mass—Term often used synonymously with fat-free mass.

liability—Legal responsibility.

ligament—The connective tissue that attaches bone to bone.

lipoproteins—Large molecules responsible for transporting fats in the blood.

long-range plan—A plan that includes goals to be accomplished, what is needed to accomplish the goals, how the organization will move from where it is to where it wants to be, and what processes should be followed to implement the program.

lordotic curve—Describes the condition of lordosis; a forward, concave curve of the lumbar spine when viewed from the side.

low back problems—Strong discomfort in the low back area, often caused by lack of muscular endurance and flexibility in the midtrunk region or improper posture or lifting.

low-density lipoprotein cholesterol (LDL-C)—This is the form of cholesterol that is responsible for the buildup of plaque in the inner walls of the arteries (atherosclerosis). Thus, high levels of LDL-C are related to a high risk of CHD.

lumbosacral—Area encompassing the lumbar vertebrae and the sacrum.

macrocycle—A phase of training that lasts about 1 year.

malnutrition—A diet in which there is an underconsumption, overconsumption, or unbalanced consumption of nutrients that leads to disease or an increased susceptibility to disease.

maximal aerobic power or **maximal oxygen uptake ($\dot{V}O_2$max)**—The maximal rate at which oxygen can be used by the body during maximal work; related directly to the maximal capacity of the heart to deliver blood to the muscles. Expressed in $L \cdot min^{-1}$ or $ml \cdot kg^{-1} \cdot min^{-1}$.

maximal—The highest level possible, such as maximal HR or oxygen uptake.

menisci—Partial, semilunar-shaped disks between the femur and tibia and the knee.

mesocycle—A phase of training that lasts for several months.

microcycle—A phase of training that lasts about 1 week.

minerals—Inorganic atoms or ions that serve a variety of functions in the human body.

mitochondria—Cellular organelles responsible for the generation of energy (ATP) through aerobic metabolism.

mitral valve—Heart valve located between the left atrium and left ventricle.

Mobitz type I AV block—On an ECG, P-R interval progressively increases until the P wave is not followed by a QRS complex. The site of the block is within the AV node.

Mobitz type II AV block—On an ECG, a constant P-R interval, with some but not all P waves followed by QRS. The site of the block is the bundle of His.

motion segment—Fundamental unit of the lumbar spine; made up of two vertebrae and their intervening disc.

motor unit—The functional unit of muscular action that includes a motor nerve and the muscle fibers that its branches innervate.

muscle fiber—Muscle cell. Contains myofibrils that are composed of sarcomeres; uses chemical energy of ATP to generate tension, which, when greater than the resistance, results in movement.

muscle group—A group of specific muscles that are responsible for the same action at the same joint.

muscular endurance—The ability of the muscle to perform repetitive contractions over a prolonged period of time.

muscular strength—The ability of the muscle to generate the maximum amount of force.

myocardial infarction (MI)—Death of a section of heart tissue in which the blood supply has been cut off, commonly called a heart attack.

myocardial ischemia—A lack of blood flow to the heart tissue.

myocardium—The middle layer of the heart wall; involuntary, striated muscle innervated by autonomic nerves.

myofibril—Found inside muscle fibers and composed of a long string of sarcomeres.

myosin— The thick contractile filament in sarcomeres that can bind actin and split ATP to generate cross-bridge movement and the development of tension.

negative caloric balance—A condition in which less energy is consumed than is expended, resulting in a decrease in body weight.

negligence—The failure to provide reasonable care, or the care required by the circumstances. The person, program, or both are legally liable for injury that results from this failure.

nicotine gum—Gum containing nicotine that is used for smoking cessation. Nicotine is absorbed through the oral mucosa, providing sufficient plasma nicotine concentrations to curb the craving to smoke.

nitrates—A class of medications used to treat angina pectoris, or chest pain.

nutrient density—The amount of essential nutrients in a food compared with the calories it contains.

nutrient—A substance that the body requires for the maintenance, growth, and repair of tissues.

obesity—Condition in which one has an excessive accumulation of fat tissue. Also may be classified by the weight-to-height relationship (see section on body mass index).

oligomenorrhea—Irregular menses.

open-circuit spirometry—The method of measuring oxygen consumption by breathing in room air while collecting and analyzing the expired air.

oral antiglycemic agents—A class of medications used to treat non-insulin-dependent diabetes mellitus; they stimulate the pancreas to secrete more insulin.

ossification—The replacement of cartilage by bone.

osteoarthritis—Most common form of arthritis (90-95% of all cases); affects joints whose articular cartilage is damaged or injured.

osteopenia—Condition in which bone has been lost but has not yet reached osteoporotic levels.

osteoporosis—A disease characterized by a decrease in the total amount of bone mineral and a decrease in the strength of the remaining bone.

overload—To place greater than usual demands on some part of the body (e.g., picking up more weight than usual overloads the muscle involved). Chronic overloading leads to increased function.

overweight—Condition in which one is above the recommended weight-to-height range but is below obesity levels (see section on body mass index).

oxygen consumption ($\dot{V}O_2$)—The rate at which oxygen is used during a specific level of an activity; oxygen uptake.

oxygen debt—The amount of oxygen used during recovery from work that exceeds the amount needed for rest. Also called oxygen repayment and excess postexercise oxygen consumption.

oxygen deficit—The difference between the steady-state oxygen requirement of a physical activity and the measured oxygen uptake during the first minutes of work.

ozone—An active form of oxygen formed in reaction to UV light and as an emission from internal combustion engines; exposure can decrease lung function.

P wave—On an ECG, a small positive deflection preceding a QRS complex, indicating atrial depolarization, normally less than 0.12 s in duration with an amplitude of 0.25 mV or less.

pars interarticularis—Part of vertebra between its upper elements (superior articular process and transverse process) and its lower elements (inferior articular process and spinous process).

percent body fat (%BF)—Percentage of the total weight composed of fat tissue. Calculated by dividing fat mass by total weight and multiplying by 100.

percentage of HRR (%HRR)—The HRR is calculated by subtracting resting HR from maximal HR. The %HRR is a percentage of the difference between resting and maximal HR and is calculated by subtracting resting HR from the exercise HR, dividing by the HRR, and multiplying by 100%.

percentage of the maximal HR (%HRmax)—HR expressed as a simple percentage of the maximal HR.

percentage of the maximal $\dot{V}O_2$ (%$\dot{V}O_2$max)—Ratio of submaximal oxygen uptake to maximal oxygen uptake, multiplied by 100%.

percentage of $\dot{V}O_2$R (%$\dot{V}O_2$R)—$\dot{V}O_2$R is calculated by subtracting one MET (3.5 $ml \cdot kg^{-1} \cdot min^{-1}$) from the subject's $\dot{V}O_2$max. The %$\dot{V}O_2$R is a percentage of the difference between resting $\dot{V}O_2$ and $\dot{V}O_2$max and is calculated by subtracting 1 MET from the measured oxygen uptake, dividing by the subject's $\dot{V}O_2$R, and multiplying by 100%.

percutaneous transluminal coronary angiography—A procedure in which a catheter is inserted in a blocked artery and a balloon is inflated to open the artery.

performance—The ability to perform a task or sport at a desired level. Also called motor fitness or skill-related fitness.

perimysium—The connective tissue surrounding fasciculi within a muscle.

periodization—A process of varying the training stimulus to promote long-term fitness gains and avoid overtraining.

periosteum—The connective tissue surrounding all bone surfaces except the articulating surfaces.

phospholipids—Fatty compounds that are essential constituents of cell membranes.

physical activity—Bodily movement produced by skeletal muscles that requires energy expenditure at a level to produce healthy benefits.

physical fitness—A set of attributes that people have or achieve relating to their ability to perform physical activity.

positive caloric balance—A condition in which more calories are consumed than are expended, resulting in weight gain.

postpubescent—After puberty changes.

power—Ability to exert muscular strength quickly.

powerlifting—A competitive sport in which athletes attempt to lift maximal amounts of weight in the squat, deadlift, and bench press exercises.

P-R interval—The time interval between the beginning of the P wave and the QRS complex. The upper normal limit is 0.2 s. This segment is normally used as the isoelectric baseline.

P-R segment—Forms the isoelectric line, or baseline, from which S-T segment deviations are measured.

preadolescents—Less than 11 years of age, also called children.

premature atrial contraction—On an ECG, the rhythm is irregular and the R-R interval is short; the origin of the beat is somewhere other than the SA node.

premature junctional contraction (PJC)—On an ECG, the ectopic pacemaker in the AV junctional area causes a QRS complex; frequently seen with inverted P waves.

premature ventricular contraction (PVC)—Wide, bizarrely-shaped QRS complex originating from an ectopic focus in the His-Purkinje system. The QRS interval is longer than 0.12 s in duration, and the T wave is usually in the opposite direction.

prepubescent—Children prior to puberty.

prediabetes—A condition in which an individual has impaired fasting glucose and/or impaired glucose tolerance. Without treatment, prediabetes typically evolves into type 2 diabetes.

pressure points—The point of application of pressure over major arteries to control bleeding.

PRICE—The suggested treatment for minor sprains and strains: protection, rest, ice, compression, and elevation.

proteins—Nutrients composed of amino acids that serve a variety of functions in the human body.

pubescent—During change from child to adult.

pulmonary function testing—Procedures used to test the capacity of the respiratory system to move air into or out of the lungs.

pulmonary valve—A set of three crescent-shaped flaps at the opening of the pulmonary artery; also called the semilunar valves.

pulmonary ventilation—The number of liters of air inhaled or exhaled per minute.

pulse oximeter—Device used to measure the percent saturation of hemoglobin in the arterial blood.

Purkinje fibers—The muscle-cell fibers found beneath the endocardium of the heart; the impulse-conducting network of the heart.

Q wave—The initial negative deflection of the QRS complex on an ECG.

QRS complex—The largest complex on an ECG, indicating a depolarization of the left ventricle, normally less than 0.1 s.

Q-T interval—The time interval from the beginning of the QRS complex to the end of the T wave. The Q-T interval reflects the electrical systole of the cardiac cycle.

R wave—The positive deflection of the QRS complex in the ECG.

radiation—The process of heat exchange from the surface of one object to the surface of another object that depends on a temperature gradient but does not require direct contact between objects, for example, heat loss from the sun to the earth.

rate-pressure product—The product of HR and SBP; indicative of the oxygen requirement of the heart during exercise. Training lowers the rate-pressure product at rest and during submaximal work. Also called the double product.

rating of perceived exertion (RPE)—A scale, by Borg, used to quantify the subjective feeling of physical effort. The original scale was from 6 to 20; the revised scale is from 0 to 10.

Recommended Dietary Allowance (RDA)—The amount of a nutrient found to be adequate for approximately 97% of the population.

recruitment—Stimulation of additional motor units to increase the strength of a muscle action.

Registered Clinical Exercise Physiologist®—A person with a M.S. degree in Exercise Science (or equivalent) who possesses good clinical experience in the use of exercise in rehabilitation.

reinforcement—Positive reinforcement involves adding something positive to increase the frequency of the target behavior. Negative reinforcement also increases the frequency of the desired behavior, but it is the removal of something negative, like losing weight because of a regular walking program. Reinforcement can be administered by oneself (self-reinforcement) or by other people (social reinforcement).

relapse prevention—Relapse prevention was developed by Marlatt and Gordon (17) to identify and deal successfully with high-risk situations by educating the client about the relapse process and using a variety of strategies to foster an effective coping response.

relative humidity—A measure of the relative wetness of the air; the ratio of the amount of water vapor in the air to the maximum the air can hold at that temperature times 100%. High relative humidity in a warm environment provides important information about the potential for losing heat by evaporation.

relative leanness—The relative amount of body weight that is fat and nonfat. Also called body composition.

repetition maximum (RM) —The maximum amount of weight that can be lifted for a predetermined number of repetitions with proper exercise technique. For example, a 5RM is the most weight that can be lifted five but not six times.

repetition—One complete movement of an exercise, which typically consists of a concentric (lifting) and eccentric (lowering) phase.

rescue breathing—Artificial respiration; used to promote oxygenation of blood in an unconscious victim who is not breathing.

resistance arm (RA)—Perpendicular distance from the axis of rotation to the direction of the application of that force resisting movement.

resistance force (R)—The opposing force that is resisting another force.

respiratory quotient (RQ) or **respiratory exchange ratio (R)**—The ratio of the volume of carbon dioxide produced to the volume of oxygen used during a given period of time ($\dot{V}CO_2/\dot{V}O_2$).

respiratory shock—A condition in which the lungs are unable to supply enough oxygen to the circulating blood.

resting metabolic rate (RMR)—Number of calories needed to sustain the body under normal resting conditions.

reversibility—A corollary to the principle of overload; loss of a training effect with disuse.

restrictive lung diseases—A number of diseases that restrict a person's ability to expand the lungs.

rheumatoid arthritis—Debilitating arthritis of unknown cause that can affect few or many joints (pauciarticular and polyarticular, respectively).

risk factor—A characteristic, sign, symptom, or test score that is associated with increased probability of developing a health problem. For example, people with hypertension have increased risk of developing coronary heart disease.

rotational inertia—Reluctance to rotate; proportional to the mass and distribution of the mass around the axis.

rotation—The movement of a bone around its longitudinal axis.

R-R interval—The time interval from the peak of the QRS of one cardiac cycle to the peak of the QRS of the next cycle.

S wave—The first negative wave (preceded by Q or R waves) of the QRS complex in the ECG.

salt tablets—Supplements that generally are not recommended as a means to increase salt in the diet; if used, they must be taken with large amounts of water.

sarcomeres—The basic units of muscle contraction. Contain actin and myosin; tension is developed as the myosin cross-bridges pull the actin toward the center of the sarcomere.

sarcoplasmic reticulum (SR)—The network of membranes that surround the myofibril; stores calcium needed for muscle contraction.

saturation pressure—Water vapor pressure that exists at a particular temperature when the air is saturated with water.

school-aged children and youth—Kindergarten through 12th grade, about 5 to 18 years of age.

sciatic nerve—Nerve originating in sacral area; it is involved in low back problems that can result in loss of feeling and control in the legs.

scoliosis—An abnormal lateral curvature of the spine.

secondary prevention—Steps taken to prevent the recurrence of a heart attack.

second-degree AV block—On an ECG, some but not all P waves precede the QRS complex and result in ventricular depolarization.

set—A group of repetitions performed without stopping.

sino-atrial (SA) node—A mass of tissue in the right atrium of the heart, near the vena cava, that initiates the heartbeat.

sinus arrhythmia—A normal variant in sinus rhythm in which the R-R interval varies by more than 10% per beat.

sinus bradycardia—The normal rhythm (i.e., the sinus node is the pacemaker) and sequence, with slow HR (below 60 beats $\cdot$ min^{-1} at rest). The occurrence of sinus bradycardia may indicate a high level of fitness or a mental illness such as depression.

sinus rhythm—The normal timing and sequence of the cardiac events, with the sinus node as a pacemaker; resting rate is between 60 and 100 beats $\cdot$ min^{-1}.

sinus tachycardia—The normal rhythm and sequence, with a fast HR (above 100 beats $\cdot$ min^{-1} at rest). The occurrence of sinus tachycardia may indicate illness or stress.

sliding-filament theory—The theory that muscular tension is generated when the actin in the sarcomere slides over the myosin because of the action of the myosin cross-bridges.

specificity—The principle that states that training effects derived from an exercise program are specific to the exercise done (endurance vs. strength training) and the muscle fiber types involved.

speed—Ability to move the whole body quickly.

sphygmomanometer—A blood pressure measurement system.

spondylolisthesis—Condition in which the vertebral body and transverse processes slip anteriorly (forward) on the vertebral body below; it is common for L4 to slip over L5.

spondylolysis—A stress fracture in the pars interarticularis.

spot reduction—The myth that exercise emphasizing a particular body part will cause that area to lose fat quicker than the rest of the body.

S-T segment—The part of the ECG between the end of the QRS complex and beginning of the T wave. Depression below (or elevation above) the isoelectric line indicates ischemia.

S-T segment depression—A condition where the S-T segment of the ECG is depressed below the baseline; may signify myocardial ischemia.

S-T segment elevation—A condition where the S-T segment of the ECG is elevated above the baseline; may signify the early (acute) stages of an MI.

stability—The ease with which balance is maintained.

standard deviation (SD)—A measure of the deviation from the mean (average) value generalized to the population. One SD above and below the mean represents about 68% of the population, 2 SD is about 95%, and 3 SD is about 99% of the population. For example, if the mean $\dot{V}O_2max$ = 25 ml $\cdot$ kg^{-1} $\cdot$ min^{-1} and SD = ±3 ml $\cdot$ kg^{-1} $\cdot$ min^{-1}, then you would expect 68% of the population to have $\dot{V}O_2max$ values between 22 (25 – 3) and 28 (25 + 3) ml $\cdot$ kg^{-1} $\cdot$ min^{-1}, 95% of the population to be between 19 and 31 ml $\cdot$ kg^{-1} $\cdot$ min^{-1}, and almost all the population to be between 16 and 34 ml $\cdot$ kg^{-1} $\cdot$ min^{-1}. A special term called the standard error of estimate (SEE) is used to indicate the standard deviation of any estimate derived for a prediction formula.

steady-state oxygen requirement—When the oxygen uptake levels off during submaximal work, the oxygen uptake value is said to represent the steady-state oxygen (ATP) requirement for the activity.

strength training—A method of exercise designed to enhance musculoskeletal strength, power, and local muscular endurance. Strength training (also called resistance training) encompasses a wide range of training modalities including weight machines, free weights, medicine balls, elastic cords, and body weight.

stroke—A vascular accident (embolism, hemorrhage, or thrombosis) in the brain, often resulting in sudden loss of body function.

structural curve—Curve that cannot be removed in normal movement because of chronically shortened musculotendinous units and/or ligaments; in this case a functional curve becomes structural.

submaximal—Less than maximal (e.g., an exercise that can be performed with less than maximal effort).

sulfur dioxide—A pollutant that can cause bronchoconstriction in people with asthma.

summation—The additive effect of force generated during higher rates of stimulation without complete muscle fiber relaxation between stimuli.

sweating—The process of moisture coming through the pores of the skin from the sweat glands, usually as a result of heat, exertion, or emotion.

synarthrodial joint—Immovable joint.

synovial membrane—The inner lining of the joint capsule; secretes synovial fluid into the joint cavity.

systolic blood pressure (SBP)—The pressure exerted on the vessel walls during ventricular contraction, measured in millimeters of mercury by a sphygmomanometer.

T wave—On an ECG, the wave that follows the QRS complex and represents ventricular repolarization.

tachycardia—HR greater than 100 beats · min^{-1} at rest. Tachycardia may be seen in deconditioned people or people who are apprehensive about a situation (e.g., an exercise test).

tachypnea—Excessively rapid breathing that may be a sign of overexertion, shock, or hyperventilation.

target heart rate (THR)—The heart rate recommended for fitness workouts.

tendon—A band of tough, inelastic, fibrous connective tissue that attaches muscle to bone.

tetanus—Increase in skeletal muscle tension in response to very high-stimulation frequencies. The resulting contractions fuse together into a smooth, sustained, high-tension contraction.

thermic effect of food—The energy needed to digest, absorb, transport, and store the food that is eaten.

third-degree AV block—On an ECG, the QRS appears independently, P-R varies with no regular pattern, and HR is less than 45 beats · min^{-1}.

threshold—The minimum level needed for a desired effect. Often used to refer to the minimum level of exercise intensity needed for improvement in cardiorespiratory function.

thrombosis—A blood clot in a blood vessel.

Tolerable Upper Intake Levels (UL)—The highest intake of a nutrient believed to pose no health risk.

torque (T)—The effect produced by a force causing rotation; the product of the force and length of the force arm.

total cholesterol/HDL-C ratio—High ratios of total cholesterol to HDL-C indicate a high risk of CHD.

total cholesterol—Because LDL-C is usually the primary factor in the total amount, a high level of total cholesterol is also a risk factor for CHD.

total fitness—Optimal quality of life, including social, mental, spiritual, and physical components. Also called *wellness* or *positive health.*

total work—The amount of work accomplished during a workout.

training intensity—A measure of the effort experienced in a workout, usually expressed as a percentage of maximal HR or oxygen consumption.

tranquilizers—A class of medications that brings tranquillity by calming, soothing, quieting, or pacifying.

trans fats (trans fatty acids)—Hydrogenated fats created to be solid at room temperature and to be used in cooking. The intake of these fats lowers HDL-C and raises LDL-C.

transfer of angular momentum—Transfer of angular momentum from one body segment to another can be achieved by stabilizing the initial moving part at a joint.

transtheoretical model—A general model of intentional behavior change in which behavior change is seen as a dynamic process that occurs through a series of interrelated stages. Basic concepts emphasize the individual's motivational readiness to change, cognitive and behavioral strategies for changing behavior, self-efficacy, and the evaluation of the pros and cons of the new behavior.

transverse tubule—Connects the sarcolemma (muscle membrane) to the sarcoplasmic reticulum; action potentials move down the transverse tubule to cause the sarcoplasmic reticulum to release calcium to initiate muscle contraction.

treadmill—A machine with a moving belt that can be adjusted for speed and grade, allowing a person to walk or run in place. Treadmills are used extensively for exercise testing and training.

tricuspid valve—A valve located between the right atrium and right ventricle of the heart.

triglycerides—The primary storage form of fat in the human body.

tropomyosin—A protein (part of the thin filament) that regulates muscle contraction; works with troponin.

troponin—A protein (part of the thin filament) that can bind the calcium released from the sarcoplasmic reticulum; works with tropomyosin to allow the myosin cross-bridge to interact with actin and initiate cross-bridge movement.

two-compartment model—Model that divides the body into fat and fat-free component parts.

type 1 diabetes—Type of diabetes mellitus in which insulin is not produced. It is caused by damage to the β-cells of the pancreas.

type 2 diabetes—Type of diabetes mellitus in which the insulin receptors lose their sensitivity to insulin.

type I or **slow oxidative fiber**—A slow-contracting muscle fiber that generates a small amount of tension with most of the energy coming from aerobic processes; active in light to moderate activities and possesses great endurance.

type IIa or **fast oxidative glycolytic fiber**—A fast-contracting muscle that can produce energy aerobically and that generates great tension; adds to type I fiber's tension as exercise intensity increases.

type IIb or **fast glycolytic fiber**—A fast-contracting muscle fiber that generates great tension; produces energy by anaerobic metabolism and fatigues quickly.

universal precaution—Safety measures taken to prevent exposure to blood or other body fluids.

ventilatory threshold—The intensity of work at which the rate of ventilation increases sharply during a GXT.

ventricular fibrillation—The heart contracts in an unorganized, quivering manner, with no discernible P waves or QRS complexes; requires immediate emergency attention.

ventricular tachycardia—An extremely dangerous condition in which three or more consecutive premature ventricular contractions occur. Ventricular tachycardia may degenerate into ventricular fibrillation.

very low-density lipoprotein (VLDL)—High levels are a high risk of CHD.

vital capacity (VC)—A person whose VC is less than 75% of the value predicted for her or his age, sex, and height should be referred to a physician for further testing.

vital capacity—The greatest amount of air that can be exhaled after a maximal inspiration.

vitamins—Organic substances essential to the normal functioning of the human body. They may be subdivided into fat-soluble and water-soluble categories.

waist-to-hip ratio (WHR)—Waist circumference divided by hip circumference; often used as an indicator of android-type obesity.

water vapor pressure gradient—The gradient between the water vapor pressure on the skin and the water vapor pressure in the air.

weightlifting—A competitive sport in which athletes attempt to lift maximal amounts of weight in the snatch and the clean and jerk exercises.

wellness—Positive health that is more than simply being free from illness.

wet-bulb globe temperature (WBGT)—Heat stress index that considers dry-bulb, wet-bulb, and black globe temperatures.

wet-bulb temperature—Air temperature measured with a thermometer whose bulb is surrounded by a wet wick; an indication of the ability to evaporate moisture from the skin.

windchill index—The temperature equivalent, under calm air conditions, attributable to a combination of temperature and wind velocity.

Z line—Connective tissue elements that mark the beginning and end of the sarcomere.

Figures

Figure 3.1 Reprinted from the 1994 revised version of the Physical Activity Readiness Questionnaire (PAR-Q and YOU). The PAR-Q and YOU is a copyrighted, pre-exercise screen, owned by the Canadian Society for Exercise Physiology.

Figure 5.2 Reprinted, by permission, from B. Balke, 1963, "A simple field test for the assessment of physical fitness," *Federal Aviation Agency Report* 63: 7.

Figure 5.4 Reprinted from *Y's Way to Physical Fitness*, 3rd edition, with permission of the YMCA of the USA, 101 N. Wacker Drive, Chicago, IL 60606.

Figure 5.5 Reprinted from *Y's Way to Physical Fitness*, 3rd edition, with permission of the YMCA of the USA, 101 N. Wacker Drive, Chicago, IL 60606.

Figure 5.7 Reprinted, by permission, from E.T. Howley, 1988, The exercise testing laboratory. In *Resource manual for guidelines for exercise testing and prescription*, American College of Sports Medicine, edited by S.N. Blair et al. (Philadelphia: Lea & Febiger), 409.

Figure 5.8 Adapted, by permission, from *Instruction manual, Monark model 818E* (Varberg, Sweden: Monark Exercise AB), 18.

Figure 5.9 Reproduced with permission, Human Blood Pressure Determination by Sphygmomanometer, © 1994, Copyright American Heart Association.

Figure 8.1 Reprinted, by permission, from American College of Sports Medicine, 1998, "The recommended quantity and quality of exercise for developing and maintaining cardiorespiratory and muscular fitness, and flexibility in healthy adults," *Medicine and Science in Sports and Exercise* 30:406-413.

Figure 9.2 Adapted, from W. Liemohn, 2001, *Exercise prescription and the back* (New York: McGraw-Hill Companies), 11. Adapted with permission of The McGraw-Hill Companies.

Figure 9.3 Adapted, from W. Liemohn, 2001, *Exercise prescription and the back* (New York: McGraw-Hill Companies), 40. Adapted with permission of The McGraw-Hill Companies.

Figure 10.1 Reprinted, by permission, from Goodman and Gilman, 1975, *The pharmacological basis of therapeutics* (New York: Macmillan), 25.

Figure 10.2 Reprinted, by permission, from G.L. Jennings et al., 1991, "What is the dose-response relationship?" *Annals of Medicine* 23: 317.

Figure 10.3 From R. Pate et al., 1995, "Physical activity and public health," *Journal of the American Medical Association* 273(5): 404.

Figure 10.8 Reprinted, by permission, from Howley, E.T., 2001, "Type of activity: resistance, aerobic and leisure versus occupational physical activity," *Medicine and Science in Sports and Exercise* 33:S364-369.

Figure 11.1 Adapted from A.H. Mokdad, M.K. Serdula, W.H. Deitz, B.A. Bowman, J.S. Marks, & J.P. Koplan, 1999, "The spread of the obesity epidemic in the United States, 1991-1998," *Journal of the American Medical Association*, 282(16), 1519-1522.

Figure 12.1 Reprinted, by permission, from J.H. Wilmore and D.L. Costill, 1994, *Physiology of sport and exercise* (Champaign, IL: Human Kinetics), 81.

Figure 12.2 Reprinted, by permission, from D. Wathen and F. Roll, 1994, Training methods and modes. In *Essentials of strength training and conditioning*, edited by T.R. Baechle (Champaign, IL: Human Kinetics), 408.

Figure 12.4 From S.K. Powers and S.L. Dodd, *Total fitness, exercise, nutrition, and wellness*. Copyright © 1996 by Allyn and Bacon. Reprinted by permission of Pearson Education, Inc.

Figure 12.5 Adapted, by permission, from V.H. Heyward, 1991, *Advanced fitness assessment and exercise prescription* (Champaign, IL: Human Kinetics), 124.

Figure 13.1 Adapted, from W. Liemohn, 2001, *Exercise prescription and the back* (New York: McGraw-Hill Companies). Adapted by permission of McGraw-Hill Companies.

Figure 13.2 Adapted, from W. Liemohn, 2001, *Exercise prescription and the back* (New York: McGraw-Hill Companies). Adapted by permission of McGraw-Hill Companies.

Figure 13.5 Adapted, from B. Pansky, 2001, *Review of gross anatomy* (New York: McGraw-Hill Companies), 391. Adapted by permission of McGraw-Hill Companies.

Figure 14.8 Adapted, by permission, from American College of Sports Medicine, 2000, *ACSM's guidelines for exercise testing and prescription*, 6th edition (Philadelphia: Williams & Wilkins).

Figure 15.6 Reprinted, by permission, from S.J. Fleck and W.J. Kraemer, 1987, *Designing resistance training programs* (Champaign, IL: Human Kinetics), 90.

Figure 16.2 Adapted, by permission, from J.O. Hollszy and W.M. Kohrt, 1995, Exercise. In *Handbook of physiology* Section II Aging, edited by E.J. Masoro (New York: American Physiological Society).

Figure 16.3 Adapted, by permission, from M.A. Rigers and W.J. Evans, 1993, "Changes in skeletal muscle with aging: effects of exercise training," *Exercise and Sport Sciences Reviews* 21:65-102.

Figure 24.1 Reprinted, by permission, from J.E. Donnelly, 1990, *Living anatomy*, 2nd edition (Champaign, IL: Human Kinetics), 199.

Figure 24.2 Reprinted, by permission, from J.E. Donnelly, 1990, *Living anatomy*, 2nd edition (Champaign, IL: Human Kinetics), 202.

Figure 24.6 Adapted, by permission, from M.J. Goldman, 1982, *Principles of clinical electrocardiography*, 11th edition (Los Altos, CA: Appleton & Lange).

Figure 24.23 Reprinted, by permission, from E. Stein, 1992, *Rapid analysis of electrocardiograms: A self-study program*, 2nd edition (Philadelphia: Lea & Febiger), 150.

Figure 28.2 Reprinted, by permission, from A.J. Vander, J.H. Sherman, and D.S. Luciano, 1980, *Human physiology*, 3rd edition (New York: McGraw-Hill, Inc.), 212 and 216.

Figure 28.3 Reprinted, by permission, from A.J. Vander, J.H. Sherman, and D.S. Luciano, 1985, *Human physiology*, 4th edition (New York: McGraw-Hill, Inc.), 263.

Figure 28.4 Reprinted, by permission, from A.J. Vander, J.H. Sherman, and D.S. Luciano, 1985, *Human physiology*, 4th edition (New York: McGraw-Hill, Inc.), 268.

Figure 28.5 Reprinted, by permission, from D.G. Sale, 1987, Influence of exercise and training on motor unit activation. In *Exercise and sport sciences reviews*, vol. 15, edited by K.B. Pandolf (New York: McGraw-Hill, Inc.), 99.

Figure 28.19 Adapted, by permission, from J. Schwade, C.G. Blomqvist, and W. Shapiro, 1977, "A comparison of the response to arm and leg work in patients with ischemic heart disease," *American Heart Journal* 94: 206.

Figure 28.21 Adapted, by permission, from E.F. Coyle et al., 1984, "Time course of loss of adaptations after stopping prolonged intense endurance training," *Journal of Applied Physiology* 57: 1861.

Figure 28.23 Reprinted, by permission, from P.-O. Astrand and K. Rodahl, 1986, *Textbook of work physiology*, 3rd edition (New York: McGraw-Hill), 200.

Figure 28.24 Adapted, by permission, from A.R. Lind and G.W. McNichol, 1967, "Muscular factors which determine the cardiovascular responses to sustained and rhythmic exercise," *Canadian Medical Association Journal* 96: 712.

Tables

Table 3.2 Reprinted, by permission, from American College of Sports Medicine, 2000, *ACSM's guidelines for exercise testing and prescription*, 6th ed. (Philadelphia: Lippincott, Williams and Wilkins).

Table 3.3 Reprinted, by permission, from American College of Sports Medicine, 1995, *ACSM's guidelines for exercise testing and prescription*, (Baltimore, MD: Lippencott, Williams & Wilkins), 25.

Table 4.8 Reprinted, by permission, from American College of Sports Medicine, 1980, *Guidelines for graded exercise testing and prescription*, 2nd edition (Philadelphia: Lea & Febiger), 20.

Table 5.2 Reprinted, by permission, from E.T. Howley and B.D. Franks, 1986, *Health fitness instructor's handbook* (Champaign, IL: Human Kinetics).

Table 5.5 Reprinted, by permission, from G. Borg, 1985, *An Introduction to Borg's RPE Scale* (Ithaca, NY: Mouvement Publications), 7.

Table 5.6 Reprinted, by permission, from B.D. Franks, 1979, Methodology of the exercise ECG test. In *Exercise electrocardiography: Practical approach*, edited by E.K. Chung (Baltimore: Williams & Wilkins), 46-61.

Table 5.8 Reprinted, by permission, from P.-O. Astrand, 1979, *Work tests with the bicycle ergometer* (Varberg, Sweden: Monark Exercise AB), 24.

Table 5.9 Reprinted, by permission, from E.T. Howley, 1988, The exercise testing laboratory. In *Resource manual for guidelines for exercise testing and prescription*, American College of Sports Medicine, edited by S.N. Blair et al. (Philadelphia: Lea & Febiger), 410.

Table 6.4 Adapted with permission. © American Society of Contemporary Medicine and Surgery. *Comprehensive Therapy* 1980; 6(9): 12-27.

Table 6.5 Adapted with permission. © American Society of Contemporary Medicine and Surgery. *Comprehensive Therapy* 1980; 6(9): 12-27.

Table 7.1 Reprinted, by permission, from B.D. Franks and E.T. Howley, 1989, *Fitness facts: The healthy living handbook* (Champaign, IL: Human Kinetics), 39.

Table 7.2 Reprinted, by permission, from B.D. Franks and E.T. Howley, 1989, *Fitness facts: The healthy living handbook* (Champaign, IL: Human Kinetics), 40.

Table 8.1 *Canadian Standardized Test of Fitness Operations Manual,* 3rd ed., Fitness and Amateur Sport, Health Canada, © 1986 Reproduced with permission from the Minister of Public Works and Government Services Canada, 2002.

Table 8.4 Reprinted, by permission, from R.E. Rikli and C.J. Jones, 2001, *Senior fitness test manual* (Champaign, IL: Human Kinetics), 143.

Table 10.5 Adapted, by permission, from T.E. Bernard, 2001, Environmental considerations: heat and cold. In *ACSM's resource manual,* 4th ed. (Philadelphia, PA: Lippincott, Williams, and Wilkins), 209-216.

Table 10.6 Reprinted, by permission, from L.E. Hart and J.R. Sutton, 1987, "Environmental considerations for exercise," Cardiology Clinics 5: 246.

Table 12.1 Adapted, by permission, from Pollock et al., 2000, "Resistance exercise in individuals with and without cardiovascular disease," *Circulation* 101:828-833.

Table 15.2 Reprinted, by permission, from American College of Sports Medicine, 2000, *ACSM's guidelines for exercise testing and prescription,* 6th ed. (Baltimore: Williams & Wilkins), 223.

Table 17.1 Adapted, by permission, from American College of Sports Medicine, 2000, *ACSM's guidelines for graded exercise testing and prescription* (Philadelphia: Lippincott, Williams & Wilkins), 106.

Table 20.1 Reprinted, by permission, from N.L. Jones et al., 1987, Chronic obstructive respiratory disorders. In *Exercise testing and exercise prescription for special cases,* edited by J.S. Skinner (Baltimore: Lea & Febiger), 175-187.

Boxes

Box 5.2 (p. 69) Reprinted, by permission, from American College of Sports Medicine, 1995, *ACSM's guidelines for exercise testing and prescription* (Baltimore: Williams & Wilkins), 42.

Box 5.5 (p. 82) Reprinted, by permission, from E.T. Howley, 1988, The exercise testing laboratory. In *Resource manual for guidelines for exercise testing and prescription,* edited by S.N. Blair et al. (Philadelphia: Lea & Febiger), 406-413.

Box 5.6 (p. 83) Reprinted, by permission, from American College of Sports Medicine, 2000, *ACSM's guidelines for exercise testing and prescription,* 6th ed. (Baltimore: Williams & Wilkins), 78.

Box 5.7 (p. 86) Reprinted, by permission, from B.D. Franks and E.T. Howley, 1989, *Fitness leader's handbook* (Champaign, IL: Human Kinetics), 87.

Box 5.8 (p. 91) Adapted, by permission, from E.T. Howley, 1988, The exercise testing laboratory. In *Resource manual for guidelines for exercise testing and prescription,* edited by S.N. Blair et al. (Philadelphia: Lea & Febiger), 413.

Box 11.4 (p. 201) Adapted, by permission, from M.D. Johnson, 1994, Disordered eating. In *Medical and orthopedic issues of active and athletic women,* edited by R. Agostini (Philadelphia: Hanley & Belfus, Inc.), 150.

Box 14.1 (p. 264) Reprinted, by permission, from N. Oldridge, 1988, Qualities of an exercise leader. In *Resource manual for guidelines for exercise testing and prescription,* American College of Sports Medicine, edited by S.N. Blair et al. (Philadelphia: Lea & Febiger), 240.

Box 14.2 (p. 268) Reprinted, by permission, from B.A. Franklin et al., 1990, *On the Ball* (Carmel, IN: Benchmark Press).

Box 14.6 (p. 275) Adapted, by permission, from M.D.Giese, 1988, Organization of an exercise session. In *Resource manual guidelines for exercise testing and prescription,* edited by S.N. Blair et al. (Baltimore: Lea & Febiger), 244-247.

Box 14.7 (p. 276) Reprinted, by permission, from B.D. Franks and E.T. Howley, 1989, *Fitness leader's handbook* (Champaign, IL: Human Kinetics), 143.

Box 21.2 (p. 341) Reprinted, by permission, from the International Osteoporosis Foundation, 2002, *Millennium One-Minute Osteoporosis Risk Test* [Online]. Available: www.osteofound.org. [October 2002].

index

about the authors

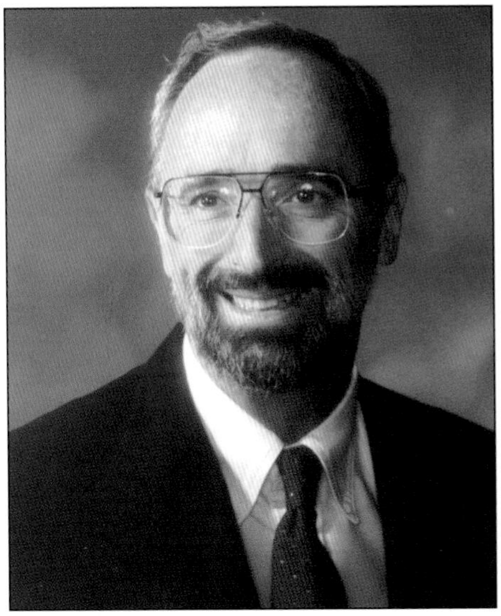

Edward T. Howley, PhD, is a professor of exercise science at the University of Tennessee, where he has frequently been honored for his excellence in teaching. He received the university's Alexander Prize for Teaching and Scholarship in 1999, the College of Education John Tunstall Outstanding Professor Award in 1995 and 1987, the University of Tennessee Alumni Association Outstanding Teacher Award in 1987, and the George F. Brady Teaching Award in 1979 and 1986. Most recently, he received the Alumni Achievement Award from the School of Education at the University of Wisconsin and the Gatorade Sports Science Institute's Excellence in Education Award.

Howley holds a PhD in physical education from the University of Wisconsin at Madison and certification as a program director from the American College of Sports Medicine (ACSM). He is currently the president of ACSM and has previously served as president of their Southeast Chapter. He has been active in ACSM's certification committee activities and was an associate editor of the sixth edition of the ACSM's Guidelines for Exercise Testing and Prescription.

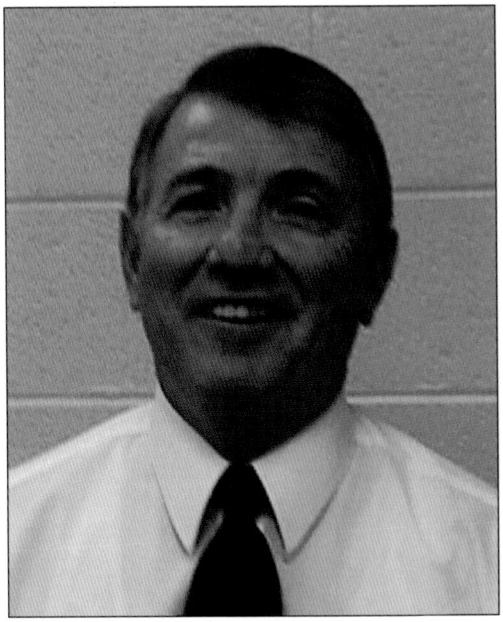

B. Don Franks received his PhD in exercise science from the University of Illinois at Urbana-Champaign (UIUC) in 1967 while working under fitness pioneer T.K. Cureton Jr. He served on the UIUC faculty until 1970 and later taught at Temple University in Philadelphia and at the University of Tennessee at Knoxville. He was senior program advisor for the President's Council on Physical Fitness and Sports in 1995. Previously, he was professor in and chair of the department of kinesiology at Louisiana State University. Currently, he teaches kinesiology at the University of Maryland at College Park.

Franks is a fellow of the American College of Sports Medicine, the American Academy of Kinesiology and Physical Education (AAKPE), and the Research Consortium of the American Alliance for Health, Physical Education, Recreation and Dance (AAHPERD). He is also a former president of AAKPE and the Research Consortium of AAHPERD, where he advocated a health-related approach to physical fitness and helped to develop the first Health-Related Physical Fitness Test. Franks has received many honors, including the AAHPERD Physical Fitness Council Honor Award and the President's Council on Physical Fitness and Sports' Distinguished Service Award.

About the Contributing Authors

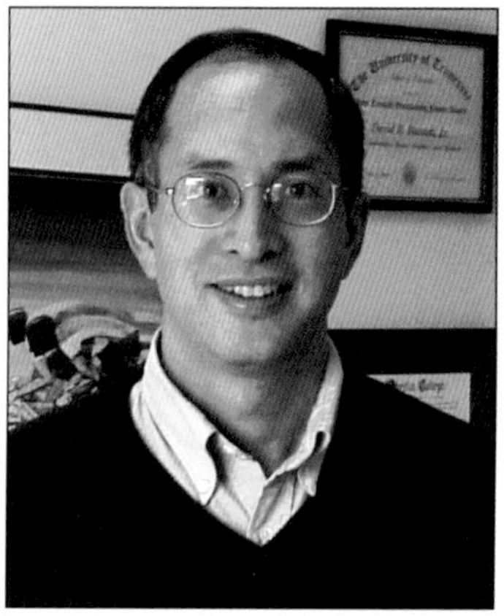

David R. Bassett, Jr., received his BS degree in biology from Oberlin College, his MS degree in biology from Ball State University, and his PhD in physical education from the University of Wisconsin, Madison. His research interests include physical activity assessment, maximal oxygen uptake, and the role of physical activity in the prevention of hypertension. He is currently a professor in the Department of Health and Exercise Science at the University of Tennessee, Knoxville. He is a fellow of the ACSM and associate editor of the journal Medicine and Science in Sports and Exercise. For recreation, he rides a bicycle, runs, and swims.

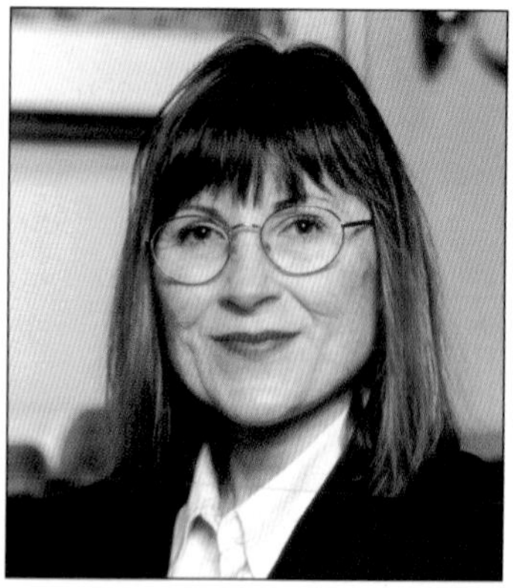

Janet Buckworth is an associate professor of sport and exercise science at Ohio State University in Columbus. She has written and presented extensively on exercise psychology and behavior change, and has been the principal investigator on several studies on exercise adherence. Dr. Buckworth became certified as a Health/Fitness Instructor in 1995, and maintains an active role in many organizations, including the American College of Sports Medicine and the Society of Behavioral Medicine. In addition, she holds two master's degrees, one in clinical social work, and is a Fellow in the American College of Sports Medicine.

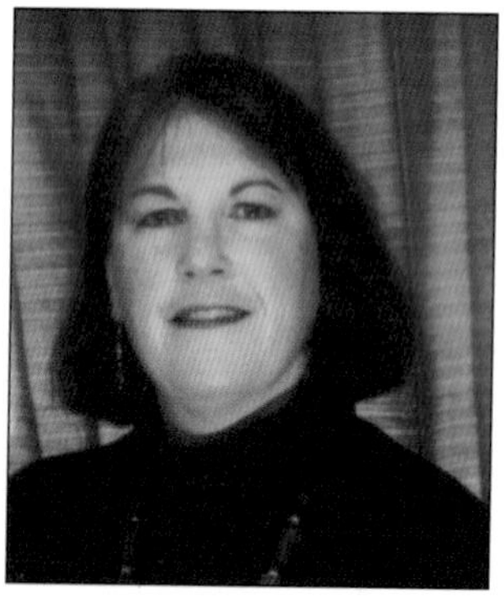

Sue Carver is presently the director of an outpatient physical therapy clinic in Little Rock, Arkansas, with Physical Therapy Clinics, Co. She graduated from Emory University with an MPT degree. She earned an MS degree in physical education with a specialization in athletic training from IU, and a BS degree in HPER from West Chester State College. She served as the Women's Athletic Trainer at the University of Tennessee from 1978 to 1982. Volunteer experiences include athletic trainer for the track and field at the 1996 Summer Olympic Games in Atlanta, the 1988 U.S. Olympic Track and Field Trials (Indianapolis), the 1985 National Sports Festival (Baton Rouge), and the Olympic Training Center (Colorado Springs) in 1984.

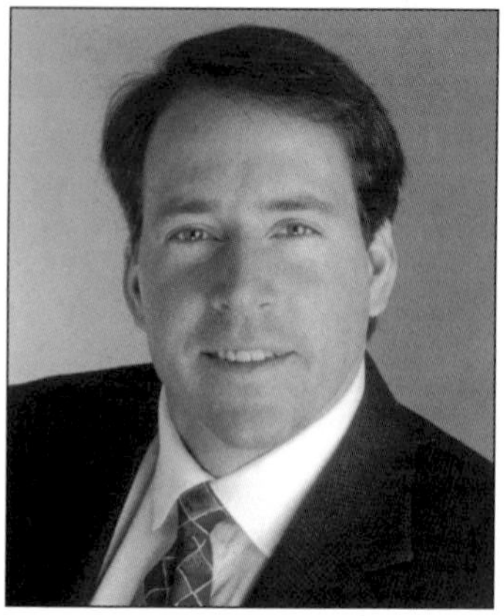

Avery D. Faigenbaum, EdD, CSCS, is an associate professor in the Department of Exercise Science at the University of Massachusetts in Boston. In addition to his responsibilities there, Dr. Faigenbaum is a well-recognized public speaker and author of two books and more than 100 articles on fitness and conditioning. He is also a Fellow of the American College of Sports Medicine, an ACSM-certified Health/Fitness Director, and an NSCA-certified Strength and Conditioning Specialist. Dr. Faigenbaum lives in Boston.

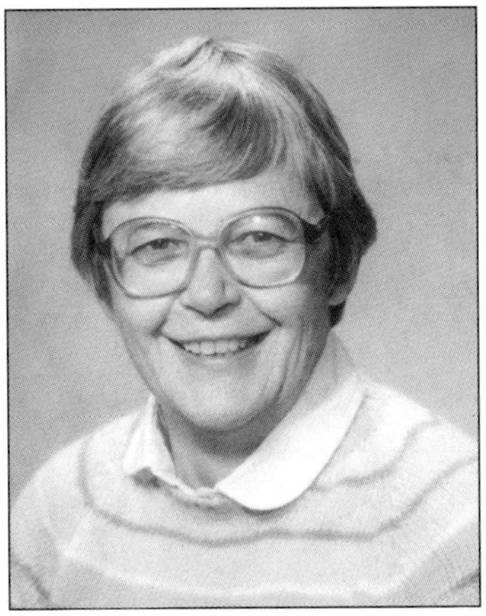

Jean Lewis received her doctorate in education (physical education with an emphasis in exercise physiology) from the University of Tennessee, Knoxville, where she is now a professor emeritus. She was involved in the establishment of undergraduate major concentrations in physical fitness and exercise physiology and has also developed courses in applied anatomy, applied kinesiology, and weight control, fitness, and exercise. Dr. Lewis was known for innovative teaching methods, which helped physical education majors understand how to apply kinesiological concepts. Recently retired, she misses the students and teaching, but is enjoying working in her garden and workshop.

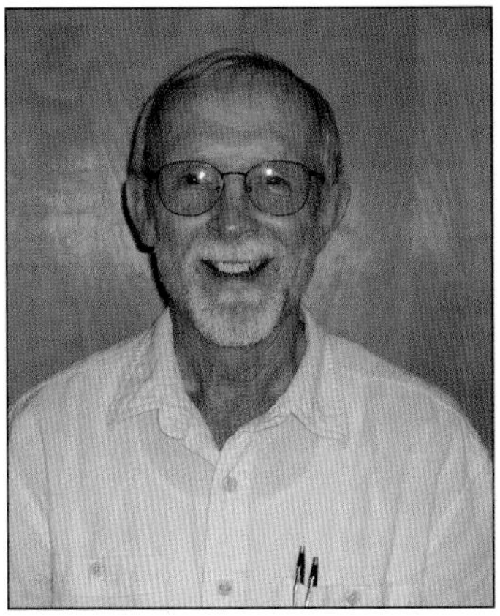

Wendell Liemohn received his BA from Wartburg College and his MA from the University of Iowa. After coaching and teaching on the collegiate level, he returned to the University of Iowa and completed his PhD. He was on the faculty of Indiana University for 7 years where his research was centered on psychomotor functioning in special populations. He has been a professor at the University of Tennessee for the past 23 years, where he started the graduate specialization in Biomechanics/Sports Medicine. He recently authored the book Exercise Prescription and the Back for McGraw-Hill; his present research is centered on the area of core stability. He is a former president of the Research Consortium of AAHPERD and is a Fellow in ACSM and in the American Academy of Kinesiology and Physical Education.

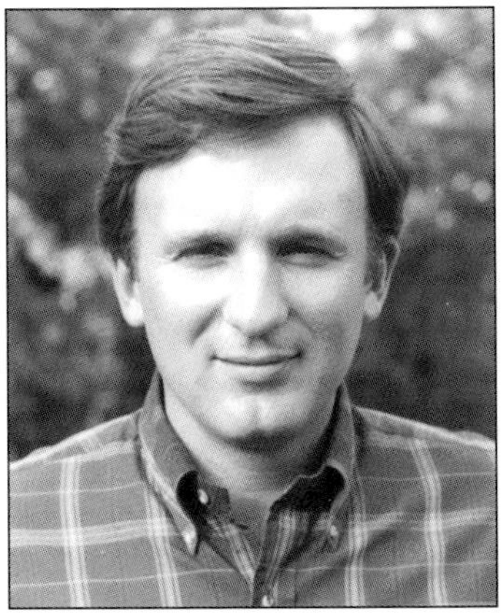

Daniel Martin earned his BS degree in physical therapy and his PhD in education from the University of Tennessee. Dr. Martin is currently an associate professor of physical therapy at the University of Florida. His research interests include exercise training and rehabilitation of lung transplant patients. His clinical activities include the rehabilitation of lung transplant patients before and after transplant and the weaning of ventilator dependent patients. He is a Fellow in the ACSM and a member of the American Physical Therapy Association. A former All-American javelin thrower at Tennessee, he now enjoys fishing in the Gulf of Mexico.

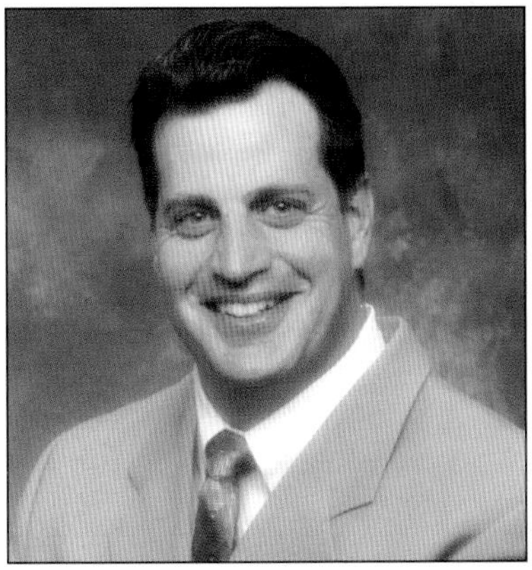

Kyle J. McInnis, ScD, is an associate professor at the University of Massachusetts in Boston. Dr. McInnis is an experienced researcher and practitioner in the area of health/fitness and chronic disease prevention. He also serves as senior co-editor of the ACSM's Health and Fitness Facilities Standards, Fourth Edition, and is a Fellow of the American College of Sports Medicine. He resides in New Hampshire with his wife Susan and their three children, Brendan, Riley, and Shane.

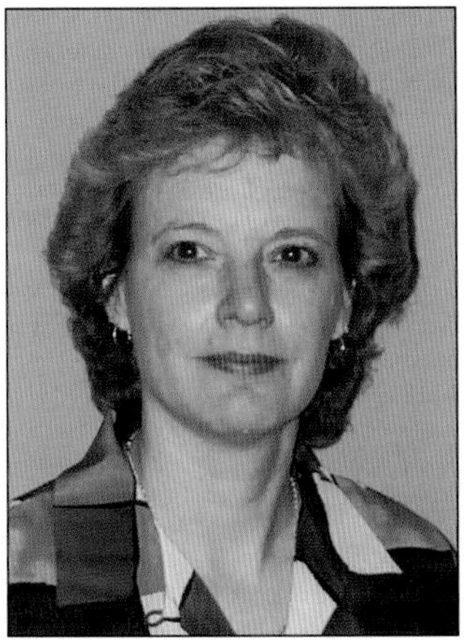

Dixie L. Thompson received BA and MA degrees from the University of North Carolina at Chapel Hill and a PhD with a specialization in exercise physiology from the University of Virginia. Dr. Thompson is currently an associate professor in the Department of Health and Exercise Science at the University of Tennessee in Knoxville. Her research interests include body composition assessment and the relationship between exercise and health in women. When not working or walking with her dogs for exercise, she can usually be found gardening, searching through antique shops, or taking in the beauty of the Great Smoky Mountains.